PENGUIN BOOKS

FLORENCE NIGHTINGALE

'So impressive. Bostridge deals impeccably with Nightingale's character . . . and with her extraordinary personal and institutional relationships' Asa Briggs, *History Today*, Books of the Year

'A biography that really stands out this year' Peter Kemp, *Open Book*, Books of the Year

'Well-judged, fair-minded and readable' Charlotte Moore, *Spectator*, Books of the Year

'A sage and fascinating life' Tim Martin, *Daily Telegraph*, Books of the Year

'The best biography I read was Mark Bostridge's *Florence Nightingale*' Philip Hensher, *Spectator*, Books of the Year

'Balanced, engagingly readable and based on impressive research . . . will surely be definitive' Jane Ridley, *Spectator*, Books of the Year

'Engrossing, a triumph, carrying the reader with the lively intelligence it deserves and making a new and authoritative portrait' Claire Tomalin, *Guardian*, Books of the Year

'Absorbing, sympathetic, enormously enjoyable to read. A masterly work' Mary Warnock, *New Statesman*

'Compulsive, thoroughly researched and eminently readable. A fine biography' *Literary Review*

'Excellent, Bostridge succeeds magnificently' *Spectator*

'A full, scholarly and compellingly authoritative biography' *Evening Standard*

ABOUT THE AUTHOR

Mark Bostridge won the Gladstone Memorial Prize at Oxford University. His books include *Vera Brittain: A Life*, shortlisted for the Whitbread Biography Award, the NCR Non-Fiction Prize and the Fawcett Prize; the bestselling *Letters from a Lost Generation*, which he also adapted for a BBC Radio Four series; *Lives for Sale*, a collection of biographers' tales; and *Because You Died*, a selection of Vera Brittain's First World War writing.

Florence Nightingale

The Woman and Her Legend

MARK BOSTRIDGE

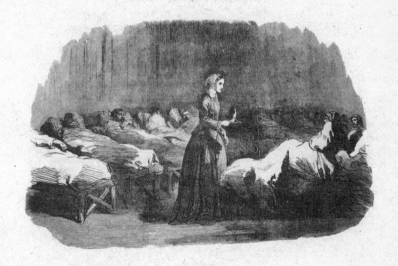

PENGUIN BOOKS

PENGUIN BOOKS

Published by the Penguin Group
Penguin Books Ltd, 80 Strand, London WC2R ORL, England
Penguin Group (USA), Inc., 375 Hudson Street, New York, New York 10014, USA
Penguin Group (Canada), 90 Eglinton Avenue East, Suite 700, Toronto, Ontario, Canada M4P 2Y3
(a division of Pearson Penguin Canada Inc.)
Penguin Ireland, 25 St Stephen's Green, Dublin 2, Ireland
(a division of Penguin Books Ltd)
Penguin Group (Australia), 250 Camberwell Road, Camberwell, Victoria 3124, Australia
(a division of Pearson Australia Group Pty Ltd)
Penguin Books India Pvt Ltd, 11 Community Centre, Panchsheel Park, New Delhi – 110 017, India
Penguin Group (NZ), 67 Apollo Drive, Rosedale, North Shore 0632, New Zealand
(a division of Pearson New Zealand Ltd)
Penguin Books (South Africa) (Pty) Ltd, 24 Sturdee Avenue, Rosebank, Johannesburg 2196, South Africa

Penguin Books Ltd, Registered Offices: 80 Strand, London WC2R ORL, England

www.penguin.com

First published by Viking 2008
Published in Penguin Books 2009

1

Copyright © Mark Bostridge, 2008

The moral right of the author has been asserted

Typeset by Rowland Phototypesetting Ltd, Bury St Edmunds, Suffolk
Printed in Great Britain by Clays Ltd, St Ives plc

A CIP catalogue record for this book is available from the British Library

ISBN: 978-0-140-26392-3

www.greenpenguin.co.uk

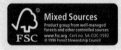

Mixed Sources
Product group from well-managed
forests and other controlled sources
www.fsc.org Cert no. SA-COC-1592
© 1996 Forest Stewardship Council

Penguin Books is committed to a sustainable future
for our business, our readers and our planet.
The book in your hands is made from paper
certified by the Forest Stewardship Council.

For Robin Baird-Smith

I study Flo as if she were a language and as she is a deep one I have not mastered it by any means.

Mary Mohl to Parthenope Nightingale, 16 February [1853]

Contents

List of Illustrations

In the text

i (title page) 'The Lady with the Lamp', from the *Illustrated London News*, 24 February 1855.

ii (page 22) Florence Nightingale's birth registered in the Protestant Dissenters' Register at Dr Williams's Library.

iii (page 211) Lithographed drawing of Athena the owlet from 'Life and Death of Athena, an Owlet from the Parthenon' by Parthenope Nightingale (1855).

iv (page 225) A plan of the interior of the Barrack Hospital, Scutari, drawn by Parthenope Nightingale, showing the nurses' quarters.

v (page 265) An engraving of Florence Nightingale's face juxtaposed with one of 'Bridget McBruiser', from S. R. Wells's *New System of Physiognomy* (1866).

vi (page 300) A nurse's brassard from Scutari.

Plates

1. William Nightingale in 1839.
2. Fanny Nightingale, with Florence and Parthenope, *c.* 1823.
3. An Italian wetnurse with a baby, probably Florence Nightingale, 1820.
4. Lea Hurst in Derbyshire. A photograph from the 1860s.
5. Embley Park in Hampshire.
6. Florence with her cousin Marianne Nicholson, *c.* 1839. A sketch by Parthenope Nightingale.
7. Hilary Bonham Carter, a self-portrait.

60. Statue of Sidney Herbert by J. H. Foley at its original site, in front of the old War Office in Pall Mall.
61. Mrs Thatcher as the Lady with the Lamp from a May 1988 issue of *The Economist*.

Picture Credits

Grateful acknowledgement is made to the following institutions and individuals:
Claydon House Trust: i, 2, 3, 4, 9, 10, 20, 41, 48, 50, 60.
Florence Nightingale Museum: ii, iii, v, 1, 5, 6, 7, 14, 15, 19, 21, 22, 23, 24, 26, 27, 28, 29, 32, 34, 35, 36, 37, 43, 44, 45, 46, 47, 52, 53, 54, 55, 56.
British Library, London: 8, 11, 40.
National Portrait Gallery, London: 13.
Wellcome Library, London: 31.
Balliol College, Oxford: 39, 42.
Lomas Family Nightingale Collection: 58.
The Economist: 61.

Nightingale Family Tree

FLORENCE NIGHTINGALE'S FAMILY
An Abbreviated Family Tree

William Smith 1756–1835 m. Frances Coape 1759–1840

- Martha Frances (Aunt Patty) 1782–1870
- Benjamin 1783–1860 m. Anne Longden c. 1802–1834
- Anne 1785–1854 m. George Thomas Nicholson of Waverley 1787–1852
- Frances 1788–1880 m. W. E. Nightingale* 1794–1874
- William Adams 1789–1870

Children of Benjamin m. Anne Longden:
- Barbara 1827–1891 m. Eugene Bodichon 1810–1885
- Benjamin Leigh 1828–1913

Children of Frances m. W. E. Nightingale:
- Frances Parthenope 1819–1890 m. Sir Harry Verney 1801–1894
- **FLORENCE** 1820–1910

- Samuel 1815
- Marianne d. 1909 m. Douglas Galton 1822–1899
- George Henry d. 1851
- William d. 1888
- Lothian 1827–1893 m. Mary Romilly
- Laura 1824–1862 m. John 1817–1884
- Thomas 1819–1829

Children:
- Evelyne Isabella m. Camillo Fenzi d. 1883
- Laura Gwendolyne m. Douglas Trench Gascoigne
- Charles Lothian
- Douglas Lothian
- John Lothian
- Edith
- Iona
- Laura
- Mary
- Malcolm

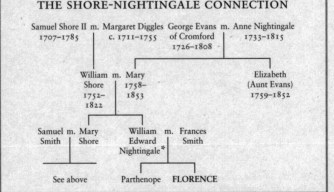

THE SHORE-NIGHTINGALE CONNECTION

Samuel Shore II m. Margaret Diggles 1707–1785 c. 1711–1755

George Evans m. Anne Nightingale of Cromford 1726–1808 · 1733–1815

- William Shore 1752–1822 m. Mary 1758–1853
- Elizabeth (Aunt Evans) 1759–1852

- Samuel Smith m. Mary Shore
- William Edward Nightingale* m. Frances Smith

- See above
- Parthenope
- **FLORENCE**

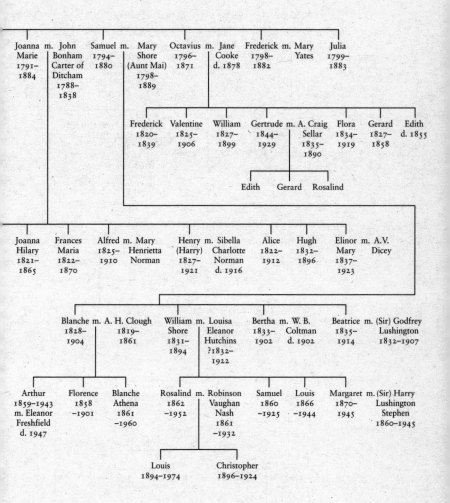

Joanna Marie 1791–1884 m. John Bonham Carter of Ditcham 1788–1838

Samuel 1794–1880 m. Mary Shore (Aunt Mai) 1798–1889

Octavius 1796–1871 m. Jane Cooke d. 1878

Frederick 1798–1882 m. Mary Yates

Julia 1799–1883

Frederick 1820–1839

Valentine 1825–1906

William 1827–1899

Gertrude 1844–1929 m. A. Craig Sellar 1835–1890

Flora 1834–1919

Gerard 1827–1858

Edith d. 1855

Edith   Gerard   Rosalind

Joanna Hilary 1821–1865

Frances Maria 1822–1870

Alfred 1825–1910 m. Mary Henrietta Norman

Henry (Harry) 1827–1921 m. Sibella Charlotte Norman d. 1916

Alice 1822–1912

Hugh 1832–1896

Elinor Mary 1837–1923 m. A.V. Dicey

Blanche 1828–1904 m. A. H. Clough 1819–1861

William Shore 1831–1894 m. Louisa Eleanor Hutchins ?1832–1922

Bertha 1833–1902 m. W. B. Coltman d. 1902

Beatrice 1835–1914 m. (Sir) Godfrey Lushington 1832–1907

Arthur 1859–1943 m. Eleanor Freshfield d. 1947

Florence 1858–1901

Blanche Athena 1861–1960

Rosalind 1862–1952 m. Robinson Vaughan Nash 1861–1932

Samuel 1860–1925

Louis 1866–1944

Margaret 1870–1945 m. (Sir) Harry Lushington Stephen 1860–1945

Louis 1894–1974   Christopher 1896–1924

*Born Shore, William Edward succeeded his great-uncle Peter Nightingale and assumed the name Nightingale by Royal Sign Manual in 1815

Prologue

As the cortège passed Buckingham Palace, the sentries presented arms and the guards stood to attention. In the streets people stopped to stare, men respectfully removing their hats as they did so. At Waterloo station, the plain oak coffin was lifted on to a waiting train, and at Romsey, in Hampshire, the train's destination, the coffin was placed on a funeral carriage, drawn through the town by two dark horses. Children ran after it, or sat on the small bridge over the river Test to catch a prize view as the carriage went by. Nine-year-old Eva Sedgefield of Station Road, the daughter of a nurse, remembered all her life the disappointment she had felt at being deemed too young to follow the procession, unlike her four older sisters.

Florence Nightingale had died, aged ninety, on 13 August 1910. Her funeral was held a week later. 'Though there was no suffering, there was increasing weariness,' reported Elizabeth Bosanquet, her companion, of her final hours, '& she was latterly quite unable to give her attention to conversation. She dozed a good deal & during Friday night ... the watchful nurse noticed a very slight change in her breathing while asleep ... This semi-comatose condition continued till she quietly passed away at 2 p.m. & we sent for the relations ...' For much of her last decade, as her faculties failed, Nightingale had been oblivious to events going on around her, and unaware of the sudden renewed attention that the outside world was paying to her name. The century had begun with what was for many the astonishing revelation that Florence Nightingale was still alive. Irene Cooper Willis, a future Nightingale biographer, remembered her own surprise on hearing the news. It was at the time of the Boer War, a conflict that brought irresistibly to mind thoughts of the Crimean War, half a century before, and with them memories of Tennyson's *Charge of the Light Brigade*, a favourite classroom recitation, and the heroic legend of the Lady with the Lamp. Once again, baby girls, in their droves, were christened Florence. Nightingale became the recipient of honours, including the Order of Merit – though Edward VII was at first loath to give the award to a woman. None of this attention, however, had caused her family to waver from its commitment to ensure that Florence Nightingale's wish for a private funeral was fulfilled. The offer of a national funeral and burial in Westminster Abbey was declined. Instead, she would be buried quietly in the family plot in the churchyard of St Margaret's, East Wellow, the thirteenth-century church close to the Nightingales' former Hampshire estate at Embley Park.

After leaving the town, the cortège rode along a winding road bordered by hedgerows to the churchyard. On its way, where the road skirts the boundary of Embley, the carriage turned in through the main gate and past the old Nightingale home. The family were concerned by the presence of photographers and cameramen, recording the procession from selected vantage points along the route. At the graveside, following a short church service, it became even more difficult to reconcile Florence Nightingale's wish for privacy 'with the universal desire to show honour to her', for the churchyard turned out to be filled with a large crowd, mostly local people, come to pay their respects. Among them was a Crimean veteran from the 23rd Foot, eighty-four-year-old Private John Kneller. He told reporters something of what they must have been hoping to hear: that, after losing an eye in the trenches before Sebastopol, he had been sent to the Barrack Hospital at Scutari, where he had often seen 'Florence Nightingale carrying her lantern on her nightly visits to the place'.

In light rain, a bearing party of eight guardsmen, from the Grenadier, Coldstream and Scots Guards, lowered the coffin into the ground beside Nightingale's parents. 'I could have wished that it had not rained and that the crowd had been less,' Louis Shore Nightingale, a cousin and executor, wrote afterwards, 'but they behaved well and were mostly country people as one would have wished.' The inscription on the headstone, decorated with a cross, reads simply: 'F. N. Born 12 May 1820. Died 13 August 1910.'

———

Like those mourners at the graveside, we have all partaken of the story of Florence Nightingale's heroic exploits at Scutari and in the Crimea –

many of us at our mother's knee – and of how she battled against the obstructive army and medical officials to ensure that the sick and wounded were nursed in civilized conditions and with proper care. In Britain, she has long been a nationally sanctioned heroine. Until recently, she was the only woman whose image had adorned the Bank of England's paper currency. For nearly two decades, between 1975 and 1993, her portrait, adapted from Barrett's painting *The Mission of Mercy*, could be found on the ten-pound note. As the historian Raphael Samuel observed, the Lady with the Lamp is one of the stock images of our island story.

Throughout the world, the sentimental appeal of the legend has consistently endured, despite frequent attempts to debunk it. 'Has there . . . ever been a name more sweetly compounded for the lavishing of sentiment,' Laurence Housman once asked, 'than that of Florence Nightingale? Among the objects commercially available in Britain, at the height of the Nightingale mania of the mid-1850s, was a 'Nightingale cradle', manufactured by another aptly named individual, Mr Sweet; similarly, in the United States, later in the century, 'a Nightingale' was sold as a kind of flannel wrap used to cover the shoulders and arms of a patient while in bed. Today, the basic idea underlying these inventions has entered common parlance, and we talk, almost without thinking, of 'doing a Florence Nightingale' when we want to describe someone devoting themselves to nursing care (the origins of this kind of remark must date back to at least 1869, when Mark Twain wrote of a female acquaintance 'acting Florence Nightingale'). Meanwhile, Florence Nightingale regularly tops polls to find the most famous nurse, or the most compassionate person in history.

To a greater extent even than most legends, this one romanticizes, grossly oversimplifies, and sometimes obscures, a complex historical reality. But the image of the ministering angel was also perpetuated in Florence Nightingale's own lifetime by a decision, partly dictated by her health on her return from the Crimean War in 1856, to live and work in seclusion. This cemented her legendary status in the way that her early death might have done, placing her reputation for saintly goodness and compassion beyond reproach, while diminishing the brilliance of her personality and intellect. It further disguised the fact that Nightingale's Crimea experience was only the prelude to a much more significant post-war career in public health reform. We all know the romantic story of the wartime nurse. Comparatively few of us, though, are aware of the importance of that story's sequel: of how, from her sickbed, Florence Nightingale, the possessor of one of the greatest analytical minds of her time, attempted to supervise the modernization of nursing, together with advising governments on Army health reform, sanitary improvements in Britain and India, hospital design, and much else besides. 'Good public!' she remarked in 1857. 'It knew nothing of what I was really doing in the Crimea . . . It has known nothing of what I wanted to do and have done since I came home.' Of course, she colluded in the public's ignorance, which stemmed in large part from her own reluctance to publicize her cause. However, while she claimed to dislike the 'buz-fuz' about her name – at least in part because of the damage she believed it had done to her mission in the Crimean War – she knew on occasion how to manipulate her fame to masterly effect for her own ends.

This book has a dual purpose. Its central theme is to trace the way in which Florence Nightingale's life and myth constantly interact. At another level, it is also an attempt, as we approach the centenary of Nightingale's death, to set the factual record of her life straight in a number of important respects. To this end, I have been greatly aided by the gradual appearance of ten volumes of a projected sixteen-volume edition of Florence Nightingale's selected writings, as well as by my research in the vast unpublished archive of Nightingale family papers at Claydon House, in Buckinghamshire. Thanks to David Young, formerly of the Wellcome Institute in London, who, in 1995, identified Florence Nightingale as a likely sufferer from a chronic form of brucellosis, biographers are able to write with greater authority about the long-term effects of Nightingale's illness. The work of nursing historians, on both sides of the Atlantic, over the past twenty years has provided a new context in which to view Florence Nightingale's nursing reforms. Her contribution to modern nursing is now seen as representing less of a decisive break with the past. At the same time, recognition of the extraordinary scope of her vision of a modern public health care system, encompassing not simply nursing, but based on health promotion and disease prevention, is more widely acknowledged and understood.

Surprisingly, I find myself indebted to Britain's first woman Prime Minister, Margaret Thatcher, for helping me to understand the political advantages and vicissitudes experienced by a woman operating in a male-dominated world. Florence Nightingale would have abhorred much about Thatcher's politics – for a start, she believed, 'without irreverence', that God was a Liberal – but she would undoubtedly have recognized elements of its style as akin to her own. Writing in 1990, the historian David Cannadine was the first to draw attention to the parallels between the Lady with the Lamp and the Iron Lady. 'Long before Thatcher, Nightingale both denied and exploited her femininity to gain power in a man's world. Long before Thatcher, Nightingale was possessed of superabundant energy, and was in a righteous rage to get things done. Long before Thatcher, Nightingale hated red tape, loathed bureaucrats, and was determined to sweep away incompetence and inefficiency wherever she found it.' In 1989, on a visit to Turkey, Thatcher laid a wreath in the British Crimean War cemetery at Scutari. Afterwards, she spoke to reporters about one of the 'great figures of history', who 'had had an idea, who knew what she wanted to do, and wasn't going to be put off by anyone . . .' Purportedly, Thatcher was referring to Florence Nightingale, but it's tempting to believe that she was really talking about herself.

———

What to call your subject can present a problem for the biographer. I have chosen to refer to Florence Nightingale, at different points in my narrative where appropriate, as Nightingale, Florence Nightingale or, most often, as Florence. This latter form of address may strike some as overly familiar, and others as politically incorrect, but at least it avoids the formidable 'Miss Nightingale' favoured by some of my predecessors. As she herself once commented, albeit in another context, 'Might we not leave out the "Miss"?'

Part One
Daughter of England
1820–54

My people were like children playing on the shore of the the eighteenth century. I was their hobby-horse, their plaything; and they drove me to and fro, dear souls! never weary of play themselves, till I, who had grown to woman's estate and to the ideas of the nineteenth century, lay down exhausted, my mind closed to hope, my heart to strength.

FN, 'Cassandra', c. 1850–53

Woman stands askew. Her education for action has not kept pace with her education for acquirement.

FN, *The Institution of Kaiserswerth on the Rhine*, 1851

To be alone is nothing – to be without sympathy in a crowd – <u>this</u> is to be confined in solitude.

FN, untitled draft novel, c. 1850–53

1. The Ridiculous Name of Nightingale

Take a walk south from the Porta Romana in Florence today, along the Via Senese, then turn westwards, and you will soon find yourself climbing a steep path along a narrow winding road. High stone walls, mossy and mottled with age, obliterate the view in either direction, but tall cypress trees line the route, and olives and vines run down to the walls on both sides.

Towards the summit, at a bend in the road, a large house comes into view. The Villa La Colombaia is now a convent junior school with an imposing modern stone façade, but parts of the house date back to the fifteenth century. On its garden side the original low building with shuttered windows, arranged around a courtyard, is still in existence. A gravel walk through an elegantly laid-out garden leads to a magnificent view over the city, of Brunelleschi's white ribbed dome amid a sea of red rooftops.

It was from this 'Maison de Campagne', on a spring day in 1820, that twenty-six-year-old William Nightingale wrote to his brother-in-law Ben Smith about the expected imminent arrival of his second child. The city of Florence itself seemed deserted – everyone was travelling to Rome for Holy Week – but William and his heavily pregnant wife Fanny were taking advantage of the fine weather to ride up and down the hillside, he on a pony, she in a carriage driven by grey horses.

As William wrote his letter, his first child, Parthenope, born just a year before in Naples, was wriggling about on his knee, proving 'so rumbustical I can hardly scribble'. He was confident that the new baby would be a boy, though apologetic that he could not report 'by the same post the arrival of a young Ulysses, the protector of Parthenope . . . He is expected every minute not to say moment, but delays his arrival I know not why . . .'

It would be a further five weeks before William Nightingale was able to announce the birth of another daughter.

'I found a house at Florence on the hill/of Bellosguardo,' wrote Elizabeth Barrett Browning in *Aurora Leigh*. Walk on a short distance from the Villa La Colombaia, and the legendary beauty of this small area outside the city gates, which has attracted so many well-to-do and famous visitors through the centuries, is immediately apparent. A stone monument at the roadside records some of the distinguished names who have lived or stayed at Bellosguardo: among them, Galileo, who retreated here after his appearance before the Inquisition, James Fenimore Cooper, Nathaniel Hawthorne, the Brownings, Henry James, Clara Schumann and, the penultimate name on the list, above that of Violet Trefusis, Florence Nightingale.

It is Henry James who provides the location of Florence Nightingale's birthplace with the link to a neat little biographical irony. For it was while staying, in 1887, at the Casa Brichieri-Colombi, another of the grand villas on the road leading to the brow of Bellosguardo, that James wrote the first draft of *The Aspern Papers*. James's novella, with its story of a would-be biographer who attempts to prise some letters of a famous American poet, Jeffrey Aspern, from an old woman, only to discover that she has burned them one by one, has been described as a moral fable for historians and biographers. It dramatizes the biographer's primordial fear: the destruction of the manuscript evidence, so vital to the craft, literally obliterated in a cloud of smoke.

The contrast with the fate of Florence Nightingale's manuscripts could scarcely be greater. While not a scrap of the Aspern papers is left for posterity, Nightingale's biographer has to struggle hard not to be buried under a veritable mountain of material, to the extent that he may find himself occasionally wishing that the odd bonfire had actually taken place. Florence Nightingale was an inveterate hoarder. She preserved not only letters, diaries, personal notes and jottings, but also copies and drafts of letters – and corrections of drafts. Identical, or almost identical, phrases in her letters sometimes make her seem like an actress rehearsing lines for a favourite role. At her death, paper was scattered through practically every corner of the first floor of her house at 10 South Street, even 'inside piano stools, behind coal scuttles, under sofas'. She had enough letters in her drawers, she had written in 1895, 'to cover Australia'.

Today, the collection at the British Library, the second largest among personal archives after that of Gladstone, fills almost 200 bound volumes, and this represents merely the tip of the iceberg. At Claydon House in Buckinghamshire, the home for thirty years of Nightingale's sister Parthenope, Lady Verney, there is another massive collection, which includes Florence Nightingale's letters to her parents and sister, and correspondence between members of the extended Nightingale family network, over a period of more than a century. The London Metropolitan Archives are a third major Nightingale repository, connected with the running of the nursing training school founded in Florence Nightingale's name at St Thomas's Hospital, in 1860. In addition to these, there are some 200 smaller holdings of Nightingale papers around the world. Although there are significant gaps in the records – some sanctioned by Nightingale's family and executors, who destroyed certain letters after the appearance of the two authorized biographies by Sir Edward Cook and Ida O'Malley – Florence Nightingale's life is one of the best documented of the Victorian age, certainly the best documented of any Victorian woman. And previously unknown letters continue to materialize, most dramatically during the Second World War, when it was only quick thinking on the part of some individual that prevented Nightingale's forty-seven surviving letters to one of her Crimean War colleagues, Reverend Mother Mary Clare Moore, from being burned during the attack by a V-2 rocket which destroyed the Convent of Mercy in Bermondsey.

It might, though, have all turned out rather differently. As a young woman, in her first professional appointment, in 1853, as Superintendent of the Upper Harley Street Establishment for Gentlewomen during Illness, Florence Nightingale had conceived of a time when she might start keeping her letters, '& after my death gratify the public with them'. Post-Crimea, however, and fame and influence made her more wary of the likely incursions of posterity, causing her to make radically different plans. 'Destroy', 'Return', 'Burn' are words which appear regularly from this time, scrawled across the upper left-hand corner of her letters. In 1860 she begged Henry (later Cardinal) Manning to burn her letters to him, adding that 'I have alas! met with such treachery in my poor life that any carelessness on the part of those I <u>know</u> to be friendly to me might easily be turned to bad account'; and four years later she recorded in a private note that she had 'taken effectual means' that 'all my papers' would be destroyed after her death. A clause in Nightingale's will of 1896 confirmed this arrangement. She 'earnestly entreated' her friends and executors that all her letters, papers and manuscripts, with the exception of those relating to her work for India, be destroyed 'without examination'. Five years later she changed her mind. She still believed that the majority of her papers should be destroyed, but she was bequeathing them to her cousin Henry Bonham Carter, leaving him with the difficult decision of what to preserve. Evidently he couldn't bring himself to effect their mass destruction either.

Why did Nightingale change her mind? She was certainly not oblivious to the threat posed by biography. 'I earnestly wish that no . . . biography of me should be given by my family or friends,' she insisted in 1862 when the onset of severe spinal pain made her 'impatient for death'. Thirty years later, she joked, 'Well might Sir Cornwall Lewis say: "A new terror is added to death",' after learning that her letters to Sidney Herbert had been lent to his biographer, Lord Stanmore, without her consent. Yet she allowed plenty of material that was damaging to her own reputation to survive.*

In the end its survival may simply be attributed to the fact that, towards the end of her life, Nightingale lacked the time and energy to embark on such a massive process of sorting and disposal. Alternatively, it could be seen as an expression of a lifelong inner conflict between a natural desire for recognition, and a deep religious conviction that she must walk invisible and avoid the snares and delusions of self-love. Or it may be that writing itself was so much a part of her identity that ultimately she could not bear to see her literary remains consigned to the flames.

For writing was Florence Nightingale's lifeblood. This was a woman, after all, who even while in the depths of delirium in the Crimea, in May 1855, insisted on being brought pen and paper, and only with these in her possession did she become calm. In her later years, as one visitor, the writer (and former Nightingale nurse) Flora Masson, remembered, a pencil and a notebook lay always close at hand. The editors of Nightingale's selected letters have observed that 'Experience appears to have taken on a reality only when it had been ordered and fixed in writing'; and sometimes the intensity of the moment seeps through into the very act of writing as she stabs at the page with her pen or pencil.

---

* This doesn't include the family letters at Claydon, the preservation of which Nightingale might well have baulked at. Her sister Parthenope, with her instincts as a historian, was scrupulous about ensuring their survival.

From an early age she was a compulsive autobiographer. Between the ages of eight and ten, Nightingale wrote down her earliest memories in a series of notebooks, as part of a French exercise, which she called 'La Vie de Florence Rossignol'. In this, and in other childhood journals, she combined vivid impressions with a precise recall of incident and event.

Later, in her twenties, when reacting against the regime of enforced idleness imposed on women of her class, Nightingale rejected writing as only a substitute for living. 'I think one's feelings waste themselves in words,' she told a sympathetic friend who had suggested that she become a writer. 'They ought to be distilled into actions, and into actions which bring results . . .' Yet after she returned to England from her brief burst of heroic action during the Crimean War, and was confined to her bed or couch as an invalid, she found that words themselves became a conduit to action, as she set about communicating in writing her plans for change and reform to a band of collaborators. A vast amount of day-to-day business was conducted by the exchange of notes between Nightingale in her bedroom upstairs at South Street and Dr John Sutherland, and other members of her secretariat, downstairs. Sutherland, her chief assistant and adviser on sanitary matters, sometimes received as many as half a dozen notes a day (he was also partly deaf, so this mode of communication served a further useful purpose).

These notes are testimony to a prodigious amount of work in progress, but it is in her letters that Florence Nightingale is revealed in all her extraordinary versatility and intellectual power. At least 14,000 are known to exist: the earliest dates from 1827 when she was seven years old; among the last, eighty years later, in December 1907, is one acknowledging, through an amanuensis, a message and gift of flowers sent by Count Metternich on behalf of Kaiser Wilhelm II. 'That power of writing a good letter whenever one likes' she considered 'a great temptation'. She cursed the Penny Post and wished it were in California, writing that one of England's misfortunes was its 'confoundedly cheap postage'. As a young child she had a weakness in her hands and didn't begin to write in cursive script until the age of ten (her printed lettering in her first letters is like sampler stitching); but her mature handwriting, often in the special HB pencil obtained directly from the War Office, is, thankfully, 'firm and beautiful'.

Many of Nightingale's letters display her brilliant powers of exposition and grasp of detail. She could, for example, 'dash off 10 pages of advice on steam boilers, 13 pages on the use of Parian cement for hospital walls, 12 pages on floor polish, and 6 pages on tea-making'. She also knew how to adapt her style of writing to a particular correspondent in order to achieve her aim, and could resort to flattery, cajolery, scolding, even bullying when it suited her purpose. Most of all, she knew how to deploy a pungent phrase, and her often devastating use of wit and irony is one of the great pleasures of much of her writing, in particular of her letters.

But while these letters are a tremendous resource for the biographer, they also contain an in-built trap. For Florence Nightingale's epistolary world is one of black and white values with few intermediate greys. It is all too easy to be beguiled by her heady sense of the dramatic, and to be drawn unwittingly into accepting her point of view without assessing the true merits of the case. And this applies as much to family matters as it does to the wider social and political arena, for instance, of nursing reform or the health of the Army. Benjamin Jowett once chastised her for a tendency to exaggerate, a fault she claimed to share in common with many other members of her mother's family, the Smiths.

Finally, the sheer quantity of material brings its own problems in tow. For many years in the latter part of her life Florence Nightingale spent at least twelve hours a day writing (letters were often composed 'by candlelight', at four or five in the morning, before London was awake). It is a staggering rate of productivity. How, though, can any individual biographer hope to encompass, let alone resolve, all the contradictions and paradoxes contained in her writings over the span of a very long life? Let Henry James have the last word here, and one that I have taken as a warning. In *The Aspern Papers* he writes darkly of 'the most fatal of our human passions, our not knowing where to stop'.

———

William and Fanny Nightingale were in Italy on an extended honeymoon tour. Like many other English travellers of the time they were taking advantage of their new-found freedom to explore the continent now that the Napoleonic Wars were over. But there was another reason, too, why a prolonged absence from England must have appeared a good idea. The Nightingales had no suitable home to move into – or, at least, not one that met Fanny's exacting standards. Furthermore, by happy accident their time abroad would ensure that they avoided the upheaval caused by what Fanny's youngest sister Julia blithely referred to as 'the

ruin of the family'. For within a year of the Nightingales' departure
from England, Fanny's father, William Smith, the distinguished Member
of Parliament for Norwich, faced financial disaster when his wholesale
grocery business, the foundation of his fortune, collapsed. On the brink
of bankruptcy, Smith would lose his country seat at Parndon in Essex
and his London home near St James's Park, together with much of his
magnificent art collection and library. For the last fifteen years of his
life, William Smith and his wife Frances would live in straitened circumstances, often dependent on their children's support.

William Smith's personal fortune disappeared almost overnight, but
the collapse of his business did not alter his commitment to his political
and humanitarian principles. In terms of a life pledged to the service
of ideals, and fired by a strong religious faith, William Smith is his
granddaughter Florence's most obvious progenitor. At the height of the
parliamentary debate on the abolition of slavery in 1797, one of the
great causes of his political career, Smith had derided the argument of
expediency, declaring that 'no system of commercial policy should be
allowed to exist for a moment, which was repugnant to moral duty';
and it was moral duty combined with a rational belief derived from his
Dissenting background that encouraged Smith to adopt another major
crusade, that of religious freedom. He lived 'as if to prove how much a
man of ardent benevolence may enjoy of this world's happiness, without
any steeling of the heart to the wants and calamities of others', was one
assessment after his death. '. . . If he had gone mourning all his days, he
could scarcely have acquired a more tender pity for the miserable, or
have laboured more habitually for their relief.'

The Smiths came originally from the Isle of Wight, where seventeenth-
century records show them to have been of fairly humble stock and
members of the congregations of Independent chapels. By the mid-
eighteenth century, the family had become prosperous members of the
merchant class. Samuel Smith, William's father, has a small foothold in
Jacobite folklore as one of those who, despite his strong Hanoverian
sympathies, provided financial aid to the penniless Flora Macdonald
when she was imprisoned in the Tower following the failure of the '45.
Samuel was proprietor of the Sugar Loaf, a successful wholesale grocery
business off London's Cannon Street, in St Swithin's Lane, which
imported tea, sugar and spices from around the world. In 1754 he
consolidated his fortune by marrying Martha Adams, daughter of a

wealthy Dissenting family, who brought with her a substantial dowry and the promise of a great inheritance from brewing and distillery. She bore four children in quick succession before dying in childbirth, at the age of twenty-five, in 1759.

Of these four, only William, born in 1756, survived infancy. He was doted on by his father, who planned for him eventually to take over the business in Cannon Street. Zoffany's dual portrait of Samuel and the young William portrays them as richly dressed merchant princes, the father teaching the son a lesson in geometry. William's 'future destination' was for trade, his father told him in 1769, 'but learning is not incompatible with it – on the Contrary it facilitates the conducting of it and gives a person a superiority in his sphere of action'. William Smith did indeed enter the family firm, but by his mid-twenties he was straining for political action, and as part of the mercantile class he had little choice but to buy his way into Parliament. In 1784 he paid £3,000 to be returned as Member for the rotten borough of Sudbury. He lost that seat in 1790, but soon found another at Camelford. Smith remained MP there until 1802, when he was elected to Norwich, a seat he would hold, with the exception of one year, 1806 to 1807, until 1830. Initially, he was loyal to Pitt, but within a decade he had transferred his allegiance to the Whigs and become a follower of Charles James Fox.

William Smith's enthusiasm and support for any number of diverse interests and causes throughout a long career are among his most appealing qualities. For example, his devotion to art made him an active participant in the affairs of the British Institution (later the National Gallery), as well as a patron of Norwich artists like John Sell Cotman and John Opie; his scientific interests led to his intervention with the government on behalf of Charles Babbage and his computer; and his political involvements encompassed both the more adventurous and the mundane, the Greek Committee to raise support for the Greeks' struggle for independence against the Turks, as well as British Fisheries and the Thames Tunnel Company.

Three projects of reform, however, remained the most cherished objectives of Smith's working life: the abolition of slavery, the extension of religious liberty, and the reform of Parliament itself. He was an early advocate of a programme of moderate Whig reform, proposing a household franchise together with an end to corruption and the undue influence of the Crown. If he was a minor player in the events leading to the

Great Reform Act of 1832, the same could hardly be said of Smith's role in the abolitionist campaign. Here he worked closely and decisively with William Wilberforce, Thomas Clarkson, and other members of the Clapham Sect, to heal what his granddaughter Florence Nightingale was one day to call 'the open sore of the world'. As a child, Florence often heard the battle for the abolition of slavery fought over again in conversations among her aunts and uncles; and it was a subject reflected in Florence's childhood scrapbooks, into which she copied and illustrated William Cowper's anti-slavery poems 'The Morning Dream' and 'The Negro's Complaint'.

William Smith's association with the Clapham Saints, the 'prosperous and pious' evangelical sect dedicated to the abolition, first of the slave trade, and subsequently of slavery itself, went back many years. In his teens Smith had lived with his father at the family home in Clapham and later, as he began married life, he moved to Eagle House, a large property on the west side of the Common. The Thorntons were close neighbours, and Henry Thornton, later a prominent economist and governor of the Bank of England, who was to become a leading member of the sect, was one Smith's childhood friends. Although Smith had left Clapham by the time Wilberforce, Zachary Macaulay and other Saints colonized the village as their headquarters, the ties with the Thornton family remained strong, and were an important factor in making Smith an ally of the evangelicals in their fight for abolition.

Smith's commitment to the anti-slavery movement was inspired by a deep religious conviction that it was 'impious' for one man to deprive another of his freedom, and one of his first steps in support of the cause was to boycott the import of slave-produced sugar, even though such action hurt his own business interests. He worked tirelessly, mobilizing public opinion, examining witnesses and furthering the parliamentary case for abolition. Politically, Smith acted as an essential bridge between the conservative Saints and his own party, the Whigs, and it was Fox who, as foreign secretary in 1806, moved the motion for the abolition of the slave trade, just days before his death. To his great disappointment Smith, who was briefly out of the Commons, having lost his seat in the previous year's election, was unable to contribute his own vote for abolition, which was carried with a triumphant majority in February 1807.

An end to slavery itself was one of his major goals for the next quarter of a century. Writing in the 1820s to his son-in-law, William

Nightingale, to ask for his help 'to procure an Anti-Slavery Meeting', Smith observed that his own 'Head, Heart & Hands, have been turned to this subject for the last 40 years . . . and, go on to perfection, it will & must – nothing can stop it'. His confidence was not misplaced. Smith lived just long enough to see Parliament commit itself to the emancipation of slaves in the British colonies.

The stout member for Norwich, with his 'heart-stirring laughter', was popular among members of the Clapham Sect. Wilberforce himself, Thomas Clarkson and Zachary Macaulay expressed deep affection for him as if he was one of their own. But as in politics, so in religion, Smith and the Saints were divided. Despite their best efforts to convert him to their Evangelical beliefs, Smith remained an avowed Unitarian.

He had become a Unitarian in the late 1780s, under the influence of Thomas Belsham. Belsham, later minister of London's Essex Street Chapel, one of the more respectable Unitarian congregations, was the outstanding preacher of a revived Unitarianism, which saw it transformed from an intellectual movement into an important denomination, small in numbers but strong in appeal. The fundamental tenets of Unitarianism – rejecting the doctrine of the Trinity, denying the divinity of Christ, as well as disputing such beliefs as original sin and the atonement – were a product of a new rationalism, influenced by the ideas of Hobbes, Locke and Newton, that did not sit easily with traditional Christianity, and which consequently had a profound impact on Dissenting thought.

It was a dangerous time to be a Dissenter. The sympathy shown by some Dissenters to the reforming ideals of the French Revolution made them the favoured scapegoats of the mob at a time when Roman Catholics were being treated with a greater degree of tolerance. In the summer of 1791, the Birmingham home of William Smith's friend Joseph Priestley, Unitarian theologian and chemist, the discoverer of oxygen, was burned to the ground in one such attack, his books and scientific instruments destroyed.

Sydney Smith, only half-jokingly, called William Smith 'the head of the Unitarian Church', and 'the dissenting king'. In 1813 William was responsible for drawing up and guiding through Parliament the Unitarian Toleration Act, which made the denial of Christ's divinity no longer a crime. But his fundamental belief in the individual's right to religious liberty without state persecution had by that time led him to assume a broader responsibility for his fellow Dissenters. Between 1805 and

1830 he served as chairman of the Dissenting Deputies, a committee of Presbyterians, Independents and Baptists, originally established to take care of the civil affairs of Dissenters, and towards the end of his time in office, Smith campaigned successfully for the repeal of the Test and Corporation Acts, one of the great symbols of prejudice against Dissenters.

Smith's own religious observance reflected his liberal stance. He was certainly not narrow or bigoted, was happy to attend the established church 'when no chapel of his own persuasion was near', and prepared to hear any preacher of note whatever his theological views. That spirit of free inquiry into religious matters, so central to William Smith, was also to be his most significant legacy to his granddaughter, Florence Nightingale.

In 1781 William Smith married Frances Coape, from an old and wealthy Dissenting family from Nottinghamshire. Frances was deeply religious as well as being something of a bluestocking, with a strong taste for theological disputation. Few escaped her sharp tongue, which made no allowances for rank or distinction. She and William were a loyal and devoted couple. They had twelve children: two died in infancy, but the remaining ten all lived well into old age. Martha (known as Patty) was the eldest, born in 1782, followed by Benjamin (1783), Anne (1786), Fanny (1788), Adams (1789), Joanna (1791), Samuel (1794), Octavius (1796), Frederick (1798) and Julia (1799). To accommodate this growing family, and to signify his new social and political position, William purchased Parndon Hall, near Harlow in Essex, in 1785. With an estate of 260 acres, and a house gradually enlarged to some twenty rooms, twice its original size, Parndon provided, if not an elegant, then at least a convenient residence for entertaining the Whig elite, and for housing William's sizeable library. In London, close to Parliament for the session, William bought 6 Park Street, a handsome Adam house overlooking Birdcage Walk, which housed his expanding art collection. By the mid-1790s, Rembrandts, Cuyps, Gainsboroughs hung alongside Smith's prized possession, Sir Joshua Reynolds's portrait of *Mrs Siddons as the Tragic Muse*.

Frances Smith was more spartan in her ways than her husband, and tried to impress her frugal habits on her children, though for many of them their father's extravagance was a way of life to which they became accustomed, and which as adults they would find difficult to match. As Patty reminisced in the 1840s: '. . . Horses, Pictures, Travelling, Masters, Artists, Society & all that belonged to the Parliamentary life – have ever made me feel the mere routine of riches.' More to Mrs Smith's taste were simple family holidays, travelling around England, Scotland and Wales in the sociable, an open carriage with facing side seats; or with herself and William in the phaeton and the children and maids crammed into the chaise. She kept a series of journals on these tours of the country, which express her delight in recording her observations of everyday matters: the local industry, for instance, like the copper mines of Cornwall, or a visit to the Lancashire cotton mills 'where the cotton is carded, roved, and spun by one large master-wheel'.

The upbringing of the five Smith girls was privileged in more than just material terms. Florence Nightingale's education, supervised by her father, is often singled out for having been advanced by the standards set for women in the first half of the nineteenth century, but in its own small way, her mother Fanny's schooling was also ahead of its time. Like other Dissenters of the period, William Smith took pains with his daughters' education. They were taught entirely at home by visiting teachers, except for Joanna, who went to school for a while, and the evidence suggests that opportunities for learning were taken very seriously. Joanna's diary for 1806 gives a broad outline of the main curriculum when it states that 'Music, French, Italian and Drawing for Fanny, I, and Julia this year has cost £47.15.0.' There was also the luxury of their father's library, the delights of which Patty, nicknamed 'Bookworm', regularly sampled. Access to its 2,000-odd volumes undoubtedly contributed to Patty's intelligence and wit, for which she had won something of a reputation by her twenties.

The children's martinet mother was always ready to crack the whip when necessary. 'Julia dwells much on my mind,' Mrs Smith wrote when her youngest child was thirteen. '. . . I wish she would translate Dante, 2 cantos a week . . .' Something of her carrot and stick approach can be seen in a letter she wrote to her eight-year-old son Octavius in 1804:

. . . You are in general a very good Boy at rising in the morning, and I well remember that you are usually the first to tap at my door with 'Mama. Mama it is Octavius' and if Octavius continue to be so early, and to improve in regularity, mama will increase in her love to him . . .

All the children benefited from their father's position at the centre of current events, though on one occasion it proved too close for comfort for Smith himself. On 11 May 1812 he was in the lobby of the House of Commons when a shot rang out and a small figure fell at his feet. Raising the wounded man, he discovered him to be the Prime Minister, Spencer Perceval, mortally wounded by an assassin's bullet. That evening, 'very much affected', Smith returned to Park Street, 'with his hands covered in blood', as Fanny noted in her diary, and one of the dead man's gloves in his pocket.

Proximity to other national occasions produced happier memories. Patty could remember as a child seeing George III being driven in state to St Paul's in 1789 to give thanks for his recovery from his first attack of madness; six years later, she witnessed the arrival of the Prince of Wales's bride, Princess Caroline of Brunswick, dressed in green satin laced with gold and wearing a beaver hat. As a young woman in the summer of 1811, Patty described to her sister Fanny the 'crush at Carleton House', the Prince Regent's London home, where the 'most elegant rooms' were decorated in purple velvet and gold. The summer months brought interesting visitors to Parndon. A 'little dark man' at dinner turned out to be Samuel Taylor Coleridge, who, Joanna recorded, was 'a most extraordinary man, holds forth like a book, in such language as I never heard before'.

The voices of the five Smith daughters have come down to us vibrant and clear in their letters to each other, bickering and bantering like Jane Austen's five Bennet sisters (in contrast to their five male siblings, whose correspondence has largely disappeared). As she approached womanhood Fanny, with her rich brown, wavy hair, slim figure and vivacious personality, was widely acknowledged as a beauty. 'She is daily improving in her appearance,' her mother wrote when Fanny was twenty-one, adding with a sniff of disapproval, 'to which her own eye is not blind.' At sixteen Fanny had attended her first ball where, her sister Anne reported, 'she was very much admired and got very beauish partners'. Fanny had celebrated her 'entry into the beau monde' by dancing until two o'clock in the morning. Dancing – along with going out in the carriage for 'a good deal of shopping' – was still one of Fanny's favourite activities almost a decade later. In the winter of 1812 she went to a ball for 120 people and danced seven dances, one of which consisted of some fashionable steps known as 'Lady Frances Pratt's Fancy'. But life was not all fun and self-indulgence. She attended a dinner for 'the poor children' and presented them with new bonnets for Christmas, and occasionally she taught in a local school. There was a serious, not unintellectual, side to Fanny that can sometimes be glimpsed beneath the carefree surface.

However, despite her attractiveness, Fanny, by her late twenties, was still unmarried. She was certainly not devoid of suitors, but all of them seem to have fallen short of the standard she had set for a prospective husband. Her brother Ben, clearly alert to how particular his sister could be, commented on one eligible candidate: 'I considered him and his 8000 a year to your special predilection – Dance with him, don't snub him – but let the speculation of your eyes speculate not harshly . . .' Perhaps the sophisticated company of her father's friends had spoilt Fanny; or perhaps it was simply that she could find no one to live up to her father's example of decency and kindness. Whatever the reason, in 1816 she made a sudden, ill-fated decision to marry James Sinclair, the third son of the Earl of Caithness. Sinclair was almost a decade younger than Fanny, a captain in the Ross-shire Militia, with no prospects beyond his army pay, and already a large accumulation of debt. Both families were against the match. The Earl of Caithness, writing to Fanny's father about this 'very thoughtless young man', regretted that 'it is quite out of my power to remove the obstacles that stand in the way to the union of your aimiable [sic] daughter with our son'. To Mrs Smith, Caithness's letter was decisive. For James Sinclair to marry at all would be 'highly improper', she told Fanny, who had fled to Brighton to nurse her broken heart:

We have laboured under a temporary illusion, and we have persuaded your Father to go farther than he ought to have done . . . and all this you should thoroughly consider and the understanding God has given you will enable you to overcome the regret you feel and to agree that it is better for all parties that the affair should terminate.

Before signing off, Mrs Smith could not resist a parting shot of her customary priggishness: 'I hope you do not . . . lie abed till near ten o'clock, for that will prove an effectual mode of defeating every good your present situation might afford.'

It was left to William Smith to put matters more considerately. He begged Fanny to 'look as well to what you have escaped, as to what you have lost'. But even he could not overcome the unsuitability of young Sinclair for his daughter:

His profession, his family would have suited you – but his Understanding, his Want of Energy could not. With regard to his love for you, which you call disinterested, I own, I call it passionate – no more. The difficulties he clearly overlooked . . . which with most men, of no larger income than his, [are] usually a reason for giving up a woman, rather than pursuing her.

The affair ended. At twenty-eight, Fanny's marital prospects looked bleak, and she must have envied the happiness of two of her sisters. Anne, two years her senior, was already celebrating the second anniversary of her marriage to George Nicholson, son of a prominent Dissenting family from Guildford, and a promising young lawyer in the Inner Temple; while that Christmas of 1816, Joanna, Fanny's junior by more than three years, was married to John Carter, the newly elected MP for Portsmouth.

Another suitor, though, hovered in the background. This was William Nightingale of Derbyshire, who had recently changed his name from Shore.

On one of the family's carriage trips across country, fourteen years earlier, in 1803, the Smiths had paid a visit to the William Shores of Tapton Hall, in Ecclesall, near Sheffield. The Shores, an old Sheffield family who could trace their descent back to the fifteenth century, had started the town's first banking business in 1774. Their prominence as a Dissenting family, and latterly as a Unitarian one, together with their support for parliamentary reform, had caused their paths to cross with those of William Smith. William Shore's oldest brother, Samuel, was a trustee of Sheffield's Upper Chapel, and a generous subscriber to the Essex Street Chapel in London, which William Smith attended; he was also a member, like Smith, of 'The Friends of the People', a society pledged to pursue constitutional reform on 'temperate principles'.

William Shore lived with his wife, Mary, and their two surviving children, a son, also called William, and a daughter Mary (known as Mai). In her journal describing her 1803 visit, Frances Smith observed that William, 'a lad of about ten years of age, has had £100,000 left to him by a Mr Nightingale, with the whimsical prohibition of neither benefiting himself while under age, nor suffering his daughters to inherit. Should he not have a son it goes to his sister.'

The Nightingale connection descended through Mrs Shore. Born Mary Evans, her mother Anne had been a Nightingale and it was Anne's brother Peter, Mary Shore's unmarried uncle, who had made the bequest to the young William Shore. The 'whimsical prohibition' was the least of Peter Nightingale's eccentricities. He had acquired a reputation in his home village of Lea in north Derbyshire as 'Mad Peter Nightingale', the daredevil sporting squire, who rode in midnight steeplechases, and was a hard drinker and gambler. Nonetheless Peter was a man of solid business acumen. Earlier generations of Nightingales had been lead smelters and merchants, and Peter built on their investments to become a man of some substance on the profits of lead and cotton. He also speculated wisely in property, purchasing the Cromford Estate, close to Richard Arkwright's new cotton mills, before selling it on at a sizeable profit. When the Smiths called on the Shores in 1803, Peter Nightingale had only recently died, in the tumbledown half-farm, half-manor known as Lea Hall.

Mary Shore had inherited something of the Nightingale wildness, having been headstrong and difficult as a young girl. Her son, William, however, thin and lanky like his Shore forebears, was of an altogether calmer and more easygoing temperament. The Nightingale inheritance, which would be his at twenty-one, would turn out to be something of a mixed blessing. Of course, the security it provided meant that he never had to learn a profession, and could follow the life that best suited him, that of a country gentleman, with cultivated, dilettante interests. Equally, though, it inclined William towards indolence, which increasingly, as the years passed, would leave him with a sense of aimlessness.

William Edward Shore had been born in Sheffield on 15 February 1794, and educated at Higham Hall in Epping Forest, which Fanny Smith's brother Octavius also attended, and where the headmaster, the Reverend Eli Cogan, was a Unitarian minister. At the age of seventeen in 1811 he matriculated as a pensioner at Trinity College, Cambridge, where he was a contemporary of Fanny's brother Sam. However, his position as a Dissenter meant that, under the University statutes, he was unable to take a degree. The expectation of a fortune led him to mark time. He spent 'a term or two' in 1813–14 at Edinburgh University, attending classes in literature and also, more unusually, in medicine, and was on a tour of the Western Highlands in early 1815, staying with the family of the Laird of Rothiemurchus, when he came of age and succeeded to his inheritance. 'Mad Peter' had tied one additional condition to his bequest: William must 'assume and take upon himself . . . the sirname [sic] of Nightingale'. While his Scottish friends joked about 'the ridiculous name', William Shore proceeded to become William Nightingale by royal licence.

William was first introduced to the Smith family as a schoolfriend of Octavius's, and appears to have quickly become something of a favourite with other family members. Stray references in Smith letters show him to have been a welcome visitor at Parndon as early as 1811, though confusion over William's adopted surname meant that latterly he was 'sometimes called Knightingale or just plain Night'. At what point he ceased to be just a friend of her brother's, and became a serious prospect as a husband for Fanny is unknown; but in the wake of the Sinclair débâcle, his suitability may have been brought startlingly into focus. In the spring of 1817, while Fanny was in Brighton, her elder brother Ben acted as a courier for their 'affectionate correspondence'. True, William was six years younger than Fanny, but then she clearly had a penchant for younger men. There was no worry about money either. The Nightingale fortune meant that Fanny would be kept in the manner of living to which she had become accustomed. William was besotted with her too. For more than half a century, he would prove attentive, patient and extraordinarily compliant to her will.

The news of William and Fanny's engagement in the spring of 1818 was greeted warmly by both Smith and Shore parents. 'I am always saying to myself,' wrote Mr Shore to Fanny, ' "I don't wonder she has got possession of William's heart for I am sure she has won mine".' William's kindness thawed even Fanny's mother, though this did not prevent her mixing her congratulations on their wedding day with a heavy dose of gloom: 'May God in his infinite mercy keep you both, may you go hand in hand happily through this life, but may you never forget that there is a better.'

Fanny 'thinks Nightingale the best man she ever saw & says she has nothing left to wish under heaven', Julia wrote to Patty Smith, who was abroad with their brother Ben, and would miss the wedding. 'It is very clear that he is of the same opinion with her. You never saw anything like the brightening up of his face, he seems so thoroughly happy . . .' They were married by the Reverend William Dealtry at St Margaret's, Westminster, on 1 June 1818, a boiling hot day. William Smith's 'roaring' at the reception afterwards was 'quite disgusting', reported

Julia, though 'whether he was drunk with wine or joy I cannot tell'. One thing marred the happiness of the occasion. Although they were staying in London, neither of the Shore parents was invited to the ceremony. Mai Shore, William's sister, had been present, but she had apparently been made to feel uncomfortable at being unsuitably dressed in the church. 'Don't you think your Mother & I ought to have been at the wedding?' Mr Shore asked his son plaintively. 'I have heard it strongly insisted on by people who are correct judges.' With no evidence of disagreements or tensions, the exclusion of the Shores is something of a mystery. Was William Nightingale perhaps worried that his parents, of traditional Dissenting stock, would embarrass him at a fashionable London wedding? Deprived of a seat in the church, Mr Shore rode to the Uxbridge Road, where he waited for two hours in the hope of seeing the couple pass on their way to Parndon, where they were spending their first week of honeymoon.

From Parndon, the Nightingales travelled on to Kynsham Court, in Presteigne in Herefordshire, a house built in the middle of the previous century, and owned by Lord Oxford. Briefly occupied by Lord Byron six years earlier, Kynsham was a modest country seat in a beautiful setting, perched on a thickly wooded hillside high above the valley of the River Lugg. William had entered already into protracted negotiations to buy Kynsham, and, like him, Fanny was enchanted by the house. She was a good deal less impressed by either of the houses on the Nightingale estate at Lea, both of which required a considerable amount of renovation before they could be inhabited as family homes.

For the time being, though, the question of where they were to live was put to one side as Fanny and William set out for the continent. With them went Fanny's maid, Frances Gale, known as 'little Gale', a woman in her early thirties, so stunted in growth that she was often referred to as a dwarf. Gale was devoted to Fanny and had cried so much at the prospect of her mistress's departure that the Nightingales had decided that she should accompany them. After some months in Rome, by the late autumn the party had reached Naples, where they decided to settle. Fanny had quickly become pregnant following her departure from England. The need to produce a male heir was paramount so that the Nightingale inheritance could be passed on directly to the next generation, and Fanny had passed thirty at her last birthday.

On 19 April 1819 a baby girl was born. '. . . It was a little disappointment not being a son,' Gale admitted in a note to Fanny's sister Joanna, a sentiment seconded by the child's grandfather William Smith, who as usual tried to put the best construction on matters: 'As for the sex, perhaps it might have been better; but I am disposed to give the little Female a most cordial welcome – & there are advantages to a Mother in having the eldest born of her own sort.' Five weeks later the baby was christened Frances Parthenope, Parthenope being the Greek name for her birthplace ('what a hard name says one, what a fine name says another'). Gale pronounced her 'quite a <u>Buty</u>'.

Less than a week after the birth, however, William Nightingale fell ill, and was diagnosed with malaria. He had scarcely begun to recover when one of Fanny's breasts became seriously inflamed. They had been intending to move on to Castellammare, but suddenly had to alter their plans and remain in Naples, which was hot and deserted in the summer months. 'The cruelty of the case,' William explained in some misery to Joanna Carter, 'is that Fanny is by no means sure that she may not lose her milk & this would be the greatest of misfortunes that could happen. We have not a soul to console us but doctors and servants . . . a dreadful mélange of medical society, & a shop full of medicine will be our souvenirs of Naples.'

On top of this, 'a cargo of bad news' reached them from England, that William Smith's business had failed, and that he was facing ruin. Julia reported that 'We shall have, selling Parndon & <u>everything</u>, somewhere about £1000 a year (more or less) left.' William Smith was in a 'torment', she wrote a little later, as Parndon went up for auction and Park Street was let, while 'my poor mother is the only one who moans without ceasing . . .'

The end of the year found the Nightingales still in Naples, waiting for the weather to change so that they could travel. The intense summer heat had given way to violent siroccos, and latterly to heavy torrents of rain. The good news was that Fanny was pregnant again. She feared that she would be unable to suckle the new baby, as one breast was 'so injured that it may never recover', but she was hopeful that the child would be a boy. In February, with Parthenope swaddled up into a neat parcel like an Italian bambino, the family at last made their way to Florence. Towards the end of March, William leased the 'Villa called Colombaja, in the Parish of St Illari Podesteria dell Galliozo', hired Umiliana Pistelli as wetnurse, and waited for the birth.

Florence Nightingale was born on 12 May 1820, and christened in the grand salon of the villa on 4 July by another visitor to the city, Dr Thomas Trevor, the Prebendary of Chester, and an old Trinity friend of her father's. Ahead of the family, Gale was sent back to England on a special mission. At Dr Williams's Library in London's Cripplegate, she recorded Florence's birth in the Protestant Dissenters' Register, thereby linking her to the religious traditions of her forefathers.

Fanny and William Nightingale would have no more children. Whether by accident or design, this absence of a larger family was to have serious repercussions, in years to come, on the smooth running of their domestic life, when their younger daughter decided to renounce her duty, and break away from the constraints of home. When that time arrived, Florence Nightingale, with the mathematical precision and dramatic sweep so characteristic of her, would find bitter reason to record that the size of a family lies in inverse proportion to its potential as an instrument of repression and imprisonment.

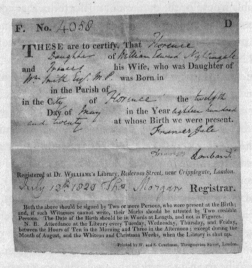

2. Pop and Flo

Ill health was Florence Nightingale's almost immediate response to the English climate. She had thrived in the warm Italian weather, but a return home, to her father's Derbyshire estates, when she was just a year old, marked the beginning of a sickly childhood. That first harsh winter left her with a bronchial cough and a persistent sore throat, accompanied by severe loss of weight. Other afflictions in her early years would have their roots in a more mysterious source. The weakness in her hands that made writing difficult was mirrored in the condition of her ankles, where a similar problem developed. Until well into her teens she would be forced to wear steel-lined boots as a corrective and preventative measure.*

The Nightingales made a slow progress back to England during the winter of 1820–21. In Paris, at the Hôtel de Breteuil in the rue de Rivoli, they were met by Mai Shore, William's sister, and by Fanny's brother Ben, and two sisters, Patty and Julia. Julia had never been out of England before, and years later she recalled the excitement of the visit, and her relief too at being away from the rest of her family while the agonizing process of selling the Smith family homes was taking place. The sight of the fat old king Louis XVIII, bundled into a coach in the Bois de Boulogne, remained a vivid one, as did her first introduction to her young nieces. Parthenope was 'a pretty piquante little creature very like a kitten, lisping Italian', while in the arms of Balia, her Florentine nurse, Florence appeared simply 'fat and chubby'.

William Smith had acted as an impressive support to his daughter and son-in-law during their disheartening months of illness and isolation in Italy, despite his own worsening circumstances. In the depths of their misfortunes he had sent out English groceries as a diversion from their

---

* Theories that Florence Nightingale's childhood illnesses may have been the result of lead poisoning emanating from the smelter close to the Nightingales' Derbyshire home, or that the water supply to Lea Hurst from the Holywell at the side of Leashaw was contaminated with lead, remain purely speculative.

Neapolitan diet, and he had also been handling the negotiations for the purchase of Kynsham, in Herefordshire, on their behalf. William and Fanny had set their hearts on making this house their main residence, and during a dry and dusty summer in Naples had dreamt of its surrounding lush woods and cool streams. Back in England, Fanny and the girls spent part of the autumn of 1822 at Kynsham while William Nightingale dealt with matters in Derbyshire. The following spring they were there again, but in 1824 the family was dividing its time between Lea and Eden Farm in Bromley in Kent, signalling that the protracted attempts to buy the house from the Harley family had finally fallen through. It was a huge disappointment.

Instead, William Nightingale concentrated on rebuilding a house on the Lea estate to suit the family's requirements, while continuing to look for a second home further south where they could spend each winter. Peter Nightingale had lived at Lea Hall, at the far eastern end of the village, and it was here that the Nightingales stayed on their return from Italy while they made further plans. The origins of the Hall date as far back as the fourteenth century, and its south front, rebuilt some 400 years later, incorporated the remains of the medieval manor. Peter Nightingale, inheriting the Hall in 1754, gave it an impressive new northern front – still standing today – consisting of five bays with Doric pilasters and an entrance crowned by a pedimented Gibbs surround. Although dilapidated after decades of use as a farmhouse, Lea Hall was perhaps the finest small seat in the county. William Nightingale, though, had a more ambitious scheme. At the opposite end of the village, raised on high ground among trees above the River Derwent, stood an early Jacobean house, overlooking 1,381 acres of magnificent parkland, which 'Mad Peter' had purchased in 1771. It had two storeys with mullion windows, faced north, and was built of Ashover Grit quarried from nearby. William fancied himself as an architect, and in 1822 set about enlarging it from his own designs. Combined with a further programme of smaller alterations in the 1860s, these would effectively treble the size of the house. A second, parallel range was added behind the old main range of the house, together with a new wing to the north, adapted from a former outbuilding. A host of other features were included: gables, crenellations, clustering chimneys, more mullion windows, while a small domestic chapel, jutting out from the original house, was incorporated into the new building. Although it is doubtful that the chapel, with its decorated chancel window, was ever used by the Nightingales for their religious observances, it may have provided a meeting place for Florence Nightingale's Sunday afternoon Bible class in the 1840s.

William Nightingale surveyed his creation with pride. Smaller details for the interior did not escape him. He was responsible for the design of all the fireplaces, the Hoptonwood stone staircase in the main hall, even several of the chairs. The park, separated from the garden by wrought-iron gates, was landscaped, taking advantage of the spectacular natural topography. The novelist Mrs Gaskell, a visitor to Lea Hurst in 1854, peering nervously from a high dormer window – 'one seems on the Devil's pinnacle of the Earth' – was entranced by the view:

First a garden with stone terraces and flights of steps, and old stone columns with globes at the top of them in every direction – the planes of these terraces being perfectly gorgeous with masses of hollyhocks, dahlias, nasturtiums &c – Then a sloping meadow losing itself in a steep wooded – (such tints!) descent to the river Derwent, the rocks on the other side which form the first distance are of a misty purple. Beyond interlacing hills forming three ranges of distance – the first dun brown with decaying heather, the next in some mysterious purple shadow, & the last catching some pale watery sun-light.

In the early 1830s, pleased with his efforts after he had helped to lay out a new terrace, William looked around him and saw 'A perfect 3 months summer residence & equally perfect 10 days winter one'. He decamped, at his wife's insistence, to London at the height of every season, and to Embley Park, the house he bought in Hampshire in 1825, for the winter months, from September to November. But Lea Hurst remained what he called 'my solace and my home'; and this was a feeling that united him with his younger daughter, Florence. Parthenope, it is true, was inspired by the romantic associations of the moorland villages, chiefly by neighbouring Dethick, where Sir Anthony Babington had lived at the old hall while plotting the escape of Mary, Queen of Scots, and would later use the legends, dialect and scenery of Derbyshire in her second novel, *Stone Edge*, published in 1871. But for Florence the connection went deeper. As a baby, in the absence of a male heir, she was known as 'the young squire' by local people, and as she grew older, her concern for the villagers would provide her with an important sense of purpose. At 'the Hurst' she could lead a life of relative tranquillity and independence, within easy reach of the sick poor, unlike the busy routine at Embley where the accent was on entertaining and display, and where a visit to the needy villagers of East Wellow was a significant carriage-ride – or a whole day's walking – away. Lea Hurst held a special place in Florence's affections all her life.* The sound of the continuous roar of the Derwent from the casement window in the nursery would recur in her dreams for years to come. Words from the local dialect – for example, the Derbyshire word 'scratting', meaning scratching or clawing – occasionally surfaced in her writing.

The Nightingales' Derbyshire home was also to play its small part in the early development of the personal mythology encircling Florence's name, both during and in the years immediately following the Crimean War. When these first pilgrims sought the shrine of their 'true but modest heroine', they did not go to Embley, but to Lea Hurst, where popular stories had told them that Miss Nightingale had ministered 'to the wants of the poor in her own neighbourhood'. In this scheme of things, Lea Hurst seemed to represent her rejection of everything 'vain, hollow, and evanescent', and to confirm her status as 'a heart unseduced by the temptations of fashion and the pleasures of the world'.

The antiquarian Llewellynn Jewitt took *A Stroll to Lea Hurst* in 1855, in the first romantic glow of Florence Nightingale's fame. He noted the picturesque situation of the house itself, but what struck him almost as much was the extent to which the landscape of wood, hill and rock was dotted with small houses, furnaces, and tall chimneys attached to lead mines and smelting mills. This was an area, he reported, in which 'a large number of persons are constantly employed in mining and agricultural occupations'.

Agriculture was, by then, in long-term decline in Lea. William Nightingale grazed sheep on his parkland for many years but, like his great-uncle and the generations of Nightingales immediately preceding him, he made his substantial profits from lead. Until as recently as the early 1980s, the burnt-out remains of the old Lea lead smelter were clearly visible on the road that leads from the old Hall to Lea Bridge, testimony to the industry that was the hub of the village from the sixteenth century right up to 1935, when the works finally closed down.

---

* The Nightingales, too, were popular with the villagers. The family's return to the Hurst each summer was greeted by the playing of the local band at the entrance to the estate.

William Nightingale operated the mine until 1856, when he leased it to a smelter from Holloway.

Holloway and Dethick combined with Lea to form a hamlet, which in Florence's childhood numbered about 675 inhabitants. The Lea cotton mill had provided the other main occupation of the area until Thomas Smedley, originally an associate of Peter Nightingale's, had moved to the manufacture of hosiery. In the mid-nineteenth century, under Smedley's son John, Lea Mill became a flourishing concern, and continues so today, with its record as the longest uninterrupted wool-spinning factory in Britain. John Smedley was also a leading light in the revival of Methodism, which was very strong in north Derbyshire by mid-century, and which had an especially fervent following among the quarrymen and mill-workers in Lea itself. The local chapel, endowed by a Nightingale at the end of the seventeenth century, was used by the Methodists, and eventually became a Methodist church. At the beginning of the 1850s, William Nightingale commented on 'the new phase of Methodism in these parts', adding that 'Smedley has begun preaching himself. His Mill will be converted into a Sanctuary.'

Try as she might, Fanny Nightingale could not accustom herself to Derbyshire's inhospitable winters, nor to the lack of opportunities for large-scale, fashionable entertaining. She worked hard to acquaint herself with local society, such as it was. 'Poor Fanny,' remarked her sister Julia, 'she would be very neighbourly if the people would let her.' But by the time the stone lintel engraved with the year 1825 was erected above the front door at Lea Hurst, recording the completion of the alterations, a search had long since begun to find a second home, in the warmer south. In the summer of that year, Embley Park, near Romsey in Hampshire, 'a capital and convenient Mansion House' of the late Georgian period, with 3,700 acres attached, came up for sale. With only five bedrooms, the house was small in comparison with the Hurst. Its gardens, though, were ornate: '1,300 acres planted. The Grotto finished with stones and shells having in front a basin with gold and silver fish, a pyramidical fountain, and an American garden and cottage attached'; and it offered 'drives commanding Southampton Water and the New Forest'.

On a July day, Patty Smith watched as Fanny, William and the two children, accompanied by a land valuer, left the Hurst to inspect Embley. 'This looks as if N[ightingale] were quite in earnest,' Patty reported, though, 'at the same time if his idea of the income [from the estate] is anything like correct, the sacrifice will be enormous in point of money, tho very likely the gain very great in point of pleasure.' She paused to add that the change of air might prove beneficial to the children: latterly Parthenope's cough had been incessant, while 'little Flo' had grown very thin.

In the final months of 1825 the family was settled at Embley. This plain Georgian house would in time offer plenty of scope for extension and redevelopment, and there was the promise of rewarding contacts among well-connected neighbours of a standing that Fanny could only have dreamed about in Derbyshire. It would not have escaped her notice that Broadlands, the family seat of Lord Palmerston, was just a couple of miles away. In future years the Nightingales would be welcomed as regular guests there, especially after Palmerston's marriage in 1840 to Lady Emily Cowper, the widowed sister of Lord Melbourne, when an invitation to dinner and a stay overnight might be accompanied by the instruction that 'Mr N.' bring his gun, as 'L.P. intends to beat a cover tomorrow if it should be fine'.

While Lea Hurst was close to William's family in the north – and on the doorstep of the Cromford home of Aunt (Elizabeth) Evans, his mother's sister, a short walk or pony ride across the moors – Embley brought Fanny geographically nearer to her two married sisters. Joanna and John Bonham Carter (like the Nightingales before them, the Carters had changed their name, in 1827, on inheriting the property of a cousin, Thomas Bonham of Petersfield) lived at Fair Oaks, ten miles away in Winchester. In the next county, near Farnham, at Waverley Abbey, built by the ruins of the Cistercian monastery, lived Fanny's second sister Anne and her husband George Nicholson. The world of Florence Nightingale's childhood was dominated by an almost constant migration between different sets of relatives, paying visits to uncles, aunts and cousins, and receiving them in return at Lea Hurst or Embley. Christmas was usually spent with the Nicholsons in the splendour of Waverley, while the summer months might bring a visit to London to see Fanny's younger brother Octavius, who ran the family distillery business at Thames Bank, and his wife Jane. Sometimes Parthenope, known as Parthe or Pop, or Florence, called Flo or sometimes Bo or Bos (a nod perhaps to Charles Dickens's pseudonym in *Pickwick Papers*), would go separately to stay with cousins; at others they would be sent off together. When Fanny and William were away, relatives would often come to stay with the sisters. The arrival of the railway eased the strain of this life of persistent travel on hazardous roads: by the mid-1840s the Ambergate line was cutting across the fields that lay at the back of Lea Hurst.

The complicated network of uncles, 'multitudinous aunts' and the 'great clan of cousins' deriving from Fanny Nightingale's numerous siblings was to be a prominent feature of Florence's early life, and beyond. By her fourteenth birthday, she could already count nearly two dozen aunts and uncles by blood and marriage, and twenty-seven first cousins; and although as a young woman she would be the author of some scathing reflections on the institution of the family, this broader family unit was always of great importance to her. All her life she set great store by the affectionate relationships within her extended family circle, and some of her relations would eventually have their more practical uses as well, when they were swept into the vortex surrounding her career and fame. It was a remarkable brood, including artists, high-ranking army officers, explorers, radical MPs and activists for women's, and even animal, rights among its members. 'What energy & phil-anthropy there is in that Smith blood,' wrote a Miss Aiken as Florence Nightingale was making her way to Scutari, in the autumn of 1854. Jane Carlyle was less enamoured of the Smith genes, commenting on their 'hard, cold . . . uniformity . . .'

A difficult situation, involving two of these uncles and aunts, had emerged on the Nightingales' return from the continent, and had briefly threatened to mar relations between Fanny and William's respective families. While accompanying the Nightingales home from Paris, Ben Smith and Mai Shore had met for the first time and had fallen in love. They rapidly announced their engagement, without having first sought the permission of Mai's parents. Mai's father was furious and opposed the match, blaming William for having encouraged the couple. Mr Shore died in September 1822, 'angry with his son to the last'. Mai was put 'upon her guard against Ben', and forbidden to see him. Ben, wrote William of his brother-in-law, was 'so completely the opposite of sim-plicity, good-taste & what may be suited to a peaceable life that no good can come of his union with anyone, but a woman as high-spirited & determined as himself'.

That woman was destined to be Annie Longden, a milliner's daughter from Alfreton who, by the end of 1826, was pregnant by Ben. The birth of a daughter was followed by four more children before Annie's death from consumption in 1834. Yet Ben never married her. Fanny Nightingale shook her head in disapproval at the prospect of scandal, her mother Frances described Ben as being 'in thralldom', and Patty Smith dismissed Annie, quite erroneously, as a professional courtesan. Ben later succeeded William Smith as MP for Norwich, and was prominent in the campaign for the repeal of the Corn Laws. He 'was such a large nature with a touch of genius in him', his niece Florence remembered in old age. But although he continued to be invited to Lea Hurst and Embley, Ben's children, 'the tabooed family' as they were known, found themselves ostracized by many of their father's relatives. In years to come, as Ben's eldest child, Barbara Bodichon, became an influential leader of the Victorian women's movement, she and her cousin Florence might have often found common cause on matters of female education and employment; but the slur remained, and though the two women probably corresponded, it seems unlikely that they ever met.

After the break with Ben, Mai Shore was a frequent visitor to Lea Hurst, where she soon won Florence's devotion. They became 'very good friends', and as Florence grew older she would come to regard her aunt as a kindred spirit. Mai's awareness of her own 'miserable education' had contributed to the development of an inquiring mind and speculative intelligence. 'She's got an oddness like nobody else,' commented Fanny Nightingale, who derided her sister-in-law's lack of fashion sense, but remained nonetheless close to her. Mai's marriage prospects were thought to be slim, and her decision, therefore, to marry another of Fanny's brothers, Samuel, came as a considerable surprise. It also gave seven-year-old Florence an unpleasant jolt. She declared her dislike of Uncle Sam and opposed the marriage 'with all her might'. At the wedding in Sheffield Cathedral on 26 June 1827, she knelt between the couple to keep them apart for as long as possible. Aunt Mai's devotion to her niece was no less clearly expressed. With startling candour, she was later to confess that Florence was 'as precious to me as any thing I possess, except my husband, for I scarcely feel my own dear children were so'.

Aunt Mai's marriage had other important ramifications. Under the terms of Peter Nightingale's will, the estate would pass to Mai on her brother William's death should he have no son. With Fanny approaching forty and no sign of an heir, it must have been some small comfort to know that the Nightingale inheritance would remain within the Shore–Smith families. In 1831 Mai's second-born was a boy, known as Shore, the apple of young Florence's eye and, from his early years, her special charge.

The lives of three other family women – two unmarried aunts and her paternal grandmother – are likely to have been powerfully suggestive to Florence Nightingale both of the possibilities open to her sex, and of the limitations encountered by some of them. In 1850 she included Aunt Patty among 'the numbers of my kind who have gone mad for the want of something to do'. Patty, the oldest of the Smith children, was also the closest to her father. Fiercely intelligent, she had been his amanuensis for many years, and had established her own independent friendships with some of the Clapham Saints, including Hannah More, and the Wilberforces, who were especially fond of her. A 'Chronology' of public and family events, written by Patty in old age, shows a depth of reading and awareness of contemporary politics, and reveals more surprisingly her interest and involvement in Elizabeth Fry's prison reform and hospital initiatives. Patty's eccentricities were something of a joke within the family: a rampant snob, she was teased about sleeping with a copy of the peerage under her pillow. But indifferent health, loneliness and a descent into genteel poverty took their toll on Patty's state of mind. In 1818 she travelled in Italy with her brother Ben, who described her as 'a troublesome companion', and wrote of her fits of uncontrollable weeping. In middle age Patty retired to the coast at Tenby – 'a place for bad health and long life' – residing there in almost complete seclusion, a subject of ongoing concern to her family.

By contrast, Julia Smith, the youngest of Fanny Nightingale's siblings, remained very much at the centre of family life, but managed to negotiate the space between the private and public spheres more successfully than her older sister. Known as 'Stormy Ju' by her niece Florence because of her excitable temperament, Julia was a human dynamo, dividing her time between the care of sick relatives whom she apparently believed always to be on the point of death, and the public causes she supported. She never married, perhaps because of the failure of an early romance with Julius Jeffreys, the inventor of the respirator, who left England in the 1820s to take up a medical appointment in Bengal. Instead, she helped to raise the five children of her brother Ben. She took up her father's banner by becoming active in the British and Foreign Anti-Slavery Society, and was among the women who played a part at the World's Anti-Slavery Convention, held in London in 1840. She later also joined the women's section of the Anti-Corn Law League. Women's education was Julia's other great interest, and provided the basis of her friendships with other Unitarians like Harriet Martineau and Elisabeth Reid. Julia would be a student, member of council, and lady visitor of the college which Reid founded for women in Bedford Square in 1849. The diarist Crabb Robinson described her as 'the most generous of the Smith race . . . She and Mrs Reid carry radicalism to a romantic excess, but their moral worth more than outweighs a little extravagance in matters of opinion.'

The third of these women, Grandmother Shore, was an individual of simpler tastes and habits. Following her husband's death she continued to live at Tapton Hall, on the outskirts of Sheffield, where Florence was a frequent visitor as a young girl. Mrs Shore had practically no education: she couldn't spell, and the Bible and her prayerbook were her only reading. But her native intelligence, her originality and, most of all, her piety – unlike her husband and son, she was a member of the Church of England – left their mark on her granddaughter. On rising in the morning, and after dressing in a plain, unshowy fashion, Mrs Shore would say her prayers before coming down to breakfast. After dining at midday, she would return upstairs, kneel down by her bed and pray aloud.

'We children,' recalled Florence, many years later, 'knew that grand-mother went up to say her prayers & we could hear her voice in the passage, speaking to God with such passion and earnestness – as if he were in the room, which he certainly was.'

Florence's earliest surviving letter, from the autumn of 1827, is addressed from Embley to Grandmother Shore. It is a businesslike affair, which mentions a trip to Buxton, reports on all the family comings and goings, asks for a solution for the rats, threatening to make a hole in the drawing room, and sends special greetings to Mrs Shore's dog Nelson. An early love of animals is reflected in other letters of this time to her grand-mother: in one Florence describes visits to the recently established Zoological Society, and provides an exact catalogue of the creatures on display there – 'two leopards, two bears, two parrots, two emus (which are very large birds), two rabbits, one lion, two cockatoos . . .' In another, she recites an epitaph, written with Parthe's help, on the death of a tom-tit which has been buried with due ceremony in the garden.

One of the most striking features of her early letters is their sheer delight in language. Florence asks her sister to try a new word game: 'Take any word, and see how many words you can make out of the letters . . . I took "breath" and I made forty words.' She writes a sentence to Aunt Patty in a juvenile pastiche of Chaucerian English. This confidence in verbal expression is combined with growing powers of analytical precision and close observation in her descriptions, whether it be of a beautiful, sea-blue jelly fish, 'large as half a tea tray', or of a distant Shore cousin, staying at Embley, who has fallen ill: 'She does not look much better. She goes to bed early. She sleeps better. She was not very well yesterday. She does not go out on cold days.' The incipient talent for organizing information into categories is evident in the lists and tables Florence sometimes includes in her letters, and is also reflected in the meticulously documented collections of shells and coins she kept from an early age. Shell-collecting was an especial passion, and on seaside holidays she scoured the shore at low tide, looking for rare specimens, which she took home to polish to a high sheen with oxalic acid. She also visited local shops, armed with her copy of Woodarch's *Introduction to the Study of Conchology*, delighting on one occasion at her purchase of a '4-pence operculum' and '2-pence Bulla'.

Her linguistic ability was not confined to her mother tongue. At the age of nine Florence was able to write a report in French to her mother about the contents of a church sermon. No doubt her fluency was a result of her close proximity to a native French speaker, her maid, Selina Clemence Coulbeaux. Clemence's father had been a coachman to Louis XVI during the French Revolution, and Clemence's own adventures during her escape from France to England formed the subject of some of the French exercises Florence was writing at this time.

Occasionally, a streak of impatience surfaces in her letters when Florence's hunger for written communication is left unsatisfied. 'Answer me my letter if you please,' she writes with a hint of imperiousness to Grandmother Shore. 'Please give me an answer,' she begs in a postscript to an aunt. Away from home, staying with the Bonham Carters at Fair Oaks, she berates Parthe for her epistolary shortcomings. 'Why don't you write? Naughty girl! I should think you had plenty of time and I write you such long letters, and you, but very seldom, write me two or three lines. I shall not write to you if you don't write for me.'

Parthenope remembered her younger sister at this time as 'overflowing with fun and wild spirits of every kind', constantly 'enquiring into the why & wherefore of everything'. Florence liked to be the leader in their games, on one occasion dressing up as a Turkish queen, leaving Parthe and their cousin Fred Smith to take the parts of her ladies of honour. From an early age, if later anecdotes are to be trusted, Florence tended to direct and organize those around her. An old woman, one of the Nightingales' tenants at Lea, remembered the two sisters collecting firewood for her. 'When the two little Misses used to pick up the wood & bring it to me,' she recalled, 'Miss Floey used to sit on the stairs & tell the other Miss how it should be set by.'

Such a strong-willed child could also be an obstinate one. Fanny Nightingale was a stickler for discipline, as her mother had been before her, and was determined to maintain high standards of behaviour. Florence's letters assure her mother that she is 'a little more yielding' or 'more good-natured'. As a reward for going a week without being disobedient, she is given a 'smelling-bottle with a gilded top'. Another of Fanny's gifts, presumably to encourage her younger daughter to perfect her handwriting, was a writing slate in a wooden frame, inscribed 'from Mama'. When Mrs Nightingale was away from home in January 1830, Florence dutifully sent her a list of promises:

I promise to take [a] run before breakfast to gate ... ½ an hour's walk before dinner, long walk after, or if cold & damp long walk before & ½ an hour's after ... to do 20 arms [exercises] before I dress, 10 minutes before breakfast & 10 after exercises, if ill done 10 more ... to practice 1 hour a day ... to draw ½ an hour regularly ... not to lie in bed ... to go to bed in proper time ... to read the Bible & pray regularly before breakfast & at night ... to visit the poor people & take care of those who are sick ... to take medicine when I want it ... to go regularly after breakfast on Sundays to church when there is anyone to go with me ... to read my books you put out for me ...

Her reading included moral tales that exhibited the clear influence of Rousseau's teaching, with their concern for cultivating rational thought and moral judgement, works like Arnaud Berquin's *L'Ami des Enfans*, presented to Florence when she was seven, appropriately enough, by

Aunt Mai. Other books in Florence's childhood library, stories 'showing
the shortness of life, and suddenness of death', owed more to the evangelical pedagogy of the time. Maria Edgeworth's books for children
were particular favourites, and among the non-fiction titles were
Scripture Riddles and *The Child's Companion*, containing arithmetical
puzzles along the following lines: 'If there are six hundred millions of
Heathens in the world, how many Missionaries are needed to supply
one to every twenty thousand?'

The trace of evangelicalism in this early reading probably owed something to Sara Christie, a young woman in her late twenties engaged by
Fanny Nightingale as a governess for her daughters in the autumn of
1827. Miss Christie was an evangelical and came to the Nightingales
on the recommendation of the Thornton family. The new governess's
religious sentiments, however, were not a cause of concern to Fanny, as
she reserved 'the religious instruction of my children to myself', and
started each day by reading the Bible with them before breakfast. Fanny's
planned curriculum was carefully outlined to Miss Christie. Emphasis
was placed on well-informed conversation to encourage Parthe and
Florence 'to search for themselves', while formal instruction was to be
limited to two or three hours a day. Fresh air and exercise would be in
plentiful supply. Accomplishments were to be 'subsequent to the useful',
though Miss Christie's own musical talents were welcomed, and Fanny
acknowledged that the girls would have 'considerable advantage' in
drawing because of 'the taste of all the family'. For their grandfather,
William Smith, the chief arbiter of that taste, it must have been a source
of pleasure to watch the development of the artistic abilities of his
granddaughter Parthenope. Soon Parthe would be revealing those gifts
in sketchbooks overflowing with drawings and watercolours of domestic
scenes and family members.

The temperamental differences between the two sisters could hardly
have been greater. While Parthe revelled in irresponsibility and childish
fun, Florence was more self-absorbed and thoughtful, with a tendency
to self-righteousness. Neat and methodical, Florence was often irritated
by her older sister's carelessness and lack of discipline. Introducing her
new charges to Miss Christie, Fanny admitted that Parthe 'has not shown
any decided tastes excepting for flowers & poetry'. But seven-year-old
Florence, she continued, 'is a child of much more character. She is a
shrewd little creature with a clear head which makes her thoroughly

mistress of all she attempts by dint of thought & diligent application . . .'

The question of why she and Parthenope, only a year apart in age, of the same parents, and raised in the same circumstances, should be so different was a conundrum that Florence wrestled with for much of her adult life. Even as a child she was much preoccupied by the divide separating them, and constantly defined her own character in opposition to that of her sister. '. . . I find so much disposition in her to detach herself from her sister in everything,' observed Emily Taylor, a school-mistress friend of Miss Christie's, who had been taken aback by the fierce individualism of Florence's announcement that 'Parthe and I are so different, that we require different treatment.'

Different treatment appears to have been exactly what she received at Miss Christie's hands. Lessons were a great success. Florence wrote to her mother, 'I do figures, music, (both Piano-forte, & Miss C[hris]tie's new way too,) Latin, making maps of Palestine (and such like about the Bible) & then we walk, & play, & do patchwork, & we have such fun.' However, increasingly, while Parthe was allowed to continue in her carefree ways, Florence earned sharp reproofs. On one occasion she was obliged to sit still beside Miss Christie, 'till', as she recorded sadly, 'I had the spirit of obedience.' In early 1831, after some months away nursing her dying brother, Miss Christie returned to find that Florence's 'self-love' still presented a problem. She reported to Fanny, 'I have been compelled to give up assisting her in dressing entirely, in consequence of seeing that every little aid I rendered ministered to her great deception, that she is to be <u>served</u> from some inherent necessity in the construction of everything and everybody about her . . .'

The effect of Miss Christie's regime on Florence was marked. In just a few years she had changed from 'a voluble little body' into a child who was increasingly morose and withdrawn. Moreover, she had begun noticeably to retreat into an imaginary world. Aunt Joanna Bonham Carter was among those sufficiently perturbed by this behaviour to comment on it to Florence's mother. On a visit to her Bonham Carter cousins, Florence had paid no attention to the diversions and little treats that had been prepared for her. 'She does not care at all about . . . castles or ruins or little pretty drives, [of] which we have had many here,' Joanna lamented. Whereas Parthenope – 'in spite of all her noise' – had grown in everyone's affections, her younger sister had remained languid and silent, locked away in her own thoughts. 'I do not like Florence's concentrated imagination,' wrote Emily Taylor, who was consulted about the child's 'peculiarities', 'and think it may be a real injury, turned upon herself & here & there one chosen object . . .' In the future Florence should be discouraged from 'all self-reflection that does not lead to good & pleasant outward results'. After all, Miss Taylor concluded, there was no likelihood that the child would ever be 'giddy or trifling'.

In the spring of 1831, Sara Christie left the family to marry William Collmann, a German widower, and the question of the future education of Parthe and Flo became a pressing one. There was briefly talk of sending them away to a school where, it was thought, other children – not cousins – might 'operate upon them beneficially'. It proved impossible to find a new governess who could unite the teaching of social graces with academic excellence. Finally it was decided that a Miss Hawkes would give the girls lessons in music and drawing: Florence showed 'no taste' for the latter, but enjoyed singing and was learning to play the piano 'with exquisite delicacy & feeling tho' without power'. At the same time William Nightingale himself would assume responsibility for his daughters' academic tuition.

As for Miss Christie, Florence remembered her in years to come with fondness mixed with an awareness of her shortcomings: 'She was just and well intentioned, but she did not understand children . . .' At the end of January 1832 came the tragic news of the death of the former governess in childbirth (her newborn son survived). Florence was filled with sorrow, but paused to reflect that if Miss Christie had not married, and had not had a baby, she would still be alive.

For the next seven years Florence thought of little else but the 'cultivation of my intellect'. The importance of the instruction that she received at her father's hands cannot be overestimated. Its breadth and range put her on an equal footing with male contemporaries, as well as ensuring that she would never think twice about engaging in discussion or debate with the opposite sex.

But it also brought other longer-term problems in its wake. Equipped with an education which would not have been found wanting at the male bastions of Oxford or Cambridge – and Florence imagined running away to college dressed as a man – it was unlikely that she would be satisfied with the conventional path mapped out for 'young ladies' of her class. William Nightingale's insistence on equal education for women was unusual, at least outside Unitarian circles, and highly commendable. Yet in the case of his younger daughter, who quickly proved herself a gifted scholar, he seems not to have foreseen the possible consequences of pursuing such an advanced programme. For Florence, education would never be just an end in itself, as it was for her father. Good sense, good manners, good conversation: these qualities, she came to the conclusion years later, were all that fathers really wanted from their daughters.

The seriousness with which Mr Nightingale undertook the task of educating his daughters was reflected in the long hours of study expected of them. Florence would sometimes rise at three in the morning to prepare her Greek, and both girls recited the lessons of the previous day to their father at breakfast, where he was already deep in his own reading. (It was a standing joke in the family that William Nightingale was unable to get through any meal 'without covering the table-cloth with literature'.) The curriculum owed much to Mr Nightingale's own courses at Trinity. Florence's commonplace book for August 1836, in which she kept notes of lessons, shows that at sixteen her instruction included the rudiments of chemistry, geography, physics and astronomy. She also studied mathematics, though as yet only at an elementary level, grammar, composition, philosophy, and read 'history of every date & every colour'. She became fluent in French and Italian. 'My father was a good & always interested Italian scholar', she wrote. 'Never pedantic, never a tiresome grammarian, but he spoke Italian like an Italian, & I took care of the verbs.' By the age of nineteen she was also studying German (though she never mastered it as a written language), and at thirty would begin learning Hebrew in order to read the Old Testament in the original. Florence's mastery of Latin and Greek was particularly impressive. In her mid-teens she was translating Homer and portions of Plato's *Phaedo*, *Crito* and *Apology* (presumably she also read the *Republic* during this period, with its proposal in Book V that women should be given the same education as men, to equip them for the same military and governmental tasks as men). Four decades later, having kept up her Plato in the intervening years, she would earn Benjamin Jowett's gratitude for her stalwart criticism of the introductions to the second edition of his translations of the *Dialogues*.

In early adulthood, Florence's reputation for learning spread beyond the confines of her immediate circle. The Quaker Caroline Fox, a cousin

of Elizabeth Fry's, left a record in her journal of one occasion from the
late 1840s when Florence's bluestocking conversation at the dinner table
left two male guests marvelling at the extent of her education.

Warrington Smyth [a mineralogist and lecturer at the School of Mines] talked
with great delight of Florence Nightingale. Long ago, before she went to
Kaiserswerth, he and Sir Henry de la Beche [President of the Geological Society]
dined at her father's, and Florence Nightingale sat between them. She began by
drawing Sir Henry out on Geology, and charmed him by the boldness and breadth
of her views which were not common then. She accidentally proceeded into
regions of Latin and Greek, and then our Geologist had to get out of it. She was
fresh from Egypt, and began talking with W. Smyth about the inscriptions, &c.,
where he thought he could do pretty well; but when she began quoting Lepsius
[the German Egyptologist], which she had been studying in the original, he was
in the same case as Sir Henry. When the ladies left the room, the latter said
to him, 'A capital young lady that, if she hadn't floored me with her Latin
and Greek!'

Parthenope, too, was full of admiration for the manner in which
Florence 'worked patiently to the pith and marrow of every subject'.
Her own recitations at the breakfast table, she admitted, were 'always
rather slurred', and she simply did not share her sister's powers of
disciplined application. She had 'not the means or the energy', as her
father rather bluntly informed her, for the sciences, while her proficiency
in languages suffered from one clear drawback, that her grammar 'came
off very short'. Ladylike accomplishments of poetry, painting and
imaginative composition were much more to her taste and ability and
these, united with undoubted qualities of charm and intelligence, marked
her out as a natural companion for her mother. By the time the two girls
reached their mid-teens a pattern had been set. While Florence and Mr
Nightingale formed a college of two in the library, Parthenope gravitated
towards her mother in the drawing room, involving herself with household affairs and family arrangements.

Parthenope might be forgiven if she occasionally felt resentful or
jealous of her father and sister's exclusive companionship, especially
when he contrasted her 'infantine' pursuits with Florence's more serious
concerns. Certainly William Nightingale was conscious that he might be
neglecting his elder daughter. As he wrote to her, in the spring of 1835,
'I sometimes fancy that you & I have not made half so much of each

other's society as we might have done . . .' The truth, however, seems to have been that directing a talent as prodigious as Florence's was not only intellectually satisfying – his powers of speculative thought were nicely complemented by her mathematical precision – but also a welcome change from all his dilettante idling. For Florence herself, the disturbing traits of childhood were, for the time being, submerged in a great enterprise of learning; and perhaps she also derived satisfaction and pleasure from filling the position of surrogate son.

This special bond between father and daughter had inevitable consequences for Florence's relationship with Mrs Nightingale. It placed Fanny at a distance and confirmed her in the role of authority figure, of the parent whom Florence looked up to, with a strong degree of respect and even awe, but to whom she could never really get close. Fanny's beauty and social poise had always contributed to making her seem unapproachable, and in a letter written by the eight-year-old Florence to her cousin Henry Nicholson, one can just catch the hushed reverence beneath the precise reportage: 'Mama went to the ball the 11th of January, came home between 5 and 6 o'clock and stayed in bed till after our dinner. She had on a dark green gown, white sleeves and diamonds.' Yet despite an underlying lack of closeness, Florence would never be less than loving and courteous towards her mother, and remained throughout her adult life extraordinarily solicitous of Fanny's welfare, and keen to shield her from any slight or hurt. Florence Nightingale's later, well-known, fulminations against maternal influence are expressions of the anger of the young woman who had failed to win her own mother's acquiescence in the most important objectives of her life, but they should not be taken as an exact representation of her true feelings for her 'dearest mum', complex and ambivalent as these often were.

The American writer Nathaniel Hawthorne, working in England in the mid-1850s, met Fanny Nightingale at a breakfast party in 1854, and although she was by then in her sixties, he was struck by her 'very fine countenance' and thought her 'altogether more agreeable to look at than most of the English dames of her age'. He also considered this 'lady born and bred' as 'very intelligent – that is, very sensible – but with no saliency of ideas'. This amounted to a shrewd summary of her character. The brief jottings in Fanny's pocket diaries show her bent on intellectual self-improvement, though the way in which her mind glides over any given subject – the plot of Verdi's *Nabucco* or a lecture by Faraday on electromagnetism which she had attended at the Royal Institution – makes these entries seem like notes for informed conversation, reminiscent of George Eliot's remarks in *The Mill on the Floss*, about 'the tone of good society', floating on 'gossamer wings of light irony', a product of the fashionable milieu which does indeed get 'its science done by Faraday'.

To be part of the best society in England was Fanny's chief ambition, and one on which she expended a considerable amount of energy. She already had the foothold in the artistic and political worlds provided by her father's connections, though there was no getting away from the fact that both the Nightingales and the Smiths were of fundamentally mercantile stock (when Florence Nightingale became famous, Aunt Patty was appalled to find that newspapers were describing William Smith as having been 'in trade', though this was obviously true). The Nightingales had swiftly acquired all the appurtenances of the high station in life to which they aspired: two large houses, an armorial ensign, even livery, with 'trimmings and tassles', for their servants. The household, trained by Fanny to run on smooth lines, played a vital part in the achievement of social success. Florence was much impressed by her mother's practical abilities as 'a most excellent manager', noting that 'order & beauty spring up under her steps'; and, of course, her own skills of household management, later employed in a wider, more dramatic setting, owed not a little to the example set by Fanny Nightingale.

The parish, both at Lea and at East Wellow, the neighbouring village to Embley, was another centre for Mrs Nightingale's activities. Florence remembered that her mother hardly ever went out in the carriage without taking parcels of dripping to distribute among the villagers. In fact Fanny's charitable impulses went beyond the small acts of kindness practised by a Lady Bountiful, of the type later dismissed by her younger daughter as 'poor peopling' or, even more contemptuously, under the general heading of philanthropy, seen by Florence as 'a kind of conscience quieter' or 'soothing syrup'. Fanny Nightingale was in large part a creature of convention, but her strain of social benevolence was stronger than has often been suggested. A coffee house at Whatstandwell, a couple of miles from Lea Hurst, and a reading-room for the nearby village of Crich were two social experiments in which she was involved, but her main efforts lay in the education of the local children. Soon after her arrival at the Hurst, Fanny employed James Buchanan to organize the infant school at Crich. Buchanan, an ex-weaver from New Lanark, had been head of an experimental school in Westminster, founded by Fanny's brother Ben, before his Swedenborgian beliefs got him into trouble. He was an eccentric fellow. Local people were alarmed to see him, Pied-Piper-like, leading a troop of children along the road, playing a flute. In 1827, after a year at Crich, Buchanan returned to London, but the Derbyshire venture stayed afloat, supported by generous injections of cash from the Nightingales, and by Fanny, Parthenope, Florence and other family members staying at the Hurst, who acted as a form of supply teaching. Eventually it merged with the school at Lea under a clergyman, Henry Bagshawe, who taught two classes of children, one of farmers and shopkeepers, the other of labourers. Fanny continued to be actively involved, and each year the school feast was held at the Hurst. At Wellow, where the local school was better established, Fanny's role was less instrumental, though she was responsible for providing all the books and materials. Education remained an interest. In 1840 she was shown round the Norwood Asylum with her sister Julia. Distressed by the sight of '1100 of the most wretched children deserted by their parents', she was nonetheless pleased to note the impressive condition of the asylum school.

Fanny seems to have been an anxious person at the best of times, and the demands of household, parish and society, coupled with worries about the health of her children, of whom she was acutely protective, took its toll on her nerves, producing what her husband termed a 'habit of general derangement'. He was always attentive – 'perfectly at your Highness's service, willing to obey you as faithfully as any knight errant . . .' – and ready to indulge her enjoyment of 'the goods of this world'. Looking back towards the end of her life, Fanny admitted that William had been 'a better husband to me than I deserved'. Nevertheless, the marked difference in their lifestyles, with her love of the metropolis and his longing for the peace and solitude of the country, led to them spending sometimes weeks apart, and increasingly, in years to come, as Florence was later to note, he would 'be at the home' where she was not, 'if he could'.

A typical letter from William at the Hurst to his wife in London describes his 'perambulations thro the many tenements of those whose walls & roofs & doors & windows are my "to-do or not-to-do" . . .'

The stirring little dairy-farmer preparing his fat calf for the slaughter with wife of tidiness . . . & dress of indescribable neatness – then again the house too dirty or too unsightly to admit me across the threshold with women unlike humanity – oh! the contrasts of human things – beauty & ugliness – roughness & softness – the attractive & the repulsive. What an infinite society is here. [I]f every house was but a little more neat & nice than it is – & every man, woman & child a little cleaner & more picturesque in outward show . . .

He had a reputation as a good landlord to his tenants (of whom there were about 100 on his Derbyshire estates), though this ineffectual philosophizing might make one question how effective an appointee he was to the local Board of Guardians of the new Poor Law commission in 1834. Having been a magistrate for several years – Florence often watched her father ride off with twenty-four other shiremen to the courts at Winchester for the local sessions – he also served a term in 1831 as Deputy Lieutenant of Hampshire. The big prize, however, was a seat in Parliament. William had refused invitations to stand for the unreformed Commons, but the 1832 Reform Bill convinced him that a new era was dawning. In the summer of 1834, encouraged no doubt by Fanny, with her dreams of becoming a political hostess, he accepted the candidature of Andover on behalf of the Whigs. The news reached Florence at Cowes on the Isle of Wight, where she was on holiday with Parthenope, 'buying shells by the wholesale'. It took her unawares, convulsing 'our quiet little world', disrupting her sleep and making her feel that something 'very extraordinary, or dreadful, had happened . . .' She wrote to her mother, after attempting to rouse her spirits with thoughts of Tory tyranny and the patriotic conviction that her father must be given up to the interests of the country: '. . . I hope now Papa will not lose his election though I had rather he would not stand at all . . . The alternative of living in London & breaking up our pleasant country life & our intercourse with the poor people or being separated from Papa . . . is what I dread.'

Her fears, though, proved unfounded. While Palmerston, soon to be reconfirmed as foreign secretary in Melbourne's new cabinet, wrote of his confidence in William Nightingale's prospects (and Parthenope prematurely addressed letters to her father as 'WEN MP'), William himself was more doubtful. 'We must win – but [there is] such an array against us.' Election bills portrayed him as the reform candidate ('And this Nightingale is very much noted/To be to reformers much devoted, / And he is noted very much above all, /Because he is so very tall'), although ironically, attacks by local Dissenters on the established church deprived him of a sizeable number of votes. 'Flo's lively feelings' on his behalf strengthened his nerves during a visit to Andover by his wife and daughters, but constitutional shyness made him instinctively recoil from the hurly-burly of party warfare, and his campaign suffered further from his refusal to bribe the voters. The result of the poll, in January 1835, found him lying in third place.

William Nightingale's failure to win the seat must have been a source of regret to his father-in-law, William Smith, who had devoted so much effort to working for parliamentary reform. Five months after the election, on 31 May 1835, Smith was dead. He had continued working right to the end, collecting 'information for the Wilberforces within 3 weeks of his death', and attending a slavery meeting just days before. A benign grandfather, he had not forgotten Florence in his final illness, bequeathing her one of the finest shells from his own collection. Frances Smith outlived her husband by five years; appropriately, the last glimpse of her in her daughter Fanny's journal describes her clasping her hands and raising them in prayer.

So William Nightingale would not be 'a great man like Uncle Carter', his brother-in-law, who had been re-elected for the seventh time as MP for Portsmouth. Instead, he returned to his quiet life, directing his daughters' education ('pray, pray, no governess', Florence had begged Fanny when separation from her father looked a possibility), and filling his days as best he could. Were it not for 'Books, Books, Books . . . the puzzle would have been to know, how [to] pass the time', was his familiar refrain. Fanny was less resigned to her husband's absence from the Commons. When her brother Ben was returned to Parliament, to his father's old seat of Norwich, in 1838, she hoped that William might be encouraged to think of standing again; but although he continued to campaign for the Whig cause, and was for a time chairman of the High Peak Association 'for promoting the purity of elections', he was too disillusioned to run the risk of being bruised by the experience of another election.

Fourteen-year-old Florence may have been delighted to have her Papa at home with her once more, but as her own dreams of an active life grew as she reached maturity, so too would her private disparagement of her father's lack of ambition. She saw this as 'the habit of his life', ingrained by circumstance. Life had never been a struggle for him, and while he was full of 'good impulses', he had never been 'forced to look into a thing, to carry it out'. 'Touch lightly, don't push' – these were the rules that governed his existence.

Increasingly, she would be pained by his lack of occupation, which ran like a neat counterpart to her perceptions about the frustrating lives of women of her class, only for William Nightingale this was a life of choice, not one ordained by sex or station. 'When I see him eating his breakfast, as if the destinies of the nation depended upon his getting done,' she wrote in 1851, 'carrying his plate about the room, delighting in being in a hurry, pretending to himself week after week that he is going to Buxton or elsewhere in order to be in legitimate haste, I say to myself how happy that man would be with a factory under his superintendence with the interests of 200 or 300 men to look after.' There can be no doubt that Florence Nightingale loved her father with intensity unmatched by her feelings for any other individual. Even in old age, she would look back and long for his caress. As time wore on, however, that love would be tempered by disappointment, loss of respect – and latterly by a degree of contempt.

Florence Nightingale's childhood produced two stories which entered popular currency during her lifetime, passed on as illustrations of an early inclination towards nursing and of her compassionate nature. One is the tale of how she used to nurse and bandage her sick dolls. This appears to emanate from information garnered by Mrs Gaskell on a visit to Lea Hurst in the autumn of 1854, at the time of Florence's departure for Scutari, which described Florence's '13 dolls *all* ill in rows in bed, when she was quite a little thing'. The story was given a light embellishment by Parthenope in her draft memoir of her sister, written post-Crimea, which stated that 'when she had the [w]hooping cough her thirteen dolls had it too & were found with 13 pieces of flannel round their 13 necks'. Sir Edward Cook, Nightingale's official biographer, was probably right to be sceptical about the value of such stories, warning about the temptation 'to magnify some childish incident as prophetic of what is to come thereafter', and making the obvious point that Florence Nightingale was far from being the only girl who had been fond of nursing dolls.

The other incident is more straightforwardly verifiable and possesses a more detailed provenance, though, once again, its significance has undoubtedly been exaggerated. As a writer in *The Nation* commented, two years before Florence Nightingale's death, 'No story was more welcome to an audience than how she began her career of mercy by binding up a dog's paw.' In its many retellings, the essential outline of the tale remained the same. Cap, a shepherd's collie, was discovered by Florence on the downs near Embley. Stones thrown by schoolboys had broken his leg, and the shepherd had intended to put him out of his misery by hanging him. However, with the guidance of the local vicar, Florence administered to the wounded animal, placing hot cloths as fomentations to reduce the swelling, thereby saving his leg and ensuring that Cap would continue as a working farm dog.

The vicar in the story was Jervis Trigge Giffard, a family friend and frequent guest at the Nightingales' dinner table. A relation by marriage of the Bonham Carters, Giffard was the incumbent of St Margaret's, East Wellow, Embley's local church, until the autumn of 1839. He later confirmed that the episode involving Cap had taken place in 1836, when Florence was sixteen. A reference to the dog in a letter of Florence's from nine years later shows that Cap must have gone on to enjoy at least a fairly long life, though her sight of him running about 'his pleasure grounds on three legs' suggests that her cure may not have been a lasting one. In 1867, Giffard, by now the Rector of Long Ditton in Surrey, published his 'Reminiscence' of the event, apparently with Florence's tacit approval, under the title *Constance and 'Cap' The Shepherd's Dog*, saving until the end the revelation that 'The Constance of this tale was no other than, FLORENCE NIGHTINGALE.' To Giffard, the moral of his book was that people who are kind to animals are most often those who are considerate to their own fellow-creatures, though rather than as an omen of her future nursing career, the story might more plausibly be seen as an early indication of the love of animals, and concern for their welfare, that was to be a constant feature of Florence's adult life. In this she was following the lead of her grandfather William Smith, who had espoused animal rights as an MP, and also of her mother's brother Adams, another fighter in the cause, who founded a Society for the Protection of Animals. Florence always appreciated the companionship of pets, believing that they acted as civilizing influences on human beings, and was the owner, at various times, of a pony called

Peggie, dogs, including Peppercorn, Teazer and Captain, a large number of cats, at least three owls, including Athena, who ate her pet cicada, Plato, on her European travels in 1849–50, chameleons and a parrot. Birds, 'a sort of mysterious being living between earth and heaven', were an especial source of wonder, and in later years, when she was confined to her bed or couch, the view from her windows of the assorted bird life was an uplifting one. She was much exercised about the decline of the bird population in the city, as well as countless other instances of animal neglect, from the treatment of horses and donkeys in London streets to the condition of a cow with a bad cough, grazing on pasture near Lea Hurst.

Inevitably perhaps, the story of Florence and Cap became an enduring part of the Nightingale legend. It was handed down to succeeding generations as part of the late nineteenth-century tradition of heroic biographies for girls – in some versions becoming entangled with the story of Nightingale nursing her dolls, so that the doll had to be nursed back to health after the dog had ripped a hole in it – or in the form of a popular illustration of the episode, copies of which reputedly hung on the walls of cottages on the Embley estate. One newspaper report of Florence Nightingale's funeral in 1910 even pointed out 'the creeper-covered thatched cottage, in which she nursed back to health the poor shepherd's collie' as still standing, and described some of the shepherd's descendants coming out of the house as the cortège passed, in order to pay their respects.

The belief that it is possible to uncover the seeds of adult greatness in the child is an entirely understandable one, even though such an activity must nearly always prove fanciful. A further childhood incident, recalled by the Nightingale family after Florence's death as revealing 'her special tendency' – that she bound up the hand of a boy cousin injured in a game, and found that 'she liked it' – may be no more authentic than the stories of the dolls or the dog. However, it does at least locate an early interest in nursing on Florence's part in its most probable context, that of her family's concern for their health, together with the opportunities that arose for caring for them. This may provide the background to Florence's own assertion in 1851, that 'the first idea I can recollect when I was a child was a desire to nurse the sick'.

Fanny Nightingale's preoccupation with health matters is evident from the remedies and prescriptions included in letters to her sisters and sister-in-law, or scribbled down on the back of stray bits of paper (it is perhaps no coincidence then that one of the earliest examples of Florence's handwriting is a prescription for the popular remedy James' powder, '16 grains for an old woman, 11 for a young woman, and 7 for a child', contained in a tiny notebook made out of her father's and mother's old letters). Fanny was zealous in her treatment of family illness, consulting the manual *Practical Suggestions Towards Alleviating the Sufferings of the Sick*. With its insistence on proper ventilation, the importance of sunlight and the absence of unnecessary noise, *Practical Suggestions* rehearses some of the ideas for sickroom management espoused by Florence Nightingale's own *Notes on Nursing*, three decades later. During her own more severe attacks of illness or debility, Fanny would go to stay in Leamington Spa to be treated by Dr Henry Jephson, renowned throughout the world for his water treatments. Closer to home, she could always turn for medical advice to Jervis Giffard, who, prior to becoming a clergyman, had studied medicine in Paris under the anatomist and surgeon Baron Guillaume Dupuytren.

For Florence, an inquisitive child with well-developed powers of observation, family illnesses were a source of endless fascination, and from about the age of nine she made a habit of noting down details of the condition of individuals who were ill or in need of care. Uncle Octavius's lumbago, the number of Pop's teeth removed at the dentist, the swelling in Gale's leg after the doctor had 'causticed' it – all captured her attention. So too did the natural processes of life and death. In June 1829 her cousin Thomas Bonham Carter, known as Bonny, her senior by just a year and 'Such a dear kind boy!', died after a six-month illness. In a letter of 16 May to Aunt Mai, Florence recorded that Bon had 'made a good night', but that he was past all hope and the doctors had given him up. Three weeks later, she described his last days: 'His complaint had got so much the better of medecine [sic], doctors, nursing and all . . . One day he said to his papa, when in great pain, "I will bear it as well as I can, but if I were strong, I think I should leap about the room with this pain."'

Aunt Mai's 'babes' – her three daughters, Blanche, Bertha and Beatrice, ranging in that order from eight to eighteen years Florence's junior, and her son William Shore, born in 1831 when Florence was nearly eleven – offered a more positive focus for Florence's interest. From the moment that 'my boy Shore', as she called him, was placed in her arms as a delicate four-month-old infant, she came to regard his welfare, physical, mental and spiritual, as her particular responsibility. With 'a baby of her own' she felt free to prattle away on the subject of babies in general in weekly letters to her cousin Hilary Bonham Carter, the oldest of a large family – and hence equipped with solid experience of baby care – who were now living in Ditcham near Petersfield. 'I am very sorry to hear that your Baby is still so poorly [Hugh Bonham Carter, who died shortly afterwards, at less than two years of age], but our Baby is much better for he has got two teeth through,' she wrote in March 1832. That summer she could not disguise her pride when one of Gale's sick headaches meant that she was put in sole charge of Shore during his stay at Lea Hurst.

In February 1836 the Nightingales were plunged into crisis when Parthenope fell seriously ill with a severe chest inflammation. An unclosed blister was applied and she was bled frequently, but for almost a week a full recovery looked uncertain. Her parents kept a vigil at her bedside, supported by Aunt Julia, while Gale slept in her room. 'Dear Flo is a most kind nurse,' her mother wrote as Parthenope began to rally. The illness of a sister had called 'forth all the latent good which in common occasions lies so deeply buried', a sentiment shared by Aunt Mai on Parthenope's behalf when she noted that the experience had given Parthenope 'thought & reflection, & married her heart to Flo, of whose nursing she speaks very affectionately'.

At some point in her life, Florence was to write years later, 'every woman is a nurse'. In her own case, care for members of her family combined in her mid-teens with a growing awareness of the sickness and poverty in the surrounding neighbourhoods of the Hurst and Embley. Visits to the sick poor had been part of the routine carved out for Florence at an early age by Fanny and Miss Christie. Fanny's letters from the 1830s demonstrate the extent of the family's involvement in the care of the sick near the Hurst, organizing, and paying for, medical consultations for the cottagers, and maintaining what amounted to case notes on those with prolonged or serious conditions. Some sections of Florence's childhood journal reveal knowledge of the dark and desperate underside of lives of deprivation that seems to reach well beyond her years. In an entry for May 1830, for example, she had recorded the death of Mrs Petty, a woman from East Wellow, who had killed herself and her youngest child while her husband vainly tried to beat down the door. Increasingly, Florence devoted more of her time to these visits, dispensing food, blankets and clothes to the needy, and offering advice and comfort to the sick and dying. Fanny Nightingale recalled that when Florence was a girl of fifteen or so, 'she was often missing in the evening'. On these occasions her mother would take a lantern and go up into the village and find Florence 'sitting by the bedside of someone who was ill, & saying she cd not sit down to a grand 7 o'clock dinner . . .' Writing from Lea Hurst, in the summer of 1836, Parthenope informed her grandmother, Mrs Shore, that 'Flo has been very busy paying visits in the village. The people about here are very fond of her, & she likes them & is always sorry to leave them.' When Aunt Julia, a woman of strong philanthropic impulse, was staying at the Hurst, she often accompanied her niece to assist her; and it was perhaps while making these calls that Florence regularly encountered Dr Thomas Poyser. Poyser, a leading practitioner from Wirksworth, the Derbyshire market town, later made the proud boast that he had given Florence her first hints in nursing and medicine, 'when as a girl she used to attend the sick poor near his home' (a claim that may be borne out by Florence's insistence in 1860, the year of Poyser's death, that he be sent a copy of Notes on Nursing straight from the press).

In the course of the next decade, attendance on the sick poor would often prove a lifeline for Florence in an existence lacking a sense of purpose. However, in January 1837, the arrival at Embley of the influenza epidemic that was sweeping southern England suddenly brought her nursing skills to the fore. Florence was the only member of the household, apart from the cook and Shore, to remain untouched by infection and, amidst 'the general chorus of coughing resounding from garrets to cellars', she relished all 'the agitation & hurry' of caring for her patients. To Parthenope, who had escaped illness by being left behind with the Nicholsons after Christmas, she wrote depicting herself at the centre of a commotion:

Your merry tidings come fraught with double gladness to our nursing ears which has nothing but Calomel, Blisters, Coughs &c, and our mouths which only open periodically to advise senna & Salts, Saline Mixture, & Gruel with Ipecacuanha Wine & Spirits of Nitre . . . The tea-pot in which is made the Senna Tea is still installed in the kitchen as our daily drink when we ask for tea & the parish which come for meat & wine are answered with fever draughts & reducing compounds.

The news from the parish, described as 'one mass of illness', was dispiriting. 'They have used up all the leeches & cannot get any in the country for love or money'.

Casting her mind back at the end of a month's nursing, Florence was amazed at the fruits of her own industry. She had acted as 'nurse, governess, assistant curate and doctor' while continuing with her studies, and allowing a pile of manuscripts to rise up 'like mushrooms' under her pen. 'At all events,' she admitted, 'I have killed no patients, though I have cured few.'

By early February, the worst of the flu was subsiding. It was just then, on 7 February 1837, a date that would always hold a hallowed position in her personal calendar, that Florence Nightingale experienced a call from God to his service.

Florence Nightingale's religious beliefs were of paramount importance throughout her long life, and nothing less than the motivating force behind all her work. Fundamentally, her personal system of belief, which she was to work on and refine in the course of her twenties and thirties, derived from two separate strands that ultimately she saw as complementary to each other. One was an essentially rationalistic approach, looking for evidence of divine law in the workings of the universe; the other was an inward seeking after union with God.

Traces of Florence's empiricism – not surprising in a child so given to reflecting on the world around her – were, according to her later account, evident from a very early age. At six she conducted an experiment to see if her prayers were being answered. She wrote down what she had asked for, specified a time by which her prayer might have been answered, continued to pray for it, and then looked for the results of divine action. She was disappointed. 'I have papers upon papers, "by the 7th of July, I pray that I may be" so and so. When the 7th of July came, I looked, and I was not.' Although there is plenty of evidence that as an adult Florence continued to pray for specific wants and desires, she remained largely of the view that rather than petitioning God, humankind itself should act to right the wrongs of the world.

Alongside this rational approach, a more spiritual quality was already manifest in the way Florence sought the divine presence in the natural world surrounding her. At ten years old, after sailing up the Thames in a small rowing boat, accompanied by the governess to Octavius Smith's

children, and '2 men to row us', she wrote home, expressing her sense
of wonder and contentment at the beauty of the setting sun:

We went up to Battersea Bridge . . . The sunset was particularly beautiful. On
one side, the golden clouds shed such a beautiful tinge on the water, and on the
other, it looked so dark and stormy, and there were 2 sweet little ends of a
rainbow on each side of the sky, & 2 windmills against it, & little boats gliding
up and down the river, Oh! so beautiful and there were 2 steam boats just seen
in the distance, that had passed us, with the smoke curling up. I felt so happy,
mama, I thought I loved God then . . .

Her mother oversaw Florence's religious education. William Nightingale, who was to be a sympathetic correspondent on religious matters
with his younger daughter in years to come, appears, however, to have
been the less devout of the two Nightingale parents. Given to endless
speculation about the nature of this world and the next, he had decided
that Bentham's utilitarian principles taught moral truth more effectually
than the teachings of all the Christian divines. It was to Fanny that
Florence reported her ongoing progress in reading the Bible, and to
whom she described the contents of the church sermons she had heard.
In May 1832, in the midst of the pandemic of Asiatic cholera, which
was arousing great fear as it spread across Europe from Russia and
India, Florence wrote of the cholera sermon that had been given at the
church near Embley. The congregation had been told of the uncertainty
of life and of the need to prepare for heaven: 'a very good sermon', she
thought, though its resignation in the face of the disease was precisely
the kind of response that would be anathema to Florence as an adult.

The story that Fanny Nightingale dropped the Unitarianism of her
upbringing in favour of the Church of England originated with Cook,
who probably received it from Rosalind Vaughan Nash, Aunt Mai's
granddaughter and a beloved cousin of Florence Nightingale's later
years. It has been repeated by biographers ever since, sometimes with
the added surmise that Fanny changed her allegiance for reasons of
social prestige. In fact the surviving evidence suggests something much
less clear-cut. In a letter from the late 1820s about her children's religious
instruction, probably addressed to Miss Christie, Fanny states straightforwardly that she is 'not of the church of England'. Moreover, she
objects 'to the common routine which is taught to its members, & wish
all doctrinal points to be left alone till our pupils are of an age to judge

for themselves'. Another letter from the same period reveals that Fanny went to some lengths, unsuccessfully as it turned out, to employ a Unitarian governess.

This open-mindedness on doctrinal points is what one might have expected from a daughter of William Smith, that beacon of religious toleration and free inquiry into differing creeds, and it may be of a piece with what we know of the Nightingales' religious observance. At a time when they were regarded as Unitarians, William and Fanny were married in an Anglican church; as we have seen, Florence was both baptized in the Church of England and entered in the births register of Protestant Dissenters; and, furthermore, although while at Embley the family would go to St Margaret's at East Wellow, at Lea Hurst they attended the local Dissenting chapel. Simple convenience may have played its part, but issues of social status were also undoubtedly involved. Despite winning legal tolerance, Unitarianism lacked respectability and remained suspect, politically and religiously, and as the owner of Embley, William Nightingale was expected to act as patron of the local parish church.

In a sense the religious affiliations of the Nightingale parents are irrelevant to Florence's own increasingly heterodox system of belief. Nominally, she would remain an Anglican, though she ceased to attend church regularly as early as the beginning of her thirties, and was fiercely critical of the bland compromises and political infighting of the Church of England, as well as disagreeing with many of its doctrines, especially those associated with hellfire and damnation. Having rejected 'rites and ceremonies', Florence's spiritual philosophy would take on a variety of hues from a wide range of sources: Roman Catholicism, including the medieval mystics and other devotional writers, the German Protestant school of historical criticism, Lutheranism and the teachings of John Wesley, for whom she always expressed considerable respect.

The teachings of the Unitarians were present in Florence's religious education as she was growing up, most obviously through her close relationship with Aunt Mai. Aunt Mai continued to frequent the Essex Street Chapel, while Mai's husband Samuel Smith reportedly read the works of Joseph Priestley out loud to his family. The influence of Priestley's Necessarian philosophy – which argued that the universe was ruled by immutable laws originated by God, and that these laws were within man's understanding and could be used by him to advance God's plan – would later leave its mark on the determinism of Florence's great work of religious philosophy, *Suggestions for Thought*; but more generally, Unitarianism never seems to have impressed Florence very much. She thought it 'dull' because of its 'pure Monotheism', and observed that while Unitarians had eliminated Christ and the Holy Ghost as objects of worship, they had not succeeded in making God 'more loved or loveable'. In view of the Unitarian concentration on 'deeds not creeds', it has always been tempting to claim Florence as one of their number, even though she spoke in terms that were clearly contrary to Unitarian beliefs, affirming the doctrine of the Trinity, for instance, and stating that all people, like Christ, are 'incarnations of God'. Where Unitarianism did assert a powerful influence on Florence was in the general ethos it provided. Its optimism and belief in social progress, its concern with the nature of moral obligations within a society, and the ways in which it placed its trust in good works and public service, were all to leave their mark on Florence Nightingale's subsequent career.

The impetus, however, for Florence's call to God's service in the winter of 1836–7 came from none of these sources. Instead it appears to have stemmed from a reading of an inspirational work by an American Congregational Minister, Jacob Abbott, author of many popular religious books for children. Sixty years later she recounted how *The Corner-stone, or, A Familiar Illustration of the Principles of Christian Truth* had 'converted' her in 1836. This, and another book by Abbott also read by Florence at this time, *The Way to Do Good*, emphasizes a practical life of charitable acts built on the cornerstone of faith in Jesus Christ. 'Let it be your distinct understanding that when you abandon your life of ungodliness and sin, and come and give yourself to the service of God, your work is <u>entered upon</u> not <u>concluded</u>.'

Florence's work had begun among the local villagers and during the flu epidemic. But on 7 February 1837 an altogether more momentous event occurred when '. . . God spoke to me and called me to His service.' What form this service was to take, the voice did not say.

The precise nature of such an experience must, by definition, remain shrouded in mystery.* That it was an inward revelation rather than a hallucinatory sensation seems likely given Florence's own disdain for

---

* However, the tradition that Florence first heard her call while seated on a bench under the cedars of Lebanon at Embley is easily discounted. Late in life, she recalled that the experience had taken place in the much more mundane situation of her bedroom.

the supernatural, and her innate suspicion of the states of ecstasy and rapture described by the great sixteenth-century mystic Teresa of Avila. That the experience may correspond to the description of the first phase of the mystical life described as the 'awakening', in which an individual undergoes an initial shift in consciousness, signalling the surrender of his or her personal will to that of God, is also possible. Alternatively, it may not rank as a mystical experience at all.

What is certain is that such voices, or 'impressions', were to be a significant feature of the rest of Florence's life. Scattered through her private notes and diaries are further instances of God addressing her. In a letter to her mother, written in 1851, at a time of particular stress, she used the image of a voice calling her as a metaphor for an inner compulsion. Her family, she wrote, might dismiss it as 'the passing fancy of a heated imagination', but 'little do you know how long that voice has spoken, how deep its tones have sunk within me . . .'

Voices could inspire or guide, or offer insight. But danger and confusion threatened when the voice of self was mistaken for that of God. For Florence, whose will was so strong and dominating, this was something she would be especially on guard against. However, as Parthenope later testified, with a mixture of bewilderment and awe, once Florence had seen distinctly what she thought to be God's will, 'it was the most resolute & iron thing I ever knew'.

3. Pink Satin Ghosts

During 1836 the Nightingales had started to make plans for a continental tour of France and Italy. It was hoped that the health of the entire family might benefit from the Mediterranean climate, and that Parthenope and Florence would be able to finish their education while seeing something of the wider world. In their absence from England, Embley would be given a facelift. The house was to be enlarged, with the addition of six bedrooms and new kitchens, and also extensively remodelled, to transform it from a Georgian mansion into something more pretentious in the Elizabethan style.

Preparations for their departure in the autumn of 1837 were intensive. A detailed itinerary was laid out for the year and a half they were to be away, incorporating soundings from other members of the family as to the best hotels and inns at which to stay along the route. The girls received copious advice about books to read in anticipation of the sights they would visit ('Consult the Edinbro' Gazeteer in 6 vols,' advised Miss Johnson, a former governess to the Coape family, 'concerning every place thro' which it is proposed to pass'). Passports, difficult to obtain without personal recommendation and very expensive, were applied for through the good offices of Lord Palmerston. And Mr Nightingale set to work on the design of a large travelling carriage. It would be drawn by four to six horses and contain room for up to twelve people.

In the summer of 1836, while these plans were still evolving, and just months after she had recovered from her serious illness, Parthenope underwent a significant rite of passage. In a dress of white satin ornamented with tiny pink hyacinths, she was presented at Court during the King's birthday celebrations. This was to be the last such occasion of William IV's reign before his death the following June and the accession as Queen of his eighteen-year-old niece Victoria. Fanny's aunt Maria Coape recognized it as 'a formidable step', but wondered 'why did not Flo enter the world at the same time?' It would, though, she admitted, be 'good food' for Patty Smith, with her obsession with social status, '& keep her quiet I trust for some time – so <u>one</u> good result is sure'. It was perhaps to mark the event that a double portrait of Parthenope and Florence was commissioned from the Bonham Carters' drawing master, William White. Twelve years earlier, Alfred Chalon (soon to start work on the first painting of the new Queen, dressed in her coronation robes) had painted a watercolour of Fanny and her daughters, with 'little Flo' leaning against her mother's knee. White's painting shows Parthenope and Florence, now almost grown up, as the epitome of young ladyhood. Parthenope holds a book that, judging from its elegant gold clasps, may be a Bible, while, in a reversal of roles, Florence has for once forsaken the library to take up one of the accoutrements of the drawing room: neatly dressed in mutton sleeves and apron, she concentrates on working at a piece of worsted, the kind of occupation that she would soon grow to despise. If, as was commonly said, neither of the Nightingale daughters were as beautiful as their mother, Florence was certainly the more comely of the two sisters. She was tall for her sex. Fanny's diaries kept a precise record of Florence's height – springing up from 5 feet 5¾ inches at fifteen to nearly 5 feet 8 as an adult – and her slender figure in youth often struck those who met her ('your sister's figure one should know at any distance', Lady Palmerston told Parthenope). There was 'the peculiarly graceful way in which her small head was set on her shoulders', while her shy, gentle manners and 'silvery' voice reinforced the image of her as 'extremely feminine'. Florence's hair was a rich brown colour, with golden red lights (a Smith inheritance) that darkened with age; her eyes were grey, while her nose was prominent (another feature common to many Smiths). Until middle age, before, as she once wryly observed, she started gnashing them at Government ministers, a perfect set of teeth was revealed when she smiled.

On the afternoon of 8 September 1837, the Nightingales sailed from Southampton on board the steam-packet *Monarch*, reaching the ancient port of Le Havre de Grace at dawn the next day. Accompanying them were Thérèse, their French maid, and Gale, who, despite her fragile health, had created dreadful scenes when it was proposed to leave her behind. Florence was unable to sleep during the crossing for excitement, and had been up into the early hours, talking to a member of the crew about his experiences on the *Amphitrite*, a female convict ship bound for New South Wales, which had been wrecked on sands near Boulogne in August 1833 with the loss of all its women and children.

For three months before leaving England, Florence had redoubled her efforts working among the poor, with 'a strong feeling of religion'. But the precise nature of her call, an answer to the question of what plan God might have in store for her, remained obscure, and she hoped that her European travels might provide fresh insight. She had elected to keep 'the journal' of the tour, she informed her cousin Marianne Nicholson, 'none of the idles inclining that way', though Parthenope, with pencils and paints always at hand, maintained a visual record of architectural features, figures and landscapes in a total of seventeen sketchbooks. Florence's journal exhibited various emerging facets of her personality. One was her precision and command of detail. She noted the exact time of arrival and departure at each stop and the distance covered, and this served as a framework for the rigorous accumulation of factual material about every place visited, its laws and customs, its political system, together with any available population statistics, and observations about its charitable institutions (like a school for the deaf and dumb which she inspected in Genoa). Then there was her deep interest in the people she encountered, and her concern for the impact of social and political conditions on their lives, whether it be old soldiers of the Napoleonic wars, like the caretaker who showed them over the castle at Blaye, and seemed to have fought everyone and yet feel rancour towards no one; or the villagers of Bosuste on the French–Spanish border, a battleground in the recent Carlist wars for the Spanish throne, whose suffering had made them indifferent even to their own destruction. And in Florence's spellbound response to her new surroundings, in her descriptions of the spires of Chartres Cathedral rising like a black town against the sky, or the long reflections of the stars in the Gironde, there is a sense of her longing for a glimpse of an unseen world.

At Rouen the party set off in their carriage. The commodious interior was equipped with devices to make it easy to read, write, eat and rest in comfort. Postillions rode the horses, and the seats on the roof enabled Parthenope and Florence to take turns to sit alongside their father and enjoy the scenery in good weather. Such well-upholstered travelling was common among wealthy families – in the next decade both the Ruskin and Dickens families made their way to Italy in this way – though Harriet Martineau for one deplored the practice of dragging 'a caravan about the continent', and was anxious concerning the effects of 'the destruction of the bodily and mental regularity of habits so essential to juvenile health'. This mode of transport was slow, no more than thirty-five miles a day, to allow the horses to be rested and baited. Inevitably, the mixture of fatigue and excitement took its toll on the passengers. 'We have some of us been rather cross & disagreeable,' Parthenope wrote home in the early stages of the journey. 'I do not mention names . . .'

There was quite a bit to be cross about in these early months, as they rumbled through 'the dull plains' of southern France along roads that were almost impassable, and put up at hotels where the food was inedible and the beds verminous. But at Nice, where they arrived ten days before Christmas, the atmosphere suddenly lightened. The town had been attracting English visitors since the late eighteenth century and there was by now a well-established colony of them, evidenced by the English Protestant Church and the shops selling a variety of English wares. Fanny was remembered from her honeymoon tour, two decades earlier, and the Nightingales were quickly drawn into a friendly circle of people with whom they made expeditions and attended dances. Florence relished the dancing, though it was only to the accompaniment of a pianoforte, as the music of a band was not permitted during Advent, and 'Nothing but quadrilles & waltzes were danced alas!' Parthenope had set her sights one evening on a Mr Plunkett, Florence told Marianne, but had returned on a subsequent night to find that he wasn't dancing, to her 'great dismay', as she had 'intended to have him for herself'.

'Italy' was the single word that headed the second volume of Florence's journal, one loaded with powerful significance for her. Italy was the country of her birth, and a country, moreover, still dominated by the legitimist system instituted by the Congress of Vienna and the Holy Alliance, which denied it the prospect of unity under the national Italian movement and kept the Italian states under direct or indirect Austrian rule. Interspersed with her carefree existence in Italy in the weeks ahead were periods when the realities of the misery suffered by the country under a repressive regime were brought home to her. In Genoa she would recoil in horror at the sight of the fortress recently built by the King of Piedmont, from which the whole town could be blown up in the event of insurrection. Florence's passionate belief in the cause of Italian freedom in the decades ahead was to be gained at first hand in the course of 1838.

On the surface, though, Genoa, which the Nightingales reached on

13 January, possessed for Florence the captivating appeal of 'an Arabian Nights dream come true', and she entered enthusiastically into the glittering social life that the city offered. There was always competition to be her partner at the balls she attended, and when the family moved on the following month to Pisa, the entertainments grew more lavish still: a great court ball given by the Grand Duke of Tuscany, and a luncheon party that ended with the inspection of the Duke's camels. Music had become Florence's first love. She had found the French unmusical, but was in raptures over the opportunities for music that the great Italian cities afforded. At Genoa Florence had decided that she would like to watch Donizetti's *Lucrezia Borgia* every night of her life – it was 'so beautiful, so affecting, so enchanting . . .' – and the annotated libretti from her stay there show that she managed to see the same production on no fewer than three occasions. In the city of her birth, where they arrived in the last week of February, she went 'music mad'. She not only received singing and piano lessons, and was introduced to the famous soprano Angelica Catalani, she also persuaded her mother to take her to the opera several times a week. Mozart was her favourite composer, and *Don Giovanni*, with its neat polarization of good and evil, would remain her favourite opera. Yet, however much music excited her imagination and allowed her to give vent to powerful emotions (even if Elaisa's last sobs in a performance of Mercadante's *Il Giuramento* were 'rather <u>too</u> terrible and <u>too</u> true'), it could not answer her overriding need for facts and information. As if to satisfy this she drew up tables in a notebook and carefully analysed the score, libretto and performance of every opera that she heard.

In rainy Florence, the Nightingales settled at the Albergo del Arno overlooking the Ponte Vecchio, whose elaborate rooms and decorations testified to its previous existence as a palace. Cultural pleasures stretched out before them and were eagerly sampled, and there were more fashionable diversions, including Fanny Nightingale's At Homes to attract the elite of Florentine society, and 'balls to infinity', given by the city's English community; but in quieter moments, Florence's reading was causing her to reflect more deeply on the development of Italian nationalism. Two books, Guerazzi's historical novel *Assedio di Firenze* (1836), which Florentines were banned from reading as it described the siege of Republican Florence by the Medici and Michelangelo's part in its defence, and Sismondi's massive *L'Histoire des Républiques Italiennes au Moyen Age* (1817), 'the Iliad of history' as Florence later called it, opened her eyes to the story of the movement for independence. Sismondi's work, in particular, with its final chapter on 'the causes which had changed the Italian character since the enslavement of their republics', attracted the latent social scientist in Florence; its brilliant sociological analysis named religion, education, legislation and the prevailing notion of honour as decisive factors in the Italians' gradual loss of their liberties since the end of the Middle Ages.

The Nightingales would meet Jean-Charles Leonard Simonde de Sismondi on the next leg of their journey. From Bologna to Venice, the party made its way across northern Italy and the lakes region, arriving in Geneva in September 1838. William Nightingale had boarded in the city for almost a year before his marriage, and still had many friends from those days. The introduction to Sismondi, living as an exile in the republican city-state in which he had grown up, came through Fanny Allen, a childhood friend of Mrs Nightingale's. Fanny Allen's sister Jessie had married Sismondi in 1819, and the web of Allen connections had aligned the historian to the English intellectual beau monde, making Sismondi at different times the brother-in-law of Sir James Mackintosh and Josiah Wedgwood II, and uncle of Charles Darwin. In person Sismondi was unprepossessing, being stunted and ugly, though as Fanny Allen commented, 'It is not possible to withhold one's affection from such a man as that, if he were as ugly as the Beast in the old tale.' Florence observed him feeding the mice in his study while writing his *Histoire des Français*, the vast project at which he worked for some ten hours a day for twenty-three years, completing the twenty-eighth volume in 1842 shortly before his death.

The Sismondis were generous and hospitable, accompanying the Nightingales to an evening with Alphonse de Candolle, the great Swiss botanist, and escorting them up the Salève on donkeys and a sledge covered with straw and drawn by four oxen. On another occasion Sismondi, sitting on a table and surrounded by company, gave an impromptu lecture on Florentine history, carefully recorded by Florence in her journal. His ideas on political economy interested her even more, and on long walks round the city she took in as much from his conversation as she could. It all 'seems to be founded on the overflowing kindness of his heart', she noted. 'He gives to old beggars on principle, to young from habit.' The publication of Sismondi's *Nouveaux Principes d'économie politique* in 1819 had established him as one of the earliest critics of the classical system. In this book he attacked the dehumanizing consequences of industrialization, the brutality of competition, the crude division of labour and the unjust distribution of profits.

Sismondi was at the centre of the Italian exiles living in Geneva, and through him Florence met a number of the figures involved in the movement to win the freedom and unity of Italy: Ricciardi, a Neapolitan aristocrat, who had been shut up in a madhouse until his health and spirit were broken; Fillippi Ugoni and Madame Calandri, both driven into exile after their model schools at Brescia, Pisa and Florence were closed by the Austrian government; Madame Ferrucci, a poetess from Ancona, who earned the family income for her husband and daughter by giving Italian lessons to the Swiss; and Confalonieri, a veteran of the insurrection of 1821, who 'still walks as if he had chains on his legs'. Shortly after the Nightingales' arrival in Geneva, news had come that the new Austrian Emperor, Ferdinand I, intended to celebrate his coronation in Milan by granting an amnesty to all former political offenders. At a party at Sismondi's house, attended by Florence, the joy among the exiles at the thought of finally returning home was overwhelming. Only the next day, however, did they discover that there was a condition attached to the amnesty, which none of them could accept: that they must undertake never to conspire against Austria again. It was plain, Florence wrote in her journal, that the Emperor's good intentions were 'whited sepulchres', and that Metternich had only published the amnesty to make the many individual disappointments more bitter.

The simmering drama of political events cut short the family's stay in Geneva. Louis Napoleon Bonaparte, nephew of the great Emperor and pretender to the French throne, had taken refuge in Switzerland, and in the autumn of 1838 the French government demanded his surrender. When the Swiss refused, French troops began to march on the frontier. As trenches were dug in the streets, and the Swiss troops positioned the cannon on the ramparts, the Nightingales hurriedly made preparations for their departure, delayed only by the shortage of horses, as every horse in Geneva had been requisitioned for the artillery. But on 1 October they finally set off, bound for Paris, with Sismondi running after the carriage to bid them farewell, tears streaming down his face. Reaching Fontainebleau a week later, they were relieved to learn that the crisis had subsided. Through the mediation of the English government, Louis

Napoleon was leaving Switzerland and, with the agreement of the French, going to live in England. The Genevese, reported the Sismondis, were dancing in the streets.

In Paris the Nightingales settled at 22 Place Vendôme. Among the letters of introduction they had brought with them was one from Aunt Patty to a Mrs Clarke, and her daughter, Mary, an Englishwoman who was beginning to preside over one of the most brilliant intellectual circles in Paris. Mary Clarke had learned her skills as a *salonnière* from the great Madame Récamier, who had sublet the Clarkes an apartment in the convent building that was her home, the Abbaye-au-Bois in the rue de Sèvres on the Left Bank. Here, *la jeune Anglaise*, as Mary was known, was a sparkling addition to Madame's *salon*, and an especial attraction for its older members, like the poet Chateaubriand. After seven years, the Clarkes had recently moved to a new home in the rue du Bac. 'Miss C no longer shares apartments with Madame R.,' wrote Patty, 'but she is in herself very clever & wd be glad to see you.'

The Clarkes lived at 112 (now 120) rue du Bac, a large *hôtel* separated by a courtyard from the narrow, bustling street, and overlooking the garden of the Missions Etrangères at the rear. Their apartment was on the fourth and fifth floors, just above Chateaubriand's, and it was in the set of small sitting rooms on the lower floor that Mary Clarke did her entertaining. On Saturdays she was At Home to any acquaintance who cared to drop in, while during the week she held more select breakfast or dinner parties. Florence first encountered Miss Clarke at a children's soirée, and she rapidly became the Nightingales' 'best friend' in Paris, accompanying them to concerts, the theatre (where they saw 'a most extraordinary actress', the young Rachel) and art galleries. She invited them to evening gatherings where they mixed with some of the literary, political and scientific names of the moment, and met their hostess's two male intimates, the medieval scholar Claude Fauriel, and the orientalist Julius Mohl, responsible for attending to the frugal refreshments of tea and biscuits. Mary Clarke also introduced them to Madame Récamier's circle, and at one 'curious séance' at the Abbaye-au-Bois, at which Chateaubriand was also present, Florence reported that they had listened to a reading of some 'Memoirs of the Revolution', in which the reader mentioned having come across Chateaubriand's sister-in-law in a delirious state on her way to the guillotine. Madame

Récamier sat in a dark corner so that 'she might be at liberty to indulge the emotions which these readings often arouse'.

Mary Clarke was forty-five, but still girlishly impulsive (her mother had once warned her to turn her tongue seven times in her mouth before speaking). She dressed unconventionally, while her tousled hair had given rise to a gibe by the statesman and orator François Guizot that she and his Skye terrier must share the same coiffeur. Patty Smith thought Miss Clarke was 'quite right to live in Paris where these sorts of self-neglect are quite forgiven in women past a certain age', but the lifestyle of the Parisian *salonnière* displayed Mary's vivacity and intellect to good effect, allowing her to talk freely in a way that would have been unthinkable in the stuffier London society of the time. For, above all, Clarkey, as the Nightingales were soon calling her, was uninhibited and unpretentious. As Florence later wrote, 'She never had a breath of posing or "edifying" in her presentation of herself, even when it would have been most desirable. She was always undressed – naked in full view. A little clothing would have been decent.'

Mary Clarke craved love, but life had also taught her that personal misery resulted in the first place from a lack of occupation, and it was in this respect that she was most frequently to give Florence her understanding and support over the course of the next fifteen years. Born in London into a family that was part Scottish Whig, part Anglo-Irish, Mary had spent her early life shuttling between the south of France and England, where her older sister Eleanor, married to a wealthy MP, lived at Cold Overton in Leicestershire. Farmed out to her sister for a year, when she was fifteen, to 'improve her conventional manners', Mary had found herself stifled by English family life and particularly by the 'dripping twaddle' of what passed for conversation. As an adolescent she took refuge in dreams, but by the time Mary and her invalid mother moved permanently to Restoration Paris and started to offer their drawing room as a meeting place for bright young liberals, Mary had formed an ideal of herself as a solitary female intellectual, based on the model of Madame de Staël. She studied painting, and did some writing – in the mid-1820s she planned a history of women – but it was reading and conversation that predominated.

She itched, though, to fulfil herself in some wider sphere. 'How delicious it would be to live in the public eye,' she wrote, 'and work for the public good, and have a busy life, instead of sitting by the fire

imagining . . .' In 1827 she had excitedly seized on the news that Elizabeth Fry had received the Government's permission to visit prisons
and suggest measures for their improvement: 'There's the beginning of
women's rise to power and government – not through love and men's
ridiculous passions, but by sheer moral force and intelligence.' In Mary's
own life, however, the lack of a consuming passion was deeply felt. By
the end of the 1830s, her relationship with Fauriel, some twenty years
her senior, remained frustratingly unrequited, while the future of her
friendship with Mohl was as yet unresolved.

To what extent did Mary Clarke glimpse the latent power in the
eighteen-year-old Florence Nightingale? It's impossible to say, though
she clearly derived pleasure and stimulus from the company of both Parthe
and Flo, refreshing her 'mind with these young things who are like May
breezes to me . . .' And the Nightingales looked forward to welcoming
Clarkey at Lea Hurst during her next visit to her family in England.

Meeting Mary Clarke, with her fearless flouting of convention and
her claims for equality with men on account of her intellect, provided
Florence with a new lesson in the opportunities that might be open to
an educated young woman. In other respects, though, Paris seemed dull
after 'beautiful Italy'. The city rarely emerged from under a veil of cold
fog or icy sheets of rain, and Florence and Parthenope were forced to
take warm vapour baths to protect themselves against the plummeting
temperatures. The season that had begun in November was brought to
an abrupt halt early in 1839 by the death of King Louis-Philippe's
daughter, Princess Marie. 'We have quite enough going out without this,
and know a great many people,' Florence wrote to Grandmother Shore,
but the activity that interested her most at this stage was her visits to
the Chambre des Députés, for which her father had obtained tickets,
where she heard Guizot and Thiers in debate amid an uproar which
seemed 'very unstatesmanlike'.

Fanny Nightingale had been closely observing the effects of their
European tour on her daughters. In a letter to her sister Julia, written
before they left Geneva, in the autumn of 1838, she had compared them
to the 'dull insipid travelling damsels with whom we fall in', and admitted
only to surprise that the Nightingale girls were 'not more worshipped'.

Parthe . . . speaks French so well that even the French tell her occasionally that
she has no accent . . . She certainly is the world's pet, and yet, strange to say,

nothing more. Florence is much admired for her beauty and she, too, is reckoned very clever and amusing, but her stately manners keep people at a distance, so I do not expect that love passages will be frequent in her life.

Her remarks could hardly have been more prescient.

'You should never have brought your daughters abroad,' one citizen of Genoa had warned Fanny. 'They will find England so dull after it.' For a time, however, after the family's return home on 6 April 1839, boredom for Florence was kept at bay by the excitement of the London season. The alterations to Embley remained unfinished and, with the house full of workmen, the Nightingales retreated for three weeks to a gamekeeper's lodge on the estate before moving to London, to stay at the Carleton Hotel in Regent Street, where Fanny was occupied 'from morning till night, hiring servants & chusing papers & carpets & curtains for our new rooms'.

Wearing a white dress purchased in Paris, Florence was presented at the Queen's drawing room at the beginning of May and admitted that she 'was not nearly so much frightened as I expected ... The Queen looked flushed and tired, but the whole sight was very pretty.' The current intrigue and scandal surrounding the Bedchamber Crisis, the first serious upset of Victoria's reign, only contributed to the sense of occasion. A letter from Florence to Selma Benedicks, a young Swedish woman she had befriended in Italy, was full of up-to-the-minute political gossip: the resignation of Melbourne's Whig ministry 'and its re-establishment in the same half week' after Sir Robert Peel, the Tory leader, 'threw up the affair in disgust' when the Queen refused to accede to his wish to dismiss some of her Whig bedchamber women. Victoria, Florence was happy to note, had been 'enthusiastically cheered' at the opera, following some months of unpopularity, and was 'perfectly idolized among our party for her firmness and spirit'. On 19 May, as lamps were lit throughout London in celebration, Florence and her mother attended the Queen's birthday drawing room.

Music remained Florence's abiding passion, and being able to share it with Marianne Nicholson only intensified her pleasure. Marianne, together with her parents and younger sister Laura, had joined the Nightingales at the Carleton, where their rooms reverberated noisily to the sound of piano, voice and the pounding of dancing feet. Florence had 'quite lost her voice in that horrid Parisian climate', but Marianne possessed exceptional musical gifts, including a thrilling soprano, and 'one unlucky piano never stopped' as she, Florence and Laura practised for hours at a time, with '4 masters between them'.

A sad loss, however, overshadowed the Nightingales' homecoming. Soon after their arrival in Florence, the previous spring, they had learned of the 'rapid change for the worse that had taken place in poor Uncle Carter', and days later had received news of his death at the age of fifty from cancer. His eldest son, Jack, had joined them briefly in Paris at the end of that year, and on arriving home they had been quickly reunited with his widow, Joanna. She was bereft, left with eight children, the youngest just two years old, inadequate to the demands of managing on her own, and relying heavily on the support of the eldest girl, Hilary, now eighteen.

At the end of 1838 Hilary had started a year's schooling at Rachel Martineau's small boarding establishment in Liverpool. Like Parthenope, Hilary was a talented artist. 'Everything that catches their eye as beautiful, either in form or colour, they sketch . . . with unbelievable rapidity . . .,' Fanny Allen observed of the two cousins. Yet despite later opportunities to study painting, under the artists Jeanron in Paris and Mulready in London, Hilary was never able to forgo the onerous family duties that had been vested in her long before her father's death, and consequently her art suffered. According to Mary Clarke, who assumed the role of surrogate mother to Hilary after the two women were introduced at Lea Hurst that summer of 1839, Hilary needed three years' 'hard labour' to make the leap from accomplished amateur to artist. 'She is at the threshold, but . . . what a pity she has so many childer to look after.'

Hilary's natural solicitude marked her out as the perfect confidante for Florence, especially when it came to family problems and spiritual matters. 'Only think dearest,' Florence had written to her from Italy, 'it is now really how long since I have seen you . . . six months, tho' it seems more like six years. The more I write, the more I want to see you.' In 1842 they would be separated again. This time it would be Hilary, accompanied by her mother and five of her brothers and sisters, who embarked on a continental tour in the Nightingales' enormous carriage.

If Hilary appealed to Florence's serious nature, it was Marianne who brought out an unbuttoned, fun-loving side; the Florence Nightingale who, according to Anne Dutton, another friend at this time, enjoyed gossiping about politics, personalities and, most of all, music. Marianne was beautiful, brilliant – and a little dangerous. She was well known for her 'prying propensities' and 'indiscreet questions', and even her close family acknowledged that her reputation as something of a troublemaker was not entirely undeserved. Among her chief attractions was her sharp wit. As Florence was to write after one uproarious occasion, 'She made my old bones shake with laughter, & they have been stiff in consequence for twenty-four hours.'

Henry Nicholson, Marianne's elder brother, was one of several family members who joined the Nightingales at Lea Hurst in June to welcome Mary Clarke to England. Henry, just twenty, had lost an eye in a shooting accident a decade earlier, and was now up at Trinity, Cambridge, reading mathematics. He and Florence soon became absorbed in logarithms, while around them, 'a scrummage between moving and not moving' to the renovated Embley was taking place. The builders remained in residence, but William Nightingale finally decreed that the move had been delayed for long enough. Unfortunately, the family arrived at the house on a stormy September day. Parthenope, resting at Harrogate to regain her strength after a summer of illness, was regaled with a catalogue of the misfortunes that had awaited them at Embley. The drive was under water, rain was seeping into the corridors and through the ceilings, and, Florence joked, 'the fishes are beginning to stick in the elms'. They sat on mattresses by the servants' fire, with no candles and only 'raw meat' and bread to eat, while Hogg, the steward, murmured 'almost with tears in his eyes, that I should see your mam wandering about the passage in the dark and the master sitting by the servants' hall, it's very strange!'

'The house does not strike us as very large though there are so many new rooms,' Florence informed her sister, a point of view that might confound the modern visitor, confronted with an extensive gothic sprawl. The new west wing had added four bedrooms to the first floor and two large rooms on the ground floor. The larger of these was the drawing room, the admiration of all. 'I might distend at length on the harmony & unity of the colouring, the richness of the moulding & the beauty of the conception . . . The oak ceiling and pendant is beautiful & the paper quite the thing . . .' The east wing consisted simply of three rooms on top of each other; that on the second floor was to become Florence's bedroom. Embley was now large enough to receive at one time, 'five able-bodied females with their husbands and belongings'. The redesigned domestic quarters occupied a bay extending the entire length of the house: new kitchens, pantries, and servants' rooms reached by a small winding staircase. The running of the household would in future be the responsibility of as many as fifteen servants, including the indispensable Gale. Throughout the property, William Nightingale had incorporated a number of idiosyncratic features: the cast iron drainpipes bore his insignia, the flower urns his coat of arms, and the new library shelves disguised a secret entrance into his study next door (though Florence considered silence the best comment on these and Uncle Octavius was 'vicious' about them). 'We are working hard at the House creeping from room to room,' Florence wrote to Parthenope some weeks later, confessing that tiredness almost prevented her from listening to Harriet Martineau's *Deerbrook*, which they were reading aloud in the evenings: '. . . The whole drift of the book is I think so mistaken – all the ladies falling in love first too, how nasty! & then that eternal love how sickening!'

There was a respite from the smell of varnish and new paint that Christmas when a large family party gathered at Waverley, the Nicholsons' home. But the festive atmosphere was almost immediately shattered by news of the death of Fred Smith, the eldest son of Uncle Octavius and Aunt Jane, and Florence's own 'early play fellow', who had been travelling in Western Australia as a member of George Grey's exploratory expedition. After being shipwrecked, Grey and his team had started a 300-mile trek back to their base, 'the strongest going forward by forced marches to send help to the rest'. Fred had died near the shore in a solitary spot, just seventy-six miles short of the destination. 'They found the poor fellow, apparently having been dead about 2 days,' Sam Smith reported to his sister Fanny, 'but so extenuated that the cause of his death is too certain . . . His only sustenance apparently must have been shell fish, the little canteen in his pocket was perfectly <u>dry</u>.'* Staying with Aunt Mai at

* Grey's expedition – his second to Australia – found little of note, though he published a successful account of it in *Journal of Two Expeditions of Discovery in North West and Western Australia*, in 1841. While certain of Fred Smith's relatives thought that Grey had 'sacrificed his followers to his own hard-hearted greediness after distinctions', they also admitted that he had only included Fred at the young man's own insistence. Florence evidently held no grudge. In 1859, at the suggestion of Grey, who had recently completed a term as Governor of New Zealand and was concerned about Maori depopulation, she conducted a study of mortality rates in aboriginal schools. This was published in 1863 as *Sanitary Statistics of Native Colonial Schools and Hospitals*.

Combe Hurst, her home on Kingston Hill, at the beginning of February, Florence paid a visit to the Octavius Smiths at Thames Bank. Aunt Jane, she wrote, 'looks woefully, so thin and says that she is <u>never</u> out of pain', though her manner was 'perfectly placid' and 'she shed no tears'.

While Florence's letters to her immediate family remained calm and unruffled, brooding discontent lay just beneath the surface. Only perhaps to Mary Clarke in Paris – in correspondence that no longer survives – was she able to express something of the dissatisfaction she felt about her way of life, in terms apparently so bitter that Clarkey complained of her 'nailed tongue'. Foreign travel and fashionable diversions had certainly taught her something about the need to be on guard against a desire to shine in society, but they had offered no further intimation about the nature of her call. It was almost three years since she had experienced the compulsion of that inner voice, yet she had achieved no further insight into its true meaning or significance.

In Aunt Mai she was discovering a valuable ally to whom she could turn not merely for sympathy, but also for practical assistance in rescuing her from frustration. At first light, before the rest of the household stirred, Florence and her aunt cemented their bond in reading and study. German and the history of the Thirty Years War were their particular focus, though Florence craved something more: the kind of certainty she believed that only mathematics could provide. Studying Euclid's *Elements of Geometry* with her young cousin Beatrice only whetted her appetite still further, and before long Mai had interceded with Fanny 'to ask if you see any objection to a mathematical master if we can find a clean middle aged highly respectable person'.

Fanny saw no end of objections. She questioned the desirability of allowing Florence to neglect more conventional occupations, her piano playing, for instance, in favour of such unorthodox study. Mai quickly countered with the estimate of the Nightingales' music master, who did not think that Florence 'would ever be a fine player' though there was no doubt that she would always be able to play 'so as to give herself & friends pleasure'. This failed to satisfy Fanny. Of what possible use could maths be to a young woman, and where would these maths lessons take place? Mai began to lose patience:

I feel that if Flo were my own daughter, I should be very restless to see her immediately hard at work. [T]hose industrious tendencies which she spends on music & needlework, would, I think make a strong interest for life if devoted to mathematics pursued into science. For instance, Sam thinks she might well study mathematics as applied to optics.

The house in Blandford Square belonging to Fanny's brother Ben was at first proposed as a suitable meeting place, then hastily withdrawn when it became known that Aunt Patty, the Smith family's epitome of intellectual womanhood, was in a state of nervous collapse there. To spare Florence 'the risk of an outbreak from Patty', it was finally agreed that she should stay at Thames Bank, comfort Aunt Jane, who was expecting another baby, and look after the other children, while taking maths lessons in Uncle Octavius's library. She felt it a blessing, Florence told Fanny, that 'a creature so nearly spiritualized as Aunt Jane should cling to me in her distress'. Mr Gillespie, a Presbyterian minister who had once tutored Fred, was respectable enough, though Florence thought him 'a most awful man' except when he reminisced about her cousin. He also gave her so much work that she could hardly find time for it except at nights. Meanwhile, she devoted herself to Aunt Jane, sending home for an air cushion for her to sit on in the carriage, and listening as her aunt confided in her. 'I had rather have a son die of exhaustion and exertion,' Jane admitted, 'than see one before my eyes always at home without any other object but living from breakfast to dinner,' a view with which in less tragic circumstances Florence might well have found some sympathy.

In studying maths, Florence was following the eminent example of Mary Somerville, who had overcome far more stringent parental opposition – including their fears that she would deplete the household candle supply and go 'raving mad about the longitude' – to become the first woman internationally regarded as a serious scientist in her own right. Somerville's *Mechanism of the Heavens*, a condensed version of Laplace's cosmological mathematics, published in 1831, had become the first book by a woman to be used in the Cambridge Mathematics Tripos, and this, together with its successor, Somerville's magisterial *On the Connexion of the Physical Sciences*, would encourage Florence and her cousin Henry to spend hours 'poring over the moon's path mathematically'.

The story of Somerville's struggle to educate herself would have been especially familiar to Florence, for Somerville was a 'cordial friend' of Patty Smith's, and a dining companion, in the 1840s, of Fanny Nightingale's on her rare visits to England from her home in Italy. A decade later, when Florence faced objections from her family to pursuing the dictates of her own vocation, she recalled Mary Somerville, sitting up 'by night working in blankets, to indulge an appetite for science' as one of those who 'have had a call within them which, in the beginning, gave pain to those they loved, but ended in their joy'.

Florence 'has taken to mathematics', her sister reported in July 1840, 'and like everything she undertakes she is deep in them and working very hard'. She was quick to pass on her knowledge to her cousins, 'doing a little Algebra' with the young Nicholsons, Laura and Lothian, and later coaching their older brother William for his Sandhurst exams, though Mr Nicholson impressed on her the importance of remaining discreet about this, as William would become a laughing stock if it became known that he was receiving tuition from a woman.* After working hard at Thames Bank, Florence rewarded herself with two visits to the opera in London with Marianne. She was also present at one of Liszt's concerts on his British tour, before returning to Lea Hurst for the summer.

Not the least of Mary Somerville's achievements – and essential to maintaining her reputation – was that she demonstrated the compatibility of high intellectual accomplishments and conventional femininity as a wife and mother. The question of whether Florence would similarly ever be able to combine a vocation with a husband was posed for her for the first time in human form that August when she received a proposal of marriage. Marmaduke Wyvill came from an established North Riding family and was the grandson of Christopher Wyvill, prominent as leader of the Yorkshire Association's programme for moderate parliamentary reform in the 1780s. The Wyvills (related by marriage to the Milneses, the family of Florence's eventual suitor, Richard Monckton Milnes) were old friends of the Smiths, and among the English families at Nice when the Nightingales stayed there at Christmas 1837.

* There appears to be no documentary evidence to connect Florence with J. J. Sylvester (1814–97), the mathematician, distinguished for his theory of invariant algebra, who is sometimes said to have tutored her. It is not, however, unlikely that she may have been one of his private pupils during the decade between his return to England from the United States in 1843 and her departure for Scutari in 1854, especially as Sylvester was friendly with Florence's uncle Ben Smith and his children.

Florence had become friendly with Miss Henrietta Wyvill, and noted in passing that Henrietta's brothers, Marmaduke and Christopher, were 'very fair in their way'.

She had probably not given Marmaduke Wyvill another thought, but a visit by him to Lea Hurst in the summer of 1840 apparently confirmed what he described to William Nightingale as 'the very great love & affection that has been inspired in me for your second daughter Miss Florence Nightingale & which I flatter myself she equally shares'. Addressing Florence herself, he adopted a more tentative tone and signed off with a dramatic flourish: 'If I am not mistaken by your manner & looks, then happiest am I of all mortals, but trembling do I wait to hear that you will confide yourself to my care & allow me to become your protector and guardian . . .'

Marmaduke was never a serious contender for Florence's hand and had perhaps mistaken pity on her part for true feeling. That October from Waverley, where she had returned with the Nicholsons after a rainy holiday in the Lake District, she admitted to Parthenope that she had heard 'some things' about Marmaduke 'which make me sorry for him, but glad for myself'. Yet however transitory the episode, it must have underscored her fears about her future, particularly in regard to what she would come to refer to – in that 'vulgar expression' – as the 'lottery' of marriage. It may be no coincidence that a surviving fragment of a novel or short story by Florence about an unsatisfactory marriage dates from around this time. The 'Biography of Ellen M' was based possibly on an incident from life, though it is presented fictionally. Far from being an educated young woman, Ellen is a 'fascinating savage', hardly able to read or write. She marries an older man, 'a clever man of literary taste', and then suffers from his neglect because they have nothing in common. The moral of the story appears to be that a woman must be allowed an independent life of the mind and scope for individual action.

Mrs Somerville, married, second time around, to a husband who supported her right to an independent intellectual life, appeared to be an exception to the general rule. 'Ladies' work has always to be fitted in,' Florence wrote to Hilary Bonham Carter at this time, her mind perhaps on the unsystematic nature of her own maths studies, squeezed in when family life permitted. 'Where a man is, his business is the law.' More and more, in the decade ahead, she would incline to the view that a woman with 'a work of God to do in the world' had no realistic alternative but to remain unattached and single.

The key to her discovery of the nature of that work would ultimately be found in the condition of the poor at the beginning of the 1840s. A series of bad harvests had created a period of enormous distress, exacerbated by the Corn Laws, keeping wages low and prices high. The resulting squalor in which ordinary people lived and the near starvation they endured were impossible to ignore. Reports of problems in the towns and villages close to Lea Hurst, filtering through at the end of 1839, provided a snapshot of the economic downturn: miners paid only half their usual wages, foreign employees dismissed, and the theft of sheep on a sharp increase. Even Smedley's mill, the largest employer in the district, was said to be 'slack' and laying off workers.

Everywhere she went Florence witnessed evidence of these new levels of deprivation. On a visit to the Nicholsons at Waverley, she wrote to her mother of the 'dreadful deal of want of work here' and the rise in begging that had occurred as a consequence. She was appalled by her own impotence in the face of such immense suffering, but the need to offer assistance, even if this took the form of little more than sympathy, was as strong as ever. 'My mind is absorbed with the idea of the sufferings of man,' she wrote in the summer of 1842, 'it besets me behind and before, a very one-sided view, but I can hardly see anything else and all that poets sing of the glories of this world seems to me untrue. All the people I see are eaten up with care or poverty or disease.'

With her growing ability to digest and master detail, she set out to inform herself about current efforts at social reform, designed to improve the living and working conditions of the poor. Parthenope later recalled the bundles of reports, the official blue books of parliamentary commit- tees and royal commissions, on the table of Florence's room at Embley. She certainly read Edwin Chadwick's *Report on the Sanitary Conditions of the Labouring Classes of Great Britain* when it was published in 1842, and followed closely Chadwick's subsequent struggle to establish the machinery for a centralized public health authority. In the spring of 1844, she waited anxiously to hear that Lord Ashley's Ten Hours Bill, to shorten the working hours of factory women, had been carried despite the attempts of Peel's Tory Government to forestall the humanitarians by launching a compromise measure. 'The horrors which have come out about the sufferings of women in factories,' Florence noted, 'have made Peel's own people vote against him' (in the event, it was not until 1847 that the Ten Hours Movement could claim complete victory).

While the gulf between the two nations, rich and poor, was growing, 'the glassy surface of our civilized life', as Florence called it, continued as before. The years 1841 and 1842 repeated the by now established cycle: Lea Hurst in the summer months and Embley for the winter, peripatetic visits to extended family, and a prolonged stay in London after Easter for the season. The Carleton, or alternatively Fenton's Hotel, in St James's, provided a London base for the Nightingales until 1842, when for the first time the family occupied a set of rooms at the Burlington Hotel on Cork Street. Christmas and New Year were generally spent at Waverley. New Year 1842, 'an uncommonly gay time', was celebrated with a masked ball for eighty guests, followed the next evening, Twelfth Night, by a family performance of *The Merchant of Venice*. Henry Nicholson, cast in the role of Shylock, had rushed to London to study Macready's performance of the character as preparation; Marianne played Nerissa, charming everyone in an after-piece entitled *Perfection*. Parthenope painted the scenery while Florence, naturally enough, took on the job of stage manager, making Uncle Adams learn his part as the Doge by going at him like 'a sledge-hammer' throughout the week of rehearsals.

Florence's longing to escape from her mundane everyday existence made her leap at any opportunity to relieve human misery, however limited and localized. In early 1843 such a case – 'of doing the office of love on earth', as she rather grandiosely described it to her mother – presented itself. The previous November, Hope Reeve, wife of *Times* leader writer and correspondent Henry Reeve, had died after giving birth to a baby daughter. The Reeves, a Unitarian family from Norwich, were old friends of the Smiths, and the impact of this sudden tragedy, consigning the care of the baby (also called Hope) to the bereaved father and his dead wife's sister, Helen Richardson, aroused Florence's sympathy. She sought Fanny's permission to be allowed to visit Helen in London and offer what support she could. When her mother demurred about the length of time necessary for her stay, Florence responded with a new note of tart asperity in her voice: if she could only persuade Helen to put off her sister's death until next year, 'as I have sanguine hopes of doing when I get to town you will certainly see me on Saturday. She can have no possible objections . . . to put off her mourning for her till another year.'

But a week's visit lengthened into one month and then threatened two. This time it was Parthenope who raised the stronger objections. In a letter to her mother in the middle of February 1843, marked 'Private', Florence complained that 'Parthe's letters are my misery, & if you cannot stop her, I suppose I must come home . . .' The slightest hint, though, that Parthenope might be open to interceding on her behalf for a longer stay produced a letter calculated to win over the hardest heart. 'Helen is sitting opposite to me to make me say that she dares "not look you in the face[,] it is not to leave her alone now". I sh'd be missing the only opport'y I ever had of doing real good . . . My dear, I cry unto you, do this thing for me for no one else can do it. You will have me all your life, for I shall never die & never marry.' Florence won her sister over, but this was a disturbing demonstration of Parthenope's possessiveness, which before long she would learn to fear.

Florence's health was a recurrent problem at this time. She described herself as having been 'very ill' in the summer of 1842; and although she reported the following year that a daily glass of port wine was doing wonders in banishing her sore throats, at Christmas 1843, staying with the Nicholsons, she succumbed to another of the inflammatory attacks that had plagued her since childhood. This illness was serious enough to keep her at Waverley for more than two months, and by early March 1844 her recovery was still incomplete. Sleepless nights reduced her strength and each time she left her room she ran the risk of catching cold. During her long convalescence she described, at her father's request, her 'experience of the Sick Room'. She had been reading Harriet Martineau's *Life in the Sick-Room*, but could not agree with her that as the body's strength decays, 'the stronger the conviction of an independent & unchangeable self'; however, she had reached the same conclusion as Martineau, that, as the Stoics had said, 'pain is no evil'.

Her recovery was aided by the company of Hannah Nicholson, Uncle Nicholson's unmarried sister, who was also at Waverley. Aunt Hannah, as she became known, was viewed by Florence as 'one of the most perfect of human beings', and evidently showed her honorary niece great kindness as she emerged from the low spirits accompanying her illness. Soon Florence was 'going into good Miss Nicholson's room every evening', coming away impressed 'with the truth of her piety'. Although the Nicholsons were from a prominent Unitarian family, Aunt Hannah was an Evangelical. To a troubled young woman, uncertain about God's purpose for her in life, she provided a sympathetic ear, and following her return home in the spring of 1844, Florence would pour out her problems to her.

At Waverley that winter of 1843–4, however, there appears to have been a subject of more immediate concern, which had nothing to do with Florence's illness or matters of her soul. In a letter to her mother, Florence referred to Aunt Hannah as being like 'an evergreen branch in the midst of discontents'. What were these discontents, and might they have had something to do with a proposal of marriage from Henry Nicholson to his cousin Florence?

The story of Henry Nicholson's wish to marry Florence Nightingale, his rejection by her, and the subsequent strained relations between the Nightingales and Nicholsons, especially between Florence and Marianne, who is said to have accused her cousin of leading her brother on, has been repeated by many biographers, though there is no direct surviving evidence to confirm it. Cecil Woodham-Smith, in the most fleshed-out account of the episode, even resorted to doctoring unrelated material in order to lend credence to the story. Yet, while the detail may be absent, there is sufficient circumstantial evidence to suggest that the broad outline is true, though the chronology remains uncertain. In 'Cassandra', Florence's autobiographical essay on the family, she analyses the ways in which people choose their marriage partner, and suggests that an intimacy between cousins, thrown together in childhood where an 'acquaintance has grown up naturally and unconsciously', is one of the most common. But the essay also underlines her theoretical objection to such marriages: intermarriage between relations was 'in direct contravention of the laws of nature for the well-being of the race', and commonly resulted in 'madness, degeneration of race . . . and cretinism . . .'

Her closeness to Henry cannot be doubted. All adult correspondence between them appears to have been destroyed – possibly another sign of the wish to preserve a discreet silence about a relationship that had ended badly – though a brief postscript in a letter from the sixteen-year-old Florence to Parthenope speaks of her regret on one occasion at not seeing Henry ('fâites-lui mes compliments et exprimez-lui mes regrets de la manière la plus touchant'). Like Marianne, Henry could be depended upon to provide interest and diversion, and his absence could be a cause

of sadness, as in the autumn of 1840, during one of Florence's visits to
Waverley, when she admitted that his departure had cast a shadow over
her stay. Their shared interest in maths had brought the two cousins
closer. While Florence must have envied Henry his three years at Cambridge, she shared in the excitement when he proved himself in the
highly competitive final year examination of the Mathematics Tripos,
though as a Dissenter he continued the family tradition by not gradu-
ating. 'Henry is 31st wrangler, my dear,' she wrote to Parthenope,
'. . . Uncle Nicholson brought the news home from Guildford on Saturday night but would tell no one till Henry came in, who was very much
surprised. He has been so jolly ever since that it has been nothing but a
succession of what a roll! as every name in the paper of honours was
examined.' Like his father before him, Henry went on to study law, and
in the spring of 1844 he was called to the Bar.

It may have been the imminent change in Henry's circumstances that
made him raise the subject of marriage with Florence, perhaps only
speculatively, while she was at Waverley for Christmas 1843. Continuing
references to him in her correspondence suggest that he didn't receive
an outright refusal from her: as late as 1846 she was on good enough
terms with Henry to pay him a visit at his chambers in Lincoln's Inn.
But might she unwittingly have encouraged him to expect that eventually
she would agree to be his wife? Years afterwards, Aunt Patty would
recall how Florence's 'kind-hearted pity for rejected suitors led to mis-
construction which she probably never suspected & would have dis-
dained if she had'. Henry Nicholson may have been one of these suitors.
He is a shadowy figure, made all the more so by his sudden death by
drowning, as a result of a freak accident while travelling in Spain in his
early thirties. It is tempting to imagine that his frequent absences abroad
in his final years were an attempt to remove himself from the scene of a
romantic disappointment. He remained unmarried.

Shortly after the death in 1854 of his wife Anne, Fanny Nightingale's
sister, George Nicholson remembered 'with pain' the 'diminished intimacy which in later years has been too evident between our portions of
the family'. By that time, Marianne's relationship with Florence, once
such a fertile source of enjoyable companionship for both women, had
all too clearly diminished, and Florence's refusal of her beloved brother
Henry offers the strongest reason for the end of their friendship. That
Marianne may have had a hand in pushing the two of them together is

suggested by one undated letter, from 1844–5, in which Florence asks Parthenope to write to Henry 'as the only note I have written to him for months, he <u>immediately</u> informed Marianne of, whose imagination <u>immediately</u> did wonders with it'. Although in 1847 Florence and Marianne were still communicating in friendly terms as of old, by the following year Florence was instructing Parthenope to 'read and burn' Marianne's letters; and a few years later, she would refer dismissively to her cousin as 'that foolish Marianne'.

None the less, the souring of this, the most important friendship of her youth, was mourned by Florence with an aching sense of loss. She had once believed, as she confessed to Hilary, that her love for Marianne would never change, that 'no unkindness could affect it' and that it would be a love forever. 'I was not a worthy friend to her. I was not true either to her or to myself in our friendship. I was afraid of her: that is the truth . . .' The passionate tone of these remarks has encouraged some commentators to jump to the conclusion that Florence's feelings for Marianne were of an erotic nature. Florence certainly recognized a danger in the intensity of feeling thrown up by such friendships. As she was to warn nursing probationers at St Thomas's, years later, 'Some of our youthful friendships are too violent to last . . .' Equally, though, it is easy enough to misunderstand and misinterpret the conventions of epistolary language between two young upper-middle-class women of the period, so often rich in endearments and high-flown sentiments. Florence would miss Marianne's 'delightful grace and talent in making life easy'; but she was right to be afraid of her, as future events would show.

'Pray write to me, dear Aunt Hannah, the struggle is too hard, life is too long. I am weary before I have gone a third of the way . . .' Hannah Nicholson had entered Florence's life as an adoptive aunt, and before long had a closer kinship pressed upon her, that of a surrogate mother, to whom Florence signed her letters 'your affectionate and grateful child'. Much to Florence's disappointment, they were rarely to meet; instead, they embarked upon a regular correspondence, lasting for much of the rest of the decade, in which the older woman demonstrated a tender concern for the younger one's state of mind and kept a watchful eye on her spiritual development. The 'mysterious power' of Aunt Hannah's sympathy seemed to provide her with 'daily air' with which to breathe. Florence responded to her entreaties to place her trust in God, and to find permanent peace in place of her endless 'restless anxiety', with 'long outpourings' in which she expressed her overwhelming gratitude to her. These letters are strongly in the evangelical mould. They express dissatisfaction with her way of life, but are also filled with self-reproach. She berates herself for her wilful sinning and her pride, and wonders whether she will ever love God as she ought, for 'only the pure in heart shall see God' and 'there is no pure thought in me'.

As Florence's spiritual mentor, Hannah Nicholson – 'to whom all unseen things seemed real, and eternal things near' – was able to guide and direct her, especially by influencing her understanding of how to draw closer to God by finding a sense of the eternal in the temporal. Yet a fundamental difference separated the two women. To Aunt Hannah, mystical union with God was an end in itself, but for Florence that union promised something more: a source of strength for carrying out one's calling in the world. Later she would comment explicitly on this distinction in *Suggestions for Thought*, the substantial work of spiritual philosophy she completed on her return from the Crimean War: 'The "kingdom of heaven is within," indeed, but we must also create one without, because we are *intended* to act upon our circumstances.'

Aunt Hannah's prescription for Florence's ills, that reconciliation with God would necessarily bring contentment with her lot, reveals both the narrowness of her own vision and how little she understood the young woman who would one day write to her, imagining the 'happiness of working ... with no alloy of vanity or love of display or of glory, but with the ecstasy of single-heartedness'. However, at a time when Florence was clinging dependently to Hannah Nicholson for spiritual succour, she was also beginning to find another kind of consolation, in the workings of her imagination.

The divide between an imaginary and an outward world, in which the former appears more real than the latter, is very much a preoccupation of Florence's twenties, often described in her correspondence with family and friends. 'Are not our imaginations the real world we live in,' she asked Selma Benedicks, her Swedish friend, 'and what we are pleased to call "real life" only the shadows ...'; and to Parthenope she admitted that it was 'a queer feeling ... not to be quite certain of which is the true & which the imaginary'. Moonlight, in particular, exercised a peculiar fascination for her, seeming to lift the veil on an unseen existence that normally remained hidden from the senses, representing the divine world beyond this earthly one. A more personal outlet was served by the imagination as well. Reading the recently published *Life of Dr Arnold* by his former pupil Arthur Stanley, Florence expressed her disappointment that Arnold had been content with 'the plain prosaic <u>now</u>' instead 'of always planning what might be done in the dramatic positions of the fancy'. Plans made in her own dramatic positions of the fancy were to become increasingly important to her as she faced opposition to carrying them out in the real world. She would live 'a strange ideal life alongside the apparent one' through which she could play out 'her desires & intentions'.

For the present, though, that outward life consisted for much of the time in entertaining and being entertained in a fashionable world populated by 'pink satin ghosts'. When Aunt Hannah expressed her fears about the possible ill-effects of the 'attractions' of London, Florence wrote assuring her that, far from being a centre of dissipation, 'London is really my place of rest.' There at least she could have the mornings to herself. '[A] country house is the real place for dissipation – sometimes I think that everybody is hard upon me, that to be forever expected to be looking merry & saying something lively, is more than can be asked, mornings, noons, & nights, of anyone – then I remember everybody's patience with me, & am very much ashamed of myself.'

The remodelled Embley had been designed partly with the intention of enticing the great and the good. Much effort was expended on the organization of house parties, as surviving records, with their carefully prepared guest lists and letters accepting or declining invitations, show. Florence had sarcastically remarked on the new state bedrooms for 'the Duke and Duchess and the Contessine', though Fanny was unsuccessful in luring members of the aristocracy to Embley to fill them (a fact that would later lead Frederick Calvert to complain that the Nightingales' friends were of insufficient social standing when his brother Harry Verney married Parthenope). Fanny could only gaze in wonder at the procession of 'innumerable Howards, Cavendishes, Greys, Percys', decked out in their finery, that she encountered on a visit to Chatsworth in 1842. The Nightingales' guests, by contrast, tended to be political acquaintances like Charles Shaw-Lefevre of the House of Commons, and Baron Rolfe, the judge who presided over the trial of the Chartist Feargus O'Connor in 1843. The Sitwells of Renishaw Hall in Derbyshire (where Florence and Parthenope stayed on several occasions) were often at Embley, and over the years a sprinkling of European intelligentsia were also invited, including the German historian Leopold von Ranke, who accompanied Mary Clarke on one of her annual visits, Charles Darwin, the botanist Richard Hooker and, most exotically, Alexander von Middendorf, the Siberian traveller. Relationships with old Smith family friends, like 'Mighty Tom' Macaulay (whose conversation Florence remembered as 'a procession of one'), and Lady Byron, the estranged wife and widow of the poet, were kept up. Lady Byron's father Sir Ralph Milbanke had been a prominent abolitionist and she continued his philanthropic work, attending the British and Foreign Anti-Slavery Convention in 1840, and pioneering various schemes for the education of underprivileged girls. The next two generations of the family, Lady Byron's daughter, the mathematician Ada Lovelace, and, later, her granddaughter, Anne Noel, were both befriended by Florence and Parthenope and received Nightingale hospitality. Ada Lovelace expressed her fascination with Florence in a poem, in which she wrote prophetically of Florence's future fame, 'Should war's dread strife its victims claim'.

Florence's own circle included another link with her Smith grandfather, the politician Sir Robert Inglis, once on the fringes of the Clapham Sect, with whom she sometimes breakfasted in London. The Whig historian Henry Hallam, later to be on the 'gentleman's committee' of the Upper Harley Street institution where Florence served in her first professional appointment, was another friend from an older generation. Much closer in age was Louisa Stewart-Mackenzie, who returned to her family home in Scotland from Corfu, where her father had been Lord High Commissioner, at the beginning of the 1840s. She was a vibrant, effusive young woman, a favourite sitter for Parthenope to sketch and paint; so beautiful, with her brilliant eyes and strongly defined features, that she was called the 'Ludovisi goddess' after her resemblance to the head of Juno in Rome. Florence was attracted to Louisa's generous spirit and romantic impulsiveness, and their friendship continued, at a distance, after Louisa became the second Lady Ashburton in 1858. But Florence also remained wary of her. Her concern, in 1861, that Louisa should send back to her, by return of post, any of Florence's letters still in her possession, lest they fall into unwarranted hands, may suggest that there was something about their past intimacy that made Florence uncomfortable.

The connection with the Palmerstons at Broadlands was by now an established one, solid enough for the Nicholsons to ask William Nightingale to use his influence with Lord Palmerston to purchase a position in the cavalry for their son William. Lady Palmerston herself was a fervent believer in the power of social influence and her regular Saturday parties in London during the season, full of gossip and intrigue, had made her the leading political hostess of the time. Weekends at Broadlands were more restrained affairs, but no less important in cementing alliances and maintaining Palmerston's power base. 'I should get quite fond of him, if he were not Lord Palmerston,' Florence wrote after one party. On a subsequent occasion at Broadlands, she watched as Prince Albert was taught billiards. When he missed, 'which he did every time, they said oh that does not count, you play again'.

In the summer of 1842 an invitation arrived from the Palmerstons asking whether the Nightingales would 'dine with us & help us to entertain the poet Milnes'. At thirty-three, Richard Monckton Milnes was already the author of four volumes of verse and, though raised as a Unitarian, had written his latest book, *One Tract More*, as a sympathetic defence of the Tractarian movement within the Church of England. His political career was less conspicuous. He had been MP for Pontefract since 1837, but though a Tory follower of Peel's, had failed to win office. He had a marked aversion to strong party feeling – matched by an equally strong personal dislike of Peel himself – and in 1846 would switch his support to Lord John Russell's Liberal administration.

'A most bland-smiling, semi-quizzical, affectionate, high-bred, Italianized little man, who has long olive-blonde hair, a dimple, next to no chin, and flings his arm around your neck,' was how Carlyle had summed him up. Above all, Milnes was a man of the world, a mover and shaker, who brought the very breath of society with him (his London breakfast parties were famous). This may make Florence's positive response towards him seem at first surprising, but she quickly saw beyond the dilettante manner to the man of progressive reforming in- stincts. He might loll on the furniture and say a thousand idiotic things, giving him a reputation for being 'quite a character', as Tocqueville said; but he was also a supporter of factory education, mechanics' institutes, penny savings banks, voted for the abolition of capital punishment, and later worked for causes that were supportive of women's emancipation, like the repeal of the Contagious Diseases Acts. 'We all liked him and thought him unpretending,' Fanny wrote after Milnes dined and slept at Embley for the first of many visits. 'He wants, I suppose, more excitement than we gave him to make him as entertaining as he can be.'

In his twenties Milnes had travelled widely in Europe, spending a year in Rome, where, in the Palazzo Caffarelli on the Palatine Hill, he was befriended by Christian von Bunsen, Prussian emissary to the Vatican, his Welsh wife Frances, and their family of five sons and five daughters. In addition to his career as a diplomat, Chevalier Bunsen was a leading scholar of religion and comparative philology. When, in 1841, he was appointed ambassador to the Court of St James, his home at 4 Carlton Terrace became a meeting place for some of the most brilliant historical, political and theological minds of the age. Florence first met Bunsen the following year, perhaps as the result of an introduction from Milnes. According to his wife's later account, Bunsen was immediately struck by her 'calm dignity of deportment', which he regarded as 'self-conscious without either shyness or presumption', her few words 'indicating deep reflection, just views, and clear perceptions of life and its obligations . . .'

Bunsen's influence on Florence would be twofold. On an intellectual level, this Prussian with a didactic manner and 'a red face as large as the shield of Fingal' introduced her to the works of great German thinkers like Schopenhauer and Schleiermacher, and to the historical writings of his mentor, Barthold Niebuhr. Bunsen's own studies in comparative religion – of the Jewish, Christian, Islamic and Hindu scriptures as well as the writings of Plato and the Christian mystics – would guide Florence's thinking and eventually leave their mark on the heterodox elements in her *Suggestions for Thought*. Bunsen was identified with the Church of England group loosely known as the 'Broad Church' movement, who were responsible for introducing to Britain avant-garde biblical criticism from Germany in the tradition of David Friedrich Strauss, author of *Das Leben Jesu*. Florence read Strauss's mythological interpretation of the Gospels in its original German, and while she later remarked that the German theologian had seen nothing in Christ 'but a village apothecary who walked over the hill of Bethany and disappeared the other side', the idea that the Bible should be studied critically 'like any other book' remained a central component of her thought.

In the short term, the direction that Bunsen was able to give to Florence's search for a meaningful role in life, through his humanitarian efforts, proved even more significant. In Rome, Bunsen had founded a

Protestant infirmary where patients of that persuasion could receive care without Catholic proselytizing. Once installed in London he started organizing the establishment of a voluntary general hospital for the large German population of the city. Funds were raised and a site was found at the former Infant Orphan Asylum in Dalston, East London. The German Hospital opened in October 1845, and eight months later, in June 1846, Florence paid a visit there, almost certainly the first time that she had inspected a hospital at close quarters. The Protestant Deaconesses responsible for the nursing care had been recruited from the Kaiserswerth Institute near Düsseldorf. This experiment for training nurses was part of a broader scheme devised in 1833 by Pastor Theodore Fliedner, encompassing a penitentiary and an orphanage, as well as a large hospital.

'What can an individual do towards lifting the load of suffering from the helpless and miserable?' Florence was reported as having asked Chevalier Bunsen one evening at Carlton Terrace. In October 1846, Bunsen would send Florence the yearbook of the Kaiserswerth Institute, setting her on the path that would lead eventually to her period of training there. But by the summer of 1844 she had already reached the conclusion that the answer to her question lay in nursing. In August that year the visit to Embley of an American couple, Samuel Gridley Howe and his wife Julia Ward Howe, on an extended honeymoon tour of Europe, appears to have crystallized her decision. The success of Howe's work in Massachusetts in teaching blind deaf-mutes had made him well known in Britain, and Florence had read the annual reports of the Perkins Institution and State School for the Blind, of which Howe was director.

According to the subsequent accounts of the Howe family, differing in detail but not in salient outline, Florence requested a meeting with Howe in the library, where she asked him: 'Dr Howe, do you think it would be unsuitable and unbecoming for a young Englishwoman to devote herself to works of charity in hospitals and elsewhere as Catholic sisters do? Do you think it would be a dreadful thing?'

Howe's reply acknowledged the difficulties involved in such a choice:

My dear Miss Florence, it would be unusual, and in England whatever is unusual is apt to be thought unsuitable; but I say to you, go forward if you have a vocation for that way of life; act up to your inspiration, and you will find that there is never anything unbecoming or unladylike in doing your duty for the good of others. Choose, go on with it wherever it may lead you, and God be with you.

This was clearly a pivotal moment in Florence Nightingale's life and has been portrayed as such in many biographies. However, there is another, less familiar, story connected with the episode, which highlights the singularity of Florence's ambition and of her eventual achievement. Samuel Howe was obviously highly impressed by Florence, a fact that was publicly confirmed in 1845 when the Howes' first child, a daughter, was named in her honour and became her first godchild. Yet Howe's admiration of the young Englishwoman, and his encouragement of her aspirations, was for many years a 'festering' issue with his wife (who was almost two decades her husband's junior). Julia Ward Howe would in time become highly distinguished in her own right, as a prominent member of the Abolitionist movement in the United States, a worker for women's rights, and as a writer – most famously as the author of 'The Battle Hymn of the Republic'; but, as she later revealed, during the first twenty years of her marriage her husband never approved of any act of hers which she herself valued. When, a long time afterwards, she rebuked Samuel Howe for having encouraged Florence Nightingale, a woman of similar age to herself, to pursue a career, when he wouldn't even allow his wife to publish a book of poems, he responded by saying that 'if he had been engaged to Florence Nightingale, and had loved her ever so dearly, he would have given her up as soon as she commenced her career as a public woman'.

In 1857 Julia Ward Howe's resentment at her treatment spilled over into a triptych of poems, written to celebrate Florence Nightingale's return to England as a national heroine from the Crimean War, and published in a collection called *Words for the Hour*. Her tribute to the woman of the hour is genuine enough, but underlying the praise there is biting recognition of the fact that men like her husband, who applaud Nightingale's selflessness, fail to recognize comparable qualities in the women in their own lives. Her anger at the praise directed exclusively at one member of her sex becomes apparent in the second poem, 'Florence Nightingale and Her Praisers':

> If you debase the sex to elevate
> One of like soul and temper with the rest,
> You do but wrong a thousand fervent hearts,
> To pay full tribute to one generous breast.

This ambivalence towards a woman who had rejected her 'proper sphere' in pursuit of her own genius was one that was to reverberate in Florence's relationships with both men and women, for the rest of her life.

For the time being Florence dug after her plan in silence, and waited for an opportunity to put it into practice. Soon, though, she would be entering a period of disappointment, frustration and, at times, of deep, morbid despair; one in which she imagined herself, long before anyone else did, as a traveller in a dark night, carrying a lantern, which shed just enough light for her to find a path along which to walk.

4. This Loathsome Life

Meanwhile, that autumn of 1844, she led what she conceived of as 'a regular life', taking part in the installation of Mr Empson, the new vicar at East Wellow, whose sermons she found 'decidedly instructive'. His wife was 'very cordial & ladylike', and Florence admired the way in which the vicarage garden was being transformed into something attractive. She continued to teach, spending 'many an algebraical hour' with William Nicholson in preparation for his Sandhurst exams, and discussing the problem of virtue with her class of girls at Wellow School in an effort to combat bad habits of attendance and punctuality. There was resignation, with the barest hint of reproach, in a letter to her father describing the monotony of her existence. She had given up riding, '& all sports of the field, even my gun, & have subsided into "an excellent plain cook and housekeeper"'. Most evenings, after dining early, she, her mother and Parthenope took it in turns to read to each other, covering fifty pages of the latest novel. They were progressing steadily through Disraeli's *Coningsby*, though she judged it 'more fitful than inspired'.

As so often for Florence, mundane everyday concerns were suddenly placed in a new perspective by a glimpse of something unearthly beyond them. Taking the sacrament with Mrs Hogg, wife of the Embley steward, who was close to death, she was overcome with a strong sense 'that the most real thing in the room was Him & that <u>we</u> were only ghosts, shaped into a body, into apparitions, for a few moments . . .'

She was ill once again at New Year. This time, perhaps, she welcomed the opportunity to be alone while the others joined the usual celebrations at Waverley, including a fancy dress ball at which Parthenope dressed as Lady Jane Grey and Marianne as Mary, Queen of Scots. In February, as she regained her strength, her cousin Shore arrived at Embley to convalesce from measles. Her 'dear lad' Shore was now fourteen, a pupil at a private school in Brighton, where his interest in engineering and mechanics had been developed at the expense of any more philosophical or meditative elements in his character. Florence's love for him was both maternal and that of an older sister, and it was almost as if their bond of double cousinhood contributed to the special intensity of their mutual feelings for each other. She could melt away his reserve like no one else, but was often made anxious by the thought of her responsibility for him. '. . . When I look at his pale thin face,' she told Parthenope, 'I feel a little foreboding at my heart, but when I hear his cheerful voice and spirit full of interests, I think that a spirit once born into the world can never be lost to us.' Aunt Mai, distressed by the discovery that her youngest daughter, Beatrice, was lame, and concerned that Shore was falling behind in his studies, had given her 'carte blanche' for the education of her 'little man', with the proviso 'to let no stitch drop of his classics'. There was much illness in the village, and Florence had been impressed at the amount of interest Shore had taken when they visited some of her patients. But she was worried about his lack of 'deliberate' religious feelings. 'Oh how is he to make the acquaintance with God which is so necessary?' she asked.

While Florence considered it important that she continue to exercise a power for good over her cousin – she enjoyed being a source of improvement in others – she feared the inevitable decay of that influence, as Shore grew older. His love for her played its natural part in that influence, yet she was wary of demonstrations of 'hot-house' affection from him. She preferred moderate to 'exclusive affections', and thought it 'terrible . . . how little a violent feeling does good . . .' Her ideal, and personal prescription for happiness, she had concluded, was to be 'pure & devoted enough to love without the need of being loved . . .' When Shore put out his arms to protect her from 'any imaginary evil' as she was reading him a frightening passage, in the original German, from Friedrich La Motte Fouqué's novel *Undine*, she shrank back, remaining 'as stern as a post' while looking 'attentively' for a word in the dictionary.

Old Mrs Shore had a slight stroke that summer, and to save Aunt Mai 'all anxious ideas of hurrying down' to Tapton, Florence spent several weeks nursing her grandmother. Although William Nightingale arrived with her, he soon returned to Lea Hurst, leaving Florence to contemplate the wild moorland solitude and isolation of a place where letters were sent for only once a week and newspapers seldom seen, so that all news there felt as if it was a quarter of a century out of date.

There was little more to do than sit holding her grandmother's hand, telling her stories about her grandchildren, relishing the silence 'which levels all earthly troubles'.

Mary Shore's circumstances were sadly reduced. In February 1843, the family bank at Sheffield had failed with debts of almost £14,000, leaving Mrs Shore the chief creditor. She had been forced to let some of her menservants go and had given up her carriage. Yet the old lady remained resilient. To Florence, her grandmother was 'a giant among pygmies', simple, straightforward, often ridiculous, but 'never small, base, thinking of opinion', and always full of affection. This admiration was reciprocated. Mr Nightingale reported that his mother 'idolatrized' Florence and often referred to her as 'wondrous Flo'. Perhaps she recognized something of herself in her granddaughter's energy and strength of purpose. According to Aunt Mai, Grandmother Shore might have accomplished great things had she not suffered from the want of 'early good training'.

Scarcely had Florence returned to Lea Hurst than Gale was taken ill. Now in her late fifties, Gale had been suffering from complications arising from dropsy for some time, though in the past she had always rallied. This attack was more serious, but the minute it was proposed that Gale remain in Derbyshire, she insisted on accompanying the family to Embley. Florence sat at her bedside, wiping away her perspiration, only to find her 'doing' about the house, a few hours later. The end came on 28 October. 'She died a hero as she had lived, upright in her chair, her last words being, "Don't call the cook: Hannah, go to your work."'

Sitting in the housekeeper's room, watching the 'beautiful' expression on the dead woman's face, Florence was appalled by the 'Mrs Gamp scene' that followed. Sarah Gamp had appeared as a comically drawn character in Charles Dickens's *Martin Chuzzlewit*, published in book form the year before, swiftly establishing herself as the popular stereotype of a negligent, incompetent, gin-swigging domiciliary nurse. Real-life Mrs Gamps attended on all kinds of sickness, as well as serving as uncertified midwives and layers-out of the dead. The sight of Gale being laid out was so horrifying that Florence could only conclude that 'One should never leave one's friends to nurses at those moments.' It was strange, she told Hilary, 'coming out of the room where there is only her and God and me, to come back into the cold and false life of prejudices and hypocrisy and conventionalisms; by which I do not mean to find fault with life but only with the use I make of it.'

With Gale gone, her days were suddenly occupied with household chores, and she found herself responsible for making curtains and row upon row of jars of preserves. A visit to Embley at the end of November by Dr Richard Fowler, physician to the Salisbury Infirmary, and his wife Anne, allowed her to turn her mind to higher things. Dr Fowler, a robust eighty-year-old who walked three miles a day, and insisted on equivalent amounts of mental exercise, was planning to devote the remainder of his life to writing a refutation of Berkeley on *Human Knowledge*. His sight was failing and he welcomed the opportunity to have Florence read aloud to him. She, for her part, found it a relief to be treated as 'a sensible & agreeable woman' for a change by a man who seemed 'to condense in a sentence the secrets of life'. Mrs Fowler, too, was an inspiring companion, full of reforming ideas for schools and education.

Florence took advantage of the Fowlers' visit to propose an idea of her own. The experience, several months earlier, of watching a woman near the Hurst die before her eyes through the ignorance of her nurses – 'as much as if they had given her arsenic' – had convinced her that she must have proper training in nursing. Her plan was twofold. She would spend three months at the Salisbury Infirmary, just thirteen miles from Embley, picking up what skills she could. In the longer term – if she outlived her 'immediate ties' – she might take a small house, in West Wellow perhaps, and establish there a kind of Protestant Sisterhood, 'without vows, for women of educated feelings'. The first step was simple enough and could be achieved with the minimum of fuss, but its end result would provide her with a little bit of heaven on earth.

Years later, Mary Clarke was to describe the powerful predominance in Florence's life of her imagination, with its images lined up in a row in her mind, like fine china. The slightest crack to that delicate china, however – to all those carefully assembled mental pictures – could produce an intensity of feeling which Clarkey believed verged on madness. The effect on Florence of seeing her carefully nurtured plans to train in nursing practice rejected, and even derided, was little short of devastating. Fanny Nightingale, as might have been expected, immediately questioned the propriety of her daughter mixing with surgeons and nurses. More surprisingly, Mrs Fowler threw cold water on the idea, and there was no support for it from Dr Fowler either. Even William Nightingale dismissed it out of hand as 'vanity and selfishness'. To her cousin Hilary, Florence confided the vanquishing of her precious hopes, writing that she saw no advantage 'of my living on, excepting that one becomes less and less of a young lady every year, which is only a negative one'.

In the series of private notes that were increasingly to become an outlet for the sense of dejection she could rarely express in public, she recorded a wish to die. 'Forgive me, O God, and let me die, this day let me die. It is not for myself that I say this . . . I know that by living I shall only heap anxieties on other hearts, which will but increase with time.'

On 1 December, she wrote of the suffering of her 'poor mind' and of the only remedy prescribed for it, that of 'concealment or self-command'. Four days later, she laid her nursing plans to rest, but with a renewed sense of the purpose of her life:

As for me, all my hopes for this winter are gone and all my plans destroyed. My poor little hope requiescat in pace. No one can know its value to me; no one can tell how dear a child, however infantile, is to its mother, nor how precious an idea, though it was an unformed one, but between the destruction of one idea and the taking up of another I can understand now how a soul can die . . .

God has something for me to do for Him or He would have let me die some time ago. I hope to do it by living, then my eyes would indeed have seen His salvation, but now I am dust and nothing, worse than nothing, a curse to myself and to others.

This morning I felt as if my soul would pass away in tears, but I live in utter loneliness, in a bitter passion of tears and agony of solitude. But I live, and God grant that I may live to do this. Oh if our Saviour walked the earth, how should I not go to him, and would he send me back to live the life again which crushes me into vanity and deceit? Or would he not say, Do this. Oh, for some great thing to sweep this loathsome life into the past.

Writing, three weeks later, to the Howes, now back in Boston, Florence attempted to put a brave face on her situation. She revealed the failure of her plans, referred again to Protestant Sisterhoods, and joked about proposing a Society 'for ameliorating the condition of young ladies of fortune and education', with herself as Secretary at a salary of five hundred pounds a year. It only increased her misery to feel that, with all her advantages, it was 'a very wicked thing' not to be happy. Yet she found it impossible to resign herself to a life of wasted energies and of frivolous activity without an end.

It must have quickly occurred to her just how 'unformed' her notion of training at the Salisbury Infirmary was. The Infirmary was an eighteenth-century foundation, almost as old as Dr Fowler himself, but in 1845 a new wing had been opened after it was discovered that parts of the hospital were infested with rats. With its redesigned female and accident wards, Salisbury Infirmary had much of which to be proud. One insuperable problem, however, remained, repeated in hospitals throughout Britain at this time: the lack of trained nurses. A decade later, the Infirmary's annual report was still echoing this common complaint, awaiting the widespread introduction of training institutions for nursing, and commenting that the difficulty of securing good nurses was compounded by the practice of requiring nursing staff 'to perform menial duties, which deters a higher class of nurses from becoming applicants'.

Florence's plan fell down on two counts. It wasn't simply the highly unrealistic idea that a woman of her background could ever be comfortably assimilated into the working practices of the Salisbury nurses, all of whom would have been from the lower or lower-middle classes, it was also clear that the Infirmary could have provided her with little or no training at all. There was an obvious need, she had told Samuel and Julia Howe, for 'some sort of establishment, which shall enable young women to do, what they cannot do now . . .' But where was such a place be found? It would take a number of significant developments throughout the 1840s to begin to provide an answer to this question.

———

Some of these developments would be the result of changes in the hospital itself. At the beginning of the nineteenth century, hospitals did not play a central role in health care. The rich continued to be nursed at home until the twentieth century, while the poor tended to be looked after within the family, or by such independent care as they could afford, avoiding where possible the workhouse infirmary or sick ward. The voluntary hospitals were charitable institutions for the so-called 'deserving poor': patients were admitted for treatment free of charge, but only if they carried letters of recommendation from hospital subscribers. Fever cases were excluded, and hospitals did not treat serious conditions like tuberculosis, cancer or smallpox, nor did they deliver babies.

The industrialization of Britain in the course of the century produced a major expansion in the institutional care of the sick. The combination of a population explosion, mass movement away from rural communities into towns, leading to overcrowding with disease following in its wake, together with the consequent breakdown of the ability of working-class families to care for themselves as work and family became increasingly separate, all contributed to a marked rise in the number of hospitals.*

Furthermore, by mid-century, hospital practice was itself changing as procedures connected to the new clinical medicine took root. Following the introduction of anaesthesia in 1846, surgeons began to operate more frequently, as well as to perform many new types of operations. In the same period, the old depletion therapies, like purgatives, emetics and bleeding, were being replaced by therapeutic regimes which emphasized the importance of diet, cleanliness and fresh air. Both changes, requiring round-the-clock, regular attendance, and skills of general management, increased demand for the introduction of trained nursing systems into hospitals.

The character of Dickens's Sarah Gamp, colourfully depicting the old unreformed nurse, was to provide useful propaganda for all those doctors, religious leaders, and women anxious to create new professional opportunities for their sex, who sought to replace the old independent practitioner with a new model nurse. Mrs Gamp may have been broad caricature, a byword for lax immorality and insobriety, but her instantaneous popularity underlines the fact that she embodied certain truths about the kind of hired nurse employed by both rich and poor.† Most obviously, she was representative of a world in which nursing still largely took place in the domestic sphere, and where the status of the nurse herself was closest to that of a domestic servant. True, in *Martin Chuzzlewit* Dickens gives us Mrs Gamp's hospital counterpart, Betsy Prig, a nurse from St Bartholomew's, but details from the 1841 Census

---

* By the middle of the nineteenth century, London had twelve teaching hospitals. Two of these, St Bartholomew's and St Thomas's, were medieval foundations. Westminster, St George's, Guy's, the London and Middlesex Hospitals were founded between 1719 and 1745, and the Royal Free, University College, Charing Cross, King's College and St Mary's Hospitals between 1828 and 1849.

† Although Dickens asserted that Sarah Gamp was 'a fair representation of the hired attendant on the poor in sickness', the same class of women ministered to both rich and poor. Dickens based the character on the nurse treating Hannah Meredith, the governess in the household of his millionairess friend Angela Burdett-Coutts.

– the first to distinguish sick-nurses from domestic servants – confirm
that in order to make a living most nurses would have had to move
constantly between domiciliary and institutional work. For of the 4,687
London nurses recorded in the census, only about 600 could have found
full-time employment in the general and specialist hospitals that existed
in the city at the time. These Mrs Gamps prided themselves on their
independence ('I goes out workin' for my bread, 'tis true, but I maintain
my indpency,' as Dickens's creation says), and in an era in which the
primacy of nursing in treating cases of fever or cholera was acknowledged by some members of the medical profession, competition for
patients between doctors and nurses was likely to have been common
(though some nurses, like Mrs Horsfall in Charlotte Brontë's *Shirley*,
published at the end of the decade, undoubtedly worked closely with
individual doctors and relied on being recommended to their patients).

By contrast, those women fortunate to be given permanent employment in the pre-reform hospitals could hope to acquire some expertise
from the physicians and surgeons. Essentially, though, neither the
matron, nor the three teams of women serving under her – the sisters,
day nurses, and night watchers – were required to possess any previous
training or experience before starting work in a hospital. The matron
fulfilled the role of housekeeper, responsible for hiring the female staff
and keeping the hospital inventory, while it was the sisters, or head
nurses, often widows of servants and tradesmen, who were most directly
responsible for patient care. Beneath them were the day nurses.
Described by Joseph Bell, a distinguished surgeon who had begun practising at the Edinburgh Infirmary in the 1840s, as servants or widows
who were unable to make good in domestic service and were therefore
forced to accept work in hospitals, these women were indistinguishable
from housemaids. In keeping with this, Flint South, later senior surgeon
at St Thomas's, referred to the day nurse as a 'ward maid', and charring,
including cleaning and bedmaking, made up the largest part of her
routine. Finally, the lowliest member of this hierarchy was the night
nurse. Typically, she was a poor old charwoman who, after a hard day's
work, received her supper and a shilling to sit by the fire and keep a
watch on patients during the long night hours between eleven and seven
in the morning.

Mrs Gamp's excessive drinking reflected a problem with nursing staff
that was widespread and of long standing. In 1854, a head nurse from

Westminster Hospital told Florence that 'she had never known a nurse who was not drunken, and that there was immoral conduct practised within the very walls of the ward'. This was manifestly an exaggeration, yet tales of drunkenness and sexual impropriety, especially among the night staff, abounded. Florence herself liked later to recount the story of how it was the recognized duty of the senior surgeon at the Edinburgh Infirmary to have the drunken nurses carried in on stretchers every night, while complaints of night nurses being caught in bed with patients were not uncommon. That addiction to alcohol was endemic among the class of women from whom nurses were largely recruited was inescapably true, as Florence was to discover during the Crimean War, and later, among probationers at the Nightingale Training School at St Thomas's, where insobriety provided a reason for swift dismissal. Moreover, the nursing world did little to discourage drinking; on the contrary, it formed part of its culture. Nurses might be tipped by patients – or on occasion, bribed – with threepence for 'a drop o' gin'. They could expect the standard allocation of beer or porter to drink (nurses at one London teaching hospital had to raise a petition for milk as an alternative). As late as the 1870s, when reforms were beginning to take root, two teetotal nurses, training at Westminster Hospital, were told that they would never be able to 'stick it' without the support of alcohol.

Yet nursing in the first half of the nineteenth century was not all scandal and abuses, as the theologian F. D. Maurice, chaplain at Guy's Hospital from 1836 to 1846, set out to show in a balanced assessment of the traditional hospital nurse:

She may often be drunken (I mean especially the night-nurse), sometimes, but I believe rarely, without feeling for the patients . . . But the temptations to these evils among persons brought up as they are, are . . . enormous; and I suspect you will have quite as often occasion to wonder at their tenderness and skill, and to ask how such gifts have come to them, as to lament over their deficiencies and offences . . . These women have never had a fair chance . . . The atmosphere of a hospital is less favourable to them than to any persons connected with it.

Nevertheless, these nurses remained no more than 'a good system of servants'. In the search for women of better character and education, who would look upon nursing as a Christian vocation rather than a form of casual labour entered out of financial necessity, the influence and example of the charitable nursing sisterhoods was to prove paramount. As Florence observed, if the age of zeal was past, 'may not the age of charity be at hand?'

It was indeed. The Anglican sisterhoods that began to appear in the 1840s, mobilizing pious women in the spiritual and philanthropic reclamation of the sick poor, made a vital contribution to the ideal of the new nurse. For the High Church members of the Oxford Movement, the foundation of orders of women devoted to good works formed part of a broader attempt to promote spiritual regeneration through the revival of traditional forms of worship. In 1845, the first of these sisterhoods, the Park Village community, was established near Regent's Park. A few years later, Priscilla Lydia Sellon established a second group, the Sisters of Mercy, in Devonport. Both orders imitated Roman Catholic communities, with some sisters privately taking vows of poverty, chastity and obedience. Consequently High Church sisterhoods tended to be regarded with suspicion, and even hostility, as Papist sympathizers – a suspicion confirmed by the frequency with which their members defected to Catholicism.

Other Anglican sisterhoods, of a nonconformist or evangelical outlook, took their inspiration from a quite different model, that of the Protestant deaconesses at Kaiserswerth in Germany. One of these was Elizabeth Fry's Institution of Nursing Sisters, founded in 1840, following a visit by Mrs Fry to Theodore Fliedner's growing establishment on the Rhine. Fry's contribution as a nursing pioneer, and as the provider of the first sustained nursing service to the poor, has often been overshadowed by her work for penal reform, though she had long been interested in extending her principles of care to the internal management of hospitals and infirmaries. But the idea for her training institution only bore fruit after she inspected the Kaiserswerth deaconesses at work in their school, orphanage and hospital, where they were also taught to nurse the poor in their own homes. Witnessing at first hand Elizabeth Fry's efforts among the female prisoners at Newgate, on visits to London in 1824 and 1833, had inspired Fliedner himself. Now it was Fry's turn to be impressed. The Fry Sisters, as they were known, came from the same class of society as the Sarah Gamps and Betsy Prigs, but they were carefully selected for literacy, wore a uniform, and underwent a three-month period of training at various London teaching hospitals, though inevitably the quality of the tuition afforded by this arrangement varied enormously. The Institution's provision of free care for the poor was subsidized by commercial nursing of wealthy clients, and by a limited amount of hospital work.

The idea of a meeting between Elizabeth Fry and Florence Nightingale proved irresistible to some of their early biographers. 'The first grasping of hands of these two pioneer women would serve as subject for a painter', was how Sarah Tooley imagined it in 1904. Yet there is no evidence to suggest that they either met or corresponded. A number of tantalizing personal and professional details, however, do link them. Fry was a member of the wealthy Norwich Quaker family the Gurneys, who were well known to their MP, William Smith, and to his children. Baron Bunsen, soon to direct Florence's attention to the Deaconess Institution at Kaiserswerth as a way towards fulfilling her vocation, was both a close associate of Fry's and a family connection (his son Ernest married Fry's niece). At the Institution itself, Florence's friend Sir Robert Inglis served as a trustee, while his wife Mary became its President. Anne Fowler, too, Dr Fowler's wife, would serve on the Institution's committee in the 1850s. Most intriguing of all is Aunt Patty's relationship with Elizabeth Fry, stretching back to the early 1820s when Patty Smith made her weekly 'trudge to & from Newgate' to accompany Fry. Patty's letters in old age to her sister Fanny Nightingale sometimes reminisce fondly about Mrs Fry, blessing 'her great kindness'.

Worn out by her demanding work, and weakened by tuberculosis, Elizabeth Fry died after a stroke in October 1845, little more than a month before Florence's hopes of training at the Salisbury Infirmary were dashed by her parents. As Florence considered her future, Fry's nursing initiatives are likely to have been on her mind. She would later claim Fry as one of her spiritual mothers, and in 1853 intended to employ Fry Sisters in her own scheme for a Protestant nursing sisterhood that never got beyond the planning stage. But in two important respects Fry's Institution did not meet Florence Nightingale's requirements. First, the Fry Sisters were clearly not the women of educated feelings that she aspired to join; and secondly, and more crucially, the underlying religious justification of Fry's nursing sisterhood – to devote its time to the glory of God *and* to the mitigation of human suffering, as it described itself – was not an objective that Florence could share. For while the Institution remained non-sectarian and without vows, it nevertheless continued to see care of the sick as part of a process of saving souls.

By contrast, St John's House, another Anglican sisterhood modelled

on Kaiserswerth, maintained more of a balance between its Christian
principles and a practical desire to introduce better nursing for hospitals
and the community at large. Founded in 1848 at the instigation of
Robert Bentley Todd, Professor of Physiology and Anatomy at King's
College, London, St John's House quickly established a programme of
two years or more intensive training for each sister in nursing and
hospital management, including lectures given by physicians. If it had
existed earlier in the decade, it might have suited Florence rather well:
based on a Broad Church conception, there were no vows, the sisters
could be married or single, were permitted to live at home, and could
work full- or part-time (later Florence was to draw many of the ideas
for the Nightingale School at St Thomas's from St John's House, and
the advice of its superintendent Mary Jones). As the first sisterhood to
insist on systematic hospital training, St John's House represented an
important break with the past.

For Florence, all roads seemed to lead to the Institution of Deaconesses
at Kaiserswerth. By the autumn of 1846, when she received one of
Fliedner's annual reports, it had become the focus of her efforts to train
as a nurse. She was always to remain wary, though, of sisterhoods, and
of hospitals where nursing was carried out under the cover of religious
influence. Religion was a high motivation for the calling, but it could
not be the highest. 'Practically', she considered there to be 'but little
difference between the religious scruple of the "sister" who neglects her
patients for her rule and the irreligious scruple of the nurse who neglects
her patients for her drink'. Time and experience would only confirm her
in this conviction.

———

Given the popular image of the nurse, the reaction of the Nightingales
to Florence's proposal was hardly surprising. It was unthinkable that an
educated gentlewoman should enrol herself in an occupation so closely
related to domestic service. Moreover, all notion of leaving home, outside the circumstances of marriage, and where a woman wasn't called
upon to earn her own living, subverted the prevailing ideal of family
loyalty. This basic tenet of middle-class life was all the stronger for being
largely unspoken. If Florence failed to become another man's wife, she
could expect to remain tied to the family's apron-strings in her role as a
daughter.

The Nightingales' attitude, then, was far from unique. Over the next few decades, their disapproval of their daughter's ambition would be reflected in the experience of scores of parents as Florence blazed a trail for other young women, eager to break free from domestic responsibilities to pursue a career in nursing. Few took as extreme a stance as Lucy Osburn's father, who displayed his vehement objection to his daughter entering the Nightingale Training School in 1866 by turning her portrait to the wall. Nevertheless, in the future William Nightingale would often find himself called upon to advise anxious parents professing themselves 'utterly ignorant' about whether they should consent to their daughters' desire to nurse. Similarly, from the other side of the fence, Florence would respond to many an anguished young lady wanting to nurse in the face of refusals from 'Mama and Papa'.

For the Nightingales, however, an additional consideration, aside from matters of caste, would consistently weigh heavily in their rejection of Florence's plans. It was their daughter's physical fragility and history of bad health that convinced them ultimately of the necessity of keeping her as close to home as possible. In due course, when Florence became an invalid after the Crimean War, they felt vindicated in the belief that they had been right all along. By that time, Florence's condition offered a cautionary tale to parents with daughters hoping to imitate her example, as well as telling confirmation to contemporary theorists of womanhood who argued that women were biologically unsuited to arduous work and, consequently, best suited to subordination in a domestic role.

On 18 January 1846, Florence made one further attempt at wearing down her father's resistance. She did so in the form of a letter, as she confessed to being unable to speak on the subject 'with composure or common self-command', and could not bear to have 'her poor little hope talked <u>at</u>' any longer. It was no use, she said, expecting anything constructive from her mother. Fanny treated her as a spoilt child, only to be distracted or amused. The world could only sympathize with three types of sorrow: loss of friends, of fortune, or of health, and all other suffering was regarded as imaginary. But Florence asked William Nightingale to consider that 'when the secrets of all hearts shall be told, when shall be known all that may be borne & never told by hundreds, with whom we have been living cheek by jowl all our lives, that the <u>remorse</u>, the <u>anxiety</u>, the <u>irritation</u>, the <u>shame</u>, & the <u>doubts</u> of life will be found to make up the real misery of it, & all else will rise up a mere hair's weight in the other balance'.

She wrote accusingly of having revealed the secrets of her own inner world to her family, only to have them scorned and treated with a lack of seriousness. 'I can never remember the time when my life was in the beautiful realities about me, when I did not live in a world of my own peopled with visions, & invisible spirits, & as I was reckoned a remarkably matter-of-fact child, nobody ever took the pains to make me talk of them.' Now, she could only repent of having finally broken 'the bounds of self-command' to speak out.

While she asked forgiveness of those she had pained, her closing lines, with their implied force of an ultimatum, proposed a variation on her original plan. '. . . Do you believe it impossible,' she asked her father, 'ever to consent that I should go for a few months to the Sisters who administer the Hospital of St Stephen's at Dublin, where there would not be the same objections as in an English Hospital . . . If you do believe it impossible to approve, I had rather know it at once, & then, let us never speak on this subject again.'

Evidently, the answer remained no, even with the promise of religious chaperonage, and Florence therefore retreated into silence. From now on, her family would receive, only where necessary, the barest minimum of information about her intentions. Her relationship with them would become, as she described it in one analogy, like that of the Moon and the Earth. The Moon revolves round the Earth, 'moves with her, never leaves her. Yet the Earth never sees but one side of her; the other side remains for ever unknown.'

So, privately, she continued her inquiries about health systems and hospitals, rising early to read her blue books, studying reports sent by Bunsen of conditions in Berlin, and of those in Paris from Julius Mohl, endlessly tabulating information from them. To ensure that she never overslept, she kept a watch on the floor by the entrance to her room, springing out of bed every morning before her maid entered to avoid the risk of having it smashed. At breakfast, she transferred for the rest of the day to the duties of daughter at home. The absence of a housekeeper at Embley that spring meant that Florence found herself 'up to my chin' in linen and glass, patiently checking lists, cataloguing damage and ordering replacements. 'Can reasonable people want all this?' she asked Mary Clarke. 'Is all that China, linen, glass necessary to make a Progressive animal? . . . And the best Versailles service says, And a proper stupid answer you'll get so go & do your accounts – there's one of us cracked.'

In the evening, after dinner – 'the great sacred ceremony of the day' – she was expected to sit with her family in the drawing room until ten, though her tendency to withdraw into herself was a regular source of irritation to her mother and sister. Florence could be a brilliant and witty conversationalist one moment, fulfilling her 'quota of amusement', like 'a play of the most beautiful fireworks', according to Parthenope. But then the lights would go out suddenly '& there was no further admittance'. Fanny complained, 'She is silent when she should talk.' Her father, too, observed that in his younger daughter's mind 'neither science nor wisdom makes progress . . . by interplay or war of words'. He was increasingly in awe of Florence. 'Flo astonishes me more & more,' he had written two years earlier, '– she is not like other folk of a truth, & I shall be her humble servant in many matters.' However, while acknowledging her superiority, he remained conspicuously aloof from confronting the problem of how she was ever to be permitted to find an occupation that would satisfy her talents.

In notebook after notebook, as the self-control she forced herself to maintain in public broke down behind closed doors, Florence gave vent to the misery and pointlessness of her existence. 'Oh if one has but a toothache, what remedies are invented! What carriages, horses, ponies, journeys, doctors, chaperones, are urged upon one; but if it is something the matter with the <u>mind</u> . . . it is neither believed nor understood.' No one reading these outpourings could doubt the acute distress she sometimes felt at having rejected her call; but nor, at others, is it possible to ignore her capacity for rising above this suffering, stifling any thought of resignation to her lot, and proclaiming her intention to 'overcome'.

Her pen offered one outlet, her dreams another, potentially more ambiguous, sense of release. Day-dreams could fleetingly dispel frustrated longings through heroic visions of action, but in the longer term they might simply become another form of enslavement. 'Dreaming always . . . never accomplishing', as Florence wrote, chastising herself and other women in her situation, who were 'too much ashamed of their dreams, which they think "romantic" to tell them where they will be laughed at, even if not considered wrong'.

Florence Nightingale's dreams have often been written about as if they were symptomatic of a condition peculiar to her alone. Yet, from the advice books and conduct manuals addressed by mid-century moralists like Mrs Ellis to the 'daughters of England' – counselling against 'the multiplicity of . . . floating ideas' and 'the play of . . . fancy', which encourage 'a constant pining for excitement, and an eagerness to escape from everything like practical and individual duty' – it's clear that dreaming was recognized as a widespread phenomenon among middle-class women. Restlessness and agitation were the new watchwords among female members of the bourgeois family, who possessed ample leisure to indulge in reveries of heroism and adventure; and in the decade's most infamous fictional heroine, Charlotte Brontë's Jane Eyre, they discovered a young woman who shared their own dangerous predi-lection for romantic illusions, and saw themselves reflected in Jane's fiery cry that women 'must have action . . . and they will make it if they cannot find it'. To Florence, who read the novel soon after its publication in 1847, Jane Eyre seemed like a real person: '. . . we know her – we have lived with her, we shall meet her again.'

A generation later, the young Beatrice Webb, searching for a purpose in life, recorded her own 'dreams of attainment', an indulgence she considered perfectly acceptable so long as it wasn't accompanied by neglect of family duties. But some of Webb's other remarks hint at the more deleterious effects that dreaming might have on an individual's state of mind: guilt at concealment of one's true motives from the people with whom one lives; a growing sense of unreality as one is separated from the outside world; and a sudden loss of energy in the transitions from the imaginary to reality, and back again, a sensation strongly reminiscent of the comparison Florence once made to feelings of intoxi-cation whenever her day-dreams had their tightest hold over her.

Back at Lea Hurst for the summer, Florence welcomed the arrival of Shore for another stay. In his company she felt released from the strain of perpetually having to keep up a front, though she continued to experience forebodings about his future, and doubts about her own ability to ensure that he didn't turn out a nonentity, well aware that the career of a young man who would one day inherit a large fortune was likely to be filled with pitfalls. Shore was nearly seventeen, and it was with some relief, as she told Hilary, that she laid 'aside the reins' with him. '. . . I drove him sometimes too hard, always fearing that I did not drive hard enough. But now he is old enough not to be driven any more, but to drive me.' In 1848, Shore started at the Edinburgh Academy, where he confounded Florence's worries about his academic prowess by being placed as the second best mathematician of his year; from there, a couple of years later, he entered Trinity College, Cambridge, like his father and uncle before him.

Absolving herself of responsibility for Shore formed part of Florence's deliberate attempt at detachment from personal relationships. Earthly friendships, she informed Hilary at this time, were too often like Atlanta's apple in Greek mythology: a hindrance on the path to true righteousness. 'And so, dearest, it is well that <u>we</u> should not eat too much of one another.' Writing to her Swedish friend, now widowed and remarried as Selma Björkenstam, she was more explicit about her objective of rooting out all personal feeling. 'My happiness no longer entirely depends on the tone or manner of the people about me,' she confessed in the autumn of 1846. 'I have no personal feeling left and with me walks my God, and these are the elements of my peace.' In light of remarks like these, it can be no wonder that Hilary later saw Florence as resembling the eponymous heroine of George Sand's novel *Lélia*. Lélia is full of mystical longings; she questions what she sees as the artificially defined role of women; but although she possesses a passionate nature, she remains cold and emotionally impotent.

Without doubt, the impact of Florence's dissatisfaction with life at home, and her desire to escape from it, fell most heavily on Parthenope. For Parthenope, awareness of her sister's plans threatened the security of her own unclouded existence, and immediately exposed the temperamental differences between them that had always been evident – not least to Florence herself – but which their common circumstances had somehow contrived to keep hidden. Once out in the open, these differences were often to provoke ill-feeling and bitter misunderstanding.

It did not help matters that in her daily life, Parthenope hardly connected with the real world at all. She lived in a bubble-like fantasy of her own making. 'And mayst thou always be the lark singing in the bright sunny atmosphere of art,' Florence greeted her in April 1847, on Parthenope's twenty-eighth birthday, 'and never descend, like the rest of us, to the busy scratching rabbit warren, where the inhabitants are digging and burrowing and making a dust for the bare life.' While Parthenope looked upon her younger sister as a remarkable, if strange, being from another world – a wild swan hatched to a family of ducks, to use her famous description – Florence, for her part, was at a loss to explain a character so alien to her own, with 'none of that restless longing for the future, that wanting <u>something</u> . . . that living in hope, which is the characteristic and the curse of the present day'. William Nightingale shared her incredulity, commenting that Parthenope's dreams were 'not of other wants than a good fire & good joy around'.

On occasions in the future, Florence would deeply regret the upset she was causing to Parthenope's untroubled way of life. But she also identified her sister's want of ambition, and lack of speculative thought, as all too representative of what society considered 'the true type of woman'. And as she struggled to gain her own independence, this model of femininity, 'fed on sugar-plums' and rendered powerless 'to rise to any abstract good, or general view', was one to be pitied, ideally treated with sympathy – and ultimately kept at a distance.

The comfortable and relatively carefree life at Lea Hurst and Embley helped to keep Parthenope confined to her amusements. Fanny Allen, clearly unaware of Florence's longing to make her escape, expressed the opinion that it would be difficult for either of the Nightingale daughters to find husbands they liked well enough to forsake such perfect homes; and in Parthenope's case, her close relationship as her mother's helpmate and companion probably contributed to making any thought of marriage especially difficult. When, at the end of 1847, a French suitor wrote declaring his unbridled passion for Parthenope ('d'un de ses enthousiasmes passionnés'), it may be significant that it was Fanny Nightingale who responded, dampening his ardour.

By now, Richard Monckton Milnes was a constant visitor to the Nightingale family. In October 1846, Florence told Shore that 'Mr Milnes was here three times last month and each time funnier than the last'. Precisely when she turned down Milnes's initial proposal of marriage is unknown, but he was nothing if not persistent, and over the course of several years she was repeatedly to delay giving him a final answer. Florence temporized, partly because she knew that here was a match that fulfilled all her mother's ambition for her – 'intellect, position, connections, everything' – but also because she must have realized that to reject a serious proposal as she approached thirty was effectively to close the door on the likely prospect of matrimony. Her confident announcement of ridding herself of personal feeling had perhaps been a little premature. She was in a very real quandary about what step to take next. Marriage, she remained convinced, was almost always a disappointment to a woman: 'to her – marriage is <u>the</u> thing, while to the husband it is only <u>one</u> of the things which form his life'. But if she was prevented from fulfilling her personal destiny as one of those women whom God had marked out to be single, might it not be better for her to submit to a sympathetic union with a man like Richard Monckton Milnes? She could not have known that Milnes, too, had his doubts. His name had been linked with any number of possible wives, but though he wished to be in love, he once confessed that he found it difficult to be so.

There seems little doubt that Florence was attracted to him. 'Mr Milnes is lively and pleasant,' wrote Fanny Allen, one of the Nightingales' friends keeping an eye on the progress of the courtship, 'but he is plain and common looking, so that he must make his way with Florence by his mind, and not the outward man.' This is just what he did. 'The poetic parcel', as Florence called him, wooed her with humour – he possessed a laugh once described as Falstaffian – and the pursuit of common interests, including literature. Milnes recited from his own poetry, including the verses in *Palm Leaves*, an account of his travels to Constantinople and Cairo, in which he professed his admiration for the Muslim faith, and his fears of the threat posed by westernization; on a visit to Lea Hurst, he read from the recently published *Poems* of Currer, Ellis and Acton Bell (Milnes was an early champion of the Brontë sisters, and his family estate at Fryston Hall was in the West Riding, not far from Haworth Parsonage);* and he described to Florence his meeting in Paris with George Sand. Ever since reading Sand's novel *Gabriel*, with its story of a couple who are disappointed in their hopes of a male heir and decide to raise their daughter Gabriel as a boy – a plotline whose resonance to her own life she found compelling – Florence had been fascinated by the life of the cross-dressing novelist.

She was most impressed by Milnes's deep concern for the victims of the Irish Famine. Unlike most politicians, he visited Ireland, in November 1846, to witness at first hand the terrible consequences of starvation and fever, writing to Florence from Dublin that 'For all ordinary purposes the

---

* Poetry by Ellis and Acton Bell (Emily and Anne Brontë) is among the favourite poems transcribed by Florence in a notebook now in the Florence Nightingale Museum in London. The front section, apparently dating from 1840, shows examples of her youthful taste, including verses by the enormously popular Felicia Hemans, as well as poetry by Dante, Spenser, Herbert, Wordsworth and Walter Scott. The Brontës' poetry, transcribed in about 1860, is at the back of the book, together with samples of Matthew Arnold's work.

root [of the potato] is gone throughout the Country. It is about as frequent as the Jerusalem Artichoke & used about as much . . .'

There were trips together to museums, and to meetings of the British Association for the Advancement of Science. In the autumn of 1846, Florence and Milnes attended the gathering at Southampton and joined the entertainment held afterwards at Embley. Sir John Herschel, in 'a very bad hat', was in charge of the astronomical section, and there was an explanation of the Earl of Rosse's great reflecting telescope, then the largest in the world. 'Our brain pans are so much enlarged,' Florence wrote, 'that we've been obliged to have new bonnets . . .'

The following summer, the BAAS moved to Oxford, where the two discoverers of the planet Neptune, the French astronomer Le Verrier and the British Adams, who had each worked without knowledge of the other, met for the first time. Florence sauntered about the churchyards and gardens by herself before breakfast, wishing she was 'a college man', and joined Milnes and her father for the day's proceedings. 'We work hard,' she told Mary Clarke, ' – chapel at 8:00 to one of those glorious services at New College or Magdalen. Sections from 11:00 to 3:00, then colleges or Blenheim, then lecture away at 8:00 in the Radcliffe Library, and philosophical tea and muffin at somebody's afterwards.' At Christ Church one day, they came across a three-month-old bear, chained to a door, belonging to Dean Buckland's son. They invited it in to lunch, where it became violent and obstreperous, and had to be carried out in disgrace. Outside it howled in a state of such nervous excitement that Florence had the idea of mesmerizing it. Milnes, keenly interested in this fashionable craze, attempted to do so, and within a few minutes the little bear was stretched out on the gravel fast asleep.

Florence pressed a white rose in remembrance of her time in Oxford, evidence perhaps that her feelings for Milnes were intensifying. Certainly, her reaction to the news of Mary Clarke's marriage to Julius Mohl, which she received on returning home, suggests that her thoughts on the subject of her own potential marriage were anything but settled. The death, in 1844, of Claude Fauriel, the great historian and philologist for whom she had nurtured a deep, if ultimately unsatisfying, passion, had filled Mary Clarke with 'inexpressible grief' and, for a time, only the editing of his lectures for publication had given her a renewed sense of purpose. In 1847, however, she had decided upon marriage to the man who had for so long occupied the other seat by the fireside in the ménage at the rue du Bac, Julius Mohl. A distinguished scholar in his own right, Mohl had a few years earlier encouraged the excavation of the royal palaces of Nineveh, resulting in the first discoveries of Assyrian sculpture and inscriptions. Always happiest surrounded by a wall of books (Thomas Trollope said he was like a mouse in a cheese, eating out the centre of the hollow in which it lives), Mohl would bring a new stability to Mary Clarke's life. But whereas Fauriel had been twenty years her senior, Mohl was her junior by sixteen years, and at the wedding ceremony in Paris that August, a witness was instructed by Clarkey to blow his nose loudly so that her true age remained inaudible.

Florence's long letter of congratulation to the new Madame Mohl contrasted the newlywed's 'love given in the full force of the inquiring and discriminating spirit' with more transient feelings of passion and fancy. But the main thrust of her remarks has an air of inconclusiveness, as well as fatalism, about it:

... we must all take Sappho's leap, one way or other, before we attain to her repose, though some take it to death, and some to marriage and some again to a new life even in this world. Which of them to the better part, God only knows. Popular prejudice gives it in favour of marriage ...

In single life the stage of the present & the outward world is so filled with phantoms, the phantoms not unreal tho' intangible, of Vague Remorse, Fears, dwelling on the threshold of every thing we undertake alone. Dissatisfaction with what is, & Restless Yearnings for what is not ... love laying to sleep these phantoms (by assuring us of a Love so great that we may lay aside all care for our own happiness, not because it is of <u>no</u> consequence to us ... but because it is of so much consequence to another), gives that leisure frame to our mind, which opens it at once to joy.

In the autumn of 1847, Florence's health failed once more. This time there was no question that the mental strain of her enforced role as daughter at home was beginning to tell on her physical wellbeing. Aunt Mai was sufficiently alarmed at her niece's condition to consult a doctor, who attributed Florence's 'slow circulation' to 'her tendency to depression of spirits'. He prescribed anything which might be 'calculated to make her life interesting & cheerful'.

An opportunity of this kind soon presented itself to the Nightingales. Charles and Selina Bracebridge, a couple in their late forties, who had been family friends for several years, and taken a particular interest in Florence's welfare, had decided to spend the winter of 1847–8 in Rome, and asked whether Florence might go with them. 'I cannot but think it would be good for her health,' Selina Bracebridge wrote to Fanny, though to save Florence from any unnecessary disappointment, she advised not mentioning the visit until a decision had been taken.

The Bracebridges liked to trace their descent back to Lady Godiva in the eleventh century. With greater certainty, they were direct descendants of a Warwickshire family with a mercantile background who had made a fortune in the seventeenth century from haberdashery stock. Their family seat, purchased in 1690, was Atherstone Hall, five miles from Nuneaton. Charles Holte Bracebridge, like William Nightingale, was a 'liberal country gentleman', and the last of his line, as he and his wife remained childless. A Justice of the Peace and Poor Law Guardian, he was an inveterate supporter of the cause of Greek Independence, owned land and houses in Greece and, as a young man, had taken part in a revolt against the Turks. A writer of sorts, constantly firing off letters to local and national newspapers, on any number of subjects, Charles Bracebridge had a nose for literary controversy. He subsequently involved himself in an embarrassing campaign to prove that one Joseph Liggins, a Nuneaton man, was the author of *Scenes of Clerical Life* and *Adam Bede*, not George Eliot; he also put up a staunch defence of the centuries-old charge against William Shakespeare, that he had stolen deer. Just before he went to Rome, Bracebridge was celebrating the recent purchase of Shakespeare's house in Stratford-upon-Avon, for which he had contributed funds, though Florence was at a loss to understand his enthusiasm. 'Is not one line of *Julius Caesar*,' she wrote, 'more a remembrance of Shakespeare than the house where his old clothes lay? We have himself, we have his whole mind, and what do we want with the room where he passed the night?'

As Selina Mills of Bisterne in Hampshire, before her marriage in the 1820s, Mrs Bracebridge had been a promising artist, a favourite pupil of the watercolourist Samuel Prout. Within a short time of meeting her, Florence had come to recognize Selina Bracebridge – or Σ, as she sometimes referred to her, using the Greek letter Sigma as a tribute to the older woman's Hellenic qualities and love of Greece – as a woman in whom she could place her trust. Unlike Fanny Nightingale, Σ did not tell her that society ought to make her happy; nor, unlike Aunt Hannah

Nicholson, did she preach that it was God's will that Florence should be contented with her lot. Dejected, and feeling misunderstood, Florence seized upon the precious sympathy that Selina Bracebridge offered. 'As long as one believes that one's inmost self, i.e., the ideas which make one's life, are hollow, there is no support from within or without. The praise and blame of others alike discourage one. God Himself is at a distance. But given one heart of fellow-feeling and the scene changes.'

That support was to be crucial as Selina Bracebridge, her 'more than mother', acted as a mediator between Florence and her family, constantly trying to ease her way and further her aspirations. Florence once described both Bracebridges as 'the creators of my life'; without them, as she freely acknowledged, her 'life could not have been'. Keen to stimulate Florence's interests and increase her knowledge, Mrs Bracebridge had already taken her on a visit to the museum at the Royal College of Surgeons, and to a workhouse near Atherstone Hall, so that Florence could observe the horrifying conditions in the infirmaries there.

The idea of spending three months with the Bracebridges was obviously an inviting one. But although Florence received her parents' consent to her accompanying them on their Roman holiday, she at first demurred, realizing only too well that the Nightingales were placing their trust in the idea that a spell abroad would divert her mind from her vocation. She concluded, however, that pursuit of that vocation depended on the restoration of her physical strength, and she had been assured that 'a winter in Rome will set me up for life'. By 20 October, she had finally decided in favour of the plan, while remaining full of trepidation at the prospect of such a prolonged separation from her family. 'It seems to me a very great event,' wrote Parthenope as she supervised the packing of her sister's belongings, 'the solemn first launching of her into life, and my heart is very full.'

Mr Nightingale pored over his large map of the city and proffered advice about the sights to visit. It would be a stirring time to be in Rome. A year earlier, a new Pope, Pius IX, had been elected amid confident expectations, still to be tested, that he would act as a bulwark of support for Italian independence against Austrian hegemony. 'I shall be curious to hear her good-sense view of the Pope & his doings,' Richard Monckton Milnes remarked, when he learned of Florence's departure.

On 26 October, Florence and her parents drove from Embley to Southampton at the start of her journey. Here they stayed the night while she, her maid Mariette, and the Bracebridges made the Channel crossing to Le Havre. To soften the blow of her departure, Florence had written to Hilary, requesting that she be 'a true angel of consolation' and come to Southampton to 'drink tea with us somewhere, & <u>go back</u> with my people . . .'

From Le Havre, the travellers proceeded for a few days in Paris, where Florence 'prosed & gossiped at length' with Madame Mohl, characteristically dressed in what looked like part of an old duster. The next stage of their journey took them across France to Marseilles by a combination of diligence, boat, omnibus and railroad. At Marseilles, they embarked by ship for the Civita Vecchia. As they got closer to the Eternal City, the mood grew more serious, and near the island of Elba, Florence imagined the shape of Christ emerging from the white mist.

The journey was completed, on the evening of 9 November, by a dramatic, starlit ride across the deserted Campagna Romana. Then, passing through the Porta Cavallegieri, Florence heard the sound of the fountains of St Peter's, 'softly plashing in the stillness of night . . .'

5. To Be Happy in My Own Way

Too excited to sleep, Florence was up at dawn at their accommodation in the Piazza del Popolo, washing off 'the dust of many days'. As soon as it was light, she went out and almost ran until she came to St Peter's. 'The dome was much smaller than I expected. But that enormous Atrio. I stopped under it, for my mind was almost out of breath, to recover its strength before I went in. No event in my life, except my death, can ever be greater than that first entrance into St Peter's, the concentrated spirit of the Christianity of so many years, the great image of our Faith which is the worship of grief.' So used to being cosseted and worried over at home, she was surprised to find the Bracebridges, on her return, completely unfazed by her absence.

They spent a couple of days scouting for more permanent lodgings, eventually settling on a third-floor apartment at 8 Via S. Sebastianello, a street leading off the Piazza di Spagna, the fashionable locale for English expatriates. Their rooms were spacious and sun-facing, though a treacherously steep and badly lit staircase caused a near fatal accident just before Christmas, when Mr Bracebridge slipped and fell down an entire flight, hitting his head against the wall (though he bled profusely, there was fortunately no sign of any concussion). To Florence's delight, one small room contained two busts of Pope Pius IX, evidence that their landlords were ardent Pietists. She did not have to wait long to see the object of the cult himself. Within days of arriving in Rome, she and the Bracebridges were permitted by a kindly Swiss Guard to approach the door of the Quirinal and watch as the Pope emerged to get into his carriage. He looked serene, she thought, a man in the prime of his life, well able to carry out the regeneration of a new Italy, even though it seemed surprising that such regeneration should emanate from the papacy, traditionally the centre of corruption itself. To commemorate this first encounter, Mr Bracebridge presented Florence and his wife each with a plaster medallion of the Pope – 'So now we shall have four Pio Nonos in our house.'

Florence's rose-tinted view of Pius IX as 'the father of liberty' needs to be seen in light of the popular fervour created on the new Pope's accession by his granting of a flurry of democratic reforms that would have been unthinkable under the oppressive regimes of his predecessors. The month before Florence's arrival in Rome, Pio Nono had responded to the clamour for further reform with a still more liberal step: the reorganization of the administration of the city under a council of 100 members, followed by the inauguration of a Consultative Assembly to assist in the work of government. Sharing her father's appetite for information about political systems, Florence obtained reports of the new arrangements and wrote to him, minutely analysing details of the changes. At the same time, she waited expectantly for the first signs of Pius IX's active sympathy in the struggle to free Italy from Austria, expressing impatience with the Bracebridges' scepticism about the Pope's intentions, while proclaiming his virtues in letters home.

Her time in Rome also encouraged Florence to make a careful study of Roman Catholic doctrine, and to collate the Latin breviary with the English prayerbook. She briefly attended the English Church, just outside the Porta del Popolo, but poured scorn on the service there as not so much 'a Communion of Saints' as 'a Communion of Bonnets', where attar of roses took the place of incense, and instead, started to go to Mass at St Peter's. Even though she admitted to being scandalized by the doctrine of transubstantiation, Roman Catholicism attracted her as 'the least unsuccessful attempt' by any church to represent the unseen. Catholicism's 'want of liberty', however, was sufficient reason for her to declare that she could never become a Catholic. She placed too much value on freedom of individual thought, and saw Catholicism's suppression of that freedom reflected in the view from the dome of St Peter's, where people were kneeling and praying, but with 'their priests standing between them and every altar'. (Years later, she would ridicule Pius IX's doctrine of papal infallibility because it was based on no better reasoning than 'the pope is infallible because he says so'.) She remained committed to a broad assimilation of different creeds, in the tradition of William Smith, and of her own father, whom she thanked for having taught her to look upon churches as merely 'accidental developments of the one Parent Sap . . .' Writing teasingly to her family to ask, 'Are you afraid that I am becoming Roman Catholic?' she reiterated her belief in a fundamental ecumenism:

I might perhaps, if there had been anything in me for Roman Catholicism to lay hold of, but I was not a Protestant before. Protestantism is confining Inspiration to one period, one nation, and one place . . . and within that period, that nation, and that place of inspiration, allowing you all possible freedom of interpretation and thought. Catholicism allows Inspiration to all times, all nations, and all places . . . but limits the inspiration of God to herself as its only channel. Can either of these be true? Can 'the word' be pinned down to either one period or one church?

One of the most intense religious experiences of these months was an afternoon spent in the Sistine Chapel. She and Mrs Bracebridge were completely alone, without custodian or other visitors, as they gazed at Michelangelo's frescoes. Although Florence could not believe in a literal 'Last Judgement', she was enraptured by the feeling that she was looking not at pictures, but at heaven itself. Attempting to describe the experience in a long letter to Parthenope, she bowed to her sister's superior knowledge, and acknowledged her own 'want of art'. Despite the blackening effects of time upon the colours of the paintwork, Florence marvelled at the way in which the artist had given form 'to the breath of god', and was particularly struck by the representation of the Delphic Sybil, full of anxiety and uncertainty as she strains to hear the word of God.* Another day she located the tiny church of S. Lorenzo in Lucino in order to see a crucifixion scene set against a stormy sky by one of her favourite artists, Guido Reni.

If St Peter's was the touchstone of Florence's Rome, she nevertheless resolved to take in the Rome of the Caesars as well. Equipped with Antonio Nibby's guide to ancient Rome, she explored the Forum, crawling on her knees to try to work out its outline in the midst of renewed excavations. Mr Bracebridge, meanwhile, was prey to one of the ubiquitous pickpockets. She visited the Colosseum, with its 'horrible green

* In later life Florence remained a 'worshipper' of Michelangelo's Sistine Chapel. Her drawing room and bedroom at her house in South Street were decorated with photographs and engravings of the frescoes, and in 1870 the Victoria and Albert Museum lent her its albums of 'autotype reproductions of the ceiling of the Sistine Chapel' for a weekend so that she could examine them from the confinement of her room.

gates with spikes at the tops', and watched men making 'terrible repar-
ations' with wheelbarrows. Mr Bracebridge's fluent Italian, with its
extensive range of gestures, came in useful, and as a guide, Florence
relied on an Englishman, Henry Colyar, whose knowledge of the antiquities was said to be unrivalled, and who accompanied her sightseeing on
a number of occasions. Colyar, a friend of the Empsons at Wellow,
wrote to them of 'the joy' of being in the company of 'your charming
and intellectual Miss Nightingale', adding that his 'admiration and veneration for her grew daily'.

The holiday was doing Florence good. She was greatly enjoying herself, and Mrs Bracebridge was able to report on 'dear Flo's improved
looks from Roman air and Roman life'. Florence's chief worry occurred
whenever news from home didn't arrive as frequently as she thought it
should, as if she couldn't believe that her family could cope without her.
Meanwhile, for her mother's benefit, she filled her own copious letters
('Rowland Hill . . . costs enormously,' she noted pointedly) with details
of the people they met, and of new clothes purchased at Fanny's insistence. She found Edward Lear, part of the artistic community at Rome for
the past decade, whose Book of Nonsense had recently been published,
'particularly agreeable'; but took an instant dislike to the American
writer Margaret Fuller, with her unattractive nasal drawl. Fanny was
delighted with Florence's letters, proudly reading extracts from them
out loud to the maids at Embley, as well as to the Empsons, and
exclaiming to Parthenope, 'how pleasant it is to think of her – instead
of being up to her neck in mud at West Wellow'.

The Bracebridges' own ill-health – she was plagued by severe neur-
algia, while he was a semi-invalid following his fall – sometimes curtailed
their socializing and excursions into society, though Florence hardly
regretted the solitude this imposed. She had to be 'dragged out' to make
her debut at a Roman tea party, but other occasions, like a reception
given by Lord Minto, Britain's diplomatic representative in Rome, she
took more in her stride, 'doing society in a business like way'.

One encounter can only be described as momentous. For it was in
Rome that winter that Florence first met Sidney Herbert, and what she
once described as her 'intimacy' with him began to develop. It was
nothing less, she recognized twenty years later, than 'a time pregnant to
me of all my future life'.

Sidney and Elizabeth Herbert were visiting Rome on a postponed wedding tour. The Tory administration under Sir Robert Peel, in which
Herbert had briefly served as Secretary at War, had fallen in the summer
of 1846 over the divisive issue of the repeal of the Corn Laws. Soon
afterwards, Herbert married Elizabeth à Court, whom he had known
since childhood. The break from government allowed him a life of
comparative leisure to travel and to enjoy the peace and beauty of his
home at Wilton, the family seat of the Earls of Pembroke, where, to all
intents and purposes, he was master following his elder half-brother's
exile abroad after a scandalous marriage with a Sicilian woman. Liz
Herbert was already a close friend of Selina Bracebridge's, and the two
groups of pilgrims were often in each other's company, at parties and
art galleries, or climbing the rocks at the Grotta di Nettuno. Florence
quickly succumbed to Sidney Herbert's charm – while admitting that
she could have entered more freely into his fun if she hadn't been afraid
of being laughed at – and compared Liz Herbert's beauty and warmth
to 'the sunshine of Italy'.

In his late thirties, Herbert's singular charm was universally acknowledged, together with his refined good looks and marked courteousness
of manner. This latter quality was to be crucial in his relationship with
Florence Nightingale. At times of stress in their future dealings, he never
allowed himself to be provoked into angry words, though his patience
was often to be tested. Long after his premature death, by which time,
admittedly, her respect for him had long since solidified into something
approaching veneration, she commented on the almost feminine delicacy
of his behaviour. '. . . He achieved far greater triumphs for his country
than by the spirit of anger and wrath,' she wrote, noting that it was his
'winning gentleness that subdued far more than resistance . . .'

One of Florence's later nicknames for him, 'the Cid', appropriately
invested Herbert with the qualities of the chivalric Christian hero,
though it appears that there was never any hint of a romantic attachment
between them. Indeed, at the outset, she found certain of his views
distinctly unappealing. He was, after all, a Tory (and one whose maiden
speech had attacked a motion favouring the removal of the remaining
restrictions on the admission of Dissenters to the universities), even
though he belonged to the more liberal Peelite wing of the party; and he
was vocal in decrying the image of her beloved Pius IX as a great
reformer. She was pleased to discover, on the other hand, that Herbert

shared her belief that a republic was the ultimate form of government. While in Rome, during 1848, as revolution spread across Europe, she pronounced herself an 'inborn republican', declaring that the 'monarchical principle' could only be allowed 'as a necessary evil'.

For his part, Sidney Herbert was fascinated by Florence. He 'quite appreciates her and talks of her forever', Mrs Bracebridge told a no doubt appreciative Fanny Nightingale from Rome. But then remarkable, commanding women had been a constant feature of Sidney Herbert's life. His mother, Catherine, Dowager Countess of Pembroke, was an indomitable character, daughter of Semyon Woronzow, former Russian ambassador at the court of St James (consequently Herbert's half-Russian parentage caused tensions when Britain faced Russia as an enemy at the outbreak of the Crimean War); while the woman who almost certainly became Herbert's mistress in the years preceding his marriage was Caroline Norton, a witty, flamboyant beauty, and prolific poet, novelist and pamphleteer, whose marital tribulations were to have a formative influence in the middle of the century on the legal position of married women. As Herbert's half-brother, the twelfth earl, was childless, Herbert's marriage was essential in order to produce an heir to secure the Pembroke line. According to society gossip, Mrs Norton went quietly, having promised Herbert that she would make no trouble for him (in 1884, the relationship formed the basis of George Meredith's novel *Diana of the Crossways*, in which Caroline Norton was the eponymous heroine, and Sidney Herbert, as Percy Dacier, the cabinet minister in love with her).

Liz Herbert was cast in a different mould from Caroline Norton, though she too was acknowledged, like her predecessor, as a beauty. Still only in her mid-twenties at the time of her marriage, she was admired for her courtesy, gracefulness of manner and soft, purring voice. A sharpness of mind led friends to nickname her 'Lady Lightning'. Yet, while her marriage to Sidney Herbert was a love match – and his letters early in their relationship dwell on his 'ever increasing love' for her – she tormented herself at times with the idea that she was not clever or amusing enough to be a fit companion for her husband. Furthermore, she was concerned about their religious differences, knowing all too well how disastrous any hint of her Roman Catholic sympathies would be for her husband's political career. Liz Herbert's later account describes Herbert as disliking theological discussions and any 'extremes' of belief.

He was High Church, a Puseyite in all but name, but his faith remained 'peculiarly child-like'. At Wilton, where he took his duty to his tenants on the Pembroke estates with commendable seriousness, he had recently rebuilt the parish church in an Italian Romanesque style, and, during their time in Rome, the Herberts scouted for mosaics to make it even more resplendent (on a visit to the church, Florence objected to having to take her galoshes from her feet, not because she stood on holy ground, 'but because it was <u>gorgeous</u> ground').

But Liz Herbert wavered from the Protestantism of her upbringing. She was later to write that she had always found Protestant worship 'formal, empty and cold'; but it was a growing friendship with Henry Manning, Archdeacon of Chichester, and an old Harrow and Oxford friend of her husband's, that encouraged serious reservations about Anglicanism and launched her on the road to eventual conversion to Roman Catholicism, in 1865, after Sidney Herbert's death. Manning offered her spiritual guidance until his own conversion in 1851, when he tactfully distanced himself from their relationship.

Manning, too, was in Rome that winter of 1847–8, convalescing from serious illness, and his closeness to the Herberts inevitably brought him into contact with Florence. 'He is about 35 and looks about 55,' she told her father, though Manning was in fact nearing forty, his ill-health and cadaverous looks combining to make him appear older. His strained appearance was no doubt also due to the anguished spiritual crisis he was facing, in which he remained outwardly loyal to the Church of England, while privately plagued with doubts about its claims to be a church at all. Florence correctly predicted that Manning, like Newman two years earlier, would eventually go over to Rome, making 'an easy transit from the Via della Croce' to the 'Convent della Santissima Croce', the building near the Lateran, occupied by the English *convertiti*.

There were then two prospective converts in the circle in which Florence moved in Rome. But there was also a third, more on the periphery, another of the women to whom Manning acted as spiritual mentor. Mary Stanley, a daughter of the Bishop of Norwich and sister of the future Dean Stanley of Westminster, had assisted her father in local schemes of philanthropy, and was now travelling to assuage her religious doubts. She was keenly interested in hospitals and sisterhoods, and with this in common with Florence, formed a bond with her, which strengthened once they were back in England. Older by about seven

years, Mary made Florence the object of an awkward devotion. It was
a friendship that was to end disastrously for both of them.

At the beginning of January 1848, Florence and the Bracebridges,
together with the Herberts, were presented to Pius IX (at home, after
reading Florence's vivid description, Parthenope attempted to portray
the audience in a watercolour). 'I cannot do justice to the benevolence of his expression,' Florence wrote to Fanny Nightingale, 'but I am
afraid of dwelling upon it to you usque ad nauseam.' Concerned that he
might have no one to look after him, she added, 'Have popes mothers?'
With her parents' permission, her time in Rome had now been extended
until Easter, and she found a ready companion in Liz Herbert as she
embarked upon 'a course of convents and hospitals'. The Herberts
maintained an interest of their own in nursing care, and had plans for a
convalescent home and cottage hospital on the Pembroke estates in
Wiltshire.

A decade later, the parliamentary commissioners hearing evidence for
the report on the health of the army were impressed by the expertise
Florence had accumulated through careful examination of hospital conditions throughout Europe. The foundations of that expertise were laid
in part in Rome during 1848. At San Giacomo, the hospital for incurable
diseases, wounds and surgical cases, she found a depressing situation.
The patients were all crowded into one large ward, and looked 'dirty
and despairing', while the stench was dreadful, 'the locale cold, airless,
dark'. The Santo Spirito, the vast general hospital, on the banks of the
Tiber, near the Vatican, was similarly 'a hopeless case', though here, at
least, the foundlings section was nursed by French sisters of the order of
St Vincent de Paul, starched, clean, efficient, in contrast to the grubby
Roman nurses.

While at benediction at St Peter's, on the evening of 6 February,
Florence noticed Felicetta Sensi, a poor orphan girl whom she decided
to help by paying for her admission to the school attached to the convent
of the Trinità dei Monti, at the top of the Spanish Steps. She was unable
to pay the fees for five years (about 100 scudi) immediately – eventually
finding the money from her clothing allowance – but in the process of
making the arrangements she formed a significant relationship with the
nun advising her, Laure de Ste Colombe, the *maîtresse des externes*,
known to Florence as the 'madre'.

The convent was part of the French order of Sacré-Coeur, and on one of her visits to the retreat house, high above the city, Florence had an interview with Makrena Mirazyslawki, better known as the Abbess of Minsk. The Abbess had suffered seven years of terrible persecution by order of Tsar Nicholas I, who had unsuccessfully attempted to force the nuns of Minsk to return to the Orthodox Church. Following eviction from their convent, the nuns had been starved, beaten and imprisoned in chains. Only the Abbess had survived to escape to the security of the Trinità. Her legs still bore the scars of the chains, and she hobbled with a stick, unable to move far. Florence admired the Abbess's 'rough humility', above all her refusal to parade her near-martyrdom, and composed a long account of her struggles, largely for her family's benefit, though she may have hoped to publish it at some time. In fact it lay untouched for almost six years until the onset of the dispute between Russia and Turkey gave rise to the idea of its use as a propaganda weapon against the Tsar, and it was sent to Charles Dickens. Dickens's article, 'The True Story of the Nuns of Minsk', published in *Household Words* in May 1854, acknowledges Florence – an 'English Protestant Lady' as he calls her – as a major source. It is an unlikely collaboration between two iconic figures of the Victorian age.

Florence's conversations with Madre Santa Colombe, and her wish to absorb something of the principle of devotion underlying religious service, led her to go on a ten-day retreat at the convent. The Madre had impressed upon her the central importance of submitting her own will to the will of God. Listening sympathetically to what Florence told her of her life at home, she had responded: 'It is no good separating yourself from people to try and do the will of God. That is not the way to gain his blessing. What does it matter even if we are with people who make us desperate? So long as we are doing God's will, it doesn't matter at all.'

Florence promised Parthenope 'the whole history of the Rise and Progress of my religious life as an inmate of the Trinità'; but while no such letter has survived, it's clear that what she experienced there was not a regular retreat. Part of her time was spent in observing the convent school, and she later adapted some of its methods – for instance, encouraging children at all times to voice their opinions freely – to her own teaching practice; while a transcribed passage, dated 'Rome 7 March 1848', in the frontispiece to her Bible, indicates that she also followed certain of the spiritual exercises of Ignatius of Loyola, including those that encouraged the visualization of events and identification with figures in them.

At the end of the ten days, Florence recorded the following dialogue with the Madre:

MADRE: Did not God speak to you during this retreat? Did he not ask you anything?

FLORENCE: He asked me to surrender my will.

MADRE: And to whom?

FLORENCE: To all that is upon the earth.

MADRE: He calls you to a very high degree of perfection. Take care. If you will resist you will be very guilty.

Although Florence left Rome with promises to the Madre that she would not forget her, they were never to meet again, and Florence rarely attempted to contact her (in 1856, after an eight-year silence, an evidently hurt Laure de Ste Colombe wrote reproaching Florence, and reminding her that 'the strong woman . . . finds time for everything and the care of great works does not let her neglect the least among her friends'). Yet, however fleeting their relationship, the influence of the Madre was lasting and marked a turning point in Florence's life. Here, at last, eleven years after God first spoke to her, was someone who took her call to service seriously. Moreover, scattered references in Florence's writings over the next few years underline the crucial role that remarks the Madre had made about the necessity of sacrificing one's own small reputation for God would play in Florence's overriding desire in the future to pursue her life and work in anonymity.

'If 1848 sees the foreigner out of Italy, what an age to live in!' a jubilant Florence wrote as the dramatic unfolding of events suggested that the moment of destiny for the Risorgimento had finally arrived. In January she had rejoiced at news of insurrection in Sicily. In February, revolution in Paris gave a powerful impetus to rebels throughout Italy, while in Rome, in March, Pius IX published a constitution and relinquished his temporal power. A revolutionary uprising erupted in Milan soon afterwards, and five days of street fighting by men, women and children against 15,000 Austrian troops won the Milanese their freedom. Venice rebelled, forcing the Austrians to capitulate, and immediately the whole of Lombardy and Venetia rose up in arms. The widespread mood of euphoria was reflected in torchlight processions on the streets of Rome. In the midst of vast crowds, Florence watched and cheered as the tri-colour of Italy was hoisted on the Colosseum.

'Italy is now all one nation,' she wrote home excitedly. But her optimism was premature. Concerns about safety cut short their Roman holiday at the end of March – 'but oh!', Florence wrote, 'how I should like to pull a trigger against the Austrian first' – so she was already back in England by the time the movement for Italian independence received its first grave blow. At the end of April, Pius IX destroyed the myth of a revival of Italy under the auspices of the Church with his declaration that as Pope he had to love all nations equally and that, consequently, he would not wage war on Austria. A year later, the glowing promise of the spring of 1848 seemed irremediably compromised, and by the end of 1849, Rome and Venice, the last bastions of republican freedom, had both fallen under the influx of foreign troops. To Florence, it had seemed for a time as if 'the kingdom of heaven' had arrived; but 'we must have a much larger growth of angels slowly ripening upon earth . . . before our eyes shall see it'.

In revolutionary France, through which Florence and the Bracebridges made their tortuous journey home, she could at least witness at first hand the results of the overthrow of Louis-Philippe. She admired the elegance of the Parisian barricades, each one adorned with a red streamer or green branch to make it look 'artistic'; and praised the 'devotion to ideas' of the French, and their 'Quixotism' – though this enthusiasm, too, would be short-lived once their Republic was replaced by the military despotism of Louis-Napoleon.

By the middle of April, Florence had arrived back at Embley. She returned in high spirits, buoyed by the excitement of events abroad, and by a sense that a new chapter in her life was about to open. It did not take long, however, for her to feel as if she had never been away, and for the old aimlessness to reassert itself. 'Everything here is in statu quo atmosphere like a warm bath . . . ,' she wrote discontentedly to her father, nine months after her return. 'I never open a book, nor my mouth, except to victual it.'

There were new distractions, visiting the Herberts, in town, and at Wilton, where they sought her advice on their scheme for building a convalescent home at Charmouth. Even an overnight stay necessitated a 'petition' from Mrs Herbert to Mrs Nightingale, promising that she

would take 'very great care' of her daughter. Wilton itself was far too
opulent for Florence's taste, but she worked in the local school and ran
errands for Liz Herbert, who was confined to bed during a difficult pregnancy after two miscarriages, and needed Florence's support, 'owing to
her having been brought up without the knowledge by which even a hen
lays eggs' (the Herberts' first child, a daughter, was born in 1849, a boy
followed in 1850, and Florence was present at the birth of their third 'bab',
another girl, in 1851). While the friendship of the two women deepened,
Sidney Herbert's admiration for Florence continued to increase. 'Mr
Herbert put off an engagement to dine with the Duke of Newcastle that
he might dine with Flo at home,' Selina Bracebridge was to write to
Fanny Nightingale on one occasion at the beginning of the 1850s, '&
very agreeable he was as usual – let me whisper in your ear that Flo
wore her new velvet gown made at Paris . . . her hair very nicely done . . .'

Florence never regarded herself as possessing 'a genius' for education,
despite expending considerable energy in the careful preparation of
lesson plans, but she continued to work in the local schools at Lea and
Wellow, always aware that in her parents' eyes, the teaching of poor
children was an acceptable outlet for her call to service. In the spring of
1849 she began an association with the London branch of the Ragged
School movement, dedicated to the education of destitute children, under
the presidency of Palmerston's son-in-law Lord Ashley. In London,
unlike the country, where 'everything that is painful is so carefully
removed out of sight', it was impossible to be unaware of the extent of
deprivation that prevailed in the miserable lives of the poor. 'My little
thieves in Westminster', as she called her ragged school pupils, were her
'greatest joy in London', where her distaste for society during the season
was more marked than ever. But her longing to explore for herself the
darker heart of the city, to bring comfort and aid to slum-dwellers, was
deemed wholly inappropriate. It would never do, she was told, for a
young woman in her station to go out in London without a servant.

The possibility of satisfying the ambition closest to her heart arose in
the autumn of 1848, only swiftly to vanish like a mirage. Parthenope
had been advised to go to Karlsbad for the water cure, and from there
the Nightingales planned to travel on to Frankfurt, where Clarkey and
Julius Mohl, who was a native of the city, were staying. For Florence
it was an opportunity not to be missed: from Frankfurt, with a little

persuasion, her parents might allow her to pay a fortnight's visit to Kaiserswerth, only a short distance away.

But at the last minute, news of riots in Karlsbad, followed by Florence being suddenly taken ill, forced the Nightingales to alter their plans, and Florence's dream was – literally – doused in cold water. Instead of her hopes of fitting in a little training at Kaiserswerth, she would accompany Fanny to Malvern, where they would undergo the hydropathic water cure (why Parthenope, who was the reason for the treatment in the first place, didn't go with them is a mystery, unless she was too ill to be moved, or Florence and her mother were intended to act as guinea pigs for this newfangled remedy).

The disappointment was almost too much to bear. 'My God what am I to do,' she recorded in a note that October. 'I cannot go on any longer waiting till my situation should change, dreaming what the change should be.' She struggled painfully with the idea that this interference with her plans should be the will of God, but travelled to Malvern, accompanied by the Bracebridges, who were joining Florence and her mother for the cure, having resolved, once more, to put a brave face on her situation. Booking themselves into the Foley Arms, Fanny Nightingale summoned Dr James Gully, a leading Malvern hydropath, for a consultation. '. . . Mama was so taken in by him,' Florence noted blithely, 'that I was obliged to tell him I had a father living.'

Gully was indeed charming and persuasive, the kind of man who could successfully market a patent hair restorer despite his own complete baldness. He, and his sometime partner, sometime rival, James Wilson, had been responsible for importing into England the hydropathic water cures practised in Graefenburg in Austria by Vincenz Priessnitz, establishing them as an extraordinary health craze which attracted a stream of famous visitors, including royalty, to the old spa town. Gully's book, *The Water Cure in Chronic Disease* – which Fanny rushed out to buy on arriving in Malvern – described the salient aspects of the treatment, centring on the soaking and immersion of different parts of the body to stimulate circulation and draw out debilitating toxins from internal organs and blood. An intensive regime, lasting every day for several weeks, consisted of being packed in wet sheets for hours on end, sweating in a chair over a lamp while wrapped in blankets, and – 'a new & horrible instrument of torture', as Florence described the 'douche' – being drenched in an icy shower of water from a great height.

You go down to the douche house [she wrote to Parthenope on 22 October], where you hear a series of little yells & squeals proceeding from the victims along the line & sometimes a prolonged howl. You go into your own den & descend into a deep well. Above are three pipes of 2″, 3″, 4″ bore, about ten feet above your head. And there you stand, stark staring naked (& mad too) like Eve in the Garden of Eden receiving some punishment from the angels.

Exercise was another part of the treatment: donkey rides for the less mobile, and vigorous walking for the rest. The Nightingale–Bracebridge party moved to lodgings at South Cottage, and thereby avoided being restricted to Gully's sanatorium, but the worst aspect of the water cure, according to Florence, was that 'it takes up all one's time'. She remained sceptical about the precise worth of the cure, once bitingly summing it up as 'a highly popular amusement . . . amongst athletic invalids who have felt the *tedium vitae*, and those indefinite diseases which a large income and unbounded leisure are so well calculated to produce'. However, she also commended Gully and his kind for seeking an alternative to the widespread medical dependence on prescribing drugs, and recognized that 'proper diet, exercise, fresh mountain air and different kinds of bathing' could work wonders. On several occasions in later years, when exhausted and overworked, she would again have recourse to the water cure and acknowledge its benefits – 'altho' it could not cure'.

Florence had espied Tennyson among Gully's other patients; and in November, after her return to Embley, she wrote to Richard Monckton Milnes to acknowledge several letters from him that had arrived in her absence, and to describe this encounter. 'Your friend, Alfred Tennyson was there,' she told him, 'with a skin so tender he walked backwards whenever the wind was north or east and that was generally. He was sadly contumacious, smoking vile tobacco in a long pipe till Dr Gully told him it coarsened his imagination and made him write bad poetry.'

Milnes had been following in Florence's footsteps in France: while she was travelling back to England in the spring of 1848, he had been on his way to Paris to celebrate the birth of a free republic. On his return, he published his *Life, Letters and Literary Remains of John Keats*. This was the first available biography of a poet, still little read by the Victorians and stigmatized by them for what they saw as Keats's tendency to 'unmanly' behaviour, sensuality, and self-indulgence. Although Milnes's book would in the long term rescue Keats's reputation from obscurity, in the short term it added fuel to the controversy about his character, especially concerning his supposed paganism. 'I hope Mrs Nightingale does not bother her daughter to accept of Monckton Milnes,' wrote an outraged Fanny Allen, in February 1849. 'He is not worthy of her. Have you seen his life of Keats?'

Milnes was about to turn forty, anxious to get married, and unwilling to be kept dangling by Florence for any longer. At Whitsun 1849, the Nightingales held a large party at Embley. This was the usual preliminary to the family moving up to Derbyshire for the summer and, as in previous years, Monckton Milnes was present. It seems likely that he chose the occasion to reiterate to Florence his wish to marry her, and that – according to the outline broadly pursued by every Nightingale biographer since 1931, when Ida O'Malley first identified Richard Monckton Milnes as Florence's most serious suitor – she refused him outright.

Or did she? A letter, written several years afterwards to Fanny Nightingale by Aunt Mai, suggests that, on Florence's part at any rate, the situation regarding Milnes's final proposal was by no means so clear cut, and that he misunderstood her intentions. According to Aunt Mai, Florence was slowly coming round to the idea of marriage to Milnes as 'the life next most valuable' to one of service, but Milnes 'seems not to have understood her, to have supposed her still to refuse him, & married another'. His immediate reaction to her response to his proposal, in whatever confused terms she framed it, may have been anger, or distress, or simply irritation. Certainly, when she saw him again, while passing through Hamburg the following summer, she was relieved to find that 'Richard was himself again'.

A misunderstanding between Florence and Milnes would account for the intense period of self-examination, weighing up the advantages and disadvantages of marriage to him, that she embarked on over the next two years – almost, in fact, to the point, in June 1851, when Milnes became engaged to Annabel Crewe of Madeley Manor, in Staffordshire. In a variety of notes – often in different versions using identical phrases – some barely legible in faint pencil, others in which she stabs at the paper almost out of desperation, Florence analysed the pros and cons of her situation.

I have an intellectual nature which requires satisfaction, & that would find it in him. I have a passional nature which requires satisfaction, & that would find it in him. I have a moral and active nature that requires satisfaction, & that would not find it in his life. I can hardly find satisfaction for any of my natures. Sometimes I think that I will satisfy my passional nature at all events because that will at least secure me from the evil of dreaming. But would it? I could be satisfied to spend a life with him combining our different powers in some great object. I could not satisfy this nature by spending a life with him in making society & arranging domestic things ... To be nailed to a continuation & exaggeration of my present life, without hope of another, would be intolerable to me. Voluntarily to put it out of my power ever to be able to seize the chance of forming for myself a true and rich life would seem to me like suicide.

Sinking to the depths of depression at Christmas 1850, eighteen months after Milnes's proposal, she admitted to herself that she felt overcome at the thought of seeing him again, and that not a day had gone by without her thinking of him, 'that life is desolate to me to the last degree without his sympathy. Yet, do I wish to marry him?'

Three months later, on 15 March 1851, they did meet again, in London, for the first time since their fleeting encounter in Hamburg in the summer of 1850. But the circumstances of their meeting, in a crowded, noisy room at Lady Palmerston's, were far from propitious. 'He would hardly speak. I was miserable . . . I wanted to find him longing to talk to me, willing to give me another opportunity to keep open another decision; or perhaps I only wanted his sympathy without looking any further. He was not ready with it. He did not show indifference, but avoidance. No familiar friendship. No confidence such as I felt towards him.'

Five days after this upsetting experience, she wrote to Milnes. Ostensibly she did so to ask him a favour for her cousin Blanche, whose parents did not approve of their daughter's courtship by the poet A. H. Clough; but, clearly, she was also seeking a channel back to their old familiarity. Perhaps by now she had heard the rumours, widespread around London, of Milnes's ardent pursuit of Annabel Crewe. If so, that would have lessened the shock of the announcement of their engagement, swiftly followed by their marriage on 31 July. The fact that by that date Florence was at Kaiserswerth, observing nursing practice and attending operations, after gaining her parents' consent to her spending three months there, must have provided some welcome distraction from the news. But the battle for a purposeful future was still, even at that stage, far from won, and Florence must have felt that she had lost the one man she could seriously have considered marrying for the sake of a personal destiny that might never be fulfilled. No wonder then that Aunt Mai described Milnes's decision to turn elsewhere as filling her niece with 'gloom'.

However, the old familiarity between them would quickly return, helped by Florence's liking for Annabel Milnes. She was 'very glad' to learn of the imminent arrival of the Milneses' first child, Amicia, in the summer of 1852, and stood as godmother to their second daughter, born in 1855 and named Florence in her honour. In the future their lives would interact in many ways. As a friend of the Nightingale family, Milnes remained a visitor to Lea Hurst, and to Embley, where, walking with his daughter Florence in the spring of 1869, he imagined he saw the ghost of her namesake 'more than once behind the rhododendrons'. Most significantly, he would remain in her life as a source of intellectual and political advice, and would play his part in the growth of the Nightingale legend through his verse, and in the dissemination of nursing reform in his capacity as the first President of the Nightingale Fund.

In the wake of Milnes's marriage to someone else, Florence wrote of herself as 'the idol of the man I adored'. Late in life, her recollections of their relationship were strongly flavoured by memories of their 'amaro dolce'. This may have been wishful thinking coloured by the sentiment of old age. Yet it's clear that the quality that Milnes offered her that she treasured most – and felt bereft without – was his sympathy. She admired him, not simply for his brilliance, but also because his talents 'in tongue or pen, whether political, social or literary, were inspired chiefly by good will toward men'.

Evidently, Milnes possessed strong feelings for Florence, even if he wasn't in love with her, and touching confirmation of this is contained in a private request he made to Lady Stratford de Redcliffe, wife of the British ambassador in Constantinople, as Florence set off for Scutari in the autumn of 1854, seeking her assurance that, in the event of Florence falling ill, she would make provision for care to be taken of her.

Despite this, it would be difficult to escape the conclusion that in failing to marry each other, both Florence and Milnes had had a narrow escape. While Florence had imagined combining their powers to some great end, the sheer catholicity of Milnes's tastes and interests, and his dilettante nature, made this an unlikely prospect; and, as she recognized, to play the part of Milnes's wife to the full would have meant entering into precisely the kind of life of socializing and entertaining that she so abhorred (admittedly, Annabel Milnes didn't enjoy it either, and in her first season as hostess, she had to preside over twenty-six dinner, and twelve breakfast parties). Moreover, the darker, more sensual, morally libertine, side of Milnes's character sits uneasily with Florence's fundamental asceticism, and makes them the most unlikely set of partners. How Florence might have reacted to the collection of erotica in the library at Fryston – jokingly called 'Aphrodisiopolis' by Milnes – or to Milnes's avid purchases of manuscripts and editions of the works of the Marquis de Sade, is almost too mind-boggling to contemplate.*

With the loss of Richard Monckton Milnes, the prospect of Florence marrying anyone else in the future looked increasingly unlikely. From time to time, there are stray, jokey references in her correspondence to other possible suitors. One of these was George Dawson, a charismatic and popular Baptist minister, who preached a gospel of service and brotherhood at his Church of the Saviour in Birmingham. Florence and her mother attended his lecture on 'Christianity and Democracy' in the autumn of 1848, when, according to Florence, he was described by friends as her 'futur' – despite the fact that he was already married. In 1853, a more serious candidate – referred to only as 'this man who wants to marry me' – presented himself. He appears to have been a widower with a child and to have been given short shrift by Florence, who regarded his proposal as 'almost an insult' because he showed so little interest in her 'views and feelings'. In a letter to Fanny Nightingale, describing the incident, she replied to her mother's concern about her single state by questioning whether marriage could possibly have anything to offer her:

* The poet Algernon Swinburne, whom Milnes introduced to the works of Sade, wrote in 1869 that Milnes was '*the* Sadique collector of European fame. His erotic collection of engravings etc. is unrivalled upon earth – unequalled I should imagine in heaven. Nothing low, nothing that is not good and genuine in the way of art and literature is admitted. There is every edition of every work of our dear and honoured Marquis.' Milnes was apparently very relaxed about pointing out the choicest sections of his erotic library to guests staying at Fryston before setting off for Sunday service at the local church. What Florence's attitude would have been can only be surmised, though by Victorian standards she was certainly no prude, and would later maintain, only slightly tongue in cheek, that administrative inefficiency rather than sexual immorality was the far greater sin.

That I am alone nobody can know more deeply than I do. That my life is most solitary and friendless, in the midst of friends, is a truism, how solitary I and only I can tell, but would marriage diminish that solitude? Certainly none of those marriages I have ever seen. I have seen the husbands of my dearest friends curl their lips with a curious kind of smile at how little their wives understood them, & most men know their wives about as much as they know Abraham.

If a woman was able to weather 'an attack of Terror of Old Maidenhood', she had advised Parthenope, '. . . the mad dog goes off, & she does very well'. Florence had weathered such an attack, bravely made a decision, and had now reached a point of no return.

Several years later, when Johnny Stanley, a soldier cousin of Mary Stanley's, searched for words to describe the new heroine of Crimean fame, he found them in a term that precisely reflected Florence's position, at the age of thirty-four, on the lowest rungs of the family chain. 'Miss Nightingale', he recalled for his mother's benefit, was the 'little old maid' they had once met at Dean Milman's.

Richard Monckton Milnes's disappointment, in the summer of 1849, at failing to receive an affirmative answer from Florence to his proposal can only have been equalled – if not exceeded – by Fanny and William Nightingale's regretful feelings on the subject. Fanny, especially, had hoped for this brilliant match, which might have fulfilled at one remove the ambitions she herself had once held of becoming a prominent political hostess. To be fair to Fanny, she had apparently never attempted to influence Florence in Milnes's direction. None the less, she was left with a discontented daughter on her hands, with no obvious solution to her immediate future in sight, and a rising tide of gossip about Florence's reluctance to marry. Again, the Bracebridges stepped in with a plan. They were going to Egypt and Greece for several months and suggested taking Florence with them. 'We have talked & talked day & a night, dear Mrs Bracebridge,' responded Fanny, '& are come to the decision that if you will take our dear child, for better for worse . . . she shall be yours . . . Your letter of this morning makes everything so easy, & Mr Milnes, who happened to be here, gives such an account of the delicious climate and absence of all difficulty in the progress up the Nile that I hope it will be a thorough rest to you all.'

Preparations for the trip were extensive. On the practical side,

Florence was advised to equip herself with 'linen gingham gowns, lined umbrellas for the sun, green spectacles', as well as a host of other accessories, including a small dinghy, a mattress, camphor, and oil as protection against insect bites. To obtain 'the *dernier mot* on Egyptology', she took tea with Bunsen, currently engaged on his massive work of Ancient Egyptian history; and included his books in her packing, along with works by the German Egyptologist Karl Richard Lepsius, and two recent guides to travel in Egypt, John Gardner Wilkinson's *Modern Egypt* – which included among its list of useful things to do in Egypt 'excavating the temple at Heliopolis' and 'clearing the Sphinx' – and Harriet Martineau's *Eastern Life: Past and Present*, published a year earlier. Martineau, who had travelled to Egypt with friends in 1846, wrote that 'a Nile voyage is as serious a labour as the mind and spirit can be involved in'. It was something of a warning of what lay in store for Florence Nightingale as she set off on 1 November accompanied by a young German woman, Trautwein (inevitably called 'Trout'), her maid for the period of the tour. From Folkestone, she scribbled a note to her mother, acknowledging her failings as a daughter: '. . . Bless you more than I can bless you. I hope I shall come back to be more of a comfort to you than ever I have been. Thank you all a thousand times.'

A visit to Egypt may well have been a dream that Florence had nurtured for years. As a young girl, she had read about the exploits of Giovanni Belzoni, the larger-than-life traveller in Egypt and Nubia, whose discoveries, including several tombs in the Valley of Kings and the temple of Rameses II at Abu Simbel, had taken fashionable London by storm in the 1820s. Like many other British tourists who floated up the Nile each year, Florence's fascination with the physical remains of ancient Egyptian culture – some of them still, like the Sphinx, submerged under sand – united with the strong desire to visit biblical sites with their Old Testament connections (at Heliopolis, where Moses was said to have been born, she was crestfallen not to find a bulrush). Egypt was by now, after almost four decades of French and British influence, a convenient, as well as a popular, destination for visitors. Arriving at Alexandria in the final months of the year, when the temperature had dropped to a bearable level, tourists travelled by canal and river to Cairo, where they hired their boat and crew. Blown by the north wind, they sailed upriver – or were towed whenever the wind failed – making only a few brief stops, until they reached the second cataract. Then,

turning round, they began a more leisurely return journey, beginning at
Abu Simbel and inspecting monuments along the 800-mile route.

Florence's letters home from Egypt – which were soon being copied
and handed round in a constant relay among family and friends, and
which eventually she was prevailed upon to have privately published –
are an eloquent and animated commentary on her travels, studded with
dazzling perceptions about Egyptian life, people, and customs, both past
and present. However, running through them, in her response to her
surroundings, is an undercurrent of despair, barely perceptible at times,
but at others clearly indicative of the conflicts that were overwhelming
her mind, and for which she could find no simple resolution. Unlike her
time in Rome, the trip to Egypt would not be a liberating or revitalizing
experience, though, ultimately, it was to have a defining influence on her
thought. Instead it confirmed Florence's sense of her own hopelessness,
pushing her to the edge of breakdown, as she confronted the difficulty
of reconciling duty to family and home with the idea of service to God,
and struggled with the distressing possibility that after all the years of
waiting, that special destiny, ordained by God, might not be hers after
all. It was 'a mistake as old as the world and as young as our time', she
wrote, reflecting this latter preoccupation, 'to suppose oneself called to
a power one has not, to do a thing which is not one's business'. Her
personal crisis is brought into clearer focus in the sparse diary entries –
a marked contrast to her copious letters – in the small *carnet de poche*
she purchased at Marseilles, as she prepared to sail by mail packet to
Malta. Here the veil is lifted on her suffering. She is driven to despair
by her continued dependence on dreaming, which becomes almost
satanic in the course of her struggle to overcome it, and by her efforts
to grapple with the true meaning of her call. (Another diary, covering
the identical period, often in the same bare outline, but without the *cris
de coeur*, resurfaced in 1999. It may have been used as an aide-mémoire
for letters or, perhaps more probably, as a journal account that prying
family eyes could be permitted to see.)

Florence was in relatively high spirits at the outset, enlivened by a day
observing nursing practice at 'the model establishment of the world',
the Hôtel-Dieu, as she, Trout and the Bracebridges passed through
Lyons. Once in Alexandria, where they arrived on 18 November, she
made good use of an introduction to the hospital there, provided by two
sisters of St Vincent de Paul, whom she had met on the train from Paris.

She accumulated some 'valuable lessons', attending on the sisters as they treated the Arabs, who came daily to them from surrounding villages, for diarrhoea, dysentery or ophthalmia. Another day they made an excursion to the site of the Battle of Aboukir, an unimpressive area of white sand fringed with a few dismal palm trees where, half a century earlier, Nelson had defeated and destroyed the French fleet. Florence was anxious to see the inside of a mosque, and so, disguising herself in a suffocating Egyptian outfit, which seemed to allow breathing only through the eyes, and, with the strict injunction not to show her hands, she slipped into one during evening prayers, followed at a close, protective distance by Mr Gilbert, the British consul. The 'hopeless' lives of Muslim women made her thankful she was a Christian, and while praising Islam for its charity of fellowship – unlike the charity of patronage that existed at home – she refused to believe that there was much chance for a nation whose religion placed such emphasis on the gratification of man's passions.

In the final week of November they left Alexandria, towed up the Mahmoudieh Canal by steam-tug to Afteh, where they boarded the *Marchioness of Breadalbane*, bound for Cairo. Also on board was a twenty-eight-year-old Frenchman, Gustave Flaubert. Although there is no evidence that Florence and the future author of *Madame Bovary* met, Flaubert left an unflattering reference in his travel notes to an 'English family' he had observed during the voyage, whom he thought 'hideous', and who may have been the Nightingale–Bracebridge party. He described 'the mother', with her green eyeshade attached to her bonnet, as looking 'like a sick old parrot'. Was this Selina Bracebridge? Flaubert's fantasy-fuelled time in Egypt – shaving his head, dancing about in a 'screaming red' *tarboosh*, and seeking homoerotic experiences in the Cairo baths – was to prove radically different from Florence's; but that first night they spent on the Nile, he sleeping up on deck, on a camp bed in the open air, she below, in the cramped quarters of the ladies' cabin, they shared the inspiration of a picturesque view of the moon, and of Venus, the morning star. Significantly, though, as the pyramids appeared against the sky, Florence discovered that she could not muster 'a single sensation'.

In Cairo they hired a houseboat, a *dahabieh*, for £30 a month, to take them up the Nile. They were the first Europeans to use the boat, as it had been built by a bey for his harem. The accommodation consisted of a day cabin, with a divan around the walls, on which Trout slept, and two sleeping cabins, separated by a passage containing large closets. A 'capital invention', the Levinge, into which the body was inserted and laced up tightly, like a mummy, ensured protection against mosquitoes. The nine-man crew, among them the black steersman on the poop, 'who never moves day or night', lived on open deck. Paolo, an old servant who had travelled with the Bracebridges in Syria fifteen years before, and experienced many Nile winters since, was to be their mainstay, while the cooking, in a tiny area at the prow, from provisions stored in chests and hanging from cages, was the responsibility of Mustafa. Mustafa's supplies were supplemented during the voyage by bread from village ovens, and other fresh produce, and by Mr Bracebridge's shooting expeditions on shore. The *dahabieh* was christened *Parthenope*, and in further honour of her sister, whose health had recently taken a turn for the worse, Florence made a pennant, 'blue bunting with swallowtails, a Latin red cross upon it', with 'Parthenope' in Greek lettering, sewn in white tape. 'It has taken all my tape and a vast amount of stitches,' she wrote, 'but it will be the finest pennant on the river, and my petticoats will joyfully acknowledge the tribute to sisterly affection . . .' With this tribute fluttering at the yardarm, the Bracebridge colours were hoisted halfway up the rigging. A Union Jack flew at the stern. They set sail on 4 December.

The sun went down, she noted, as if it hadn't the strength to colour the clouds, an observation which rather reflected Florence's own prevailing mood. She had declared herself 'no dahabieh bird, no divan incumbent', and when the wind dropped, she generally disembarked and went ashore with a member of the crew (passengers were banned from walking on deck for fear that they might bring in fleas). In the early days, it seemed as if the wind had blown itself out; then, suddenly, at the end of the second week, a *khamsin* (sand wind) arrived from the south-east, so strong that the sailors could not pull against it, and they were forced to remain anchored under the shelter of a bank.

  For much of the voyage, though, Florence lay in 'a sort of torpor' on the divan, reading aloud to Mr Bracebridge, or composing a 'little history of Egypt' for his benefit (Wilkinson's work she judged 'notoriously incorrect', while Bunsen's was 'very confused for common use'). Time itself appeared to have been suspended in the lethargy of their daily rhythms – an illusion assisted by the long delays in posts from England – and she experienced the eerie sensation, as they floated slowly along, that she was on a passage to another world. It was as if she had lost all feeling of distance, as the figures on the shore loomed unnaturally large. 'You seem to lose all feeling of identity too,' she wrote after a week, 'and everything becomes supernatural.'

Everything was also inordinately ugly. The unnatural 'colourlessness' of Egypt, in its two or three shades of brown, disturbed her, while its landscapes seemed positively diabolical in their petrified, mortified state: 'one almost fancies one hears the Devil laughing'. She had Trout read the story of Joseph to her, but still, for all its biblical associations, the 'dying, withered' desert remained the work of the devil, 'an earth tumbled up and down', and it was a relief to look up at the radiant sky, or to dig out a shell from the sand. Touring Egypt, with its spectral landscape of monuments and graves, was, she realized, nothing like visiting sights in Italy or the south of France. 'It is like the ghoul visiting the tombs.' At their first stop, the sepulchres of Beni Hasan – apart from the pyramids, the most ancient antiquities in Egypt – she was both awed and diminished by the thought that, 4 or 5,000 years before, men 'who thought and felt like us' had stood nearby; but she could hardly contain her irritation at the behaviour of Trout, who sat with her back to the door of one tomb, busily crocheting a polka pattern, instead of studying the hieroglyphs on the doorpost. The company of this 'wretched' woman, with whom Florence constantly bickered, was only bearable when Trout had toothache, and became 'nurse-able'.

What horrified Florence most, and seemed to confirm the unbridgeable gulf between the heights of ancient Egyptian culture, and the degradation to which modern Egypt had sunk, was the squalor and misery of its people. After a period of relative stability under Muhammed Ali, the Albanian mercenary supported by both the French, and the British, who wanted a safe passage to India, Egypt had reverted to political turmoil, and in 1849 the country was ruled, tyrannically and avariciously, by the reactionary despot Abbas, Ali's grandson. Nothing had prepared Florence for the shock of the ordinary people's 'voluntary abasement', not even the adventures of the explorers Mungo Park and James Bruce, whose descriptions of African villages she had read in order to under-stand conditions on her own travels. At Asyut, the capital of Upper Egypt, she found 'the sort of city the animals might have built when

they had possession of the earth ... a collection of mud-heaps ...';
while the village that had grown up in the ruins of the temple at Luxor,
with houses with doorways only four feet high, utterly appalled her. 'To
see human beings ... choosing to crawl upon the ground like reptiles,
to live in a place where they could not stand upright ... I longed to have
intercourse with them, to stay with them, and make plans for them; but
here one gathered one's clothes about one, and felt as if one had trodden
in a nest of reptiles.' She compared them with the underclass in London
and Edinburgh and found them wanting, declaring that whereas the
British poor were 'still human beings', the poor of Egypt were no more
than 'beasts'. Even the 'South Sea savages' that ran away from her, 'like
a troop of jackals', at Elephantine, were somehow a disappointment:
they were 'not shiny as savages ought to be, but their black skins all dim
and grimed with sand like dusty tables ... I heard some stones fall into
the river and hoped it was they and that that debased life had finished ...'

Choosing to represent the inhabitants of modern Egypt as animals
was nothing new, and was in fact an unpalatable aspect of a wider,
ongoing ethnographical debate about the racial origins of these latterday
Egyptians. By the 1840s, such comparisons were already commonplace
in travel literature. Harriet Martineau, for one, had described modern
Egyptians as 'frogs, camels, bees, ants, beavers, sheep, birds, pigs, deer,
rabbits, and apes'. But Florence Nightingale went a step further. Her
compassion had failed her. She had denied her fellow human beings
their humanity, as well as imagining the unforgivable, a fantasy of their
extinction. Of course, her words were hyperbolic, a means of wishing
away 'that horrible Egyptian present' in order to concentrate on the
magnificent richness of its past. But they were also an expression of
self-disgust at her own impotence. The discovery that she was unable to
help the poor and dispossessed in Egypt – 'the impossibility' of doing
them 'the slightest good' – must have deeply concerned her; and her
depiction of the Egyptians as inhuman, and therefore ineligible for her
care, may have been a way of mitigating that distress.

Her study of comparative religion was another way of retreating into
the past. Florence was fascinated by the parallels between an ancient,
monotheistic Egyptian religion, in which 'one God' was represented
under various names to express 'the different relations under which God
appeared to His creatures', and the familiar Christian version of the
Trinity. She was especially attracted to the worship of the goddess Isis

at Philae. According to myth, Osiris was a beneficent pharaoh, murdered by his brother Seth, and resurrected by his wife Isis. Osiris's resurrection signified the regeneration of all life, and had obvious resonances of the passion of Christ, so much so that following a visit to Osiris's chamber, Florence crept back alone a few days later, to lay her crucifix in the sand.

'Egypt is beginning to speak a language to me . . .,' Florence wrote to her family shortly after the *Parthenope* reached Abu Simbel, in the middle of January 1850. On a visit to the rock-cut temples of Rameses II and his queen Nefertari, from the second century BC, she found the solitude and silence that she craved, and experienced a moment of spiritual and intellectual epiphany, which she described in a long letter home. Gazing at the colossal figure of Rameses himself, she saw him crowned on either side by the principles of good and evil, and instantly understood that 'The evil is not the opposer of the good but its *collaborateur*, the left hand of God, as the good is His right.' The lesson she derived from this was clear. God makes laws which mankind breaks, and man's evil, equated with his error, is a necessary agent of the teaching through which God will bring each and every one of us to perfection.

Modern Egypt, she now saw, must have broken some law of nature to have fallen to such a degraded state. The issue that remained was, were all nations to sink in this way? 'Or will a nation find out at last the laws of God by which she may make a steady progression?' This idea – that mankind is called upon by God, not as a worshipper or petitioner, but as the *discoverer* of the workings of His laws – was to provide the foundation for her work in the future. Egypt, she wrote, is a country which, 'like its own old Nile, has overflowed and fertilised the world'. It also fertilized Florence Nightingale's thinking.

But, in the midst of these insights, she 'spoiled it all by dreaming'. Dreaming had become her 'enemy', the 'constant murderer of my thoughts'; she chastised herself for daring to dream 'in the very face of God', and in the diary she began for the New Year, she begged to be delivered 'from this slavery'. At times she could participate fully in the sightseeing that was going on around her, and then suddenly her thoughts wandered, and she was lost. She had been longing to visit Karnak, with its three major temples one of the most impressive sights in all Egypt, but when they arrived there in mid-February, she was barely able to take it in. 'Karnak – & where was I?' she wrote distractedly, 'all the while that I was on Propylon [the monumental entrance to the temple precinct], & half the afternoon, dreaming, Karnak itself cannot save me now – it has no voice for me.' She had been writing home almost every other day throughout the first part of that month. On 27 February, however, she completed a letter, and then didn't write again for ten days, the longest gap in her Egyptian correspondence. The reason for this silence is evident from her diary: God had spoken to her again.

'God called me with my Madre's words,' she recorded. Could she do good for God without desiring 'great things for herself'? And would she be able to suppress her own will and accept whatever God had in store for her? In the course of the next few months, these were the questions that dogged her, and which she continually agonized over, as she contemplated her future.

March 3. Sunday . . . Did not get up in the morning but God gave me the time afterwards . . . a solitary 2 hours in my own cabin, to 'meditate' on my Madre's words . . .

March 7. Thursday. Gale all night. Lying under Gebel Hereedee [south of Thebes]. God called me in the morning & asked me 'Would I do good for Him, for Him without the reputation.'

March 8. Friday. Thought much upon this question. My Madre said to me Can you hesitate between the God of the whole Earth & your little reputation? as I sat looking out on the sunrise upon the river in my cabin after dinner.

March 9. Saturday. During half an hour I had by myself in the cabin . . . Settled the question with God . . .

March 12. Tuesday. Very sleepy. Stood at the door of the boat looking out upon the stars & the tallmast in the still night against the sky . . . & tried to think only of God's will – & that everything is desirable only as He is in it or not in it – only as it brings us nearer or farther from Him. He is speaking to us often just when something we think untoward happens.

Back in Cairo, having said their farewells to the crew, who displayed their gratitude merely for not having been maltreated, Florence, with Trout and the Bracebridges, returned to Alexandria, where they spent their final day in Egypt on 6 April. The British naval blockade of the Piraeus, a result of the Don Pacifico affair, in which Palmerston, as Foreign Secretary, supported the claims of a British subject, a Jewish merchant who had lost his property during anti-semitic rioting in Athens, caused them to take a circuitous route to Athens. On board an Austrian ship, the *Schild*, they were refused permission to land at Corfu, and travelled instead by a 'panoramic' route on to Italy, still suffering under Austrian occupation, via Trieste, Ancona and Brindisi, finally reaching Athens on 22 April. Florence viewed Athens with the eyes of a classical scholar, though she was disappointed that the city resembled 'a cork model', and shocked by the small size of everything. Her imagination had exaggerated them because of their historical significance.

On a visit to the Acropolis, she bought from some Greek boys a baby owl that had fallen from its nest. Naming her Athena, after the Greek goddess of wisdom, the owlet became Florence's constant companion, riding on her shoulder, or sitting in her pocket. Athena was a peevish creature. She required a daily sand bath, possessed an annoying taste for 'tangled cotton' – to say nothing of her appetite for Florence's cicada Plato, whom she hungrily gobbled – and had to be coaxed out of her cage by mesmerism. Nor was her appearance exactly appealing. 'A few hints on washing and dressing would be of great use for her . . .' Florence wrote later that summer. 'She has rubbed all the feathers off her nose . . . and half of them off her neck . . . Σ has constructed for her a little bag, which pulls up tight around her neck and in which she sits when on my lap.'

The Bracebridges introduced Florence to John Henry Hill and his wife, Frances, Episcopal missionaries who had founded the first schools in Athens, after the expulsion of the Turks in the Greek War of Independence. Frances Hill quickly became an object of Florence's devotion, as Florence observed her giving Bible lessons in her school, respecting the traditions of the Greek Orthodox Church and making no attempt to proselytize her pupils. Mrs Hill emphasized the will of God as the guiding force in her life, and in relating the story of her work as a missionary told Florence that 'It was always God who made the initiative never she.' Her example, and 'the few words of love' she offered, were a source of comfort to Florence. Here was a woman who, outside the confines of religious order, had listened intently to what God was telling her, and had successfully acted upon her call.

Florence resolved once more to 'think only of God's will'. In marking her thirtieth birthday on 12 May, she wrote to her mother of her 'misspent' youth, and of how she had longed to reach thirty, 'the age when our Saviour began his more active life'. But the path forward remained unclear. Reading the *Memoirs* of Henry Martyn, an Anglican missionary who was chaplain to the East India Company in the first years of the century, she made a number of extracts that expressed her inner turmoil: 'To have a will of my own, not agreeable to God's is a most tremendous folly'; 'I pass so many hours as if there were no God at all.'

She also found a reflection of her spiritual and mental distress in William Cowper's autobiography of his early life, in which he wrote of the alternating bouts of torture and consolation provided by his religious faith, and described his attempts at suicide. 'Reading Cowper's life – his madness – or is he sane & is it we who are mad? There is no one whom I feel such a sympathy for as Cowper – his deep despondency, his earnest single heartedness.'

Her own despondency increased its hold. She suffered sleepless nights, punctuated by dreaming, and emerged 'physically & morally ill & broken down, a slave'. At this point, Selina Bracebridge intervened like some *deus ex machina*. Acutely sympathetic to Florence's condition, Mrs Bracebridge made a plan that she knew would alleviate her suffering: on their way home through Germany, she and her husband would stay at Düsseldorf, while Florence spent a fortnight at Kaiserswerth. There was no time to seek permission from the Nightingales for this change of plan, though in a letter to her parents from Berlin on 12 July, Florence mentioned Kaiserswerth as a possibility – 'if you don't object'. But there was no word from them.

In any case, Florence was by now too exhausted to worry much about her parents' reaction. Her greatest wish, her goal of visiting Kaiserswerth, was almost within her grasp, but at this final stage her resolve faltered. She had no 'spirit', no 'energy', she wrote in her diary after a 'miserable' week in Berlin. 'I had 3 paths among which to choose – I might have been a married woman, a literary woman, or a Hospital Sister. Now it seemed to me, as if quiet, with somebody to look for my coming back, was all I wanted.' Nevertheless, the earliest surviving photograph of Florence, taken in Berlin, suggests if not an awareness of triumph, then certainly a sense of relief at being so close to accomplishing her object. This carte-de-visite shows her pale, though surprisingly full in the face, eyes cast down reading a book, with the hint of a smile playing on her lips.

Her purpose was revived by a visit to Berlin's Bethanien Hospital, a deaconess institution established with Fliedner's support from Kaiserswerth; and, as they passed through Hamburg, she returned with admiration from a tour of the Amalienstift, a children's hospital, home for the poor, and a school for girls, directed by its founder Amalie Sieveking. In letters home, Florence wrote pointedly about the respectability of both institutions. Bethanien was like a palace, the rooms resembled those at Embley, and she wished English people 'could see how perfectly possible it is to unite the cultivated woman with the Sister of Charity'; while Sieveking was an outstanding example of an educated woman who wished to give other members of her sex 'real Christian liberty'.

Setting off early on 31 July from Pyrmont, where Charles Bracebridge was undergoing a water cure, Florence reached Kaiserswerth at eight o'clock that evening. She could hardly believe that she was there at last, but knew at once that it was home.

6. Your Vagabond Son

Kaiserswerth, now as then, lies six and a half miles below Düsseldorf, on the right bank of the Rhine, at a point where the river is at its widest. In 1850, the Institution of Deaconesses was a jumble of assorted buildings and enclosed grounds that had gradually grown up around a tiny summerhouse in the vicarage garden. It was to this place of refuge, no more than twelve feet square, that the Lutheran pastor Theodore Fliedner and his wife Friederike had welcomed their first inmate, Minna, a released prisoner, in 1833. Three years later, the Institution was formally established. Fliedner's purchase of a large house nearby enabled them to add first an infant school, and then a hospital, where the first deaconess, Gertrude Reinhardt, the daughter of a doctor, nursed male and female patients with the assistance of seven probationary sisters. By the time of Florence Nightingale's arrival at Kaiserswerth, Fliedner's foundation had expanded on to a firmer footing. The penitentiary and asylum for released female prisoners, intended as a place of transition between prison and reintroduction into society, was kept separate from the rest of the Institution, and its numbers restricted to fifteen at any one time. Those with a good record of behaviour after a year or two – procurement of brandy was often cited as marking the beginning of a slide to recidivism – could count on having jobs secured for them. A school, with training for deaconesses, and an orphan asylum existed alongside the infant school; and the hospital now contained 100 beds, divided into four wards, for men, women, boys and children (defined as girls under seventeen and boys under six). The number of deaconesses totalled 116. Of these twenty-two were still probationary, and sixty-seven scattered abroad in hospitals, parishes and poorhouses in Germany, England, America and Palestine, leaving just under fifty deaconesses at the mother house. Such was the demand for Kaiserswerth Deaconesses as Christian carers for the sick and the young that, as Florence noted, 'More are eagerly desired.'

Florence was received kindly by Fliedner and his second wife Caroline, a former student of Amalie Sieveking's from Hamburg, on the evening of 31 July and, accompanied by Trout, spent that night at the local inn. Following a tour of the community the next day, her 'hope was answered', and she was admitted to the *Diakonissen Anstalt* [Institution of Deaconesses]. Returning to the inn, she dismissed Trout, collected her belongings, and returned to spend her first night at the Institution, where the Fliedners had invited her to stay at their own home, one of a row of houses overlooking a walled garden used by the patients. After all the distress of the past weeks, she was recovering her mental and physical strength. 'I felt queer,' she recorded in her diary, 'but the courage which falls into my shoes in a London drawing room rises on an occasion like this. I felt so sure it was God's work.'

This stay at Kaiserswerth was to be all too brief, just under a fortnight, but during that time Florence managed to devote two or three days to the work of each department. On her first full day she visited the children's ward with Schwester Katerina before taking a trip with a crowd of excited children to bathe in the Rhine; and on following days she observed teaching in the schools, took part in prayers, and inspected the wards on a night watch with the apothecary sister. The deaconesses' living conditions were spartan. Meat was served only twice a week, the greater part of their diet consisting of broths and soups, cooked from vegetables grown on the forty acres of land behind the pastor's house, which also served as pasture for the Institution's eight cows and several horses. Florence didn't mind the frugal meals, objecting more to the inadequate washing facilities. 'I hope you have struggled for a tub of cold water and then the rest won't signify – but don't give up that for health's sake,' Mrs Bracebridge wrote to her from Pyrmont on Florence's third day at Kaiserswerth. 'I am sure you are right: these fancy hospitals will never answer for England – the coarse practical affair is what you must look to and, if you find sincerity and religious feeling at K., that's the school to learn it, though one hates the ugliness of nakedness.' These were exactly the qualities that were impressing Florence. The friendliness of the sisters in sharing their knowledge was remarkable, especially when contrasted with the jealous behaviour of nurses and surgeons in hospitals at home. Furthermore, in the familial atmosphere she found a sense of belonging, encouraged by the invitation to call Caroline Fliedner 'Mother'. Prospective deaconesses served a probationary term of up to three years, and once admitted they served a five-year period, after which they could renew their commitment or leave the Institution. Yet although the Institution stood *in loco parentis*, deaconesses could be released at any time should they wish to marry, return to their parents, or respond to any other claim on them. This was the fact of central significance for Florence, that Kaiserswerth existed '*free from vows or cloistered cells*'.

Religious feeling suffused everything, and nowhere was this more evident than in the hospital, where Florence noted a simple, but crucial, underlying principle: that women undertaking their office out of Christian motives of love and service would make better nurses than those who did it merely for money (deaconesses received just a small, subsistence salary after six months). Train a nurse to exert a spiritual and moral influence over her patients, and her work would not only be more purposeful and less 'toilsome', it would also contribute to the atmosphere of Christian 'gracefulness'; for wasn't sickness 'one of the means sent by God to soften the heart'? In a letter to her father, Florence admitted that the Kaiserswerth hospital was 'poor & ugly' and that it presented 'by no means a pattern of cleanliness'. Nevertheless, 'with regard to all essential points' it offered 'a model for England' because of its 'humanizing, refining, propriety-teaching' qualities, and 'the tender care' of its nurses. She was struck by several other aspects of the hospital's practice: the lecture, filled with guidance and plain instructions, given each week to the nurses by Pastor Fliedner; the rules of strict propriety, which ensured that male wards were served by male nurses, under the supervision of the deaconesses, and that no sister could enter the men's wards after 8 p.m.; and the absence of a medical man from permanent residence on site, so that the clergyman remained master of the hospital.

Florence attributed the success of the Institution to the charismatic personality of Fliedner himself, to his spirit of self-denial, and to his ability to delegate. She was less enamoured of his autocratic ways. At fifty, he was 'a man of a thousand, not agreeable, not interesting, but if you can fancy a Napoleon who has dedicated all his gifts to God, without a Napoleon's vanity, that is Fliedner's character'. Before he and Florence parted, Fliedner requested that she write something to introduce Kaiserswerth's work to an English audience. Reunited at Düsseldorf with Mr and Mrs Bracebridge, and 'feeling so brave as if nothing could ever vex me again', she began writing after they reached Cologne on 14 August, completing the thirty-two-page pamphlet at

Ghent on the seventeenth while the Bracebridges waited patiently for her to finish. Up at sunrise the next day, she wrote out a fair copy and then handed it over to Charles Bracebridge to make corrections. On 19 August, she sent it off to Fliedner with a covering letter in French (her written German was inadequate for the purpose) stating that 'As I have undertaken this little exercise in obedience to your wishes, I must be allowed to stipulate that my name may never be mentioned in connection with it . . .'

The Institution of Kaiserswerth on the Rhine, for the Practical Training of Deaconesses was Florence Nightingale's first published work; it is also a largely neglected document of mid-nineteenth-century feminism. At Pyrmont, before setting off for Kaiserswerth, Florence had been reading *Shirley*, Charlotte Brontë's second published novel, which had appeared the week before she left England. While Shirley Keeldar, the eponymous heroine, is an heiress whose wealth allows her more freedom than most members of her sex, her friend Caroline Helstone, devoid of independent income and immediate family, is forced to depend on her uncle for her livelihood; and it is through her character that Charlotte Brontë explores the dilemma for young, educated, middle-class women of finding some meaningful activity to engage them. A despondent Caroline declares her frustration, at one point, at her lack of a purposeful existence: 'I often wonder what I came into this world for. I long to have something absorbing and compulsory to fill my head and hands, and to occupy my thoughts.'

Caroline's words, and the memory of the well-born Prussian women she had encountered in Berlin, whose freedom from social restraints had struck her forcibly, may well have been uppermost in Florence's mind as she began to write her booklet. As a preamble to her main business of describing the work of the Institution, she asked why so much opportunity was given to modern woman 'to cultivate her powers', and so little to finding her '*necessary* occupation':

If . . . there are many women who live unmarried, and many more who pass the third of the usual term of life unmarried, and if intellectual occupation is not meant to be their end in life, what are they to do with that thirst for action, which every woman feels who is not diseased in mind or body? God planted it there . . . What were His intentions with regard to 'unmarried women and widows?' How did he mean to employ them, to satisfy them?

One answer – 'For every want we can find a divine supply' – lay in the office of deaconess. Since the early Christians, as Florence demonstrated by careful marshalling of her evidence, women had been accepted by the Church in the service of the sick and poor. Moreover, long before the establishment of the order of the Sisters of Mercy by St Vincent de Paul in 1633, these women had existed free from vows. It was common prejudice to believe that the office of deaconess was copied from the Roman Catholic Church, when in fact it had existed among all Christian churches, 'and earliest in those of the Protestant faith'. Florence's conclusion was that 'God has not implanted an impulse in the hearts of women without preparing a way for them to obey it.'

The pamphlet appeared in 1851, printed by the inmates of her Ragged School in St Ann's Street, Westminster. Florence's insistence on her anonymity was undoubtedly an attempt to live up to the Madre's precepts about sacrificing her reputation (as well as protecting her identity from the other sisters should she find herself among them again); but it also appeased her family, by then acutely anxious that in the interest of respectability no hint of Florence's connection with Kaiserswerth should reach the ears of the wider world. This cloak of secrecy not only contributed to the pamphlet's neglect, it also appears to have expunged the memory of her first production from Florence's own mind. In 1897, when the British Museum approached her to request a copy for its collection, she claimed never to have thought of the booklet again after the original print-run had been distributed, and a thorough search of the house in South Street eventually produced only a couple of dirty and badly torn examples.

From Cologne Florence had scribbled a message to her father on the back of an envelope, as if she was laying out a programme for her future and seeking his approval. 'I think Kaiserswerth quite all that I expected and a few months there would teach an Englishwoman all that is necessary if she had sense to apply it with the modifications necessary for England.' There was no doubt in her own mind that she had to return.

Florence parted from the Bracebridges on the morning of 21 August, after reaching London from Dover the night before, and took the train from Euston Square to Amber Gate. By three that afternoon she was back at Lea Hurst, surprising her 'dear people' in the drawing room.

While she sat on the sofa talking to them, Athena the owl popped out
suddenly from her pocket to introduce herself. Later the Fowlers came
to dinner, and the next day Florence talked to her parents in the nursery.
She had been away for almost ten months, so there was much for them
all to tell one another. On the 23rd, Professor James Pillans, the Scottish
educational reformer, arrived to stay. At this point, Florence's diary,
maintained since the beginning of the year in Egypt, peters out, as the
life of the daughter at home once again asserted itself.

Selina Bracebridge had offered to 'make no mention of your being at
Kaiserswerth in any letter to England in case you have not named it at
home'; but although Florence had been completely open about going to
Kaiserswerth, prolonged delays to the posts meant that the Nightingales
may only have learned of her decision shortly before she returned home,
certainly too late for them to do anything to prevent her visit. Her
parents' disapproval remained, but it must have begun to dawn upon
her father at least that they were fighting a losing battle. In the five years
since Florence had announced to her horrified family that she wanted to
train as a nurse, a number of nursing reform initiatives, including the
Protestant Sisterhoods, had emerged that were founded and led by
middle-class 'ladies', every bit as respectable as the Nightingales themselves. The existence of these effectively gave the lie to the notion that
nurses had inevitably to be slovenly working-class women of dubious
moral character. This was a point underlined by Mrs Bracebridge as she
joined forces with Aunt Mai to try to make Fanny Nightingale see
the situation in a new light. 'The opinion of the world . . . has much
changed . . .,' she observed. 'Young ladies of a standing in society, quite
equal to Flo's, do things now of this kind, which were unheard of
formerly, witness the Ladies at Clewer, the district visitors in London –
the Hospital in Chandos Street . . . they are not in any way looked down
upon because they devote themselves to Hospitals or Patients.' But the
Nightingales' continuing opposition to their daughter taking up nursing
did not arise simply from objections to the conditions of hospitals and
their staff. It was also based on a larger, much more inchoate fear of
Florence deserting her home and her duty, contributing to the break-up
of the family, and leaving her parents and sister to fend for themselves.
In some desperation to prevent this happening, they sought alternatives
around Embley and the Hurst, emphasizing to Florence the attractions
of local parish and school work. But they must have known how vain

their efforts were: there were never going to be projects at home of
sufficient scope and interest to keep Florence occupied.

One vital factor which made these problems altogether more intractable, and contributed over the next few years to a rising mood of
bitterness on Florence's part, and a staunch obstinacy on her mother's
and sister's, was Parthenope's physical and mental condition. During
Florence's time away, both of these, inextricably linked, had sharply
deteriorated. Hilary Bonham Carter, characteristically, had tried to lift
Parthenope's spirits in Florence's absence, imagining 'your Flo floating
up the Nile: & yourself – standing with cheerful heroism on the slopes
of Albion – letting her go again from you, & rejoicing in it too'. This,
however, was the last thing that Parthenope was able to do. She longed
to share an ideal life with her brilliant younger sister, and felt shut out
and excluded by Florence's vocation, which she could not understand
nor, as yet, play any part in; she resented her sister's absences, which
had become longer and more frequent, and envied her freedom (Madame
Mohl thought that 'Dear Flo's vocation' had bereaved Parthenope 'as
the absence or death of a lover might do'). These feelings had become
fixations in her mind, dominating her with a mounting intensity that
can only be described in terms of monomania. In the early summer of
1850, while Florence was in Greece, coping with her own mental distress,
Parthenope had been sent to London to stay at the Hyde Park Gardens
home of family friends, the Coltmans. It may seem an odd prescription
for a cure to send someone who is ill out of the country into the heart
of a busy city at the height of the season, but the reasoning behind it
appears to have been that it would help to remove Parthenope from
familiar scenes, keeping her 'intellectual . . . & physical existence equally
quiescent' while the Nightingales awaited Florence's return. Such was
their anxiety about the possible effect on Parthenope of seeing her
sister again that William Nightingale briefly toyed with suggesting that
Florence 'take another ¼ of a year before she reappears amongst us'.

But this was hardly a workable solution, and in any case, Parthenope
could barely wait to be reunited with Florence. The Waverley cousin
who wrote to Parthenope, just days after Florence's homecoming, about
'the intense satisfaction' she must feel 'to have a _real_ sister again, that
you can look at, & touch & feel, bodily as well spiritually your own!'
can scarcely have guessed just how close to the mark this description
came. Now the Nightingales reversed their earlier opinion and decided

that, in view of her long absence and its contribution to the deterioration of her sister's health, Florence should devote the next six months exclusively to Parthenope. It didn't take long, however, for this plan to be exposed as a failure as all Parthenope's old niggling resentments began to resurface: criticism of Florence's silences, of her preference for working among the villagers instead of joining in the tedious daily round of social observances, and most of all, of her undisguised intention to pursue her nursing training. 'I can hardly open my mouth without giving my dear Parthe vexation,' Florence observed later. As if to spite her sister, Parthenope refused to allow Florence 'to rub her', or take any active part in nursing her, though, as Florence told her parents, 'being allowed to take charge of Parthe in the nursing line, would have been enough to live upon . . .' Nor did Parthenope's health show any improvement under this new regime. She started drawing again, but was forced to give it up as 'it excites her too much'; not surprisingly, given that her favourite subject, over and over – in full-length studies, or head and shoulders only, in imagined or biographical scenes – was Florence herself.

The family dynamic was set for the foreseeable future: Parthenope possessive and unrelenting, Fanny protective and supportive of her, Florence looking for any opportunity to escape. William Nightingale tried to remain a passive onlooker, admitting to Fanny that 'my selfishness tells me to let all alone & leave you womenfolk to your own battles'. But the truth of this pathetic state of affairs, as he confessed wearily to his sister Mai, was that Fanny and Parthenope agreed to such an extent on every subject that his only recourse was to silence, 'for even to enunciate anything seemed to unite them to oppose'.

At the beginning of October, a visit with Aunt Mai to Grandmother Shore's house at Tapton offered Florence her first respite, since her return home, from the emotional pressure of her domestic situation. In Aunt Mai she knew she could count on a sympathetic ear for her problems, an interested one too in their shared passion for religious and philosophical debate. A week 'in this undisturbed way' with Florence, Mai told her daughter Blanche, 'was one of the greatest pleasures I could have'. Florence, who was 'handsomer than ever', had opened her heart to her – 'do not repeat anything I say of her', Blanche was warned – and had discussed with Mai the importance of returning to Kaiserswerth for a more intensive period. Her aunt supported her, and admired the way in which Florence refused to give in to disappointment. Yet she could also see the other side of the argument. 'Her bent is so decided, but in a direction so opposed to her surroundings. I cannot wonder that her people should see quite differently . . . You know her interests would be for hospitals . . . & much in connection with them she has at heart, which at present it seems impossible to realise. I feel quite indisposed to talk of her generally, for some would blame her, some would blame her people (Aunt Julia the latter), equally unreasonably.'

When, later that month, Mai went to stay with her mother's sister Aunt Evans at Cromford Bridge in Derbyshire, it was straightforward enough for Florence to prolong her absence from home by telling her parents that Aunt Mai had asked that she accompany her. In her late eighties, Aunt Evans was a spirited old lady, but also one that any member of her family dreaded being left alone with, as she liked nothing better than an opportunity to air all her old grievances, chiefly those directed against her sister, Grandmother Shore.

It was at Cromford Bridge, in the second half of October, that they received news of Henry Nicholson's death in Spain. While Aunt Mai wondered whether her old black satin gown would do for mourning 'if trimmed with crepe', Florence subjected the details of his accident, gathered by Henry's brother Sam, who had rushed to the scene of the tragedy to gather what information he could, to close scrutiny. It was difficult to come to any solid conclusions. Henry had been travelling in a diligence with a friend, and fifteen other passengers, through an area of Valencia where the roads were poor. According to one report, the diligence, pulled by mules on a narrow coastal path, was swept out to sea by a sudden 'avalanche of water'. Another account blamed the driver for falling asleep during a thunderstorm which so frightened the mules that they lost their footing and plunged the carriage down a seventy-foot drop into the water. Henry's companion, Mr Beavan, was the only survivor, having leaped from the diligence just in time.

Florence visited 'the House of Mourning' at Waverley during the last week of November. Henry had been 'the axis on which the whole family turned'. Uncle Nicholson could hardly speak of his dead son – 'I should not wonder if it were to shorten his life' – while 'the poor mother cannot quite keep "if this," and "if that had not been so" out of her mind's eye'. As for Marianne, Florence longed for Lothian Nicholson's return from his army posting in North America so that he could comfort his sister. Meanwhile, she was anxious to get Mr Beavan on his own to test the veracity of his story, which she found unconvincing in certain details. If she felt any personal remorse at the death of a man whose love for her she may once have rejected, there was no sign of it, though Aunt Patty noted how much paler and graver she looked. If anything, as Florence told her father, Henry's death had 'brightened & strengthened' her views of life. '. . . I do so agree with you <u>not to regret</u>,' she wrote to her friend Georgina Tollet, ' – to look at the thing as a whole as God's will – surely that is the way He intends – there is no <u>truth</u> in those regrets.'

At Embley, though, as the old year faded out, she was overwhelmed by her failure to break her habit of dreaming – which 'like gin drinking' was 'eating out my vital strength' – guilt-stricken at the pain she was causing her family, depressed by the loss of Monckton Milnes, and welcoming the thought of her own death, as she could see no prospect of her situation ever changing. On 30 December she recorded that 'I have no desire now but to die.'

Unconsciousness is all that I desire. I remain in bed as late as I can, for what have I to wake for? I am perishing for want of food . . . Therefore I spend my days in dreams of other situations which will afford me food . . .

Starvation does not lead a man to exertion; it only weakens him. Oh weary days, oh evenings that never seem to end. For how many long years I have watched that drawing room clock & thought it never would reach the ten & for 20 or so more years to do this. It is not the misery, the unhappiness that I feel so insupportable, but to feel this habit, this disease gaining power upon me – & no hope, no help. This is the sting of death.

In such a state, there was no disguising her condition from her family. 'I feel myself perishing when I go to bed,' she told them at Christmas. 'I wish it were my grave.'

One woman, whom Florence came to regard as a fellow-worker, contributed to strengthening her resolve. Small, shy and with a glass eye, Elizabeth Blackwell had made medical history in January 1849, when she became the first woman to qualify and register as a doctor. *Punch*, the Nightingales' favourite weekly, apostrophized her in doggerel. 'Young ladies all, of every clime/Especially of Britain,/Who wholly occupy your time/In novels and in knitting,/Whose highest skill is but to play,/Sing, dance, or French to clack well,/Reflect on the example pray,/Of excellent Miss Blackwell.'

Blackwell had gained admission, the only female student among 150 men, to an obscure medical school at Geneva, in New York State, by a fluke. The dean and faculty of the college had put her application to a student vote, confident that it would be rejected. Instead, the students voted unanimously in her favour. Blackwell graduated at the head of her class, and in Paris, in May 1849, enrolled at La Maternité, France's leading school for midwives, as no Parisian hospital would admit her as a doctor. Here she contracted purulent ophthalmia, which left her blind in one eye and with only partial vision in the other. 'She can distinguish the flame of a lamp as through thick mist,' her brother wrote despairingly, 'and can discern something when the hand is passed across the eye.' Blackwell's impairment – for which she sought a hydropathic cure under Priessnitz at Grafenberg – ended all hopes of her becoming a surgeon. In October 1850, she began a year's postgraduate training at St Bartholomew's Hospital in London, admitted as a 'Lady Doctor' to all departments – except that for women's diseases.

Exactly when, and under what circumstances, Florence met Elizabeth Blackwell is unknown. They may have been introduced by the Brace-bridges, in the late spring of 1849, while Blackwell was on a flying visit to relations in the Midlands, or during her brief stay in London before she left for Paris. More probably, the two women came to know each other once Blackwell was settled in her lodgings at Thavies Inn on Holborn Hill, in the autumn of 1850, perhaps through Aunt Julia, who had already encouraged friendship between Blackwell and another of her nieces, Florence's 'tabooed' cousin, Barbara Leigh Smith. At the beginning of 1851 Florence met Blackwell again, this time at Wilton, where Blackwell was attending on Liz Herbert during the birth of her third child, Elizabeth Maud, and where Florence's presence had also been requested, to nurse the mother in the final stage of her pregnancy. Florence and Elizabeth Blackwell had much in common. They were almost the same age – Florence was Elizabeth's senior by eight months – and aspects of their backgrounds were similar. Samuel Blackwell, Elizabeth's father, who had been born in Bristol before emigrating to the United States, was a sugar refiner, like Florence's Smith antecedents, and an anti-slavery campaigner, like William Smith; and although Elizabeth's medical ambitions had the support of her family, she knew what struggle was, not simply from having to fight to gain acceptance on account of her sex, but also because the sudden death of her father had left the Blackwells impoverished, and forced Elizabeth to take teaching work to support herself. One of the most fervent reasons behind her decision to train as a doctor was her wish to remain free of marriage and dependence on a man.

In April 1851, Florence invited Elizabeth Blackwell to stay at Embley. With signs of disfigurement still visible around her eye, Elizabeth was possibly not the most encouraging example to the Nightingales of what might lie in store for a woman embarking on hospital training. But walking together in the grounds, as Blackwell later remembered, 'in the delicious air, amid a luxury of sights and sounds, conversing on the future', Florence drew strength from the prospect of perhaps one day joining her new friend in some shared venture in women's medicine. Pausing in front of the drawing room, Florence remarked, 'Do you know what I think when I always look at that row of windows? I think how I should turn it into a hospital ward, and just how I should place the beds!' Two days earlier, Florence had been upset by her encounter with Monckton Milnes at Lady Palmerston's, when he brushed by her with a dismissive acknowledgement. Now, though, as Blackwell later recalled Florence telling her, 'she should be perfectly happy with me, she should want no other husband'. Two weeks later, Blackwell 'dined & drank tea' with her in London as they inspected the Spine Asylum and the Lock Hospital, founded for the relief of venereal patients who were excluded from other hospitals, attended a lecture on political economy, and visited the Bracebridges. Florence, 'who is about leaving, uncertain she will see me again', as Blackwell wrote to her sister Emily, talked of her hopes of returning to Kaiserswerth, while Elizabeth explained the necessity of her own return to New York. It was beyond her means to establish a private practice in London, and so she had decided to go back to New York, where she believed there was less discrimination against women doctors. The two women parted in tears, but on 23 June they managed to meet again, this time to visit the German Hospital in Dalston, Florence's 'beau ideal' of a hospital, staffed by deaconesses from Kaiserswerth, where their names appear side by side in the visitors' book. A month later, Elizabeth Blackwell left England aboard the *Constitution*.

They did not see each other again for seven years. 'Write to me . . . I beseech you,' Florence requested, as Elizabeth Blackwell endured the professional difficulties of her first New York winter, 'and tell me what you think of the things about which we used to talk.' But the two women were set on paths which already diverged, and ultimately refused to meet. For Blackwell, medicine was an arena in which women could prove themselves the equal of men; but for Florence, the idea of introducing women into a profession widely considered to be badly in need of reform made no sense at all. 'I have no faith in medicine,' she wrote in February 1851. '... As people put in the "Marriages" the name of the clergyman ... who married them, I would put in the "Deaths" the name of the doctor or doctors who killed them.' A fully instituted nursing profession, on the other hand, taking its medical orders from doctors, but otherwise led and controlled by female nurses, would give women the hospital training they required.

Elizabeth Blackwell's example, though, could only be inspiring at this time. It steadied Florence's nerve, and galvanized her into considering various practical steps she might take 'to diminish the difficulties' of her life. To preserve her state of mind and health, she promised herself to spend at least an hour each day that summer, at the local school near the Hurst, which might her leave more 'obedient' to whatever pursuits her mother and sister wished to follow for the rest of the day; she would keep to an hour-and-a-half's 'steady thinking' before breakfast, for 'Without this, I am utterly lost'; and she would try to place her relations with her parents and Parthenope 'on a true footing'. She did not hold out hope of receiving any real understanding from them, but for her own peace of mind, she had to stop herself 'vibrating between irritation & indignation at the state of suffering I am in – & remorse & agony at the absence of enjoyment I promote in them.'

I must expect no sympathy, nor help from them. I have so long craved their sympathy that I can hardly reconcile myself to this. I have so long struggled to make myself understood, been sore, cast down, insupportably fretted by not being understood (at this moment even I feel it when I trace these conversations in thought) that I must not even try to be understood ...

Parthe says that I blow a trumpet – that it gives her an indigestion – that is also true. Struggle must make a noise – & every thing that I have to do that concerns my real being must be done with struggle.

Events, however, now moved with a speed that may have surprised even Florence. That catch-all for any ill-defined physical or nervous disorder – the hydropathic water cure – had been prescribed for Parthenope's ailments. For three months, she and her mother, together with Athena, to whom Parthenope had grown devoted, as their companion, were to tour the German spas, taking countless baths, and consulting with eminent gynaecologists who, inevitably, like most specialists of the time, traced female neuroses to reproductive origins in the uterus or ovaries. While they underwent this regime, Florence would be permitted to spend another, more intensive period at the Institution at Kaiserswerth. A gap in the family correspondence means that we cannot be certain of how this decision was arrived at. Behind it undoubtedly lay a ploy on Parthenope's part to ensure that her sister's time at Kaiserswerth was placed within strict limits. If Florence accompanied Fanny and Parthenope to the continent, they would be able to persuade her to return with them, whereas if she remained with her father at the Hurst and went later, her stay at Kaiserswerth might be open-ended. But what had made them consent to Florence's going in the first place? A reference in a subsequent letter from William Nightingale to his wife about the 'danger' that had confronted Florence before her departure suggests that her family had become only too aware of the suicidal depression into which she might fall if their agreement was withheld.

She had won their consent, but not necessarily their sympathy. If we are to believe a much later account, written by Florence during the course of an outburst of bitter recrimination against her family, an evening spent in the company of her mother and sister at the hotel in Karlsbad before she travelled to Kaiserswerth ended in a violent scene, with Parthenope flinging bracelets in Florence's face, and Florence herself fainting. A semblance of calm had reasserted itself by the time Florence, accompanied by Fanny, was admitted to the Institution, at the end of the first week in July, donning the blue print dress of the deaconess. Fanny was taken round the penitentiary – though not the hospital – and shown the room in the pastor's house in which Florence had stayed on her first visit. This time, however, Florence was moved to another room, in the orphan asylum, for which, as a trainee, she paid a fee for board and lodging. Of more paramount concern to her mother was that friends and other family members should not discover her daughter's whereabouts, despite Florence's attempts to reassure her that the people whose opinion she cared about most – like the Bunsens, Lady Inglis, and Lady Byron – would think it 'a very desirable thing' that Florence should be there; while she was able to report that the Herberts, who were taking the waters at Homburg, were intending to visit Kaiserswerth themselves to find a deaconess for their establishment at Charmouth. It was 'a state secret', Hilary Bonham Carter admitted to Madame Mohl, who was mystified by Florence's sudden disappearance. Various cover stories were concocted for general consumption, including one that can have hoodwinked nobody, that Miss Florence Nightingale had gone abroad to recover her complexion. Even the Bracebridges, on their way to their own spate of twenty-four baths for Charles Bracebridge's lameness, at Blankenberghe, near Bruges, were astonished to learn that Florence was again at Kaiserswerth, but promised to keep 'a profound silence' on the matter. They arrived one August afternoon to take Florence back with them to Düsseldorf for the night, and reported finding her looking remarkably well, compounding medicines 'on the Apothecary station'. When Aunt Mai revealed to Shore the truth of Florence's secret mission, he could not hide his admiration. 'Oh what pluck she has,' he said.

A month after her arrival, Florence reported to Fanny, now back at Karlsbad, news 'I know that you will be glad to hear', that she was renewed in body and spirit, and that 'really I should be sorry now to leave life'. As previously, she worked in all Kaiserswerth's departments, as well as giving English lessons, and taking part in the twice-daily services in the church, where she sometimes led the prayers. On several occasions she went begging and sold lottery tickets in the town for the support of the Institution. There were fêtes, to celebrate the 'perpetual' birthdays of the children, moonlit walks in the garden or to a tower by the river, and long excursions into the fields outside the grounds. The atmosphere was prayerful – the children were taught to listen for the voice of God within – and everyone was encouraged to pray aloud, but the mood was generally sunny, though Florence was initially disappointed that many of the younger deaconesses she had been on familiar terms with the year before were no longer in residence, having been sent abroad on foreign service.

Along with many hours of lessons designed to educate deaconesses from humbler backgrounds in the basic skills of reading, writing and arithmetic, the regular student nurses, 'Probeschwestern' as they were called, had only one formal nursing class a week. Florence appears not to have attended this. Where her months at Kaiserswerth were to prove invaluable was in the practical, clinical experience she acquired. She dressed wounds, practised bandaging, prepared and issued medicines, applied leeches (to induce bleeding), and assisted at operations. 'Cupped for the first time under Schwester Amalie's instructions . . . and did very well,' Florence noted on 21 July. She soon grew used to being present at the bedsides of dying patients, often standing watch through the night, and asking Fliedner's advice as to how best approach the issue of salvation with a dying man (Roman Catholic patients were always permitted a priest). One patient, Karius, died 'very quietly' one evening, as she sat reading to him. '. . . When he was gone, I sat on the window sill and looked out on the busy, lighted town. Death is so much more impressive in the midst of life.'

She often went to bed 'dead beat', but longed always to be with the seriously ill, dreading the call from Caroline Fliedner that would remove her from the hospital, for her turn in the seminary. She had a particularly heavy day at the end of July when she took part in her first amputation, recording the details carefully in her journal.

9–11 a.m. The two doctors arrived, room prepared for Meurer's amputation, leg taken off as high as possible. Chloroform acted well. Dressing difficult. It was 10.30 a.m. before I left the room to tell Mother [Caroline Fliedner] it was over. A beautiful operation. Patient suffered much in the afternoon. Cold water compresses every five minutes . . . Window sills decked with flower pots by Heinrich's care.

7–8 p.m. With the patient . . . Prayed with him – Catholic. What made the operation so difficult was the adhering of the flesh to the skin from disease which prevented the reserving skin enough to fold over the wound, which was dressed with collodium strips . . . Taking up of the arteries beautiful. Sawing of the bone momentary.

A week later, however, after Meurer had appeared to be making progress, he had a sudden relapse, became delirious, starting bleeding at the nose and temples, and went into a stupor. He had caught typhus. 'In the evening the tongue and teeth were black.' The doctor saw him, 'and did not dress the stump'. Following Meurer's death on 9 August, the body was removed, his room fumigated and sprinkled with vitriolic acid and chloride of lime.

'You will find ordinary twaddling life more insupportable than ever after this taste of your own heart's choice,' wrote a friend to whom Florence had written confidentially, both about the amputation and about the permission she had recently received from her father to extend her time at Kaiserswerth for the entire period that Fanny and Parthenope were away. Fanny, who had learned about the operation from Selina Bracebridge, was hurt that Florence hadn't told her about it herself. She had omitted to mention it, Florence hastened to reassure her, only because she had assumed that her mother would see no more interest in it 'than the pleasure dirty boys have in playing in the puddles about a butcher's shop'. But although Florence had sworn to live without it, she still craved her family's sympathy, joined with their approval. A series of bad-tempered letters arrived from Parthenope. She wasn't enjoying their stay, in soaring temperatures, at Franzensbad, remained in poor health, and was clearly unprepared to be any more accommodating to her younger sister. Florence replied that she liked the hot weather, and 'am perfectly well, body & mind (though I am afraid you would much rather hear I am not)'. A fortnight later, she responded to another letter from Parthenope, attempting to match its more conciliatory tone. 'You don't think I don't know that you love me, my dear. I have had too many proofs of it.' Her 'earnest affection', her 'heartfelt gratitude', were Parthenope's, she continued in a still further letter, 'but I have also thirst for what I believe to be my right work'. She knew that Parthenope looked upon her desire to nurse as a passing fancy, and understood as well the crushing disappointment her sister must feel to see 'the idol of her imagination' – a description no less than the truth – pass through life as though fettered in a prison from which there was no escape. Yet the solution to all this seemed so straightforward. 'If you could, through love & imagination, become my champion, I & my home would be a blessed one, & you, seeing me so happy, would be happy, too.' Parthenope, though, refused to unbend, and continued to withhold her blessing from Florence's 'sense of right in my path of life'. Turning to her mother, Florence also asked for her blessing and trust, and for time to prove that she wasn't seeking estrangement from her family. It would come home to her heart, she told her mother, 'my pure, my lovely one', that her daughter was doing nothing of which she need feel ashamed. On this occasion, the response she received was more encouraging.

William Nightingale had been warning his wife all summer that, given Florence's evident need for 'some great absorption', Fanny 'must not quarrel with her present work'. She had clearly taken his advice to heart. On 7 September, with just seven more baths in the offing, to be followed by visits to Dresden, then Prague, Fanny wrote to Florence. Her letter is a moving document, partly because it demonstrates so strongly the efforts of an elderly mother to move in a direction contrary to her instinct and way of thinking out of concern for her daughter, and also because it overturns the one-dimensional caricature of Fanny Nightingale, portrayed by generations of biographers, as an uncaring parent, motivated solely by fears about what the outside world might think.

Fanny began by hoping that 'This time will have been ... a real happiness for you & a rest to your spirit ... & that there are happier & better things in store for you at home, even tho' our opinions may differ with yours as to what the right way always is, as well as the way of doing it.' She continued:

Meanwhile, believe me, we will do our best to have faith as you ask, if not always in you, always at least in the greater & wiser who cares tenderly for us & who will work out your salvation ... We are not arrogating to ourselves a monopoly of wisdom, only the anxious look out of affection ...

Yes, my dear, take time, take faith & love with you, even though it be to walk in a path which leads you strangely from us all.

I assure you, you yourself cannot have been more thankful to Kaiserswerth than we have all been at this time, as a shadow in a thirsty land for you, & [a] halt in your struggle with life, for a little season – trusting & believing as you have always said that you will come back stronger & calmer for the rest to your spirit.

Goodbye, my love. I cannot write long on such matters ... I will do my best, I will indeed, to think you right, & let you follow the manner of man you are, & you must be merciful & not lay upon us more than we are able to bear.

Florence left Kaiserswerth at the beginning of October, rejoining Fanny and Parthenope at Cologne to begin their journey home. She remained grateful, for the rest of her life, for her time there, leading the tributes to Theodore Fliedner on his death – 'in harness' – in 1864, raising funds for the Institution, and maintaining contact with Fliedner's widow and children, one of whom, Carl, born in 1853, became her godson, and eventually a doctor. Writing to Samuel Howe, the year after her return, she commented on the system at Kaiserswerth as 'first-rate', and wished that it could be introduced in England, 'where hospitals are ill nursed by a class of women not fit to be household servants'. But in later years, it was the value of the moral tone at Kaiserswerth that she emphasized, at the expense of its hospital conditions. She grew irritated by stories that she had received her training there, and went so far as to tell her colleague Dr Sutherland that despite loving Kaiserswerth dearly, she had 'never in all my life seen a hospital so ill managed, so beastly, so unhealthy'.

Fanny's words, while scarcely amounting to an endorsement, had been sufficient to give Florence some encouragement. Back at Embley for Christmas 1851, she revealed her new confidence in an imaginary dialogue with her mother. She was not going to spend her life 'dangling' about the drawing room, and would 'go & look out for work, to be sure'. Then, taking her lead from the closing words of Fanny's letter, she proposed a new character for herself. 'You must look upon me as your son,' she told her, 'your vagabond son . . .'

7. Unloving Love

Soon after her return from Kaiserswerth, Florence went down with an attack of measles. By early December she was better, but as her father had also been in poor health, with a recurring eye inflammation and a severe bout of constipation, it was agreed that they should accompany each other for a month's water cure. Instead of Malvern, they decided on the establishment run by Dr Walter Johnson at Umberslade Hall, near Tanworth-on-Arden in Warwickshire. Johnson was 'a little, strange, scrubby, boorish-looking man', without Gully's charm, who immediately irritated Florence by taking her pulse and describing it as 'a miserable little <u>weed</u>'. In spite of his unprepossessing manner, however, Johnson came to impress her with his cleverness, amused her with his anecdotes about drunken nurses he had known, and reassured her that he would be able to restore Mr Nightingale to his state of health of six months earlier.

On their way to Umberslade, in the first days of January 1852, they stopped for a couple of nights with Aunt Mai and Uncle Sam at Combe Hurst. Also staying with the Smiths was the poet Arthur Hugh Clough, who, only days before, had become unofficially engaged to their daughter Blanche. Clough's prospects at this stage looked unpromising. He had recently resigned as head of University Hall, London, loathing the drudgery of the work and finding it difficult, as an agnostic, to accommodate himself to the college's Unitarian council, with its insistence on morning prayers for the students. His prospective father-in-law, Sam Smith, an Examiner of Bills at the House of Commons, insisted that marriage to his daughter was contingent on Clough finding an income of at least £500 per annum. It was to prove a protracted search. Having applied in vain for a professorship of classics in Sydney, Clough would set off at the end of 1852 for nine months in America on another unsuccessful trawl for a job.

It wasn't so long since Arthur Hugh Clough had been regarded, first at Rugby under Dr Arnold, and then at Balliol as a pupil of W. G. Ward, as one of the golden hopes of his generation. Yet, in the atmosphere of theological conflict stirred up at Oxford by the growth of Tractarianism, he was scourged by religious doubt, and by the end of the 1840s Clough had moved further from orthodoxy, recanting his acceptance of the Church of England's thirty-nine articles, and then resigning his fellowship at Oriel as a result. In Florence's judgement, Clough's main problem throughout his life was that he could never hope to meet the high standard of conscientiousness that Arnold had imposed upon him. His first major poem, *The Bothie of Toper-na-Fuosich*, was published at the end of 1848 (the title later had to be changed when it was discovered that 'Toper-na-Fuosich' was slang for the female genitalia). This 'long vacation pastoral', set in the Highlands of Scotland, was an enterprisingly modern take on the classical epic, in updated Homeric hexameters. It sold well and made Clough's reputation, though in more conventional circles it earned a certain notoriety for being 'indecent and profane, immoral and . . . Communistic'. This notoriety was one more black mark against Clough's suitability as a husband for Blanche.

Unlike some of her cousins – Lothian Nicholson, for instance, who found him insufferably superior – Florence liked Clough 'extremely', while admitting that he was 'desperately shy, and timid like a bird'. She had first met him some time the previous year, when he was tutoring Shore, and had spoken up for him with Blanche's parents, enlisting Monckton Milnes's support in favour of his suit, with such conviction that Milnes had amusingly jumped to the mistaken conclusion that Florence wanted Clough as a husband for herself. She also went to some lengths to obtain Samuel Howe's view of the chances of Clough finding employment in America, growing impatient when faced with Clough's indecisiveness about his future. Blanche had grown up in awe of Florence, remembering her cousin, who was eight years her senior, from a child's perspective, as 'a fine young lady', and envying her for her 'white frock'; as an adult, she may have been envious of Florence's intimacy with her mother, but she appreciated Florence's efforts at playing Cupid. So, too, did Clough, who referred to her as 'the friend'. But he reserved a more critical note about her for his letters to his future wife, where he wrote of Florence's 'unsympathetic, unloving sort of temper'; and described her as 'une tête forte, lucid, and not rich, though intelligent; not creative, arithmetical, "positive", matter of fact; a little arid, not tender but of a

high steady benevolence . . . moral, but though not strict, a little hard . . .'
The 'arithmetical' part of Florence sat down with Aunt Mai and calculated the future household budget for Blanche and Clough according to
the number of children they might produce. Before long Clough would
reverse his opinion; or if he didn't exactly change his mind, he came to see
how much Florence, and what she stood for, might mean to him. He had
lost his faith long ago, and sought something else with which he could
replace it. ' "*Service*" is everything,' he told Blanche in the early days of
their engagement, a sentiment which, in the first flush of romance, hurt
and profoundly shocked her; or as he put it in a phrase from one of his
poems, which Florence afterwards used often to quote, 'Love is fellow
service.' Ultimately, over the next decade, he was to discover that this was
something that only Florence Nightingale could provide.

At Umberslade Hall that January, Florence and her father whiled
away the time, 'like two fools', playing battledore and shuttlecock when
they weren't undergoing the water treatment, which, much to their relief,
turned out to be a milder process than Gully's at Malvern. 'Papa says
capital mutton & potatoes, beautiful brown bread pudding & today a
beautiful apple Charlotte,' Florence wrote to Fanny on 8 January,
reporting a sharp fall of snow which kept them indoors. A few days
later the weather had improved – though they could only go for walks
round 'the dull . . . gentlemen's park' in the dark, to fit in with the rest
of the treatment – and Mr Nightingale's eyes were better, allowing him
sometimes to read to himself. Florence herself was 'quite full of work
& preparation', sending home for reports from Kaiserswerth and a
deaconesses' institution at Paris. At night she passed a critical eye over
the rest of the company. 'And if you were to see them,' she joked to her
mother, 'you would have some hopes for me that I should learn the
value of <u>good society</u> by its contrast. Mrs Ford sits with her hands
between her knees. Mrs Johnson does not h'aspirate her haitches.'
Florence was a first-rate mimic, and one can imagine her, in the privacy
of her father's room, doing uproarious imitations of the other inmates
downstairs to amuse him.

This period of seclusion with her father allowed Florence some leeway,
after they left Umberslade at the end of the month, to pursue her own
interests. She went to London and visited the Octavius Smiths, the
Bunsens, and Mary Stanley and her recently widowed mother. In March,
accompanied by Liz Herbert, she inspected the Anglican sisterhood at

Clewer. This had been founded in 1849, as a refuge for prostitutes, in a house outside Windsor and had been taken over three years later as a permanent settlement, run on conventual lines. Florence, though, was unimpressed by the penitentiary there, which she felt placed too much emphasis on preaching, and not enough on providing the women with the education or training that might enable them to find jobs. Clewer was 'a fancy place, where, if you could get husbands for the Sisters and send the money and the penitents to Kaiserswerth, things would go on much better'.

Much of the spring of 1852 was spent in the company of Aunt Mai, at Tapton and at Cromford Bridge with 'the old ladies'; and then at Harrogate, at the beginning of May, where she and Aunt Mai tried yet another water cure. Rejecting one lodging because of its pervasive smell of paint, they tried another, but 'bundled out again', fearful of what Fanny Nightingale might say if she heard that they were staying somewhere for only a guinea a week. Finally, they found some 'very superior' accommodation at 'Mrs Wright's, York Place'. 'We have got a window & two daughters plus a widow,' Florence informed her family. It was a holiday full of enjoyable 'larks'. One day Aunt Mai 'got her drinking over early' so they took the train to York to see the Minster. From one of the shops in the shadow of the cathedral, Florence purchased a pamphlet on 'Reasons for Leaving the Church of England', and got into stimulating conversation with the 'red hot convert' to Catholicism behind the counter, who told her that Roman Catholics were the only people who were able to make headway against the tide of atheism that was sweeping through the manufacturing towns of the north of England. Later, after taking a train on the Scarborough line, she and Aunt Mai walked along a shady country lane to Castle Howard.

It was in this contented mood, alone with her beloved aunt, that Florence composed a letter to her father, marking her thirty-second birthday on 12 May. It is a strangely formal good-bye to all that, in which she expresses relief that her youth, with all its 'unfulfilled hopes & disappointed inexperience', is past. But the rising confidence of her voice is unmistakable as she announces that she has come into possession of herself, and has escaped from the 'bondage' of 'bad habits', signifying that her dreams no longer have a hold over her, to impair her vision and float like a veil between her imagination and her perception of the real world.

*

Aunt and niece were together again that June, this time in London. Towards the end of the month, in the company of Hilary Bonham Carter and Madame Mohl, they called on Marian Evans – who would emerge later in the decade as the novelist George Eliot – at the house at 142 Strand where she was part of the complicated ménage of *Westminster Review* editor John Chapman, his wife and his mistress. It was a world in which free living coexisted alongside free thinking, and the Chapman household had become a focus for radical politics and intellectual debate. Such an atmosphere fitted Aunt Mai – praised by Marian Evans for her freedom and simplicity, and for her 'non-subjection to "formulas"' – like a glove; though Hilary, whom Evans found rather affected, and Clarkey ('whose *make-up* was certainly extraordinary') may well have felt rather less at ease. Marian Evans had nothing but praise, however, for Florence. Florence's 'loftiness of mind', she thought, was 'well expressed by her form and manners'. She also noted that Florence had read Charles Bray's *The Philosophy of Necessity*, a book, published more than ten years earlier, that had played a significant role in freeing Marian Evans herself from the evangelical piety of her early life, setting her along a path of liberal thinking in religion, and a resulting loss of faith.

This reference to Florence's reading of Bray is interesting, for Bray's adoption of a central strand of the Unitarian philosophy, expounded by Joseph Priestley and his disciples towards the end of the previous century, and called Necessarianism, mirrored Florence's own preoccupation at this time with the relationship between God and a created world run by natural and social laws. Bray had argued that the universe was governed by unchanging laws deriving from God. It was man's duty to discover the workings of these laws, and then, in effect, to work with God in the creation of an ever-improving world.

Florence had long since rejected the supernatural and miraculous underpinning of Christianity. She saw prayer essentially as a misdirection of human energy that would be more fruitfully employed in going out into the world seeking to effect change. Most fundamental of all, she proposed a form of religion in which human beings actively contributed to the realization of God's law through work. Unlike Marian Evans, Florence did not experience a loss of belief as the age's new spirit of critical inquiry rocked the foundations of the literal interpretation of the Bible. Instead, she attempted to construct a system in which science and reason became handmaidens to religion, rather than a threat to belief. And in her formulation of these ideas, no influence would have a greater part to play than that of Aunt Mai.

It may indeed have been Aunt Mai who directed her niece's attention to Bray's work. In her early fifties, Aunt Mai continued to attend the Essex Street Chapel to hear the liberal Unitarian James Martineau preach. For years now she and Florence had talked and corresponded at length on religious subjects. A letter from the mid-1840s depicts the two of them at Combe, 'having a family dawdle in the fields . . . & long theological discussions all afternoon'. As Parthenope observed, Mai's 'metaphysical mind' suited Florence best. Although Mr Nightingale was also a recipient of Florence's ideas about religion, father and daughter often failed to find common ground on the subject. At Abu Simbel in 1850, when Florence acquired her insight into the notion of good resulting from evil, an understanding of how evil could have a positive purpose in God's plan, leading to the perfecting of human beings, it was Aunt Mai whom she warmly acknowledged in her letter describing the experience, for 'all she had taught me'. This exchange of ideas continued more intensively on Florence's return to England as the two women were increasingly in each other's company. '. . . I have become more & more penetrated all winter with things that you used to talk about at Cromford Bridge,' Florence wrote to Mai following their weeks together in the autumn of 1850.

The direct impetus, however, for expressing these ideas on paper, in something close to a publishable form, arose out of Florence's mounting indignation at what she saw as the deplorable state at mid-century of the Established Church; and from her burning desire to do something to remedy the lack of religious observance and spread of atheism among working men, particularly those employed in the manufacturing towns and cities of the north, to whom she planned to offer an alternative to conventional religion.

The Church of England was certainly in a condition of turmoil. One after another, a series of crises battered it, from within and without. The restoration of the Roman Catholic hierarchy in 1850 had given it the jitters; the so-called Gorham Controversy, which had begun in 1848 as a disagreement over infant baptism, and the question of whether infants who died before being baptized were unable to be saved from eternal damnation, had expanded into a contest over whether the state could adjudicate in church affairs; and, still to come, the dismissal of F. D. Maurice from King's College, London, on heresy charges, at the end of 1853, because he had argued against the doctrine of eternal damnation, only lent further support to the view that the Anglican Church was more concerned with squabbling about orthodoxy, and in maintaining its doctrinal positions, than in spreading the gospel.

Florence was scornful about the current state of the Church in which she had been raised, but to which she rarely paid anything more than lip service. She scoffed at its ministers as theologians and 'mere tea-drinkers', declared that the Church of England was fading fast, and 'can hardly last my time', and chastised it for looking for God in the dictionary rather than in the surrounding world. 'With us, God is dead. He has been dead nearly 2000 years. He wrote the Bible about 1800 years ago – & since then, He has not been heard of.' The strife-filled relations between the Established Church and its Catholic rival impressed her still less:

. . . One would think that all our RELIGION was political [she wrote to her father in the summer of 1851] . . . The two churches seem still convulsed in a manner discreditable to themselves & ridiculous to others. The Anglican screams and struggles as if they had taken away something of hers, the Catholic sings and shouts as if she had conquered England, nevertheless neither the one nor the other has happened. I feel little zeal in pulling down one church or building up another, in making bishops or unmaking them. If they would make us, a faith would spring up in us of itself & then we should not want Anglican Church or Roman Catholic to make it for us.

For the Roman Catholic Church, though, she reserved a note of appreciation that resonated with personal significance. Choosing to ignore the growing number of Anglican sisterhoods, and insisting that the Church of England left women 'almost wholly uncared-for', she praised Catholics for allowing a place for women in their scheme of things, through their founding of nursing orders.

General concern about the effect of the Church of England's undignified internal disputes on levels of church attendance united with growing fears about the godless poor. Had the spread of urbanization, coupled with the failure of the Anglican Church to respond to the enormous demographic changes this entailed, by keeping churches open and livings filled, succeeded in alienating the working-class from traditional forms of religious observance? Charles Dickens, for one, evidently thought so. In Coketown, the fictional setting of his novel *Hard Times*, published in 1854, Dickens commented on the 'perplexing mystery of the place', where one could 'walk through the streets on a Sunday morning' and note how few of 'the labouring people' responded to 'the barbarous jangling' of the church and chapel bells. These fears were confirmed by the results of a survey of public worship conducted on Sunday 30 March 1851, and published in a report by Horace Mann at the beginning of 1854. The statistical analysis of this report – delayed because of the length of time it took Mann and his enumerators to chase up the unreturned forms and then digest the great mass of data – concluded that over 5.25 million people, the majority of them poor or working-class, who ought to have attended church did not. Added to this picture of spiritual destitution was a disturbing fact for the Church of England, immediately jolting it from its complacency: the Established Church could no longer be said to represent the majority of the population.

Florence had taken her own soundings on the problem, and not just from the bookseller in York who had engaged her in conversation. 'I like anything which associates me with any class not my own . . .,' she told her mother – who must have been horrified (which may have been partly the point) – in the spring of 1851, after she had spent a train journey quizzing the wives of Yorkshire tradesmen, down in London for the Great Exhibition, on their views of socialism. Florence had probably encountered working men of Owenite socialist convictions while working with the sick in Holloway, during her months at Lea Hurst. More importantly, from the late 1840s, she was an occasional visitor to the London bookshop run by Edward Truelove, next door to the Literary and Scientific Institution in John Street, Fitzroy Square. Truelove, a vendor of radical and 'freethinking' literature, was a follower of Robert Owen and had worked at the Owenite utopian community of New Harmony, Indiana, for a year, before returning to England in 1846 to act as secretary to the Institution. Florence, described only as 'a west-end lady', had visited the shop initially without disclosing her identity, but in the course of long conversations with Truelove's wife she became well known to the couple, and subsequently kept up a friendship with Mrs Truelove, whose generous nature embodied the spirit of her surname, over many years. Florence's object was to assess

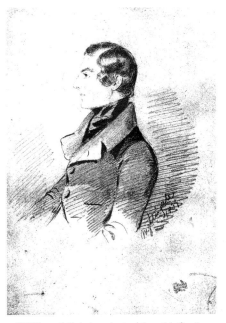

1. William Nightingale in his mid-forties. A sketch made in 1839, perhaps during the Nightingales' tour of the continent.

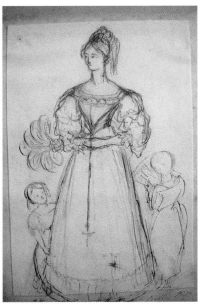

2. Fanny Nightingale in court dress, *c.* 1823, with Florence (*left*) clutching at her mother's skirt, and Parthenope. A charcoal sketch by either Patty or Julia Smith.

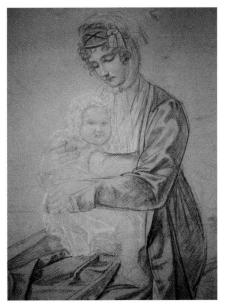

3. An Italian wetnurse with a baby, probably Florence, 1820.

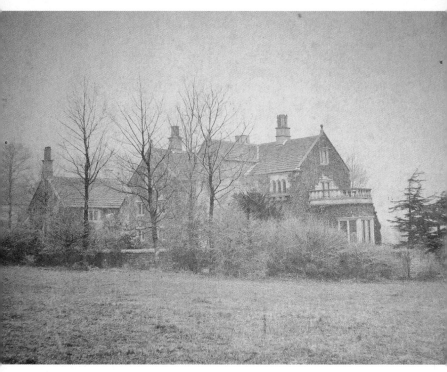

4. Lea Hurst in Derbyshire, the favourite home of Florence Nightingale's youth. A photograph from the 1860s. The gate to the parkland, through which Florence walked on her return from the Crimean War, in August 1856, can be seen to the right.

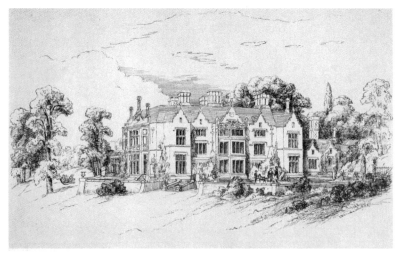

5. Embley in Hampshire. The Nightingales' second country residence, where Fanny Nightingale was able to indulge her love of entertaining and display.

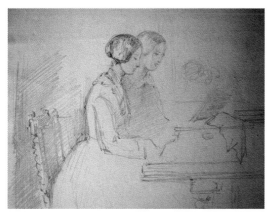

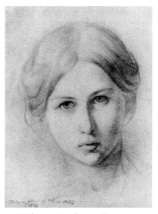

6. Florence (*left*) with her cousin, the dangerously indiscreet Marianne Nicholson. A sketch by Parthenope Nightingale, *c.* 1839.

7. Hilary Bonham Carter, loyal, faithful and put upon. A self-portrait.

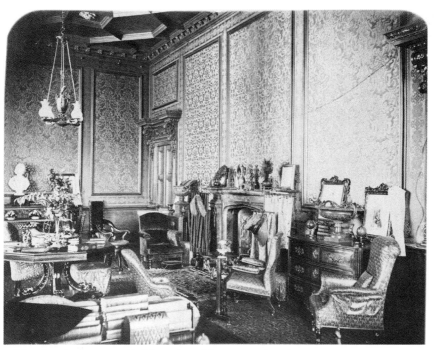

8. The drawing-room at Embley, where Florence endured many a monotonous evening in the 1840s, reading aloud and being read to. A photograph taken in the late 1870s after the Nightingales had vacated the house. The bust of Florence by Sir John Steell, her family's favourite likeness of her, is displayed at the back of the room.

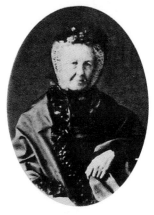

9. Mai Smith, Florence's aunt, who wrote of her niece that she was 'as precious to me as any thing I possess, except my husband...'

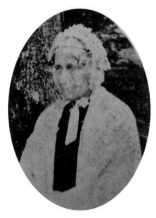

10. Mary Shore, William Nightingale's mother. Wild and headstrong in her younger days, she 'idolatrized' her granddaughter Florence in old age.

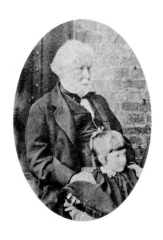

11. Sam Smith, Aunt Mai's husband, and Fanny Nightingale's younger brother, with one of his grandchildren. Uncle Sam was responsible for overseeing Florence's financial affairs during the Crimean War, and for many years afterwards.

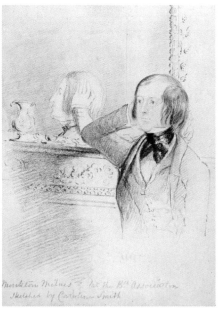

12. Richard Monckton Milnes, Florence's most serious suitor, in characteristic pose, lolling by the mantelpiece. 'Plain and common looking' according to a description by one of the Nightingale family's friends, he nevertheless attracted Florence through his wit and commitment to the social issues of the day.

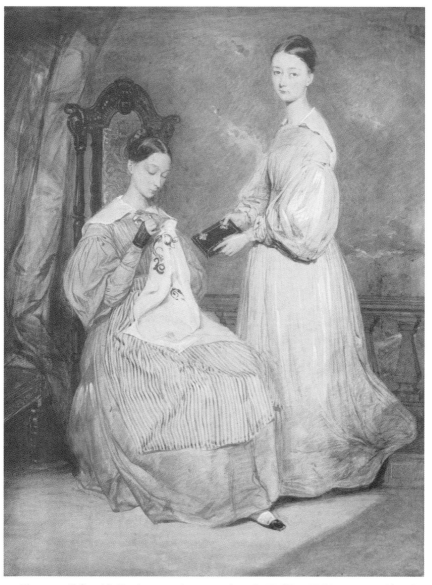

13. Florence (*left*) with Parthenope. A watercolour by William White, *c.* 1836. Already Florence is averting her eyes from the gaze of the onlooker.

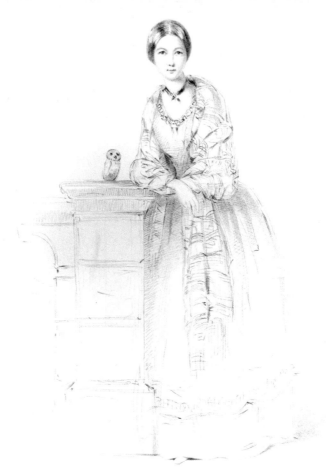

14. Florence with her bad-tempered owlet Athena, rescued from the Parthenon in 1850. This engraving, based on a drawing by Parthenope, became a popular image of Florence during the Crimean War after it appeared in the *Illustrated Times*.

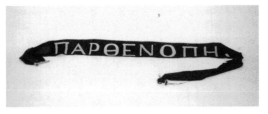

15. The pennant, made by Florence as a 'tribute to sisterly affection', which flew from the yardarm of the house-boat taking Florence and the Bracebridges on their journey up the Nile in 1849–50. The name 'Parthenope' is sewn on to it in Greek lettering on white tape.

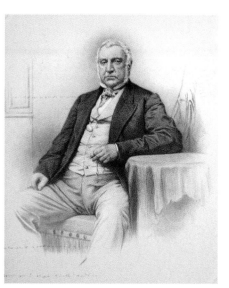

16. Charles Bracebridge, writer, benefactor, country gentleman – and inveterate trouble-maker. He is said to have been the original of the character of Mr Brooke in George Eliot's *Middlemarch*.

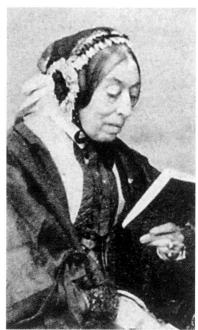

17. Selina Bracebridge, whom Florence called her 'spiritual mother'.

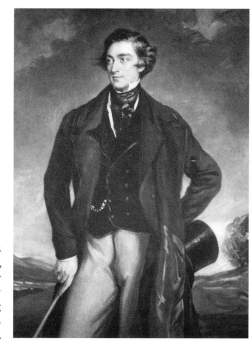

18. Sidney Herbert, who, as Secretary of State at War in 1854, sent Florence to Scutari and later collaborated with her on Army health reforms. An engraving after the painting by Francis Grant, *c.* 1847.

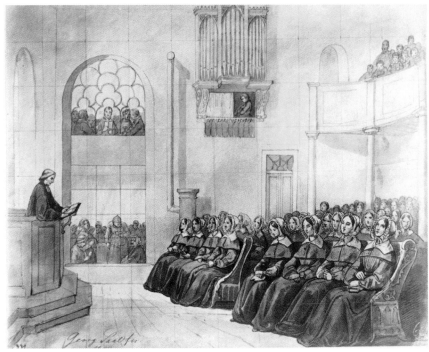

19. Pastor Fliedner reading to the deaconesses at Kaiserswerth.

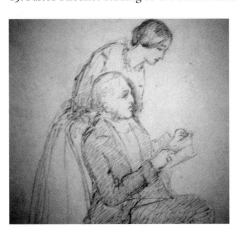

20. This drawing by Parthenope of Florence with William Nightingale captures the closeness between father and daughter. However, despite their shared intellectual interests, Florence found it difficult to forgive her father for not doing more to help her escape from the constraints of family life.

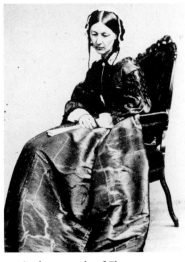

21. A photograph of Florence, c. 1853–4, while she was Lady Superintendent of the Upper Harley Street Establishment for Gentlewomen during Illness.

the kind of literature that appealed to the more intelligent working-class man. Her conclusion was that 'the most thinking and conscientious of the artisans have no religion at all'. Consequently she took on the challenge of presenting them with a new religion, to appeal to their emotions, as well as to their reasoning and intellect.

She set to work, bringing into tighter focus many of the ideas she had discussed over a long period with Aunt Mai. She drew on her experiences in Egypt, which had indicated to her that even entire nations were subject to immutable laws; she was influenced by the works of Spinoza and Hume, and of Baden Powell, the Professor of Geometry at Oxford, which confirmed her sense that, in an ordered universe, there could be no interruption to the laws of nature, and therefore, no possibility of miracles; and she consulted the work of the Scottish philosopher Sir William Hamilton, who argued that man was incapable of perceiving the divine, to confirm to herself what she *didn't* believe. Aunt Mai pressed a hard-line determinism on her, which Florence eliminated only after reading J. S. Mill's *System of Logic*, which introduced an element of free will and maintained that, although the human mind functions according to law, a human being can choose to be determined by some causes as opposed to others. From her cousin Hilary, in Paris with the Mohls, she sought information about the new positivist philosophy of Auguste Comte. In 1851, Comte began publishing a four-volume work of sociology, laying out the basis of his Religion of Humanity. For the artisan class in England, positivism was already an attractive alternative to a God-based religion, and was to prove even more so after 1853 when Harriet Martineau produced her translation and abridgement of Comte's work. Like Comte, Florence believed that the world was subject to universal laws; unlike him, she held that these laws emanated from a higher intelligence, the mind of God.

In her birthday letter to her father of May 1852, Florence offered to read him 'any of my "Works" in your own room before breakfast'. Four months later, she was keen for Henry Manning to read her 'Science of Theology', though whether he ever did so is unclear. What is more certain is that, by January 1853, when she asked Monckton Milnes if he 'would look over certain things, which I have written for the working-man on the subject of a belief in a God', she had prepared and had printed a sixty-five-page proof, dedicated 'To the Artizans of England'. She told Milnes that she had read it to 'one or two' working men, who had liked it, and she wondered whether it was likely to be read by more.

The God that Florence revealed to them was a benevolent being of infinite goodness and wisdom, wholly unlike the wrathful, punitive deity of traditional belief. It followed, therefore, that she utterly rejected the doctrine of eternal damnation as hardly consistent with a perfect God; nor did she have any time for the atonement, finding the idea that God would have sacrificed His son on the cross totally abhorrent. In place of a God whom mankind must constantly propitiate, she presented a benign alternative, a God with whom man could enter into partnership, as a 'fellow-searcher' after truth. In a modern world, where 'reason is all', it could no longer be simply a case of 'only believe'. On the contrary, if one accepts that God is always revealing himself through the discernible laws of the universe, it must be mankind's object, and his active task, to discover what these laws are. This was never more transparent than in the laws relating to health. 'With regard to health or sickness,' she later wrote, 'these are not "sent" to try us, but are the result of keeping, or not keeping, the laws of God; and, therefore, it would be "conformable to the will of God" to keep His laws, so that you *would* have health.'

Events were shortly to overtake the fate of Florence's work on 'Religion'. It never reached the working-class audience on the scale for which it had originally been intended, and one wonders, given its somewhat convoluted prose style, whether it ever possibly could have. By the time Florence was ready to expand it, in 1858, two years after her return from the Crimean War, the work's focus had widened considerably, to include social criticism on the family, 'practical deductions' directed towards the upper sections of society rather than the lower. None the less, as she recognized in a memorandum to herself at the end of 1852, she had succeeded in remodelling her entire religious belief; and in so doing, had provided the underlying principles for much of her future work.

———

But how were these laws to be discerned, let alone measured and subjected to analysis? The answer lay in the new science of statistics, which had fast become one of the passions of the age. The 1830s and 1840s had seen the beginnings of the civil registration of births, marriages and deaths, the collection of statistics by several Government offices, together with the growing refinement of techniques for conducting the census, which had been first introduced under the Population Act of 1801.

Statistical societies had sprung up widely, in London and provincial towns, while, in 1833, the British Association for the Advancement of Science had bowed to the need for official recognition, and founded its own statistical section. There seemed to be no limit to the application of this new science to practical affairs, as statisticians were called upon to direct their findings to different departments of human need: economics, politics, medicine – the first English textbook on vital statistics appeared in 1829 – social problems and, in particular, the condition of the poor. Dickens satirized mid-Victorian society's preoccupation with the 'deadly statistical clock', and poked fun at the kind of people who could see nothing but 'figures and averages'.

Florence Nightingale was one of these passionate statisticians. Her early predilection for collecting and analysing data, combined with a love of mathematical precision, had been carried forward into adult-hood, and pursued with illimitable enthusiasm and curiosity. Where other young ladies might find pleasure in a novel, she found greater enjoyment in studying a book of statistical tables. 'I can never be suf-ficiently thankful to Papa,' she wrote from Rome in 1847, 'for having given me an interest in Statistical & Political matters.' This interest in statistics had perhaps been stimulated by the arrival at Embley, during her childhood, of house guests like the mathematician Charles Babbage, a founder of the London Statistical Society, and John Rickman, the clerk of the House of Commons responsible for establishing, then overseeing, the machinery of the first four censuses. The passion for statistics was also something else that united Florence and Richard Monckton Milnes, in later life a President of the Royal Statistical Society. In 1853, the year in which an International Statistical Congress was founded, Florence prepared her first close analysis of census material, a study of the results of the 1841 census. This was the first modern census, supervised by a statistical bureau, in which householders were issued with a printed schedule for completion by families throughout England on a single allotted night. At about the same time, Florence began to tabulate the results of her own questionnaire on health administration, distributed among selected hospitals throughout Europe.

Florence's mentor in statistics, however, was a man whom she met only once, in 1860, but whose name she was consistently to adulate. Alphonse Quetelet, born in 1796, was an astronomer and meteorologist at the Royal Observatory in Belgium, but his international reputation rested on his work as a statistician and sociologist. Quetelet's ground-breaking achievement in the analysis of statistical data derived from his formulation of the concept of *l'homme type*, the average man. While there are no laws governing human behaviour, Quetelet maintained that regularities in attributes and behaviour do exist which can be characterized mathematically through laws of probability. Starting with the examination of birth and death rates by month and city, by temperature and time of day, he subsequently investigated mortality by age and profession, by locality and season, in prisons, and in hospitals. Before long he had moved on to consideration of moral qualities, gathering statistics on drunkenness, insanity, suicide and crime. His research on the French crime rate, looking at the influence of such factors as gender, education and age, concluded that society in some ways prepares individuals for their crimes. In 1835 he incorporated his findings into a book, known under its short title as *Physique Sociale*, and translated into English in 1842 as *A Treatise on Man and the Development of his Faculties*.

When did Florence first read Quetelet's work? We cannot be sure, but it seems highly probable, given her passion for statistical inquiry, that she would have become acquainted with Quetelet's ideas in some form during the period following the first appearance of his work in England (if not through the French or translated versions of *Physique Sociale*, then perhaps as a result of the treatise on probability and social science which Quetelet addressed in 1846 to the Belgian King's two nephews, Albert, the Prince Consort, and his brother Ernest). For Quetelet's theories offered Florence a firm methodological framework, corroborating her overriding belief in discernible laws, and confirming statistics as a sacred science which would permit man to read the mind of God.

———

Meanwhile, Florence kept herself busy. In line with the resolution made before her return to Kaiserswerth, she continued every day with her writing, and undertook what little practical work she could find. At the end of June, she was involved in a scheme organized by Caroline Chisholm. Mrs Chisholm, known popularly as 'the Emigrant's Friend', was the leader of what was in essence a moral crusade to resettle working people, especially unmarried girls, in Australia. Florence was running an errand for Chisholm in the countryside outside London when she came upon an Irish widow, reduced to living in a shed by the roadside, and in considerable distress because her fourteen-year-old daughter had run away and faced falling into prostitution. The girl, a Catholic, was eventually discovered to be safe, and in the course of finding a home for her with a Kensington order of sisters – as her mother was 'a poor feckless thing [who] could not keep her at home even for a night' – Florence sought the assistance of Henry Manning, renewing the acquaintance they had begun in Rome, five years earlier. As she had predicted at that time, Manning had become a convert to Roman Catholicism. 'After this I shall sink to the bottom and disappear,' he had observed in the spring of 1851, having taken the momentous step, which deprived him of many friends, and the Anglican Church of a significant levelling influence.

Florence had in fact encountered Manning in person at Amber Gate station in the autumn of 1849, a couple of months before her departure for Egypt, but had felt constrained from inviting him home to Lea Hurst for dinner by his ascetic appearance, his 'extinguished eye and spiritualized mouth'. Now, to her surprise, she found herself treating him as a confidant. For a start, she immediately realized how helpful Manning could be in providing her with an introduction to the Catholic sisterhoods in Dublin and Paris, where she still hoped to receive training. But as she felt that he wrote to her out of a spirit of kindness rather than proselytism, she was franker than she needed to be about her thwarted ambition, the opposition of her family, and, most tellingly, about her own attraction to the Catholic Church. She was already aware of the part Manning was continuing to play in bringing Mary Stanley, the daughter of a bishop and sister of a future Dean of Westminster, closer to conversion.

Florence's letters to Manning – his to her from this period don't survive – interestingly foreshadow some of the basic elements of her mature epistolary style. There is the open impatience with the slower pace of others, countered by a layer of courtesy and implied humility, together with an unrelenting sense of urgency, as if everything should have been done and dusted yesterday. There is also her magnificent, and sometimes exaggerated, sense of drama, which can sweep away the intricacies of human behaviour with a sudden sleight of hand (so, for example, describing Parthenope's anger at her for going to Kaiserswerth, she says that her sister hasn't spoken to her since, despite the survival of correspondence between them from this period, suggesting at least a more moderate version of sisterly displeasure).

From the outset Florence left Manning in no doubt of the kind of home the Catholic Church could offer her, in contrast to the Church of England, which had given her neither work, nor training. 'All my difficulties would be removed ... My work, already laid out for me, instead of seeking it to & fro & finding none. My home – sympathy, human & divine.' She belongs to 'Rome' much more than to 'Canterbury'. But, nevertheless, her 'conviction ... hangs back'. Unlike Manning, she thinks like a mathematician, not an historian, and as a result her will is inextricably connected to her reason. The difference between the two churches is that the Catholic Church 'insists peremptorily upon my believing what I cannot believe', whereas the Anglican Church 'is too careless & indifferent to know whether I believe it or not'. Over several months of writing to Manning, she remains attracted to the idea of finding work and an identity within a sisterhood, but is finally unable to give her unconditional allegiance to a faith which she can accept empirically – through her observation of 'the uniformities which exist in the Catholic Church of faith, simplicity of aim, of love & self-sacrifice' – but not scientifically. On his side, having accused Florence of everything from eclecticism and intellectual dishonesty to tiresomeness, Manning must have reached the conclusion that she simply didn't possess the essential prerequisite of the budding convert: the ability to submit the will and ego to an unquestioned authority.

He kept to his promise, however, of making what arrangements he could for her visit to Dublin. Her plans for this suddenly took definite shape in July when she received a letter from the Fowlers announcing their own intention of going to Ireland for the meetings of the British Association in Belfast. They planned to stop for several days in Dublin on the way, and asked Florence to go with them. As this facilitated her visit 'in the eyes of my people', she gratefully agreed, bombarding Manning with reminders, just in case her requirements should have slipped his mind. 'If you have forgotten,' she wrote to him at the eleventh hour, 'may I remind you to ask the Mother to admit me into the Hospital at once, which is not customary?' On 24 August, she and the Fowlers crossed by the Holyhead ferry, reaching Dublin late that night. But, for Florence, her time there was unexpectedly a wash-out. '... My mission in Ireland has entirely failed,' she informed her father from Belfast, five days later. St Vincent's, the Dublin hospital, had been closed while undergoing repairs, though she derived some consolation from the fact that what she had seen of its nursing practice had failed to impress her. The sisters neither sat up at night with their patients, nor attended operations, two duties Florence considered far too important to be left to the ward maids. Meanwhile, she found Belfast 'about as unspiritual and uninteresting as it is possible to conceive'. They returned to Dublin to begin their journey home, but were interrupted by the news that Parthenope, staying at Birk Hall near Ballater, in Aberdeenshire, with family friend Sir James Clark, the Queen's doctor, had suffered a break-down and was demanding Florence's presence. 'She has a great longing for you,' Charlotte Clark, Sir James's daughter, had written to Florence on 6 September, '& today begged me to write two letters one to Dublin, the other to Belfast, to beg you to join her here . . .'

Florence set off immediately, arriving at Birk Hall, with her maid Mariette, on 13 September. '. . . My dear Pop was very glad to see me . . .,' she reported to her mother. Sir James Clark thought Parthenope was making good progress, and diagnosed 'absolutely no disease but a marked irritability of the brain'. In this condition, she was sometimes delirious – 'The flood whirls about my head,' she wrote to a friend – and believed herself unable to walk even the short distance downstairs; while her 'fancies are more in number than the sands of the sea'. She dictated letters every day, requesting new gowns from Aberdeen, and possessed an apparently insatiable appetite for pears.

Sir James Clark had an interesting past. As a young doctor in Rome, in 1820–21, he had attended on John Keats in his dying months, caring for him devotedly (though possibly failing to diagnose his tuberculosis), and carrying out the poet's final wishes regarding his burial. Later, as a trusted physician and friend to both Queen Victoria and Prince Albert, Clark had been damaged by the controversy surrounding Flora Hastings, the Queen's lady-in-waiting, when he failed to spot the growth of the abdominal tumour that eventually killed her. Nevertheless he was a considerate doctor, with a good bedside manner and an enlightened approach to the treatment of the mentally ill. Moreover, his support and direct access to the Queen was one day to prove of especial importance to Florence in her efforts on behalf of the army's health. Balmoral, in Parthenope's opinion, 'not quite in the crème de la crème, though a charming house', was five miles away. One afternoon they came upon the Queen while out walking. Victoria's niece, Feodora, Princess Hohen-lohe, had been thrown from her horse, and was in need of attention

from Sir James. On another occasion, the young princes, Bertie, Prince
of Wales (later Edward VII), and Alfred, came to lunch at Birk Hall.
Florence thought that the Prince of Wales was 'as nice a little boy as I
ever saw – so simple, so unaffected; but Prince Alfred was more high-
spirited in comparison'. She wondered whether the impression Bertie
gave of being 'a little cowed' arose from him having been 'over taught'.

Sir James's formal diagnosis of Parthenope's illness, sent to the
Nightingales at the beginning of October, was, in effect, a condemnation
of their daughter's lifestyle. She possessed 'a fine intellect', but needed
exercise to combat her 'state of debility'. Overall his conclusions were
more worrying: 'the extreme irritability of the nervous system, the total
absorption in self, with, at times, chronic delirium' might, if left
untreated, lead in time to imbecility. He suggested that Parthenope
should be sent to stay with a kind relative who could have more influence
on her than her parents. What, curiously, Clark didn't mention in this
letter was that the most crucial and necessary step to be taken on
Parthenope's road to recovery was her complete separation from her
sister. According to Florence's later report to Henry Manning, Clark
had given her an 'awful warning'. Florence's presence at home obviously
aggravated Parthenope's condition, increasing her excitement and
fostering her monomania. It followed, therefore, that if Florence wasn't
'to yield to my sister to her destruction', she had no alternative but to
withdraw from taking any part in their common family life.

Fanny and William Nightingale seem at this point to have been para-
lysed into inaction, perhaps out of shame, or from a simple inability to
know what to do next. While they were evidently informed of what
Fanny termed 'Sir JC's fatal opinion', Parthenope was 'kept in ignorance
of the particulars of her illness'. This left the situation frustratingly
unresolved. If Florence absented herself from home, she was liable to
cause her sister distress; equally, if she remained with her family, she
would only contribute to Parthenope's continuing obsession.

It was left to Florence to take charge of Parthenope on a long and protracted journey to Lea Hurst, punctuated by several stops, at Aberdeen,
Edinburgh and York, to ensure that Parthenope didn't get overtired.
Parthenope sobbed as she was placed by her nurse into the carriage for the
drive to Aboyne; then ate a hearty mutton chop on arrival at Aberdeen;
and had to be carried 'bodily' into the railway carriage by a porter at
Edinburgh. The two sisters were back in Derbyshire on 4 October.

Once home, Parthenope made good progress. In a long poem composed as she regained her strength, she recalled the 'dim and dreary season' of her time in Scotland, and tried to come to terms with 'the busy nothings' that hitherto had made up her life.

To Florence, Parthenope exemplified the fate of the middle-class or upper-middle-class Victorian daughter, starved of mental and spiritual nourishment and condemned to spend her days in a meaningless round of trivial occupations, which ate away at her vital strength, and left her moribund from an excess of nervous energy. Parthenope's illness, as Florence explained to Manning from Birk Hall, had been brought on 'by the conventional life of the present phase of civilization, which fritters away all that is spiritual in women'.

Although so unalike in temperament and ambition, the two sisters had this much in common: they were both, in their very different ways, the victims of a lifestyle that effectively kept them imprisoned in a gilded cage. Florence's bitter frustration, alternating with hopeless despair, at her plight as an extraordinarily gifted woman, constantly thwarted in her attempts to find work and training, had also brought her at times close to breakdown. However, in the period following her return from her 1849–50 European tour, she had found an outlet for her feelings in a series of draft manuscripts centred on what she mildly refers to at one point as 'something of the difficulties of a "Daughter at Home" '. Today, the essay 'Cassandra', edited from these manuscripts by Florence herself for private publication in 1860, and subsequently released to the wider world in 1928 by Ray Strachey as an appendix to her short history of the women's movement, *The Cause*, is probably the best known of all Florence Nightingale's writings. Yet 'Cassandra' is only the later, impersonal recension of a work that had evolved on a complex journey through a number of guises: as a novel, largely consisting of a dialogue between three daughters and their parents, and as a more autobiographical piece of fiction, partly told in a male voice, before its eventual transformation into the anonymously narrated, third-person essay we are now familiar with.

'I must do something for women,' Florence had written in a note to herself in 1849 as she weighed up the possibility of marriage to Richard Monckton Milnes, a statement of intent that may well mark the beginning of a project to examine the lives of women of her class. Conventional

dating places the writing of Florence's 'novel', as it is known, to
1850–51, when Nightingale was thirty. This is the age at which the
tragic heroine of one of the drafts, Nofriani, who renames herself
Cassandra, after the doomed prophetess of Troy, dies after a life of
confinement and enforced idleness. But the conversion of one of the
daughters, Columba, to Roman Catholicism, and her decision to become
a Sister of Charity, suggests Florence continued to write the novel well
into 1852, the period when she herself confronted the question of becoming a convert. That she didn't finally abandon the manuscript until
March 1853 is indicated by the inclusion of that date near the end of
the text.

   Florence's novel is, to some extent, a wry commentary on the proliferation of advice books addressed to middle-class daughters of the mid-
Victorian era, a genre it subverts through its reversal of expectations.
Sarah Ellis's *The Daughters of England. Their Position in Society,
Character and Responsibilities*, which first appeared in the mid-1840s,
was the most popular of these. Mrs Ellis's advice to daughters was that
they should be content with their inferiority to men, put up with their
want of power and, most importantly, remember that they were part of
a family. More interesting, though, in light of Florence's arrangement
of one draft of her work around the remarks of three daughters, is
Passages from the Life of a Daughter at Home. Written by Sarah
Stephen, and published anonymously in 1845, *Passages* had struck Mrs
Gaskell as 'very painful' in its depiction of the purposelessness of the
lives of many single women. Ironically, it had been one of the books
selected for the ritual of after-dinner reading out loud, on long evenings
at Embley in 1846. It tells the story of the four Mowbray sisters, focusing
on one of them, Anna, who is dissatisfied with her life as an unmarried
daughter at home, and prefers 'self-indulgent' study to duty to her
family. At times Stephen's narrative reflects Florence's own experience
with extraordinary precision. Anna does not care for reading aloud:
'. . . she had no interest in her needle-work, and it was dreary to think
how many such evenings must be passed'. Anna's silence – the 'idle
reverie' that leads her to 'weave a vision of herself under circumstances
more suited to draw out the better part of her character' – is criticized
by Mary, her sister, who exclaims, in a startling echo of Fanny and
Parthenope, 'I do think when people have the whole day to themselves,
they might give up a few hours in the evening to their own family.'

Anna, for her part, feels guilty for not being sufficiently 'self-forgetting'. But the novelist's prescription for her is a profoundly depressing one, which by implication Florence would criticize and overturn in her own analysis of the lives of daughters. Anna is made to give up her study, which is turned into a sitting room for her sisters. In the final scene of the book, she is shown in middle age, having submitted herself to the will of God and now wholly content to forgo her desire for study and solitude in order to serve her surviving sisters.

Florence's three sisters, in the original dialogue-based fiction, have been given exotic-sounding names, Fulgentia, Portia and Columba (their two married sisters are called, more conventionally, Mary and Kate). The settings of the novel are romantic and escapist. In one draft they are reminiscent of the Renaissance palaces that Florence had visited in Italy as a teenager; in another, the action is played out against a backdrop clearly inspired by her time in the East. In a scene where Fulgentia arrives at a London ball, she is asked by her male companion 'whether she did not like Society', to which she responds with the words, 'What has "Society" done for us?' The autobiographical origins of the following passage are immediately apparent:

Oh! If we lived in a race which knew how to employ any strength instead of frittering it & repressing it, how different it would be. But now when it finds one of its members with a great power of work, it is disagreeably surprised, it does not know what to do . . .

Women's business is supposed to be to find something to '<u>pass</u>' the '<u>time</u>' . . . in drawing or music or literature or worsted work. If I & my sisters were now sitting round the table doing worsted work, we should be supposed to be very appropriately & rightly employed – especially if one were reading aloud.

The mother is to be pitied just as much as the daughter, for 'the impossible' is demanded of her. 'She is expected to . . . sympathise with & understand all her children, among whom are the most dissimilar characters – the most unlike her own.' It is this lack of sympathy that, in the end, will drive Fulgentia to her premature death:

Of my life I was thoroughly weary. The ennui of existing was too great for me. I, who could have done everything, now I can do nothing. Well, be it so! It is right I should die to shew [sic] the effects of this killing system. I am resigned, I am glad.

The large number of false starts and gaping holes in the story indicate that Florence never found a novelistic framework for her ideas that worked to her satisfaction; and despite the regrets expressed by recent commentators, it's difficult to see how the flowery dialogue and flights of fancy could ever have combined with the underlying theme to create a convincing effect. At the end of the decade, when Florence returned to the manuscripts to fashion a version for print, it was in order, as we shall see, to pare down the original into an essay form which would stand as an anonymously narrated commentary on the lives of women everywhere, rather than as an account of the personal suffering from which, by that time, she had managed to liberate herself.

She felt like 'a stranded ship', Florence told Manning, following her return from Scotland. He had spoken on her behalf to the Abbé des Genettes in Paris, who had arranged for Florence to receive some training from the Sisters of Charity in the rue Oudinot, close to where the Mohls lived. But having planned to go to them in the autumn, she was now only too aware that any suggestion of foreign travel would induce a fit of hysterics in Parthenope. Staying at Embley, 'where I am blamed by everybody', was no better a solution. So, in November, in need of 'a little strengthening' after the experiences of the past months, she went back to Umberslade; and from there to Cromford Bridge, where Aunt Evans was entering her final illness.

Parthenope was physically stronger. But September's patient, dependent and distressed in childlike confusion, had been replaced by a troubled woman seeking to unburden herself of a weight of accumulated resentment against her sister. Madame Mohl received a bad-tempered outburst from Parthenope later that autumn, attempting to put her side of the story, and complaining that Florence's repeated absences from home throughout the year had left the 'eternal poor . . . to the mercies of Mama and me, both very unwell . . .':

. . . I believe . . . [Florence] has little or none of what is called charity or philanthropy, she is ambitious – very, and would like . . . to regenerate the world with a grand *coup de main* or some fine institution . . . Here she has a circle of admirers who cry up everything she does or says as gospel . . . I wish she could be brought to see that it is the intellectual part that interests her, not the manual. She has no *esprit de conduite* in the practical sense. When she nursed me, everything which intellect and kind intention could do was done, but she was a shocking nurse. Mariette [her maid] was ten times better. Whereas her influence upon people's minds and her curiosity in getting into the varieties of mind is insatiable. After she has got inside, they generally cease to have any interest for her.

Although couched in an astringent tone, there is much here – the contempt for philanthropy, the recognition that new ideas about nursing did not amount simply to refinement in the laying on of hands – that Florence would have undoubtedly acknowledged. Clarkey's response intimated that she knew this to be so:

Flo you know has more of activity and hunger for discovery than the mere want of doing good. Some people have great delight in looking after the poor from more charity (not I), others have new ideas, and it is not really charity, but activity and invention. Their minds have a superabundant quantity of Gastric Juice which eats our Stomach, I'm told, if it has not victuals to dissolve. No one can help it, and one must be fed accordingly.

What, though, was going to cut across Parthenope's life, and alter the course of her existence? Some, like Lady Byron, attributed Parthenope's predicament to the fact that Florence was insufficiently 'self-forgetting'; others sided more with the view of Aunt Mai, who shook her head in sad disapproval at Parthenope as a 'Poor sweet loving spirit, condemned to inflict wounds in her own & other spirits, because her vision is walled round . . .' It was Fanny Allen who paid the tribute that Parthenope probably most wanted to hear. She wrote to her, quoting Milton's line, 'They also serve who only stand and wait', in support of her belief that Parthenope, like Florence, was doing God's work, and that their parents were blessed in not one, but 'a couple of swans'.

In the summer of 1854, Parthenope received a proposal of marriage from William Spottiswoode, the mathematician and publisher. His family firm, Eyre and Spottiswoode, were printing a private edition, much against Florence's will, of her letters from Egypt. Parthenope was supervising the publication, and formed a strong, flirtatious friendship with Spottiswoode, six years her junior. He was an attractive catch, highly intelligent and civilized, and persistent in his attentions, but finally she refused him. Her future, by then, hung on Florence's destiny.

*

Moves to win Florence her independence from home were gaining momentum, as both Aunt Mai and Selina Bracebridge advanced her cause with Fanny Nightingale. Mai had argued for months, as diplomatically as she could, that some kind of compromise must be reached, and had secured Fanny's agreement that at some future unspecified age Florence should be allowed her freedom to run an institution of her own devising, away from home. Mrs Bracebridge backed up her arguments. 'Ever since I have known Flo's strong desire to form an Institution,' she wrote to Mai, towards the end of 1852, 'I have always discouraged the idea.' However, she had now 'come to the conviction that nothing on earth will change it – that she will never be happy herself, or able to make her family happy . . . in her present mode of life – tenderly as she loves them . . .' Mai pointed out to Fanny how much the difficult situation in the family would be improved if Florence had the freedom 'to follow out, sometimes from home, sometimes at home, these ideas, so busy working within'. But still Fanny prevaricated. Mrs Bracebridge grew impatient, finally exploding in a letter to Mai, in which she recommended that Florence be given an independent income by her father of £300 per annum: '. . . her Parents pay this penalty for having a child of such <u>power</u> & genius – they may therefore consider it expedient to make <u>great</u> sacrifices to enable her to make an <u>Experiment</u> – which is likely to be a successful one if she has <u>means</u>, and <u>time</u> & <u>free action</u>, allowed her.'

Where could this experiment take place? The forest lodge at Embley having been mooted as a possible location, and then quickly dismissed by Florence as unsuitable, another possibility soon presented itself. Shortly before Christmas, Florence was at Carlton Terrace in London, staying with the Bunsens – and listening to Mary Stanley's excited report of her recent presentation to the Pope in Rome – when she received a telegram informing her of the death of Aunt Evans. Following the funeral, Fanny offered the vacant house at Cromford Bridge as a home for a small institution run by Florence. Once again, the offer was rejected. 'I do indeed feel deeply grateful for the sympathy with my wishes which such proposal shows,' Florence wrote to her mother. But she believed herself still too 'untrained and unprepared' to make a success of such a plan at present. Instead, she continued to press to be allowed to go to Paris to train with the Sisters of Charity. When Fanny finally relented and gave her permission, there was a huge, collective sigh of relief. Madame Mohl reassured Parthenope that there was no possibility of Florence enjoying the work so much that she wouldn't want to return. 'She would never be content to be a soeur de charité ... she would soon get tired of dressing sores. However delightful she might think it now, she would want to make all the soeurs do it better ...'

Suddenly a number of avenues were opening. Before Florence left London at the end of January 1853, she received an initial approach, through Lady Canning, from the Ladies' Committee of a small charitable institution for sick gentlewomen in Chandos Street, off Cavendish Square. Mrs Bracebridge had learned that its committee was looking for a new superintendent for the institution, which was being reorganized. Would Florence be interested? She was, and from Paris kept up a regular correspondence with Lady Canning, outlining her ideas for placing the institution on a better footing. 'I think it very likely I may help her if she offers me conditions that I like,' she told her mother at the beginning of March.

France was accustoming itself to having an Emperor once more at its head. 'Notre-Dame looks like an old actress at a fair, painted & dressed up in old finery,' Florence noted soon after her arrival in Paris, observing the preparations being made for Napoleon III's marriage to Eugénie. She declined, however, as a protest against the despotism of the new regime, to watch the great state processions from the cathedral on the day. At the Mohls, in the rue du Bac, she shared a room with Hilary – 'a very nice one with a curtain drawn across two beds' – and sat for her portrait, in Hilary's chilly atelier. She knew that her mother would be pleased to hear that within a week of her arrival she had already been 'to two balls, one concert at the Conservatory, have one invitation of dinner, one to the opera, & two to evening parties'; while Parthenope was assured that 'my black lace' was worn 'to great effect' at a ball at the Mohls.

As for more serious business, she made a detailed survey of Paris hospitals after Julius Mohl obtained a permit for her from Government offices, giving her the right to enter any hospital. On 5 February, Florence wrote to Parthenope, 'I have been to the Hôtel Dieu, under the Soeurs S. Augustin & the Hôpital Beaujou under the Soeurs Ste Marthe – both very well conducted in most respects it seemed to me – & to the Enfans Malade under the Soeurs S. Thomas ...' In mid-February, with snow deep on the ground, she entered the Maison de la Providence, the hospital run by the Sisters of Charity, in the rue Oudinot, as arranged for her by Manning. Here, she wore a convent uniform, nursed the sick under the directions of the sisters, but ate and slept in separate quarters.

The news that Grandmother Shore was seriously ill abruptly altered her plans. On 11 March, Florence announced to her family that the news from Tapton was worse and that she was returning to England to be at her grandmother's bedside. At first, Mrs Shore seemed not to know her, but when her maid opened the shutters, letting in the light, and Florence spoke her name, she knew who she was. 'The first snowdrops are out, but she will not live to see them; on Monday she was 95 and will see her snowdrops in another land.' The end was painfully drawn out. When Mr Nightingale arrived, Florence kept the room dark so that he should not become too distressed at the sight of his mother, 'diminished to a small remnant in comparison to the reality of her former self'. In the last week Mrs Shore's suffering was terrible. 'Night nor day have her cries ever ceased', though 'for 7 days no drop even of water passed her lips'. She died on Good Friday, 25 March, and the funeral took place a week later at Ecclesall Church, in weather 'so characteristic of her', violent storms alternating with bright sunshine.

Florence was shaken. 'I was much touched, dearest mother, by your care for me,' she wrote to Fanny on 5 April, '. . . Grandmama occupied a large share in my life. The world seems to me a different place with her & Aunt Evans not in it.' She appeared impervious to human comfort. She didn't need 'bodily' care, but stressed that it was 'of the first importance' that Athena was brought to London to be with her. 'I shall want her company after this . . .'

During Mrs Shore's final weeks, Florence had been inundated with approaches from Lady Canning about the Chandos Street institution. The offer of the position had been 'first on, then off, then on again, twenty times in a fortnight'. She was wearily indifferent, and had finally lost patience with 'the fashionable asses', especially as the appointment would probably require her to give up the placing she had fixed with the Sisters of St Vincent de Paul back in Paris, as the committee wanted her to go into the house immediately. She assured her family on 8 April that she had little enthusiasm for the idea, but ten days later was on her way to meet Lady Canning to discuss the proposal. 'I will call for you in my Brougham about 12 o'clock,' wrote Liz Herbert, who had been placed on the committee to broker Florence's acceptance of the position.

Lady Canning was taken aback by Florence's youthful appearance, but delighted with her quiet, sensible manner. '. . . I hope the old House-keeper or Matron will in . . . outward appearance supply her young lady's deficiencies in point of years,' she wrote to Mrs Herbert, con-firming her satisfaction with Florence. By 25 April, Florence had engaged Mrs Mary Clarke, originally matron of a union workhouse at Sheffield, where Florence had met her on a visit to Tapton the previous year, to work as housekeeper under her.

Events were now moving so fast towards a fait accompli that control of them was slipping out of the Nightingale family's hands. Florence had assured her parents that she would do nothing without their consent, but the likelihood that she would permanently leave home, in order to reside either at the institution or in its close vicinity, had Parthenope up in arms in injured protest. Worn out by this battering, Mr Nightingale retreated to the quiet of his London club, the Athenaeum, to think things out, resolved upon bringing the unhappy situation arising from Florence's 'impossible future' to an end. Only, once there, he was defeated by his own indecisiveness.

Memorandum. Apr 20

I have today reached the conclusion that Parthe can no more control or moderate the intensity of her interest in Flo's doings than she can change her physical form & that her life will be sacrificed to the activity of her thoughts unless she removes herself immediately from the scene – the only question being 'where to go'?

The above conclusion is arrived at quite as much by observing the manner in which she furthers Flo's plans, as when she objects to them.

Apr 24

Reconsidered – retirement might do more harm than good.

What then.

Drafting a letter to Parthenope, he faced a similar dead end:

Having come to the resolution that it is entirely beyond your mental strength to give up interference in your sister's affairs & being equally sure that your health cannot bear the strain, we advise you to retire from London & take to your Books & country occupations till her proceedings are settled.

Apr 23 – I doubt my own thoughts.

He described this state of affairs as slow torture, while fearing that what was to come might be the first act 'in a great Tragedy'. Should Florence remain at home, or should she be allowed to go? 'I dare not try to turn the balance by adding the lightest feather in the scale if it hangs trembling in the air . . .'

Finally, though, William Nightingale did tip the scale by awarding his daughter an allowance of £500 a year (about £30,000 in modern values), paid quarterly in advance. The days of wasting time in her mother's drawing room, instead of going out in the world to do God's work, were over. Florence at last had her freedom.

How could the strongest character in the family also be the most submissive? This was a question that Florence Nightingale asked herself when she came to consider the problems of family life, and in particular its problems for women, at the end of the decade. Her answer was that the more powerful a person is, the stronger their affections are, and it is by these affections that they are led into subjection to the weaker. The break-up of Florence's own family life, however deeply she had desired it at times, was not a matter that she took lightly, something that Madame Mohl discovered when she received an irritated response to her question about Florence's decision to leave home and live at Upper Harley Street. 'I do not wish to talk about it – and this is the last time I ever shall do, but as you ask me a plain question . . . I will give you a plain answer. I have talked matters over . . . with Parthe, not once but thousands of times. Years and years have been spent in doing so. It has been, therefore, with the deepest consideration and with the fullest advice that I have taken the step of leaving home . . .' She left no room for discussion.

Her bitterness against the institution of the family became in time a festering wound. It was a feeling exacerbated by illness after the Crimean War, a steady decline in her health which she sometimes believed had its roots in the strains imposed on her by family tensions in the years before she went away. A family that checked the development of one of its members had no right to the name; it was not a family, but 'a thumbscrew, a Procrustes' bed, an instrument either of torture or deterioration, a disabilities office'. It was also, to use a phrase of Aeschylus's that Florence favoured, an 'unloving love'.

Even when her family expressed their pride in her achievements, and basked in her reflected glory, as they were often to have good reason to do in the course of the next few years, she could not help but contrast it to their obstructive attitude in earlier times. She had their blessing, but she still craved the understanding and sympathy she believed they withheld from her. Fanny Nightingale stood in awe of her daughter, but she continued to refer to the consequences of Florence's 'eccentric turn', which had left her bereft of the family support on which any woman, at her time of life, and in her position, should expect to depend.

However, beneath Florence's flashes of white hot anger and red raw hurt, less complicated emotions are just occasionally discernible. Throughout her time at Scutari and in the Crimea, she wore a bracelet with a green enamelled heart-shaped pendant and snake's head clasp. Worn under her sleeve, it contained woven strands of hair of those for whom her affection was strongest: her father, her mother, Parthenope and Shore.

8. In the Hey-day of My Power

Florence made her formal acceptance of the position of Superintendent of the Establishment for Gentlewomen during Illness on 29 April 1853. However, before she could do so, there was an embarrassing bit of family business to clear up. At a late stage in the negotiations over her employment, Mrs George Eyre, one of the ladies of the committee, had asked Marianne Nicholson – since her marriage in the summer of 1851, Mrs Douglas Galton – whether Florence's family had given their consent. Although Marianne later strenuously denied having stirred up trouble, the story according to Mrs Eyre, of which she immediately rushed to inform the other members of the committee, was that she had it on the good authority of a cousin that the Nightingales were very much opposed to the plan. 'There was a great "scrimmage",' reported Parthenope; several ladies announced at once that the news placed Florence's future at the establishment in jeopardy, while others resolutely refused to believe it. Only a letter from William Nightingale, providing Florence with his official, patriarchal, sanction, set their minds at rest.

Florence was in no doubt that Marianne's ill-natured tongue had been responsible for the mischief. But there was an unforeseen, and from Florence's point of view, entirely satisfactory outcome of the affair, when her mother and sister united in support of her. Fanny 'behaved beautifully', a cousin recalled later, letting it be known that 'they wished ... [Florence] to go', though they were sorry to lose her; while Parthenope, incensed at her sister's treatment, and stirred by family loyalty, took up the cudgels on Florence's behalf. First she fired off a letter to Marianne's younger brother Lothian, describing Marianne's 'absolute denials' as 'dishonoured notes'. Then, when this strategy seemed to be leading nowhere, she took the case to a higher authority, that of Hannah Nicholson, Marianne's aunt. Of course, she wouldn't have chosen such a course for Florence, she wrote to Aunt Hannah, 'but ... we are honestly & lovingly anxious that she should do what she thinks right . . . I do wish to exonerate Flo with you & to ask you not to believe all you hear about her from a source which distorts her thoughts & deeds, not for the first time.' Florence, meanwhile, sat back and left it until late that summer to write to Lothian Nicholson, warning him not to become involved in 'paper wars' in support of his sister.

The history of these negotiations, Florence told Clarkey, offered sufficient material for 'a comedy in fifty acts'. She was pleased, though, to have been given the unconditional terms she had insisted upon, with the right to retire as superintendent after a period of twelve months, and positively ecstatic when, in her first week of admitting patients that August, she scored her first victory over the committee. Lady Canning apart, she had a low opinion of the general council, made up of a gentlemen's as well as a ladies' committee, and satisfactorily trounced them when it came to the issue of whether the Institution should become non-sectarian. Florence was adamant that it should, the committee equally certain it should remain Church of England. 'My Committee refused me to take in Catholic patients – whereupon I wished them good morning, unless I might take in Jews and their Rabbis to attend them. So now it is settled, and in print, that we are to take in all denominations whatever, and allow them to be visited by their respective priests and Muftis, provided I will receive . . . the obnoxious animal at the door . . .' She also prevented the committee from forcing a new chaplain on the Institution. He was too young and liable to flirt with the patients, spiritually or otherwise.

Since its foundation under royal patronage in March 1850, the establishment at 8 Chandos Street had attempted, with varying degrees of success, to offer care to a specific class of person: 'the gentlewoman, of good family, well educated', but of limited income, who in the course of 'a lingering and expensive illness' had access to neither the medical treatment paid for by the rich, nor the free service provided for the poor in hospital wards. By far the greater number of patients treated by the Institution were governesses, though admission was also open to the female relatives of clergymen, naval, military and professional men. For a woman of 'gentle birth' but low income, becoming a governess remained the only work that she could perform for pay. At the end of the 1840s, however, the number of women seeking such positions, usually in private households, vastly outsoared the demand. The 1851 census demonstrated this in blunt terms: 365,159 unmarried ladies, known as 'excess women', for just 24,770 positions. Not that securing one of these jobs necessarily resulted in a happy outcome. Governesses were generally put upon and underpaid, working long hours for salaries as low as £10 per annum (as a comparison, the nurses at Chandos Street were paid more than double this). Miss Draper, governess to the family of Lady Teignmouth, and among those treated under Florence's supervision, provides one example of the physical and mental stress often suffered by such women. Described as 'wretchedly delicate', Miss Draper had been 'incapacitated from fulfilling her duty, notwithstanding every wish and effort to do so'.

Clearly there was a need for the kind of service to be found at Chandos Street, but at times it had been a struggle to fill the beds. A large part of Florence's work, once the Institution was in its more spacious accommodation in Upper Harley Street, would consist in adapting the skills connected with running a large household to the management of a small hospital and, initially, the most urgent of requirements was to balance the budget. Within months of taking over, she uncovered a £700 short-fall and was forced to set about raising subscriptions. Subscribers of five guineas per annum could recommend a patient for admission, and if considered eligible by the Ladies' Committee, which met twice a week, the patient would be admitted free of charge for a period of up to two months. She instituted cuts in expenses, saving money, for instance, by authorizing the house surgeon, instead of the local apothecary, to dispense medication, and also by keeping a sharp eye on the weekly running expenses. Edward Marjoribanks, a senior partner at Coutts, was the treasurer, with whom, early on, Florence established a good working relationship. The promotion of the Institution through public advertisements had started before Florence's arrival; and an article on 'Benevolent Institutions', in the July 1853 issue of the journal *The Pen*, informed readers of Florence's appointment: '. . . a Lady, eminently qualified for the work, has undertaken, gratuitously, the office of superintendent.'

Many friends and acquaintances were surprised that, with her great powers, and after such a long period of preparation, Florence should have settled for such a comparatively mundane occupation. She was 'too good for her work' was a commonly expressed view. As Parthenope later wrote, 'to the apparent eye it was cutting stones with razors for that noble intellect to be engaged in reducing the bill for flour, looking after tallow candles & pounding rhubarb'. Yet, in small but decisive ways, the Establishment for 'Decayed Gentlewomen', as Aunt Patty insisted on calling it, would enable Florence to put into operation some of the practices she had observed in hospitals on the continent, while allowing her to develop the administrative and purveying skills that were to prove of vital importance at Scutari during the Crimean War. Elizabeth Blackwell, in the process of setting up a small dispensary in New York, recognized the value of the experiment. While she regretted that Florence, consistent with her position as a lady, wasn't receiving payment for her services (not only that, she was also paying Mrs Clarke's wages), she sympathized 'most heartily in your resolve to act rather than to theorize', and acknowledged the part she was playing 'in weakening the barriers of prejudice which hedge in all <u>work</u> for women'.

Florence's letter of acceptance to Lady Canning manifested her grander ambitions for her new post when she asked that the committee consider the terms under which 'volunteer Nursing Sisters shall be received into the Institution, should any such offer themselves'. She had evidently conceived the plan of offering training to suitable applicants, an idea confirmed by the grandiose scheme she had in mind for the alternative site for the Institution, once a move from Chandos Street was decided upon in the months before she started. In dismissing one possibility, of a house in nearby Mansfield Street, Florence observed that something more than a private residence was required, otherwise 'the Institution can never be anything but a poor place', and recommended taking a wing of the new hospital, or of 'the magnificent new hotel', recently erected opposite Paddington station. The committee had more realistic ambitions and opted for a three-storeyed house, with attic and basement, and a stable building at the rear, at 1 Upper Harley Street. The area of Harley Street – the upper and lower regions were united in 1866 under one address, and 1 Upper Harley Street renumbered as 90 Harley Street – was not yet the centre of the professional medical establishment that it was to become in the next decade, though as a precursor of this development, the eminent physician Sir William Jenner had set up his practice at 8 Harley Street, two years earlier.

By the time the committee had decided on the new quarters, Florence was back in Paris, visiting the Salpêtrière, with its 5,000 female inmates, sick, old and insane, said to be the best-managed workhouse in the world. Then, on 8 June, she re-entered the Maison de Providence to continue the training with the Sisters of Charity that had been interrupted by her grandmother's death. With Lady Canning's permission, she had returned to Paris while renovations to Upper Harley Street were continuing. She hadn't told anyone else on the committee about her stay in a convent, as she was certain they would disapprove, 'instead of being very obliged to me for acting as a spy to despoil the enemy of their good things'. Three weeks later, she informed her family of the reason for her silence during the interim: '. . . I have had the <u>measles</u>!' – her second attack in eighteen months. The sisters had nursed her like one of their own, she told them, and she was now spending her convalescence in the back drawing room at the Mohls' apartment in the rue du Bac. As Clarkey was visiting her relatives in England, it was Julius Mohl who cared for her with paternal kindness, though she blushed at the impropriety of the arrangement.

In mid-July, Florence returned to London. Work on the new premises was moving slowly. 'You see, this is just the time London Workmen are busiest,' Selina Bracebridge explained to her, 'every one has their house <u>done up</u> & they will <u>neglect</u> you at any time if <u>some man</u> does not step forward to bully them.' Florence obtained Shore's help with the installation of 'a lift', presumably the dumbwaiter which conveyed food to different floors, and was pleased to have carried her point 'for stained (not dry rubbed) floors & only bedside carpets'. Progress sometimes faltered, but, with Mrs Clarke's assistance, she swept like a new broom through the house. Immediately dispensing with the 'rat-eaten' furnishings from Chandos Street, she patched together pieces of carpet and 'contrived bed covers out of old curtains'. She funded the replacement of the household linen out of her own pocket, after finding vermin running about 'tame in all directions'. Under her instructions, a system of pipes, leading from a boiler at the top of the house, brought hot water to every floor; while a simple but ingenious arrangement of bells and valves, indicating which patient was in need of attention, was designed to save nurses from being 'converted into a pair of legs for running up & down stairs'. From home she brought prints for the walls, bits of furniture and books for the patients, asking Parthenope not to renew her subscription to the London Library for her ('I who never read any books but what are not to be found there'), as she preferred to take out one at Mudie's for the Institution's benefit, though not at its expense. She also bought books for Upper Harley Street, including *The Christian Year*, *Bleak House*, and a copy of Clough's poems. Among other purchases from her father's first cheque were eight 'hermetically sealed' commode pails and six bed-rests; and, no doubt reflecting her belief that the new superintendent should be smartly outfitted, a black silk gown, and a grey one, at a cost of £1 12s. and £1 8s. respectively.

Accommodation for twenty-seven patients was being prepared: ten single rooms and seventeen compartments. As for Florence's own quarters, these consisted of two rooms, newly partitioned, with a fireplace and south-facing window in each; one on the ground floor next to the dining room, the other directly above it on the first floor. With Aunt Mai, who came to London every Sunday, and whose daughter Bertha would occasionally do 'a turn' in her cousin's Institution, Florence also took rooms in St James's Square. These were intended as a bolt-hole, somewhere to rest, spend her days off, and disguise from the patients the fact that she no longer attended church regularly.

Parthenope, who had handled inquiries from the committee while Florence was still in Paris, was keen to furnish Florence's rooms in Upper Harley Street. '. . . I so well enter into your feeling of seeking to make her more comfortable than she would herself care to be . . .,' Lady Canning wrote in thanking her. The two sisters were on better terms, with Florence commenting on 'dear Pop's pleasant kindness', though Parthenope's over-zealous concern for Florence's health was a continuing source of irritation. As an economy, as well as to ensure that she was obtaining the best quality, Florence went to Covent Garden to buy her own vegetables. Parthenope was mortified, earning herself an exasperated rebuke. 'You foolish child, don't you see that the Covent Garden expeditions are just the best thing I could do? They get me out – they give me air, exercise, variety.' Meanwhile, welcome gifts of flowers, fruit, partridge and pheasant arrived regularly from Embley.

Frantic preparations continued up to the eleventh hour. 'To settle with Mrs Clarke who is to clear the candlesticks, who the grates, who the passages,' runs one of Florence's last-minute notes about the housemaids; 'to stipulate against artificial flowers either in cap or bonnet'. On 12 August, she took up residence at 1 Upper Harley Street.

Not everything went smoothly at the start. The workmen – who, Florence observed, seemed to have spent the summer striking for their own amusement – were still very much in evidence and, on one occasion, when the foreman got drunk, she had to step in to break up a fight between them in the drawing room. The system of ventilation was threatened by gas, leaking from a stove and coming out into the rooms, where it 'went off with a series of partial explosions'. With the exception of 'John, the Cook & Nurse Smith', she had quickly dismissed the servants and nurses from Chandos Street, and now had three nurses, one on each floor, with whom she was 'perfectly satisfied'. That satisfaction didn't last long. She soon felt forced to give Nurse Bellamy – who had 'nothing of the nurse but the name and wages' – a warning, and to read 'our slovenly, unhandsome nurses' a lecture on punctuality. Even Mrs Clarke, usually such a stalwart, had displayed an inconvenient tendency to retire to bed whenever anything offended her. In a letter to Pastor Fliedner in September, Florence bemoaned the old problem, that 'salaried nurses . . . have neither love nor conscience. How happy I will be when we will all be Sisters.' She added, however, that she envisaged remaining at Upper Harley Street for the next few years, as the difficulties she had encountered there provided such excellent training for her.

The patients, though, were quite another matter. She hadn't expected to find them so 'full of joy and consolation', nor indeed so manageable. Although the maximum occupancy of twenty-seven was never met, numbers had quickly risen from the seven already in residence at the beginning of September to twenty-five by mid-October. 'We are filling fast,' she told Parthenope, 'which I am glad of, as it is easier to manage thirty than three.' Among 'our new invalids' admitted at the beginning of October were women diagnosed as suffering from general debility (described as incurable), from internal inflammation, scrofula and anchylosis (stiffness resulting from the joining together of bones). She almost longed for 'a good operation case', and one presented itself early on: a Miss Goodridge, who had cancer of the breast, but was thought likely to recover after an operation to remove it. The medical men attached to the institution, especially Dr Henry Bence Jones of St George's, and the ophthalmic surgeon, Dr William Bowman, from King's College Hospital, impressed her. Florence's 'Rules for Patients' specified that 'The Lady Superintendent will, on every occasion, accompany the Medical attendant on his visits to the patients, unless . . . she deputes the Nurse to take her place.' At operations, Florence was on hand, closely observing and ready to administer the new anaesthetic, chloroform, or tie up an artery.

Florence herself inspired great devotion among her patients. She defrayed fees for some, occasionally paying them herself, covered the cost of sending one governess for a holiday to Eastbourne, and was generally sympathetic to the impoverishment and loneliness faced by many of these women. 'You are ... [the Institution's] sunshine ...,' wrote one, acknowledging her generosity. 'I could not be there without you and were you to give up your influence, all would soon fade away and then the whole thing would cease to be'; another testified to 'Miss Nightingale's kindness, attention & affection'; while a story, relayed to Mrs Gaskell, told of a patient who used to stand on the cold hearthstone when Florence was doing her rounds, in the hope that she would rub her feet for her. Word spread of the 'care & kindness' to be found in the new Establishment. In the summer of 1854, the artist Dante Gabriel Rossetti, learning of its burgeoning reputation, considered sending Lizzie Siddal for a spell of treatment there for her fragile health and increasing addiction to laudanum. The 'Sanatorium', he informed his brother William, 'contains only about 20 or 30 patients or so, and is ... most admirably managed, the object to make it as much like a home as possible'. It was too much like a home for some. One of Florence's persistent problems was that the malingerers were using the Institution as a temporary refuge, when they weren't seriously ill, simply because they had nowhere else to go. 'There is not a trick in the whole legerdemain of Hysteria which has not been played in this house,' she stated. Sundays and Thursdays, the days before the bi-weekly committee meetings when admissions were decided upon, would find patients preparing themselves 'by getting up a case', leaving their flannels off in order to develop a cough; or going without their meals to prove loss of appetite, and eating them secretly during the night when hunger pangs struck. It was a struggle to make the Ladies' Committee agree to the enforcement of a rule to limit a patient's stay to two months – except for the mortally ill – on the basis that otherwise she would have no incentive to get well. But, by the spring of 1854, Florence had got her way.

In her first quarterly report, dated 14 November 1853, she rehearsed the difficulties associated with moving to a new address, and concluded with a summary of the number of patients admitted (eighteen), of how many remained (thirteen), and of the remaining five who had been discharged. 'I had great reluctance to putting some things in my Report, which sounded like praising myself,' she told her family, 'but Σ & Mrs Herbert said it was quite necessary & egged me on ...' In reply to her father's request for her 'observations upon <u>my</u> Time of statesmanship', she revealed her propensity for intrigue and, in particular, her delight in pulling the wool over the committee's eyes:

... when I entered service here, I determined that, happen what would, I never would intrigue among the com'tee. Now I perceive that I do all my business by intrigue. I propose in private to A, B, or C the resolution I think A, B, or C most capable of carrying in Com'tee & then leave it to them – & I always win.

I am now in the hey-day of my power. At the last Gen'l Com'tee, they proposed & carried (without my knowing anything about it) a resolution that I should have £50 per month to spend for the House & wrote to the Treasurer to advance it to me – whereupon I wrote to the Treasurer to refuse it to me. L[ad]y Cranworth, who was my greatest enemy, is now, I understand, trumpeting my fame thro' London, and all because I have reduced their expenditure from 1s 10d per head per day to 1s.

William Nightingale was taken aback, and wrote to reprove her. 'I regret very much your unmitigated tone of condemnation of your committee. Your business <u>must be</u>, if you differ with them – to lead them, to teach them, to abide by them ... The whole scheme of life is to <u>work through others</u>.'

The winter of 1853–4 was characterized by almost daily conditions of thick, impenetrable fog. At 1 Upper Harley Street the house was kept warm, though smoke billowed so much from the fireplaces that Mrs Clarke and her niece Anne had to take turns in 'constantly nursing' them. One January morning, 'an insane governess' was brought in by Mr Garnier, the parish clergyman. In spite of Florence keeping a watch over her, she escaped and 'raised a mob' in the street. 'We have recaptured her,' Florence reported with an air of triumph, 'but I am now making arrangements to send her to St Luke's . . .' There was just enough variety in individual cases to keep Florence stimulated. One woman, cured of an affliction labelled 'self-mismanagement', was of particular fascination. She had been confined to her bed for three years when she came to Upper Harley Street, and believed herself incapable of taking any solid food but port wine and cream. After two months she left the Institution, completely cured, able to eat meat and take long walks. Yet this transformation was achieved almost without a grain of medicine passing her lips. The solution had been to keep the woman isolated 'from other patients & all influences which would have strengthened her illusions'.

As time wore on, however, it was becoming increasingly obvious that Upper Harley Street was not going to provide Florence with the opportunity to carry out the scheme closest to her heart, the training of volunteer nurses. A single suitable candidate, a Mrs Foster, applied for instruction in the spring of 1854, but in the absence of the means and facilities for a properly developed programme, Florence had little choice but to reject her. Instead, she paid out of her own pocket for Mrs Foster to attend the London Nurses Institution, at King William Street, in the City. Meanwhile, she began to spend her spare time visiting London hospitals to collect facts to establish a case for reforming conditions for hospital nurses. This was a subject that strongly interested the Herberts. After Florence inspected St Bartholomew's, Liz Herbert wrote asking for information, on her husband's behalf, about the 'bad pay & worse lodging' of the nurses there. Since the end of 1852, Sidney Herbert had once again been in Government, as Secretary of State at War in the coalition led by Lord Aberdeen.

At the end of May, the Institution faced its most anxious case in Florence's time as superintendent, when an operation to remove a cataract went disastrously wrong. No blame attached to Dr Bowman, but the woman was left blind and, according to Florence, faced the prospect of insanity. 'I had rather, ten times, have killed her,' she wrote. There was some doubt that she would be free to attend Blanche's wedding to Arthur Clough at Embley on 13 June, though in the end she was present to join in the celebrations for a couple whose path to matrimony had been interspersed with setbacks. '. . . There have been difficulties enough to make one sometimes turn faint,' wrote the bride's mother, Aunt Mai, 'but I think it is impossible to live side by side with these two, without feeling that it would be wrong not to let them join their fates.' Clough had at last found a job, as examiner in the Education Office in Downing Street, remunerative enough to satisfy Sam Smith's conditions. Back in London after the wedding, Florence let her family into a secret. Through the recommendations of Dr Bowman, who was highly impressed with her abilities, she had been approached by King's College Hospital for the post of Superintendent of Nurses in the reorganization that was being planned there. 'They have asked me to send in my conditions,' she told her mother. 'This must, of course, be mentioned to <u>no one</u>.'

All the old objections were immediately raised as Fanny and Parthenope attempted to dissuade her. Even Mrs Bracebridge did not approve
of a move to King's because of its 'Physical & Moral' atmosphere. '. . . I
do trust that Flo will be brought to see the undesirableness . . .,' she
wrote in agreement with Fanny. Florence, however, was having none of
it. Away from home, out of the line of direct interference by her family,
she was more of a free agent and had, in any case, decided to leave
Upper Harley Street to pursue her goal of nurse training. In her final
quarterly report, dated 7 August, which marked her first anniversary at
the Institution, she noted the satisfactory results 'as to good order, good
nursing, moral influence & economy', and ended

I therefore wish, at the close of the year for which I promised my services, to
intimate that, – having as I believe, done the work as far as it can be done, – it is
probable that I may retire, if, in pursuance of my design & allegiance which I
hold to it, I meet with a sphere which is more analogous to the formation of a
Nursing School. I would wish to give notice of three months, to be extended, if
possible, to six months . . .

Lady Canning's letter, written the next day on behalf of the committee,
expressed sorrow at the loss of Florence's 'devoted services', but recognized that 'the great work you have always had at heart', to improve
hospital nursing, 'cannot be carried out in such an institution as this . . .'
By the end of Florence's period of notice, they hoped to have found
another Superintendent to continue her work – 'tho' we are without the
slightest hope of meeting with your equal'. Florence's decision to leave
was kept a secret for the time being, while she attended interviews with
the 'leading Men' at King's. They didn't intimidate her; on the contrary,
she thought that they themselves seemed frightened, in the course of
paying her meaningless compliments, of what they might be letting
themselves in for. 'If I don't turn up in one Hospital,' she confidently
predicted to Parthenope, 'I shall be in another.'

Florence never forgot the Upper Harley Street Institution. A year after
her return from the Crimean War, she returned there on a committee
day, 'where all received her with the greatest reverence & affection'. And
she continued to follow its subsequent incarnations – as the Hospital for
Invalid Gentlewomen, and eventually, from its new address at 19 Lisson
Grove, as the Florence Nightingale Hospital for Ladies of Limited Means
– with interest. In *The Times*, in 1901, she made an appeal for funds for

the Institution. 'I ask and pray my friends who still remember me not to let this truly sacred work languish and die for want of a little more money.'

On 31 August, she took temporary leave of absence from Upper Harley Street. The worst outbreak of cholera in the history of London was decimating the population of the area of Broad Street on the north edge of Soho. Over 500 lives were lost in ten days. Florence volunteered her services at the Middlesex Hospital, superintending the victims of the disease, going without sleep for two nights as the seriously ill poured in. Among the worst affected were the prostitutes, who were brought in from their 'beat' along Oxford Street. She undressed them, placed turpentine stupes on their stomachs, and managed to avoid falling ill herself (meanwhile, John Snow, the physician and epidemiologist, was setting out to show that the majority of deaths took place in the vicinity of Broad Street's water pump). As the intensity of the epidemic receded, she returned to the Institution, but was unable to shake off a heavy cold. Assured that the rest of the staff could cope in her absence, she decided to take a short break with her family at Lea Hurst.

There she coincided with the arrival of the novelist Elizabeth Gaskell. Mrs Gaskell had fallen behind with *North and South*, her latest novel. With its serialization in *Household Words* lapping at her heels, she needed urgently to make some progress with her writing, and had been invited to the tranquillity of the Derbyshire countryside to try to do so. Her acquaintance with Nightingales was relatively new, but she shared with them a Unitarian background, as well as an interest in reformed nursing with Florence. In *Ruth*, her last novel, Mrs Gaskell had argued for the dignity of the nursing profession through the main character, who ends up nursing typhus victims; and, later, she was to encourage her younger daughter, Meta, to become a nurse, when Meta showed signs of wishing to follow in Florence Nightingale's footsteps. In her mid-forties, warm and confiding, she was always hungry for stories to fill her writing, not least her voluminous correspondence. Florence's story, already in the process of being nicely burnished by her mother and sister for the novelist's benefit – Florence as their 'wild swan' in the Hans Christian Andersen tradition – utterly enticed her.

In a 'privatish' letter, written one evening during her stay, to her friend Catherine Winkworth, Mrs Gaskell described Florence's childhood in terms reminiscent of the lives of the saints: her desire from childhood always to be taking care of the sick poor, her rejection of pleasure-seeking, and her eventual study of nursing at Kaiserswerth and in Paris. 'She is like a saint,' Mrs Gaskell averred, perhaps St Elizabeth of Hungary, a medieval princess who had devoted her life to works of charity, and built a hospital at the foot of her father's castle. 'She must be a creature from another race so high & mighty & angelic, doing things by impulse – or some divine inspiration & not by effort & struggle of will . . . she seems as completely led by God as Joan of Arc.' Not many saints, perhaps, have been practised mimics, but Mrs Gaskell thoroughly enjoyed Florence's imitation of 'the way of talking of some of the poor governesses in the Establishment'. Florence's literary skills also inspired admiration. Her letters from Egypt were being prepared for private publication at Parthenope's insistence, though Florence had more than once refused to be bothered with correcting proofs (and a year later, when Florence's name was 'in every one's mouth', Fanny had to go to great lengths to ensure that the surviving proof sheets were destroyed, for fear that they might fall into unauthorized hands). Mrs Gaskell didn't care for travel, still less for Egypt, but she couldn't help being impressed when the letters were read out loud, and longed for a published copy of her own.

Yet within a short time, Mrs Gaskell's attitude towards Florence changed. She had seen an aspect of her character, the complete reverse of her own, that chilled her. Having been told by Parthenope that Florence 'does not care for *individuals* . . . but for the whole race as being God's creatures', Mrs Gaskell then witnessed an illustration of this, in the 'extreme difficulty' with which Parthenope persuaded Florence to visit a widow in the village, who had recently lost her husband, and was well known to Florence as she had nursed her son on his death bed seven years earlier. 'She will not go among the villagers now,' Mrs Gaskell wrote to Emily Shaen, another friend, 'because her heart and soul are absorbed by her hospital plans, and as she says, she can only attend to one thing at once. She is so excessively soft and gentle in voice, manner, and movement that one never feels the unbendableness of her character when one is near her.'

She and I had a grand quarrel one day. She is, I think, too much for institutions, sisterhoods and associations, and she said if she had influence enough not a mother should bring up a child herself; there should be creches for the rich as well as the poor. If she had twenty children she would send them all to a creche, seeing, of course, that it was a well-managed creche. That exactly tells of what seems to me *the* want – but then this want of love for individuals becomes a gift and a very rare one, if one takes it in conjunction with her intense love for the *race*; her utter unselfishness in serving and ministering.

Observing the elder sister's devotion for the younger, Mrs Gaskell surmised correctly that Parthenope's 'sense of existence is lost in Florence's'. Her description, though, of Parthenope as having 'annihilated herself', forgoing her own interests and tastes to take over Florence's home duties so that she could be set free to do her great work, shows how closely she had been influenced by Parthenope's version of events. This sympathy for Parthenope's position formed the basis of a friendship between the two women that would last throughout the next decade, until Mrs Gaskell's death.

Up in her turret room at Lea Hurst, well stocked with candles and coal, and with only Athena for company, Mrs Gaskell hurried on with *North and South* following the departure of the Nightingales for London in mid-October. A quarter of a mile of staircase separated her from the remaining servants packing up the house, and she found it difficult to imagine a more complete solitude. Thoughts about Florence Nightingale, and of their recent conversations, lingered in her mind as she attempted to resolve the fate of her heroine, Margaret Hale, in the novel's final chapters. Following the deaths of her parents, and a return to her former home, Margaret's dark musings about her future reflect Mrs Gaskell's own ambivalence about her recent encounter with a woman who appeared to place love of mankind above love for individuals: 'If I were a Roman Catholic and could deaden my heart, stun it with some blow, I might become a nun. But I should pine after my kind; no, not my kind, for love for my species could never fill my heart to the utter exclusion of love for individuals.' Despite, however, her cousin Edith's fears that Margaret will become 'strong-minded', Margaret is on the brink of matrimony with the mill owner John Thornton as the novel ends.

The Crimean War cuts obliquely across the pages of Mrs Gaskell's *North and South*. In the climactic riot scene, the 'thread of dark-red blood' that trickles down Margaret Hale's face is suggestive of the 'thin

red line' that became famous as a symbol of British heroism at the time
of the Battle of Balaclava in October 1854. In Florence's letters from
Upper Harley Street, the war is similarly perceived in the background.
She commented, but only in passing, on the mounting crisis in October
1853 as the Sultan of Turkey threatened Russia with a declaration of
war if Russian troops were not removed from Wallachia; and once
Turkey had declared war on Russia, and the Russian Black Sea fleet had
destroyed the Turkish naval force at Sinope harbour at the end of
November, she offered her Abbess of Minsk material for use as propaganda against the autocratic tyranny of Tsar Nicholas I. However, the
first reference in her correspondence to British troops in the conflict,
after Britain and France allied themselves with Turkey in an uneasy
partnership and declared war on Russia in March 1854, comes not in
one of her own letters, but in one addressed to her, by Liz Herbert.
Writing at the end of September, by which time Florence had already
left London for Lea Hurst, Mrs Herbert wrote of the anxiety being
experienced by the whole country as it waited for news of the outcome
of the Battle of the Alma, where the British and French were attempting
to rout the Russians and remove the threat of the Russian naval base at
Sebastopol. 'We hope to have tidings of the Battle which was to be
fought on the 20th,' Liz Herbert told Florence. 'God help us & them.'
It was while Florence was at Lea Hurst that the initial, harrowing reports
began to appear in *The Times*, shocking the entire nation, and moving
it to a frenzy of indignation, with their descriptions of the woefully
inadequate care of sick and wounded soldiers.

The spark that had ignited the Crimean War was a dispute between
Russia and Turkey over control of the holy places in Jerusalem; but this
had quickly escalated as Russia used the disagreement as a pretext for
moving troops into Moldavia and Wallachia. After a peace of nearly
forty years, following the defeat of Napoleon at Waterloo, Europe was
again being threatened by the rise of a great power: Russia in the East.
British interests were affected, as the country watched with alarm the
development of Russian sea power at its naval dockyard at Sebastopol
in the Crimea. Russia was advancing from the north, intent on securing
access to the Mediterranean. If Turkey collapsed in the face of Russian
aggression, Britain's main route to India would come under threat.

As 30,000 British troops embarked at Portsmouth, on their way to
the East, at the end of March 1854, the mood in the country was

confident and almost bullish; a liberal, western democracy, fresh from the triumph of the Great Exhibition three years earlier, which had demonstrated Britain's industrial prowess and superiority to the world, was to fight against Asiatic despotism. 'Well, here we are going to war,' Arthur Clough wrote to Charles Eliot Norton in Boston, 'and really people after their long and dreary commercial period seem quite glad; the feeling of the war being just, of course, is a great thing.' But at Varna, the small Bulgarian port on the Black Sea where a combined force of almost 60,000 British and French troops encamped in June to await orders, the first serious signs of the problems with climate, sanitary conditions and disease that were to paralyse the campaign began to strike. In February of that year, Dr Andrew Smith, the Director-General of the Army Medical Department, had sent a team of doctors to Varna to scout for suitable locations for hospitals and facilities. They had made their recommendations, most of which were ignored. The Army now paid the price. Between June and August, 20 per cent of the British expeditionary force went down with cholera, diarrhoea and dysentery; almost 1,000 men died before a shot had been fired. William Howard Russell, the *Times* correspondent, reported seeing dead bodies rising from the bottom of the harbour and bobbing around in the water, 'all buoyant, bolt upright, and hideous in the sun'.

Worse was to come. Engaging with the enemy on the banks of the river Alma, just above Sebastopol, on 20 September, the British suffered heavy losses. Those who survived, many of them weakened and exhausted by disease, were able to claim victory, though they failed to march on Sebastopol while the Russians were in retreat. The deficiencies of the medical system thrown up by mismanagement, lack of preparation, and logistical incompetence, meanwhile, were becoming ever more apparent. The sick and wounded waited, without care, for days or weeks, to be loaded on to ships for a voyage, sometimes lasting as long as a week, across the Black Sea to the base hospital at Scutari, situated opposite Constantinople, on the Asiatic side of the Bosphorus. On arrival they faced more waiting, and an agonizing journey, loaded on to carts or strapped to mules, to the hospital. What they found there became the subject of a series of eyewitness accounts, graphically related by Russell, and by Thomas Chenery, the *Times* diplomatic correspondent in Constantinople, that simultaneously launched a new era of war reportage, and of the mobilization of middle-class opinion to generate reform.

On 9 October, Russell's dispatch from the battlefield was published in *The Times*. He acknowledged a 'glorious victory' at Alma, but, alluding to the futility of nursing arrangements, emphasized that 'The number of lives which have been sacrificed by the want of proper arrangements and neglect must be considerable.' Three days later, a long letter from Chenery, 'Our Special Correspondent' in Constantinople, dated 30 September, pushed home the point by describing conditions at Scutari:

Not only are there not sufficient surgeons – that, it might be urged, was unavoidable; not only are there no dressers and nurses – that might be a defect of the system for which no one is to blame; but what will be said when it is known that there is not even linen to make bandages for the wounded? The greatest commiseration prevails for the suffering of the unhappy inmates of Scutari, and every family is giving sheets and garments to supply their wants. But why could not this clearly foreseen want have been supplied? Can it be said that the Battle of Alma has been an event to take the world by surprise? Has not the expedition to the Crimea been the talk of the last four months? . . . And yet, after the troops have been six months in the country, there is no preparation for the commonest surgical operations! Not only are men kept, in some cases, for a week without the hand of a medical man coming near the wounds; not only are they left to expire in agony, unheeded and shaken off, though catching desperately at the surgeon whenever he makes his rounds through the fetid ship; but now, when they are placed in the spacious building, where we were led to believe that every thing was ready which could ease their pain or facilitate their recovery, it is found that the commonest appliances of a workhouse sick-ward are wanting . . .

The next day, another letter from Chenery rose to a new pitch of anger, as he compared the treatment of the sick and wounded to that of 'the savages of Dahomey', and begged the question why, if the French could be assisted by their Sisters of Charity, the same standard of nursing care could not be applied to the British Army. That same day, a donation of £200 from Sir Robert Peel, son of the late Prime Minister, started a *Times* fund, which would eventually total some £11,000, to provide supplies and relief for the care of British soldiers.

Florence must have read Russell's story while staying at Lea Hurst. On 10 October, she left Derbyshire for London, four days ahead of the rest of her family, accompanied by a friend who recalled later that she spoke little on their journey, appearing to be in deep contemplation –

she was suffering from a mouth abscess, which may have been another reason for her silence – 'but mentioned the state of the Scutari Hospital & said how much she should like to go to help it'. In London she moved swiftly, utilizing what connections she could. She was contacted by Lady Maria Forester, one of many private individuals keen to organize a volunteer relief effort, who proposed offering £200 for someone to go out with three nurses. But Florence had in mind an even smaller scheme, consisting of herself and one additional nurse whose expenses she would pay, perhaps Mrs Clarke from Upper Harley Street (who did in fact volunteer to go with her). This was the proposal she outlined to Lord Palmerston, now Home Secretary, on 12 October. He in turn requested Lord Clarendon at the Foreign Office to write to the British Ambassador at Constantinople, Lord Stratford de Redcliffe. On Friday 13 October, Florence approached Dr Andrew Smith in the Army Medical Department, and received a letter of authorization from him to go out to Scutari, together with a letter of introduction to Dr Duncan Menzies, the Principal Medical Officer there.

Thus far, Florence's plans bore all the marks of a hastily improvised private expedition, and it was in this vein that she described it, in a letter to Mrs Bracebridge on 15 October, two days before her planned date of departure. Revising her original idea, she had decided to pioneer the way with a detachment of three or four women. This, she thought, would be infinitely easier 'than to march in, (even supposing it possible) with a great batch of undisciplined women not knowing what places to assign them, in so new a position as a military hospital'. The letter reveals that Selina Bracebridge was not favourably disposed to such an enterprise under this guise, but Florence asked her nevertheless to explain her undertaking to Fanny Nightingale 'without unfavourable comment'. On the previous morning, Saturday, Florence had gone to the Herberts' London home in Belgrave Square. Finding that they were out of town, she wrote to Liz Herbert to inform her of her intentions, asked for Sidney Herbert's advice as Secretary at War, and requested that she, or another lady of the committee at Upper Harley Street, write on her behalf to Lady Stratford, wife of the ambassador at Constantinople 'to say "this is not a lady but a real Hospital Nurse" . . .' The Herberts were in Bournemouth that weekend. By coincidence, on the Sunday, the day after Florence's abortive visit to Belgrave Square, Sidney Herbert wrote to Florence with a proposal of his own, asking her to superintend a

Government-sponsored group of nurses to the military hospital at Scutari. His and Florence's letters crossed in the post.

In recent years, a theory has gained ground that this scenario is too contrived and that, in fact, it conceals a prior agreement between Florence and Herbert, only confirmed by his letter, that she would accept his offer of the post. Such ideas can be instantly dismissed. Florence's letter to Liz Herbert, on 14 October, makes it abundantly clear that she is writing to her primarily 'as one of my mistresses' – that is, as a member of the Upper Harley Street committee – to discover whether she has the support of the Institution in breaking the period of notice she has given them. Moreover, there is a vast chasm of difference between the private plan Florence was ready to act on before she received Herbert's letter, and the official scheme that she subsequently acquiesced in. Nor was Herbert's request couched in terms that suggested he was certain of expecting an answer in the affirmative from Florence. He carefully laid out the reasoning behind the decision to send female nurses, explaining that the absence of a fixed hospital until that time had made the introduction of female nurses impossible; but now, with Scutari as the base, 'no military reason exists against the introduction, & I am confident they might be introduced with great benefit . . .' He paid tribute to Florence as the 'one person in England that I know of, who would be capable of organizing & superintending such a scheme', and singled out her 'personal qualities', knowledge and 'power of administration', as well as her position in society, as making her eminently qualified for the job. He was sure that the Bracebridges would accompany her, but asked, 'If you were inclined to undertake this great work would Mr & Mrs Nightingale consent?' He then proceeded to surmise – correctly as it turned out – that they would be unlikely to withhold their agreement to their daughter playing a part in work of such national importance.

Herbert emphasized the experimental nature of the expedition. At an early stage, before the Army embarked upon its Crimean mission, the possibility of employing female nurses had been mooted, and then rejected when it became obvious that 'the general opinion of military men was adverse to their employment'. Women had played an ill-defined role in military nursing during the Napoleonic Wars, when the practice of using army wives, widows and camp followers as nurses probably reached its peak, but in the years following, demand for their services had sharply declined. Herbert was under no illusions that there wouldn't be considerable practical difficulties associated with his new scheme. Finding suitable women was one problem, introducing them to the smooth running of a hospital under the eyes of military and medical men, another. But, as he observed in the closing paragraphs of his letter to Florence, if this experiment succeeded, 'an enormous amount of good will be done, now, & to persons deserving everything at our hands, & a prejudice will have been broken through, & a precedent established wh[ich] will multiply the good to all time'. It was a momentous decision, and one for which Sidney Herbert deserves full credit.

To Florence it must have seemed that her hour of destiny had arrived. Uncle Sam obtained her parents' agreement to her going without difficulty. 'Government has asked, I should say entreated, Flo to go out & help in the Hospital at Scutari,' Parthenope wrote excitedly to a friend. The extent of Parthenope's Damascene conversion to the idea of her sister's destiny was revealed in a further letter, in which she commented on the remarkable way 'in which all things have . . . fitted her for this . . . None of her previous life has been wasted . . .' On Monday 16 October, Florence and Herbert met at Upper Harley Street to formalize arrangements. During this meeting, they probably agreed on the terms of the official instructions which Herbert issued to Florence four days later, and which were supplemented by Herbert's letter to the editor of the *Morning Chronicle*, published on 24 October, publicizing their arrangements. Herbert confirmed Florence's acceptance of 'the Office of Superintendent of the female nursing establishment in the English General Military Hospitals in Turkey . . .' This simple statement, limiting Florence's jurisdiction to the base hospital at Scutari (as Scutari was the only such hospital in existence at this time), was to have serious ramifications when Florence attempted to claim control over nurses serving in front-line hospitals in the Crimea.

Florence wanted the nursing party to be limited to twenty in number, foreseeing the difficulties of finding qualified women, and of supervising a greater number. But Sidney Herbert proposed a larger number, and finally forty was the figure agreed upon. Nurses were solicited from the Protestant Institutions of Nursing. Both the Fry Nursing Sisters, and the All Saints' Sisterhood, founded in Fitzroy Square in 1851, declined to supply nurses, as they were to be subject to Florence's jurisdiction rather than that of their own committees. By contrast, the council of St John's House agreed to suspend their rules so that their members would come under the nursing superintendent's rule. The Sellonite Sisters of Mercy from Devonport, and from St Saviour's, Osnaburgh Street, in London, also waived their rules and sent sisters.

Not to be outdone, the Roman Catholic Church immediately appreciated the value to its cause of sending nurses from its own sisterhoods to Scutari, allowing it to wrap itself in the mantle of patriotism (it might be noted additionally that as many as one-third of the British troops in the Crimean War were Irish Catholics). Thomas Grant, the Roman Catholic Bishop of Southwark, contacted Herbert and offered the services of his nuns. Five women from the Bermondsey Convent of Mercy, led by Mother Mary Clare Moore, were the first to leave London, on 17 October. Unescorted, and without a chaplain, they reached Paris late that night and were ordered to await Florence Nightingale's arrival. Five more Roman Catholic nuns came from the Convent of the Daughters of the Faithful Virgin at Norwood. Both sets signed an agreement subjecting them to Florence's authority. Alert to the sensitivity of introducing Catholics, Herbert warned Florence in his instructions to guard against any attempt 'to tamper with or disturb the religious opinions of the patients' and, if necessary, to take 'severe measures' against it.

Meanwhile, the headquarters of the expedition had been set up at the Herberts' house at 49 Belgrave Square. Here, Liz Herbert, Mrs Bracebridge, Mary Stanley and Parthenope organized the recruitment of nurses. The large number of surviving applications in the National Archives, for this and subsequent nursing parties to Scutari and the Crimea, gives some indication of the wide variety of backgrounds from which the interested applicants came, as well as providing testimony to the enthusiasm with which the call for female nurses was received. All grades of household servants, even kitchen maids, applied to be sent out East, in addition to monthly nurses and hospital matrons. The above-average wages were obviously a powerful incentive to some – 12 to 14 shillings a week plus keep and uniform, rising to 18 to 20 shillings after a year's good conduct – especially, it seems, to the recently widowed. Mrs Mary Jones, for example, bereaved at fifty, attempts to convince the selection committee of her religious orthodoxy ('Am a firm Protestant') as well as her personal strength ('I walked through Wilts, Hants & Surrey this summer for amusement . . . from twelve to fifteen miles a day'). At some point during that week of harassed preparation, Selina Bracebridge went to Oxford to inspect potential nurses selected for her by Felicia Skene, who had organized a band of nurses during the cholera epidemic in the city earlier that year. From Skene's later account, it appears that these hopeful recruits were subjected to quite a grilling. Comparing Mrs Bracebridge to the Queen of Hearts in *Alice in Wonderland*, she recalled that the women were lined up along a wall and had 'sudden questions' fired at them. If the questions weren't answered satisfactorily, Mrs Bracebridge barked, 'She won't do; send her out.' Back in London, the standard of women, according to Parthenope, who had started to keep a journal, was dispiritingly low. On 20 October, having sat in Belgrave Square all day, 'seeing nurses', she recorded, 'Got 2. Such rubbish came.' Among the successful candidates was Mrs Eliza Roberts. With twenty-three years' experience as a nurse at St Thomas's Hospital – reflected in the fact that she received more than double the salary of the other nurses – Mrs Roberts was the most qualified member of the group, and would more than live up to her promise. The final number was thirty-eight, reflecting the scarcity of those with even the minimum of qualifications: fourteen Anglican Sisters, ten Roman Catholic nuns, and fourteen women, including Mrs Clarke, with civilian hospital experience and, as Madame Mohl tartly remarked, 'of no particular religion unless the worship of Bacchus should be revived'.

Sidney Herbert had presented Florence's appointment to the Cabinet on 18 October, where it received unanimous approval. The Admiralty were requested to provide passage for the nurses on board the mail packet *Vectis*, from Malta to Constantinople. In spite of their poor health and advanced years (they were both in their mid-fifties), the Bracebridges had agreed to accompany Florence to Scutari; Uncle Sam would go with them to Marseilles, Arthur Clough with Florence as far as Calais. Sir John Kirkland, the Army agent, had been ordered to provide Florence with £1,000 for all expenses. On the morning of 21 October, the day of departure, Florence and Parthenope drove to Belgrave Square from the house in Cavendish Square in which their parents had taken rooms earlier in the year, still reading and sorting letters from prospective nurses as they went. At the house, Mary Stanley was writing out a fair copy of the agreement that each of the civilian nurses was to sign, setting out their terms of employment. The hall was full of the Sellonite and St John's Sisters, together with the secular nurses. While Sidney Herbert made a rousing speech, impressing on them the need to obey Miss Nightingale in all things, Florence stood 'in the centre of the Arc of the bow of her staff'. It was just eleven days since she had returned to London with plans to offer her services at Scutari.

What was going through her mind in the little time that she had for herself, as they prepared to leave? The enormity of the undertaking can never have been far from her thoughts, though her mother remembered her afterwards, setting forth 'calm & self professed to the last'. On the eve of her departure, Florence had inscribed a prayer on the flyleaf of her copy of Thomas à Kempis's *The Following of Christ in Four Books*. In the words of Madame Elisabeth, sister of Louis XVI, as she awaited execution as a prisoner in the Temple during the French Revolution, Florence submitted herself to the will of God. 'What will happen to her, O God, I do not know; all I know is that nothing will happen that You have not ruled, foreseen and ordained from all eternity . . . I make my sacrifice one with that of Jesus Christ my saviour.'

She had longed for real life instead of the dreams of her imagination. She knew that the suffering that released her from a passive existence could strengthen or enrich her, but might also paralyse or extinguish her altogether. Florence was far from certain that she would survive her oncoming ordeal. In a farewell letter to her father, she admitted that she little expected to see England again, and then confessed that she loved him 'as I never loved any but him'.

———

One thing had been overlooked in all the upheaval surrounding preparations for their departure. Late in the afternoon of 19 October, as Mrs Gaskell was busily writing at Lea Hurst, the housekeeper Mary Watson entered her room with the news that Athena the owl had been found dead. In a letter written to Fanny Nightingale, Mrs Watson expressed the household's delight 'with Miss F going to act so noble a part in the East', and told her the distressing news.

Honoured Madam

I am sorry to inform Poor little Owl is dead. She was in the room yesterday morning, until 1 o'clock. I then took her to the little Bedroom and let her out of the cage. She seemed quite well but when I went back to her at ¼ past 5 she was dead; she was on her Back and there was [sic] a small quantity of Blood had come out of her mouth.

Mrs Watson brought the owl's corpse to London the next day, so that the dead bird could be taken to the taxidermist. 'Her mistress asked to see her again, & the only tear she shed through that tremendous week was when we put the little body into her hands.'

As Parthenope remarked later, the incident seemed to set the seal on the death of Florence's old life.

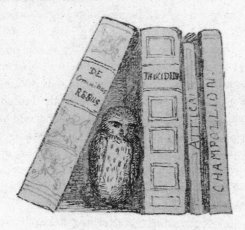

Part Two
Lady with the Lamp
1854–6

Exposed as I am to be misinterpreted & misunderstood, in a field of action in which the work is new, complicated, and distant from many who sit in judgement upon it . . .

FN to Sidney Herbert, 6 January 1856

N is Miss Nightingale, with her fair band,
Who solaced our sick in a far distant land . . .
The Panoramic Alphabet of Peace (1856)

I have lived a more public life than ever queen or actress did.

FN, undated note

9. Calamity Unparalleled

The Selimiye Barracks at Scutari impose themselves upon the skyline of modern Üsküdar, a short ferry ride across the Bosphorus, on the Asian side of Istanbul. At night, when its four prominent turrets are brightly illuminated, this gigantic structure is impossible to ignore. To Sarah Anne Terrot, one of the Sellonite sisters accompanying Florence Nightingale's expedition in the autumn of 1854, the building seemed on first sight to be 'the ugliest object visible'. Another English visitor that year – 'after climbing two or three banks, jumping two or three ditches, and picking his way round two or three mud-holes' – found himself in front of 'a large quadrangular edifice, very much like our Millbank Penitentiary'. Rebuilt for Sultan Mahmud II by the Armenian architect Krikor Balyan at the beginning of the nineteenth century, after the previous quarters were destroyed in the 1808 Janissary insurrection, and subsequently expanded by later sultans, the Barracks stands on uneven ground, two or three storeys high, overlooking a vast central parade area. Around the inside of the building run corridors facing into the quadrangle. Charles Bracebridge, accustomed before long to perambulating them, estimated their extent at 500 by 200 paces; more conventional measurement sets them at 220 by 194 yards. Hastily surrendered by the Turkish authorities to their British allies for employment as a base hospital, with a swift application of whitewash to disguise its dilapidated and unsanitary condition, the barracks provided a backdrop for some of the earliest photographs of the Crimean War: James Robertson's views of groups from the Coldstream and Grenadier Guards encamped at Scutari, in the spring of 1854, taken before they sailed up to Varna, the Allied camp on the west coast of the Black Sea. By September, many of these same men had been sent back on a painfully protracted journey to the Barrack Hospital, sick, ill-fed, and inadequately clothed.

Following the cessation of hostilities in 1856, and the departure of the final patients and medical staff, Scutari reverted to its original role as a military barracks. Today it serves as the closely guarded head-quarters of the Turkish First Army. The Barracks's chequered history over the past few decades has included its use as the base for Turkey's invasion of Cyprus in 1974, and a period as the office of the Martial Law authorities, when the basement of the building where, during the war, Lady Alicia Blackwood had taken charge of the wives, widows and infants of soldiers, living in 'a Pandemonium', became a different kind of hell as the centre for the interrogation, imprisonment and torture of political prisoners. Nowadays the cracked stone paving of the corridors, along which Nightingale and her nurses used to walk, has been replaced with a rubber-tiled floor which is waxed and spotless, while the only pervasive smell is one of soldiers' lunch. In 1973 an idea mooted by the British Government, to improve the contents of two rooms previously set aside to commemorate Florence Nightingale's memory in what is known as the 'North-West Tower', was taken up with enthusiasm by the Turkish Nurses Association, who refurnished them with relics and reproductions. Unfortunately, the wrong tower had almost certainly been chosen. Surviving evidence, including a plan of the nurses' quarters drawn by Parthenope Nightingale from her sister's and the Bracebridges' descriptions, together with a series of sketches of the hospital made by the matron Anne Morton in the spring of 1856, indicates that the true nurses' tower was the one that is situated to the left, and not to the right, of the main entrance, a part of the building currently closed to visitors.

Almost a century before the refurbishment of the museum at Scutari, the social reformer Octavia Hill was an early tourist to the site. In 1880, recovering from illness and the setbacks, personal and professional, that threatened the continuation of her work, she found renewed strength in contemplating Scutari as a symbol of Florence Nightingale's achieve-ment during the Crimean War. For Hill, the Barracks no longer stood for the calamitous neglect of the health of the British soldier, but rather as something 'so good, and solid, and in order'. A short distance from the Barracks, and also visited by Octavia Hill, is the British cemetery where the dead from the hospital, among them several nurses, are buried. It now overlooks the shipping terminal, only faintly obscured by a row of trees, but in Florence Nightingale's time the cemetery commanded a magnificent view: 'a little promontory jutting out into the Sea of Mar-mora ... seen by all ships entering the Bosphorus'. A monument to the memory of the British forces in the shape of an obelisk, designed by

Marochetti and with an inscription by Macaulay, was erected in 1857 near the main entrance. But only a few of the graves, as Hill noted, 'have any stone, name, or record'; and most of the 'heroic dead', as Nightingale called them, the 5,000 ordinary soldiers who died in the nearby hospitals, the greater proportion of them from sickness rather than wounds, lie in unmarked turf.

———

Entrusting the nursing party to the charge of the Bracebridges and Uncle Sam, Florence went ahead of them to Paris, on the evening of 21 October 1854, accompanied as far as Calais by Arthur Clough. Already concerned that the hospital nurses might prove 'feckless' – and indeed, two days later, one of them, Mary Wilson, turned up drunk at the railway station, and had to be dismissed shortly after arriving at Scutari – she had hoped to recruit sisters from the Order of St Vincent de Paul. However, despite the support of the British Ambassador's private secretary, who accompanied her to their headquarters, and letters from the British and French Governments, her application was refused. Meanwhile, the Bracebridges with the other nurses (minus the Bermondsey contingent, who were also to join them in Paris) left London Bridge station early on the morning of 23 October, bound for Folkestone, where they connected with the Boulogne packet. At Boulogne, their luggage was carried by the local fisherwomen to the Hôtel des Bains, where they sat down to 'a very tasteful display of French cookery', and were attended to by Marianne Galton, no doubt expiating her mischief-making over the Upper Harley Street appointment a year earlier by undertaking some hard graft in Florence's cause. Proceeding to Paris, they arrived late that night and were reunited with the rest of the party. The entire expedition set off the next day to Lyons, reaching Valence by boat down the Rhône on 25 October, and from there taking the train to Marseilles. Here Florence had the foresight to buy various supplies, among them several iron bedsteads as well as a pair of binoculars for herself, made of blackened brass. There was no time to rest as she made herself available to shopkeepers, the British consul, and the *Times* correspondent, as well as to her nursing staff. Her influence on them, and kindness in responding to their needs, appeared to be humanizing the rougher ones, even improving, as Uncle Sam observed, their table manners, while Florence's exhortation to them 'at the last' reportedly moved some to tears.

The paddle steamer *Vectis* sailed from Marseilles for Constantinople on the evening of Friday 27 October, loudly cheered by sailors and passengers from another vessel in the harbour rigged alongside her. Designed to carry mail at speed, the boat had a tendency to roll in high seas, and by Sunday afternoon many of the nurses were confined to their berths, suffering from sickness. Florence, a notoriously bad sailor, was one of them, in spite of having taken the precaution of obtaining medicine from Dr Poyser before her departure to alleviate the condition. 'She lies quite unable to dress or wash,' Charles Bracebridge wrote as they came in sight of Sicily, '& every time she swallows a mouthful is sick directly . . .' The weather, though, was 'lovely', and up on deck Mr Bracebridge, in full possession of his sea legs, was seated under an awning to protect him from the sun, while he spied on the three or four nurses unaffected by sickness, who were doing their best to attract the attentions 'of the impudent young surgeons', also travelling East. He liked the Sellonites very much – 'they are much more lady like than the rest' – regarded the St John's sisters as 'troublesome' because of their inclination 'to go their own way & . . . break out into finery – bracelets, brooches & velvet dangles', and had to admit that, to his surprise, the 'rabble', with the exception of the disgraced Wilson, were much improved. Among other passengers on their way to Scutari was Dr Alexander Cumming. Cumming, one of a three-man commission appointed by the Government, in the wake of the public outrage provoked by *The Times*, to report on the state of the hospitals at Scutari and in the Crimea, seemed 'a very sensible & practical man', according to Selina Bracebridge; and one, moreover, that Florence was likely to 'get on very well with . . .'

The *Vectis* anchored at Malta at daybreak on 30 October. A large group of the sisters and nurses went ashore, commanded by Mr Bracebridge, who marshalled them in procession, sisters in black vestments in front, those in white to the rear, with nurses in an intermediate position, bawling military-style instructions at them. The winds rose as they left Malta, and passing the Greek islands, the tiny boat was dashed by high waves which seemed at one point as though they were going to swallow her up. In the dark, cramped cabins, the air was foul, the floor swimming in water. Florence remained 'very suffering', while other members of the party panicked and offered up prayers. Early on the morning of 4 November, Florence, looking very worn, staggered on deck. Before her, she wrote to her family, as the party waited to disembark and receive their orders, was Constantinople, in 'thick & heavy rain', resembling 'a bad Daguerreotype washed out'. News had just reached them of the Battle of Balaclava, the first attempt by the Russians to break the siege of Sebastopol, and of the disastrous Charge of the Light Brigade. '. . . 400 wounded arriving <u>at this moment</u> for us to nurse . . . The first wounded I believe to be placed under our care. They are landing them now.'

Four days later, the Reverend Sydney Godolphin Osborne of Durweston in Dorset, a philanthropist of militant opinion, known to the Herberts, reached Scutari on an unofficial inspection, having traded his official connections for a role as an additional chaplain. A veteran visitor to workhouses and hospitals, especially during the famine in Ireland, and consequently not easily shocked, Osborne was none the less horrified by the sights that met his eyes. Walking down one of the long corridors, thickly lined with cases of cholera and dysentery, he found himself entering a 'vast field of suffering and misery', in which men lay either on the floor on thin stuffed sacking, or on the rotten wooden divans at the side, alive with vermin and every imaginable kind of filth. Witnessing the inadequate and chaotic system of hospital transports, Osborne noted the inhumane treatment of the sick and wounded following their 300-mile voyage from Balaclava, waiting on board ship, sometimes for as long as three days, to be taken ashore, or for hours on stretchers on the rudimentary landing stage as preparations were made to take them up the steep slope to the hospital. He observed the absence of 'the commonest provision' for the men once they got there, the lack of stores which he had been assured by the Director-General of the Army Medical Service, Dr Andrew Smith, back in London, had been sent out in abundance, the scarcity of medicines, and the poor level of diet. 'You may call it dinner, if you like,' Osborne was to recall later in his testimony before a House of Commons select committee, 'but I have seen meat brought up raw into the ward and put upon a board, and the orderly took a stick or a knife, and . . . cut it into rations.'

In short, Osborne found very little of what he termed 'the order of a hospital'; indeed, he wondered whether Scutari merited the title of hospital at all. There was no trace of any kind of system evident, 'and about the whole sphere of action' there existed 'an utter want of that accord amongst the Authorities in each Department which alone could secure any really vigorous effort to meet the demands, which the carrying on of the war was sure to make upon them'.

Breakdown on such a massive scale clearly begged the question of how such failure could ever have occurred, and answers would be sought in the numerous inquiries and committees convened both during the course of the war and in the years immediately following it. The British Army, uninvolved in a major conflict since Waterloo forty years earlier, had been allowed to atrophy. It was in no condition to embark on the rigours of a major conflict on enemy soil, and was signally ill-equipped to do so, as the absence of adequate hospital ships and lack of proper ambulances show. The British soldier may have been famous for his fortitude and discipline, but he suffered from poor leadership under the command of seasoned veterans, whose main qualification for their appointment appeared to be their advanced age. Lord Raglan, for one, commander-in-chief during the Crimean War up to his death in June 1855, was already sixty-five at the start of it. The weaknesses of the management and distribution of supplies were similarly of long-standing: the war simply exposed them and exacerbated their consequences with disastrous effects. It was a tragedy of epic proportions in which bureaucratic muddle and sheer human incompetence played the larger part, thrown in with a measure of bad luck (as, for instance, when the steamship The Prince, carrying medical supplies and winter coats and boots for the whole army, went down in a hurricane on the Black Sea in November 1854). All too often it was a case of the right hand being wholly unaware of what the left was doing. In London, Andrew Smith might have ordered the necessary supplies to be sent out and trusted that all was well, but in the meantime other complications had intervened. Stores might go missing, be misaddressed by the Ordnance officer, or sent to the wrong place. In September 1854, vital supplies from England were still arriving at Varna, even though it had already been abandoned by the Army in the wake of the decision to invade the Crimea; no one, though, had seen fit to inform Smith. The potential for the greatest amount of confusion in obtaining provisions for the Army existed in the antiquated Purveyor's department. The Purveyor supplied base hospitals with equipment and food through the Commissariat and a bewildering system of requisitions that had to travel through eight Government departments in London before they could be dealt with.

Until the end of December 1854, when Sidney Herbert made changes partly as a consequence of information he had received from Florence Nightingale at Scutari, the Commissariat remained a branch, not of the War Office, but of the Treasury. Thrift therefore was often at the root of the terrible hardships suffered by the troops, a fact brought into harsh focus by the refusal of the Purveyor to consider requisitioning shirts for soldiers who arrived at hospital straight from the battlefield without their packs because such items were 'unwarranted'.

The inadequacies of the hospitals themselves stemmed from the fact that there had never before been any attempt to establish permanent base hospitals on the scale which the invasion of the Crimea demanded. Smith had instituted a search through his department's records from the Peninsular War, in the hope of finding some precedent, but 'only two or three valueless documents' had surfaced. As a result, general hospitals were run according to the rules that applied to those that operated on regimental lines, despite the disparity between the function and administration of the two styles of hospital. Conflict was inevitable between the self-contained regimental system, designed for an army on the move, in which staffing, including medical officers and non-medical personnel, cooks, ward-masters, and orderlies, was the preserve of the regiment, and the administrative demands of a fixed hospital, established in existing buildings, and designed for the longer-term care of casualties once the regiment was on the move again.

The general military hospital was unpopular with soldiers, as it removed them from the company of friends and a familiar environment, and was regarded with suspicion by senior doctors, crowding men together and dramatically increasing the potential for spreading disease. Moreover, throughout the war, Army medical staff were fighting against an overriding problem: that, with the exception of the hospital constructed according to Isambard Kingdom Brunel's prefabricated design at Renkioi, on the south-west shore of the Dardanelles, which in any case remained unfinished at the end of the war, none of the other general hospitals used by the British had been designed specifically for that purpose. The largely military origins of the buildings taken over as hospitals made them inherently unsuitable. They were often in a bad state of overall structural disrepair, with suspect water supplies and almost non-existent drainage systems, while some were sited unhealthily close to Turkish burial grounds. Even the General Hospital at Scutari, a red-brick building about half a mile north of the Barrack Hospital across a patch of common ground, which had been taken over by the British in May 1854, and has often been described by historians as having originated as a hospital, was probably built by the Turks as a barracks. The British hospitals, according to one observer, provided 'a humiliating contrast' to those managed by the French, who had snatched all the prize sites for their hospitals.

Florence appears, on arrival, to have been wholly unaware of the existence of another large general hospital so close to the Scutari Barracks, evidence once more of the hastily improvised arrangements for her departure. Nevertheless, she immediately assumed responsibility for it, and quickly organized the provision there of ten of her thirty-eight nurses on a rotational basis. Three other smaller hospitals, opened as problems with overcrowding grew worse at the two major ones, also lay in the vicinity. Koulali Hospital, established at a cavalry barracks a few miles further north up the Bosphorus from Scutari, was ready by the end of January 1855. The Palace Hospital at Haidar Pasha, near the small town of Kadekoi, and, as its name suggests, a former Sultan's residence, opened earlier that month, while at Abydos, near Gallipoli, the hospital, again converted from a barracks, was accepting convalescent patients, at what was considered an unusually healthy site, at the end of 1854. Of these, neither Haidar Pasha nor Abydos was ever to come under Florence's superintendence.

The *Times* reports of conditions at the Barrack Hospital brought not only the Reverend Osborne, but a stream of other visitors, medical and non-medical, to Scutari, intent on discovering the truth for themselves. The atmosphere at times, according to one newspaper correspondent, was 'more like a fair than a Hospital'. Many accounts by these eyewitnesses are as damning as Osborne's. But how is one to explain those that run contrary to the general note of want and neglect? Assistant-Surgeon David Greig, who had sailed to Scutari on the *Vectis* with the Nightingale party, was one whose impression was more favourable, writing in his diary soon after arriving that 'There is plenty of everything, comparatively speaking.' More significantly, Dr John Hall, the Inspector-General of Hospitals and Chief Medical Officer in the East, with whom Florence would later famously cross swords, had visited the Barrack Hospital at the beginning of October and commented that 'the sick and wounded ... are doing better than I would have expected'. A month later, in the midst of rising criticism, Hall adopted a more outwardly defensive position, declaring that the 'difficulties' they were contending with at Scutari had been 'magnified and falsified to enlist the sympathies of the multitude against us . . .'

Admittedly, Hall had seen the Barrack Hospital before the desperate problems associated with overcrowding, following the influx of casualties from the Battles of Balaclava and Inkerman in early November, had begun to bite. Furthermore, to his discredit, he never returned to Scutari to reinspect the hospital for the remainder of the war. Yet the tenor of Hall's remarks – and those of others who insisted that the picture was not as black as it had been painted – was symptomatic both of a prevailing attitude and of a widespread inertia among the old guard in the British Army. It may well be true that the treatment of the ordinary soldier, and the kind of conditions he encountered at the base hospitals, were on balance no worse than those experienced by British forces in the past, in the Napoleonic Wars or earlier campaigns. However, the vital difference about the Crimean War, which Hall and his kind failed, to their cost, to appreciate, was that public opinion, the conscience of the nation, had been mobilized in the soldier's cause as never before. A principle of accountability had been established. Back in England, the Nightingales' friend Fanny Allen was one of those who recognized the immensity of this development when she wrote that she did not remember from previous wars 'that intense feeling of interest in the sufferings of the army that now appear so universal . . . The letters of the soldiers "and [of] our own correspondents" have brought things so vividly before our minds that we realize the miseries of war more . . .'

Florence Nightingale was an agent of this new notion of accountability. She also represented hopes of reform among the more junior members of the Army medical staff at Scutari. Not only was she equipped with the financial wherewithal to make a difference, she possessed the powerful connections at home to influence change, though she remained wary at all times of falling under suspicion as a Government spy owing to her line of direct communication with Sidney Herbert as Secretary of State at War. Some of the younger doctors, like Alexander McGrigor, Principal Medical Officer at the Barrack Hospital at the time of her arrival, were from the first to cooperate openly with her schemes for improvement. Equally, there were some, usually older staff, who flatly refused to have anything to do with the woman they scornfully referred to as 'the Bird'; and yet others who went behind their seniors' backs in their dealings with her, only later to be brought to account like naughty children.

Her mission was balanced delicately on a knife's edge. As a woman, she had been granted a field of action that was unprecedented in the Army's history, yet she behaved at all times with scrupulous attention to Army regulations to ensure that neither she nor her staff could be accused of infringing them. Received courteously by Dr Duncan Menzies, the Chief Medical Officer at Scutari, as she entered the Barrack Hospital on 4 November, Florence immediately demonstrated her recognition of the need for self-discipline. Menzies, coping as best he could in the circumstances, later recalled that she expressed surprise at the 'regularity and comfort' that she found in the wards. If she did indeed make this remark, it may have been as a tactical move designed to disarm him. Florence's next step displayed an even greater degree of diplomacy. Neither she nor her nurses would enter any ward, nor attend on any patients, except at the specific request of the medical officer in charge there. Mr Bracebridge's first report back to Herbert in London showed that she had calculated correctly that this would help to disperse some of the underlying resentment against her. 'Miss N.,' Bracebridge told him, 'is decidedly well received.'

The nurses' quarters consisted of a number of small, sparsely furnished rooms in the north-west tower, opening off a large kitchen or day-room, fitted with a stove at Florence's behest as the previous occupants had cooked with charcoal. Twelve nurses were crammed into one room together with Mrs Clarke and Mrs Roberts; ten nuns in another large room; a room at the top of the tower was occupied by the Sellonites; and a smaller room, reached by a staircase through this, held the St John's sisters. Mr Bracebridge and the courier slept on divans along the corners of the sitting room, while Selina Bracebridge's room doubled as an area in which Florence could receive people. Finally, 'a wee room . . . full of linseed & bad smells' was where Florence herself slept. The inhabitants were often at the mercy of the elements. On stormy days, part of the roof was liable to be torn off and the windows blown in, while, through the matting covering the holes in the floor, a heavy trickle of rain descended into the rooms beneath.

Some of the nurses, restless at their inactivity, were itching to be sent into the wards for the job they had come out to do. 'We tried to console

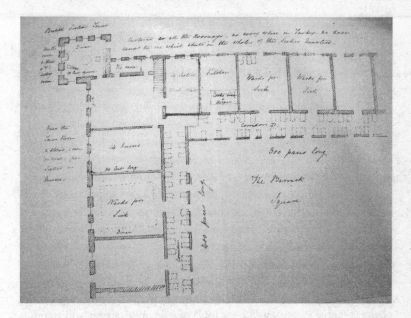

ourselves by making flannel shirts and bandages,' Sarah Anne Terrot wrote in her journal. Many of the women were set to work scrubbing the walls and floors. The rotten boards, which surrounded most of the wards, and on which men slept on the top of a thin layer of bedding, were difficult to wash, but Florence's introduction of a new standard of cleanliness was consistent with her adherence to the miasmatic theory of disease. According to this theory, widely prevalent at a time when Pasteur's first published work on fermentation, leading to the development of germ theory, was still more than a quarter of a century away, poisonous vapour arising from decomposed matter, identifiable by its unpleasant smell, could cause illness. Adequate ventilation, difficult to achieve if your hospital was overcrowded, sited in the vicinity of a burial ground, for instance, or a contaminated water supply, was the other widely prescribed means of combating the existence of miasmas.

One unpublished letter from late 1854, written by Richard Dawes, the Dean of Hereford, and preserved in the vast tranche of correspondence handed around among the Nightingales' family and friends, records that another of Florence's first actions at the Barrack Hospital was 'to take a piece of chalk & number all the beds throughout the Hospital'. This sounds characteristic of Florence's organizing powers, though the incident almost certainly belongs to the initial period after the stand-off was over. For on 8 November, the waiting ended. With numbers in the hospital beginning to rise, and in expectation of the arrival of an even more overwhelming flood of casualties from the recent engagements, the medical officers turned to Florence for her assistance. In consultation with the doctors, she began to distribute nurses around the hospital. Two of the Sellonites, for instance, were sent to a far end of the hospital, to the cholera wards. While there were no cholera patients at this time, cases of low fever, diarrhoea, dysentery and scurvy were present in abundance. With other nurses, Florence went from ward to ward, giving the men new shirts, provided by the *Times* fund, to replace their blood-saturated old ones. 'The great corridor,' Charles Bracebridge reported that first day, '450 yards long, and four rooms holding 27 each, have been filled with beds and men in double rows, leaving 4 feet to walk in the middle. This was done from 12 o'clock to 6 o'clock. They were all dressed and fed by 8 o'clock.' According to Bracebridge's figures, there were 1,730 patients in the Barrack Hospital, and 600 in the General. Soon there would be a total of four miles of beds in the two hospitals, each bed separated from its neighbour by a statutory eighteen inches.

Over successive days, the crisis deepened. Selina Bracebridge's letter to Fanny Nightingale on the tenth – as 'Flo has not a moment' – expressed a growing realization of 'the confusion & the want of method', which she found 'beyond all description'.

Yesterday I shall <u>never</u> forget. 600 wounded from Sebastopol, the sufferers of the horrible battle of the <u>5th</u>, arrived here – they began to land them at 12. It was 5 o'clock before a bit of lint could be provided except <u>what we had</u> – not a soft towel had any surgeon . . . Many of the officials lost their heads – crying out to Flo 'you must make requisition for this & that' – & not knowing what to do. <u>There is</u>, no doubt plenty of every thing, but nothing to be had.

The stream of casualties seemed never-ending. As fast as one batch of men was dealt with, another was admitted. '700 were landed yesterday, & 800 expected tomorrow,' Charles Bracebridge recorded on the thir-teenth, 'the wounded are doing well, but the sick ill, many of them die of long standing dysentery . . .' Deaths, in the two hospitals combined, numbered between twenty and thirty a day. At one o'clock each after-noon, the sombre procession of corpses, sewn into blankets and carried on stretchers to the dead house, could be observed from the windows of the north-west tower.

'The night scenes are quite Rembrandt,' Mr Bracebridge told Parthenope. 'Florence, the Medical Inspector General, S. G. Osborne ... & orderlies with candles surrounding a poor fellow on the ground with his arm off. Our Prioress [Mary Clare Moore, the Bermondsey Sisters' Superior] with a flowing veil, kneeling over a man, & mopping with a sponge his bleeding leg. Florence & Sister George [Mary Gonzaga Barrie] binding up a stump, the surgeon on one side, the orderly with a light on the other.' In all this intense activity, it was a week before the Nightingale party was able to sit down together at dinner, having engaged two cooks and found enough chairs to seat everybody. Florence's meals were eaten in spare moments: 'her breakfast, tea, or supper stands on a chair beside her while she writes. Taking a spoonful between is her way.' Mrs Clarke, meanwhile, spent most of her waking hours standing before an enormous table in the day-room, 'cutting, cooking, ordering, teamaking', and preparing nourishing extra diets for the soldiers: beef tea, rice milk, custards, and doses of arrowroot, as Mrs Clarke put it, for 'them as bees faint'.

Florence's letter to William Bowman, of King's College Hospital, on 14 November, carried a note of exhilaration at having faced the tide of sick and wounded, matched by a sense of purposefulness at the realization that they were doing some good in the midst 'of this appalling horror'. On her nightly rounds among the newly wounded she described how moved she had been by the way in which 'these poor fellows' bore pain and mutilation 'with unshrinking heroism, and die or are cut up without a complaint'. In the entire Barrack Hospital, she doubted whether there was as much as an average of three limbs per man. One practical remedy introduced by Florence at this early stage was to place a screen around a patient being amputated so that the sight of the operation would be hidden from his comrades, 'for when one poor fellow, who is to be amputated tomorrow, sees his comrade today die under the knife it ... diminishes his chance'.* She remained fascinated by interesting cases on the operating table, something that caused her

---

* Dr John Hall had warned that the use of chloroform, a relatively new drug, widely favoured by younger surgeons coming out to the war straight from medical school, could increase danger in operations on patients suffering from shock. However, by the second quarter of the war, chloroform was employed in all major cases of amputation.

letters home to be bowdlerized prior to their circulation, whenever Florence's clinical descriptions of wounds were considered to be too disgusting for widespread consumption. Such fascination also drew disapproval from the Army and medical establishments as being inappropriate behaviour, which failed to reflect 'the modesty of anyone deserving to be a woman'. Lieutenant-General Sir John Burgoyne was repeating a no doubt well-worn story when he wrote to Lord Raglan, in the spring of 1855, that 'Miss Nightingale . . . seems to delight in witnessing surgical operations with arms folded . . .'; but the claim of Assistant-Surgeon Alexander Struthers that Florence had kept a man lying on the operating table for fifteen minutes until she could be found, as she insisted on being present at every operation, was more damaging and led to a flurry of controversy in Government circles at the end of 1854, which had to be countered by Sidney Herbert himself.

By the end of November, Florence had achieved another of the goals in her onward march towards cleanliness and hygiene, after the Purveying department had shrugged off responsibility for the washing of the men as a minor detail. With money from the *Times* fund, she took a house at Scutari and converted it into a laundry. Obtaining boilers from the Army Engineer's Office (at length a drying closet, donated by Angela Burdett-Coutts, arrived from England), and utilizing the services of some of the wives and widows from the cellars of the Barrack Hospital, she looked forward to the prospect of providing every patient with a clean shirt twice a week. As the year drew to its close, the renovation of the dilapidated wing of the hospital, capable of holding 800 patients, a quarter of its total capacity, helped to reduce the risks run by overcrowding. After problems with officialdom, in the person of the wife of the British ambassador to Constantinople, Lady Stratford de Redcliffe, who had engaged workmen who subsequently went on strike, Florence took on another 200 and saw the project to completion.

But the ongoing problem continued to be the fundamental deficiencies of the Purveying department, led by the 'wretched' Purveyor-General Mr Wreford, whose guiding principle appeared to be the avoidance of expense. Attempting to obtain supplies, Florence constantly encountered obstruction and delay. Much of the time, her requisitions for stores, signed by the presiding medical officer, were met with a refusal from the Purveyor, even when she knew for certain that the items were in stock. Her impatience at this abysmal state of affairs led her to take unauthorized measures. 'This morning I foraged in the Purveyor's Store,' she reported to Sidney Herbert in December, 'a cruise I make almost daily, as the only way of getting things. No mops, – no plates, no wooden trays . . . no slippers, no shoe-brushes, no blacking, no knives & forks, no spoons, no scissors (for cutting the men's hair, which is literally alive . . .) – no basins, no towelling, no Chloride of Lime.' In desperation, she requested that Herbert bypass the official procedures and send supplies directly from London. She also enlisted the support of Osborne, Bence Macdonald, the *Times* fund administrator, and Augustus Stafford, the Northamptonshire MP, who had come to Scutari as a keen advocate of Army reform, to observe conditions for himself, for the purchase of her own supplies from Constantinople's Grand Bazaar, to be kept in a storeroom in her quarters. Additionally, there were the voluntary contributions, nearly £7,000 in money and a host of other gifts, great and small, from donors back in Britain. Linen, some of it monogrammed, some of it amounting to little more than dirty rags, arrived in profusion after an appeal by Florence was published in *The Times* in November, requesting that supplies be sent to Messrs Cuthbert of Paternoster Row to be forwarded out East. There was a touching range of homemade gifts, too. Francis Eyre of Padbury, Buckinghamshire, sent slippers to keep soldiers' feet warm in bed, with a letter saying that he and his children had devoted their Christmas to making them, while a Mrs Gollop donated her raspberry preserves and ginger biscuits. Although Florence never released anything without official authorization, she quickly became the de facto source for a wide range of goods. 'I am really cook, house-keeper, scavenger . . . washerwoman, general dealer, store-keeper,' she announced to Herbert. Yet the underlying fragility of this provisional scheme was exposed the minute she left off her purveying for a single day, and chaos ensued. The men of C Corridor were drunk, having downed their wine all in one go, as they had been given no cups from which to drink it.

The admiration for Florence's exertions of Peter Benson Maxwell, another member of the Hospitals Commission, knew no bounds. In a letter to his wife, he described her as

a fine specimen of humanity, all the softness & gentleness of her sex, all the cold clear-headedness of the Mathematician, a capital head for devising the ten thousand little details of <u>administration</u> & a thorough honesty of purpose, a resolute boldness in action that quails before no obstacle. The cool steady way in which she does everything notwithstanding occasional sour looks from officials is perfect.

The Commission itself was a lame duck, as Florence well realized. Its report, to which she contributed evidence, was published in the spring of 1855, but the Commission had been mandated to make suggestions for improvements, not carry them out. For her part, in letter after letter to Herbert, written with furious determination throughout the winter of 1854–5, Florence continued to push home the plans she perceived as necessary 'for the systematic organization of these Hospitals upon a principle of centralization'; a comprehensive system, much of it later enshrined in the findings of the Royal Commission on the Sanitary Condition of the Army, proposing radical changes to the purveying, feeding and clothing of patients, and improvements in the standards of training for orderlies and medical staff. She had expected to end her days as a Hospital Matron, she joked to Dr Bowman, but never as a Barrack Mistress. Nonetheless it remained true that she was not merely Superintendent of the Female Nursing establishment, but, by force of circumstance, Purveyor-Auxiliary to the hospitals at Scutari as well. Florence's vital importance in this role was confirmed by the serious consideration that Lord William Paulet, the new Commandant of the Scutari Hospitals from early 1855, gave to the idea of officially appointing her as Purveyor.

'What F does & what she is, is most faintly conceived of in England . . .,' wrote Parthenope Nightingale in an aide-mémoire. 'The public there generally imagine her by the soldier's bedside, where doubtless she is often to be found, but as she herself said, how satisfactory, how easy if that were all. The quantity of writing, the quantity of talking is the weary work, the dealing with the selfish, the mean, the incompetent . . .' This disparity between the figure in the public's imagination and the flesh and blood reality would only grow wider. Certainly, by the summer of 1855, as Aunt Mai was to report, Florence had ceased to do any nursing beyond her nightly rounds among the patients.

Control of the nursing establishment was becoming an increasing headache for its Superintendent. For some of the women, the experience of working at Scutari had fallen far short of their expectations, while

Florence had been confirmed in her worst fears about the unsuitability of many of them – with honourable exceptions – for the job. It was clear early on that some were either not hardy enough to accustom themselves to the climate, or were unprepared to accept the discipline and privations of the way of life, to make the sacrifice, as Selina Bracebridge put it, 'for the love of their fellow creatures'. One Sellonite, Ethelrida Pillars, swigging eau de cologne on the voyage from Marseilles to combat acute sickness, had no sooner set foot on dry land than she was on her way home again, unable to eat the food provided and apparently too ill to work. Food was a common source of contention. A nurse threatened to leave if the puddings didn't improve, while in December 1854 an anonymous St John's sister wrote to Mary Jones, her Superintendent in London, to protest at the quality of meat prepared by Mrs Clarke: '. . . We Cannot get our teeth through and the Magets get out on our plats.'

Class predictably reared its head, complicated by the fact that there was no two-tier grading of nurses (unlike many civilian hospitals at home), as did problems associated with mixing lay nurses with religious sisters. The nurses were generally respectful of the nuns, but Mary Clare Moore, the Bermondsey Superior, subsequently admitted the uneasiness she and her other sisters felt at associating with 'persons of doubtful character' who, she claimed, were 'almost daily intoxicated'. Mrs Clarke, described by Florence a little euphemistically as 'somewhat brusque', upset the nuns with her abusive language, was said to be 'seldom sober', and was regarded as something of a tyrant by the others, allegedly insulting one, Mary Ann Coyle, every time she saw her. The St John's sisters, accused by Mrs Bracebridge of having pretensions beyond their status, were also affronted by the paid nurses, declaring that they would 'not Mix with those Low womin Miss Nightingale braught out . . .'; while the rank and file only left off wrangling with each other to have a go at the St Johnites. One of the St John's nurses, Emma Fagg, who had undergone three months' training at Middlesex Hospital in 1852 before being admitted as a probationer at St John's House, was clearly something of a troublemaker. On the voyage out she behaved in a disagreeable manner towards many of the others, and refused to accept discipline from Rebecca Lawfield, placed in charge of the St John's contingent, forcing Mrs Lawfield to wait on Fagg and her friends Mrs Boyle and Mrs Bowmett. Emma Fagg never settled down at Scutari, and was dismissed for incompetence in January 1855.

The greater proportion of the nurses' duties at Scutari, namely washing, sewing and cooking, corresponded precisely with the kind of household management that many of them would have practised in their own homes, or in the homes of others, as domestic servants. Their responsibilities, as a later official circular phrased it, consisted 'of every branch of work which lies in a woman's province'. It should come as no surprise then that Florence's superintendence of her staff was in large part derived from the mistress–servant relationship to which she had become accustomed, as a 'lady', in her own upper-middle-class home. Her manner towards them at times betrayed its origin in this relationship and was liable to cause offence. The anonymous St John's nurse, mentioned above, wrote of being treated 'With the greates disrespect and unkindness by Miss Nightingale . . .' Whether Florence ever scolded her nurses with the fierceness she was said to dole out to the hospital orderlies has gone unrecorded, but Assistant Surgeon Taylor thought the members of the nursing party he saw at Scutari 'very meek-looking'. Sister Joseph Croke, member of a subsequent nursing party (and scarcely one of Florence's admirers) was later to observe that 'Miss Nightingale is sweet, amiable, gentle, most insinuating whenever she is merely doing the lady . . . but when she wants to domineer she has a way of putting completely aside all her womanish qualities.'

The nurses' uniform, intended partly as a leveller, partly as a means of instant identification, also reinforced the idea of subservience. The nuns and sisters wore their habits (black in the case of the Bermondsey and Sellonite sisters, white for the Norwood nuns), but the rest wore white caps, plain black woollen dresses, covered by unbleached linen aprons, with a scarf across the shoulders from left to right, embroidered in red thread with the words 'Scutari Hospital'. Unfortunately this costume – 'a very ugly one' in the opinion of one of the nuns – only came in a single size, so that there was the constant comic spectacle of women who were tall wearing short dresses, and those who were short, long. As the war continued, official regulations governing 'uniform upper clothing' for nurses were published, with the rules for conduct and allowances (for example, if a nurse was found intoxicated she would be dismissed immediately, but any nurse in 'constant attendance on cholera or infectious fever' might be permitted an extra allowance of her chosen tipple at dinner, at the Superintendent's discretion). Florence herself ordered the nurses' boots from London, from Moore's in Knightsbridge, which sold servants' footwear. Her own boots, with elastic sides, 'not laced', came from Mr Chollocombe at Romsey, with galoshes to wear over them, but she suffered from a want of clothes. 'She has one flannel petticoat left,' Mrs Bracebridge wrote despairingly to Parthenope in early 1855, 'one bonnet with a hole in it – her black gowns (& she wears no others) are very grubby.' She reported that Florence also needed caps with a plain border of Maltese lace. After some weeks of cold creaming her hair, Florence decided to wear it very short, for convenience and to keep it free from vermin. There was 'no time for long hair' that first winter at Scutari.

At different times, Florence estimated that between ten and sixteen of her nursing staff were effective workers; at best, well under half the total workforce. The rest she considered completely undisciplined. After an unpromising start, when she had complained about the cap she was forced to wear, and seemed 'fonder of sketching than of poulticing', Rebecca Lawfield was praised as an outstanding nurse, not for her skill ('she does not know a fracture when she sees it', wrote Florence tersely) but because of her exemplary conduct and kindness. Eliza Roberts, with more than two decades of experience, and prized qualities as a surgical nurse, proved to be 'of an infinitely superior character' to any of the others. Of the religious sisters, Mary Clare Moore was, like Selina Bracebridge, to fill the dual role of confidante and support to Florence, as well as for years afterwards acting as her spiritual guide and mentor. Born in 1814, a child convert to Catholicism, Moore had worked under Catherine McAuley, founder of the Sisters of Mercy, at Baggot Street, Dublin, and with the Mercy community in Cork City, before becoming the first Superior of the Bermondsey foundation in 1839. The Bermondsey convent, designed by Augustus Pugin, was the first to be built in London since the Reformation. The work of the community there revolved around instruction of converts and the education of the young, as well as the visiting of the sick poor in their homes, and at Guy's and St Thomas's Hospitals. Moore's administrative powers – it was said that 'she was fit to rule a kingdom' – together with her diplomacy and her calm assurance, were frequently to be called upon in the course of the war. The skills of two of Moore's sisters, Mary Stanislaus Jones and Mary Gonzaga, were also singled out for Florence's praise. With Gonzaga, whom she called 'my Cardinal' – Florence was 'the Pope' – Florence formed a lasting friendship, and her trust in her was repaid when Gonzaga later proved an effective head of Scutari's General Hospital.

Much of the rank and file, however, continued to baulk at the restrictions placed on them, and at the absence of opportunities for the real nursing work for which they believed they had been engaged. These restrictions were undeniably tight. If called to a bedside, nurses were instructed on no account to converse with the medical officer, to 'speak soothingly' to the patients but avoid talking to them unnecessarily, and in 'moments of excitement' to 'exercise extreme self-control'. There was no night nursing, and they were not allowed in the wards after 8.30 at night, though Florence later admitted that sometimes nurses had 'rushed out against' this order. Above all, they were to remember that they were constantly under observation, and that any indiscretion on their part would reflect badly on the experiment.

Writing from 'Scrutaria' at the beginning of January to Mary Jones, the St John's head, Emma Fagg, self-appointed leader of the malcontents, complained that she and others of the party had found the experience a 'great disappointment . . . we are not fatigued with our duties'. In her own defence, Florence had already expressed serious reservations to Miss Jones about her group of sisters, condemning their manners as 'flibberty-gibbet' – a phrase which so mystified the St John's Superintendent that she had to seek assistance in defining it – and accusing them of flouting her rules of female decorum, running 'scampering over the wards themselves at night, feeding the men without medical orders'. As a consequence of this, and because their dressings of wounds were inadequate, she had occupied them 'less in nursing, & more in making Stump Pillows etc. for the men than I should otherwise have done, with the view of protecting them'.

Lurking here is Florence's abiding fear that an unoccupied nurse will inevitably fall into some kind of mischief, if not directly of a sexual nature, then stemming from the usual problems associated with excessive consumption of alcohol. But her remarks also expose a wider concern that returns us to the question of how many female nurses she believed should be employed in an Army hospital. In October 1854, as we have seen, she had opted for twenty, but had then had almost double that number forced on her. Yet her time at Scutari, and later in the Crimea, only reinforced her in the view, expressed most forcibly after the war in her *Subsidiary Notes* on the introduction of female nurses into military hospitals, that 'the fewer women are about an Army Hospital the better'. Too many, and they became harder to manage, even more so if they were unfitted for nursing duties. Florence was to maintain on several occasions, when her authority on the subject was questioned, that the doctors at Scutari agreed with her. The evidence for this is conflicting. Arthur Taylor, an Assistant-Surgeon visiting Scutari in early 1855, maintained the medical officers there believed the Nightingale nurses were doing a lot of good, but that they were 'very much in the way'. Running contrary to his view is the testimony of Assistant-Surgeon Greig, who commented that for the nurses to be really effective at the Barrack Hospital there would have needed to be fifty times the number. Greig's remarks hint at the truth behind this situation, that in the absence of a larger female nursing staff, most of the work continued to be done by the male orderlies (Sidney Herbert's reform of the orderly corps, after the frustration of earlier attempts, began to produce results in the summer of 1855, with the newly created Medical Staff Corps).

Florence's close surveillance of her nurses reflected her anxiety that the slightest outbreak of disobedience could seriously jeopardize the success of the whole operation. Elizabeth Wheeler, a Sellonite, was one of the first to be sent home after a letter of hers, exaggerating the shortage of food and restoratives in the wards to which she was assigned, found its way into *The Times* on 8 December 1854. With her, on the same boat, sailed the five Norwood nuns, unceremoniously returned after having revealed themselves to be totally devoid of any nursing experience. Their chaplain, Father Michael Cuffe, accused Florence, in a stormy interview, of acting like Herod driving the Blessed Virgin across the desert ('Pray confirm Father Michael Cuffe in his position here!' she wrote dryly to Sidney Herbert afterwards. 'It is the only agreeable incident I have had!'). Ironically, though, the greatest challenge to Florence Nightingale's position and the smooth running of her experiment now came, not from the nurses, but from the British Government itself, in the person of Sidney Herbert. At the beginning of December, without prior warning and unsolicited by Florence, Herbert authorized the sending of a second party of nurses to Scutari, in direct contravention of the official agreement that no more women would be sent until Florence specifically requested them.

Since the departure of the first expedition, women keen to nurse soldiers had continued to collect at the Herberts' home in Belgrave

Square, where Liz Herbert, Mary Stanley and Parthenope, with support from Lady Canning and Catherine Gladstone, interviewed candidates. 'Pray say that we don't want any more nurses to every one you see,' Parthenope wrote to her father at this time. '307 was the last number on the list. We are glutted with the article. Linen is, I am happy to say, abating, even boots & knitted socks are slacker, but the nurses flow on with an uninterrupted stream.' Immersed in other business, Sidney Herbert's decision to send a party of forty-six to Scutari appears to have been taken hastily. He had always believed that Florence was capable of managing a greater number of nurses, and bearing this in mind he possibly misinterpreted a stray remark in one of Charles Bracebridge's letters suggesting that a further group would be welcomed. Liz Herbert, 'overwhelmed in a sea of nurses', may have added to the confusion by implying that they were waiting for Florence to state definitively that 'she does not want any more'. But the influence of Manning on the situation, bent on increasing the proportion of Roman Catholic sisters in the nursing establishment, and his hold over Mary Stanley, still trembling on the brink of conversion, was obviously decisive. Those recruited comprised fifteen Irish Catholic Sisters of Mercy under their Superior, Mother Francis Bridgeman of Kinsale, later joined by a Jesuit chaplain, Father William Ronan, twenty-four professional nurses – and nine 'ladies'. In the midst of all the other problems that were to ensue, the introduction of this new social stratum – something Florence had avoided by not engaging lady volunteers for the original party – brought difficulties of its own. In time these would be dealt with by the issue of a new regulation, that 'It having been found that some of the Nurses have believed they were to be on an equality with the ladies or sisters, it is necessary they should understand that they will remain in exactly the same relative position as that in which they were in England . . .' Mary Stanley was to lead the party, settle them at Scutari, and then return to England. On 2 December they left from London Bridge. 'No wonder you are so fond of Mary . . .' Hilary Bonham Carter wrote to Parthenope, who remained 'entirely in the dark' that this new expedition was being sent without Florence's permission until the day before it sailed from Marseilles. 'How welcome her stay will surely be to those at Scutari.' Before long her words would assume a hollow ring.

*

CALAMITY UNPARALLELED 237

At Scutari itself, things at last were on a more level footing. 'We have painfully worked through the first act,' as Charles Bracebridge said. The purveying system remained overrun and, without Florence's intervention, close at times to breakdown, but a basis for order had been imposed, despite the fact that a fresh influx of wounded was always liable to put everything to the test again. The chaplain John Sabin commented on the new 'air of comfort and enjoyment' he found at the Barrack Hospital at the end of that year. Every man had a wooden bedstead and comfortable bedding; surgeries had been built on the wide staircases; stoves were kept burning in each ward; and tin baths stood at the corners and entrances, ready for use. The strain, however, of all the effort was beginning to tell on Florence herself. She was painfully thin and exhausted, and the Bracebridges had been wondering for some time how much longer she could hold out. Word of the imminent arrival of the Stanley party placed renewed pressure on her and pushed her that bit nearer to breaking point. On 10 December, she wrote 'in great haste' to Herbert to express her alarm at the news, informing him of the impossibility of housing or keeping the women, and rehearsing the arguments against a larger workforce. But it was already too late. A week later, the *Egyptus*, the French steamer transporting Mary Stanley's expedition, anchored off Constantinople. Messages were sent across to Scutari, but it was hours before any reply came. Finally, Mr Bracebridge went on board to tell them that, owing to the War Office's mistake, not only were their services not required, there was no room to accommodate them either. The same information was relayed by Florence herself in an interview with the party's escorts, Dr Meyer and the Hon. Jocelyn Percy MP. The next day, to Percy's shock, he was handed a piece of paper 'itemizing our conversation', and asked to sign it. Percy had come out East as one of Florence's most fervent admirers; he returned to England, disappointed and aggrieved. 'Nobody is perfect not even Miss N,' he wrote. 'She is an admirable nurse but a poor superintendent and thinks she herself must do everything.'

Florence was in no mood to spare Sidney Herbert. On 15 December she had written him a letter, offering her resignation, and flinging a host of accusations at his head. He had come to her in his distress, told her that he was unable to find anyone else for the job and that if she failed him, the scheme itself would fail. She had sacrificed her better judgement and gone out with forty females, 'well knowing that half that number

would be more efficient & less trouble'. Now, however, he had introduced a fresh batch of women, raising the total to eighty-four, in the
face of the 'distinct understanding' that had existed between them. 'You
have sacrificed the cause, so near my heart,' she wrote bitterly. 'You
have sacrificed me, a matter of small importance now. You have sacrificed your own written word to a popular cry.' Although written two
days before the *Egyptus* and its cargo docked, Florence didn't post the
letter, as she informs Herbert in its final lines, until the day after the
ship arrived. She wanted to make it clear to him that this was no angry
outburst, unleashed on the spur of the moment. Rather, it was a studied
statement of her position, though there can be little doubt that she had
no intention of surrendering the superintendency, and knew that, in the
circumstances, he couldn't possibly ask her to do so. Nevertheless, she
continued to taunt him with the threat. 'You have not stood by me, but
I have stood by you,' she wrote with further recriminations on Christmas
Day, before suddenly warning him that '. . . I can bray so loud that I
shall be heard, I am afraid, as far as England.' Later that same day, she
adopted a more conciliatory tone, dropping the threats, and reverting
in a second letter to the familiar problems of the Purveyor and his stores.

She was right to be affronted at the way her work had been undermined and her authority threatened, as Herbert himself was the first to
acknowledge. '. . . There never was such a cruel thing done . . .,' wrote
Selina Bracebridge, who predicted 'the downfall of the whole concern',
and whose powers of exaggeration extended to describing the Barrack
Hospital itself as having ground to a complete standstill out of dismay
at this new development. For the time being, while the question of
whether or not to return them home was debated, the cloud of locusts,
as Mr Bracebridge ungallantly referred to the Stanley party, were put
up in temporary quarters: the nuns at a convent of French sisters at
Galata, the ladies and paid nurses at the British Ambassador's summer
residence, further up the coast at Therapia.

In her remonstrations to Herbert, Florence had noted that, with the
new arrivals, the proportion of Roman Catholics in the nursing establishment had 'increased to 25 in 84'. Given that the presence of Catholics
in the original party had already created an outcry in England among
the anti-papist lobby, this increase could only lead to further protest,
and renewed fears that nuns were taking advantage of their place at the
bedsides of dying soldiers to indulge in proselytism. Attention in the

press had been drawn to Herbert's own High Church sympathies, while Florence was accused of being a conspirator in some Romanist or Tractarian plot (to counter these suspicions Charles Bracebridge suggested publishing extracts from Florence's Egyptian letters, 'which express her great souled, large hearted religion', an idea that was sensibly quashed). If anything was likely to succeed in derailing the Nightingale mission at this point, it was sectarian division.

It was bad enough, from Florence's point of view, that Mary Stanley had been instructed to report on arrival to Dr Cumming and not to herself. Far more damaging, and likely, if the Sisters stayed, to make a difficult situation unworkable, was that Mother Bridgeman, leader of the Irish nuns, in an arrangement negotiated through Manning, had insisted on retaining the autonomy of herself and her sisters. While, at the outset, Bridgeman accepted Florence's authority in hospital matters, she maintained that her ultimate authority derived from her bishop, Dr Thomas Grant, and the higher echelons of the Catholic Church in Ireland. This was in sharp contrast to the position of Mother Clare Moore and her Bermondsey nuns. As an Irish Sister of Mercy, working in London at a time of great anti-Catholic feeling, Moore understood the importance of cooperation, and indeed had placed herself under Florence's supervision and protection, earning Bridgeman's disapproval for being 'the perfect drudge'. The Kinsale Superior and her sisters, on the other hand, would strive consistently to stand apart. In her early forties, Bridgeman had been described by Manning as 'an ardent, high-tempered and, at first, somewhat difficult person – but truly, good, devoted and trustworthy'. From their first meeting on 22 December, it was evident she and Florence were not going to get on. Mother Bridgeman, shocked by the limited space allotted to the Bermondsey nuns at the Barrack Hospital, and taken aback by the quality of the 'lunch' offered her – a remnant of musty cheese, a scrap of dirty butter, some cold potatoes, and 'something in a bottle' – realized 'that she had an ambitious woman to deal with on whom she could not rely.' For her part, Florence saw Bridgeman as having come out to Scutari 'with a religious view', as she told Herbert, 'not to serve the sick, but to found a convent . . .' Despite having Herbert's permission to return the forty-six as she saw fit, Florence believed this was a 'moral impossibility', as well as likely to visit universal opprobrium on her own head, and sought instead to distribute them among the hospitals. But how was this to be achieved while at the same time maintaining the essential balance between secular and religious nurses? Florence proposed to Bridgeman that five of her nuns be sent to the Barrack Hospital under Mother Clare Moore to replace the Norwood sisters. Bridgeman refused, countering that she had been ordered to keep her sisters as one community under herself. They had reached a stalemate.

Mary Stanley, responsible for her ladies and nurses, was more slippery, but also clearly out of her depth. 'Dearest,' Florence had written to her old friend on 20 December, 'Will you come & see me?' At their meeting the following day, in the presence of Dr Cumming and Mr Bracebridge, Florence immediately seized the upper hand, formally resigning and requesting that Mary Stanley take her place. If her aim was to destabilize Stanley, she more than succeeded. She offered, in fact, an object lesson in how to take your opponent off guard. Stanley, never the most confident of women, and far from strong, became flustered and burst into tears. She was then placed in the humiliating position of borrowing money from Florence, having exhausted her own funds by staying in the best hotels en route through France. Yet she stood her ground in choosing to remain in Constantinople until the fate of the women placed in her charge was resolved. 'I confess that I have got to be convinced that more nurses are not needed,' she wrote to Liz Herbert, whose own loyalties were becoming divided.

In the subsequent, and often partisan, retellings of the circumstances surrounding the unhappy demise of the Nightingale–Stanley relationship, the women have each found their adherents. However, the faults on both sides were more equally matched than has sometimes been admitted. Despite vehement protestations to the contrary ('Could Mrs Herbert think I was "jealous" of Miss Stanley? But that is, Oh! Such a minor matter here'), Florence undeniably resented Mary's intrusion on her authority. What made matters worse in her eyes was Mary's sudden transformation from loyal disciple – she had been introduced to nursing, as her brother Arthur recalled, by Florence's 'noble example' – to challenger to her position. A persistent flaw in Florence's character was her inability, having once perceived a wrong, to prevent her mind from restlessly pursuing her sense of grievance. Mary Stanley's actions felt like a betrayal, and Florence was unable to lose sight of the injury she felt so keenly. Although Mary reassured Parthenope that the 'mutual affection' between herself and Florence would survive their difficulties, she also reportedly told Manning how shocked she had been at the way Florence treated her, 'with an official coldness very unlike our former intimacy'.

But Mary Stanley was neither consistent, nor open about her motives while she remained in the East. 'We long for a good plain woman,' exclaimed Charles Bracebridge, who found Stanley 'dry, antagonistic ... contradictory' in his dealings with her, and believed her to be always intriguing, turning her ladies against Florence, and generally acting 'a double part'. Even members of her own family questioned Mary's reasons for going to Constantinople, and hinted that behind it all lay a desire to share in some of Florence's glory. 'So Mary has reached the height of her ambition . . .,' remarked one relative. 'Such nonsense . . . to say she did not <u>wish</u> to go.' Stanley's only serious scheme for the dispersal of her party, in the weeks that followed that initial meeting, was to suggest that some of her ladies be assigned as 'female ecclesiastes', or visitors, working under the hospital chaplains. This was in keeping with the views she had outlined, shortly before the war, in a book called *Hospitals and Sisterhoods*, in which she had portrayed nursing as a pastoral calling where sisters and ladies, too refined and feeble even to carry a coal-scuttle or water pail, supervised the work of ordinary nurses. Such a proposal was anathema to Florence Nightingale. She had other, more serious, reservations, though, about Mary Stanley. As Parthenope succinctly put it to Lady Canning, who was showing signs of going over to the Stanley camp, Mary could not be exonerated 'from accepting a position where she has to act openly as a Protestant, while in reality she was doing all in her power to serve the Roman Catholics'. Florence had not only long been aware of Mary's Catholic tendencies, she had even at an earlier stage, before the outbreak of war, been approached by Arthur Stanley, at this time a Canon of Canterbury, with the request that she use her influence to dissuade his sister from conversion (later, in defence of Mary, Arthur Stanley would drop a veiled threat that, if matters came to a head, he might expose Florence's own connections to Catholic institutions in Paris).

With *The Times*, on 9 January 1855, reporting that there was a danger of the whole Nightingale undertaking 'coming to an abrupt conclusion' unless certain religious dissensions were set at rest, there was an urgent need to conciliate Bridgeman and her nuns. In fact, four days before the newspaper report, Mother Clare Moore had been sent by Florence on just such a mission, sailing across the Bosphorus in an open boat during a violent snowstorm. It was an uneasy meeting, but they reached a settlement, later confirmed in an agreement drafted by Father Ronan, the nuns' chaplain. Bridgeman and four of her sisters would work at the General or Barrack Hospitals. The remaining ten would be sent to Koulali, when the hospital opened there at the end of January, where they would be joined by Bridgeman herself. At all times, the sisters would form a separate community under Mother Bridgeman, 'for she is their duly appointed Superior and cannot transfer her authority to any other'. They were also permitted to tend to the spiritual needs of their Catholic patients at the request of the patients themselves, or of the Catholic chaplains. Relations between Florence and Bridgeman, however, showed no signs of thawing. Bridgeman resolved to have as little as possible to do with Nightingale, seeing her only 'when she considered it might be useful', while Florence continued to view these Irish sisters with suspicion and dislike, tinged with intolerance. Bridgeman was 'Manning's nun' or 'Mother Brickbat' ('the Goddess of Humbug' was the title the sisters conferred on Florence). The clash between these two women of not dissimilar temperament might have been avoided if Florence had set out to coax Bridgeman a bit more graciously. As it was, she had made a fateful miscalculation. The existence of an independent group of Irish Catholic nurses, bent on opposition to Florence's rule, and soon in flagrant opposition to it, was to form the basis of much future discord.

Mary Stanley, who had refused to ameliorate the situation by assuming the management of Scutari's General Hospital, was meanwhile propitiated on 28 January by the establishment of herself and a selection of her ladies at the Koulali hospital, with the Bridgeman nuns, under the leadership of one of their number, Amy Hutton. Florence could not help but see intrigue behind the move, especially as Lady Stratford, the ambassador's wife, whom she had already condemned as a time-waster and as playing a game of popularity, was assisting in the arrangements. Florence remained nominally in charge of Koulali until the spring, when she asked to be relieved of the responsibility on the grounds of Mary Stanley's refusal to cooperate, and her own lack of confidence in the nursing being pursued there under the direction of the Koulali doctors. By then, the War Office had decided to take her at her word, that she was unable to exercise real supervision from Scutari of a hospital some miles away, and on 20 April formally agreed to her request.

In letters to Herbert, Florence piled on one stinging phrase after another to describe 'the lady plan', as she contemptuously referred to the type of nursing taking place at Koulali. She depicted Mary Stanley and her acolytes, 'scampering' about the wards ineffectually, 'wandering about with notebooks in their hands', and indulging 'in nothing but spiritual flirtations'. These phrases have tended to stick, though the evidence about the relative efficacy of the Scutari versus the Koulali systems remains inconclusive. Despite widespread criticism of Koulali, not least for its defective ventilation and bad sanitation, its mortality rates to March 1855 were no worse than those for the General and Barrack Hospitals at Scutari. Assistant-Surgeon Patrick Watson criticized the Stanley nurses 'who promise to do, but don't and can't perform', while Sister Aloysius Doyle, one of the Bridgeman nuns, expressed surprise at the lack of experience of the ladies she worked with. At the same time, the skilful nursing of the Irish sisters drew universal praise from the doctors (like Florence, some of them had made their own study of French hospitals on a visit abroad, in 1852), and the charges of proselytism, though alleged, were never definitively proven.

According to Selina Bracebridge, Mary Stanley's 'betrayal' had 'gone very deep into Flo's heart'. But in its wider significance, the Stanley episode marked the end of any possibility of a single unified wartime nursing establishment in the East under one head, Florence Nightingale. The nursing experiment had expanded seemingly beyond anything originally envisaged by Sidney Herbert, and as a result was passing out of Florence's direct control. In January 1855, at Lord Raglan's express wish, the female nursing corps was extended to the Crimea itself, when Emma Langston, Mother Eldress of the Sellonites, led a staff sent to the General Hospital at Balaclava. In April, Jane Shaw Stewart, one of Mary Stanley's ladies, rejected for the first party, but encouraged by Florence to gain experience at Guy's Hospital, took over the newly opened Castle Hospital on the Genoese Heights above Balaclava. Florence still appointed nurses to these hospitals but, inevitably, their management became the responsibility of others, some of whom questioned whether the terms of Florence's appointment as Superintendent in Turkey entitled her to the exercise of authority in the Crimea. This was a struggle for the future. Meanwhile, at Smyrna and Renkioi, hospitals were opened on civilian initiatives, which never came under her jurisdiction at all. By the end of the war, the total number of nurses who had served in the East had swelled the original figure of thirty-eight by almost six-fold. The larger proportion of these women nursed outside the area of Florence Nightingale's superintendence and, consequently, without reference to her standards of professional practice. By February 1855, Florence herself was requesting more nurses from the War Office. The Scottish Presbyterians were eager to send out nurses, and she was pleased to take advantage of the offer. 'But I must bar these fat drunken old dames,' she told Herbert. 'Above 14 stone we will not have – the provision of bed-steads is not strong enough.' (Unfortunately, two months later, a pair of the Presbyterian nurses, Thompson and Anderson, came back to Scutari, dead drunk after a night out with an orderly, and were sent back to England. Thompson jumped ship at Constantinople and got drunk again.)

As for Mary Stanley, her time at Koulali was short-lived. At the beginning of April, worn down by worry and ill-health, she returned to England. Before leaving Constantinople, she was received into the Catholic Church by Father Ronan. 'I regret that I cannot resign my charge into your hands myself,' she wrote to Florence, but there was to be no further meeting between them. Back in England, towards the end of 1855, she unwisely became a focus for the disaffected, lending support to the cause of Charlotte Salisbury, a nurse at Scutari, dismissed for dishonesty, and even assisting her in bringing a libel action against Florence. The action failed. In London, Jane Carlyle encountered 'Mary Stanley of Crimean notoriety . . . a very considerable goose I think . . .'

Florence could neither forgive nor forget Mary's 'treachery'. When there was talk of Queen Victoria presenting a jewel to Florence 'as proof of regard & one at the same time to Mary Stanley', Parthenope let it be known that '. . . Such an association would be a source of very great pain to my sister.' Somewhat naïvely, a year after her departure, Mary applied to Florence to return to the East. Florence received her offer with incredulity. 'Do not be taken in by Miss Stanley,' she warned Parthenope. 'I say this with a heavy heart for you know what her defection has been to me. It has nearly broken mine, but she is not "a weak fool". She is practising upon "weak fools". I have proofs of her duplicity . . . which would stagger you.' What these were, she did not specify.

The rest of Mary Stanley's life was filled with good works, among them schemes of visiting and nursing the sick poor, and of training soldiers' wives as nurses during the Franco-Prussian War. After her death, in 1879, Arthur Stanley gave voice to the overarching theme of his sister's life. 'The feeling that her public labours were for the most part unacknowledged', he wrote, had cast something of a shadow over her existence. By then, the power of the Nightingale icon had ensured that the figure of Mary Stanley had largely dissolved from the pages of nursing history.

The British Army was passing through the hospitals at Scutari. They 'formed one of the most ghastly processions that ever poet imagined', William Howard Russell wrote in late January, describing a group of casualties beginning the long journey to Scutari from the heights above Sebastopol. 'Many of these men were all but dead. With closed eyes, open mouths and ghastly attenuated faces, they were borne along two by two, the thin stream of breath visible in the frosty air, alone showing they were alive.' One estimate suggests that admissions to the base, and regimental hospitals at the front, reduced the 30,000 men holding the British sector in December by as much as two-thirds from January through to March. The Coldstream Guards provide an illustration of this devastating statistic. In February 1855, the Guards' force stood at just 100 men from its original strength at the end of the previous year of 480. With no major military action during this period, disease had become the real enemy. The Crimean winter was harsh, though, ironically, at the beginning of 1855, Britain was experiencing its coldest weather on record, the lowest temperature, 1 degree Fahrenheit, being colder than any recorded in the Crimea. The decisive factor, however, in the ensuing high mortality rates was the combination of the climate with the Army's ill-preparedness for the cold: its lack of warm clothing, deficient diet, and the inadequate provision made for long-term accommodation in the camps.

At Scutari, where, at the beginning of January, there were 2,500 men in the Barrack, and 1,122 in the General Hospital, it was too late for many of them to be saved. 'They stretch out the hand & say "sister" & "mother",' wrote Charles Bracebridge, 'they never groan & turn, but most are scarcely sentient & go off like animals.' The greatest proportion of admissions at the two hospitals, and the highest incidence of death in the winter months, was from bowel disease, including diarrhoea and dysentery. Fever, of an ill-defined nature (though not typhus on any large scale), highly contagious in the overcrowded wards, accounted for a large number of deaths, along with chronic rheumatism and diseases of the respiratory tract, like pneumonia. Other, more sporadic conditions, giving rise to only a small number of deaths, included frostbite. Only four cases of cholera were recorded as admitted in these months, and all died. From September to December 1854, the total mortality rate at Scutari had been 10 per cent of all admissions, a figure that Florence was later to analyse as being only slightly higher than the percentage mortality in civilian hospitals. Between January and March 1855, however, the mortality rate in the Scutari hospitals soared to 33 per cent, with 3,354 deaths; in February, when the emergency reached its peak, a staggering 52 per cent of those admitted died. '... The mortality is frightful,' Florence confirmed to Herbert on 5 February, shortly after receiving men from the *Golden Fleece* whose condition 'exceeded in misery' anything she had seen; 'thirty in the last twenty-four hours in this [the Barrack] Hospital alone. One day last week it was forty ... We bury every twenty-four hours.'

Her own efforts were tireless. Sometimes she was on her feet for twenty hours at a stretch, distributing stores, directing her staff, and attending on the most seriously ill with an utter disregard for her own health. A rare respite from work was her walk, once a week on Sundays, around the clifftop path to a local house, to take a vapour bath. Her sense of purpose remained undiminished. Dropping a quick line to her mother, at the beginning of February, to reassure her that Scutari was not experiencing an outbreak of cholera – 'Can you suppose that such a Scavenger as I am have not a sack of Chlor.[ide] of Lime at the corner of every Corridor ... ?' – Florence wearily asserted her intention, of working 'for these miserable Hospitals as long as I have power to do so'. Several days later, in a further, unfinished letter to Fanny Nightingale she was more resolute, seeing herself as 'an Originator', who had bridged the chasm to reform, but believing, as yet, that it would be left to others to do 'greater things': the reform of the Army, the Army Medical Board, and the military hospitals, 'those three sinks of jobbery & official vice'.

In England, public criticism of the conduct of the war had culminated in the collapse of Lord Aberdeen's coalition government. In the

Commons, the passing of the Radical MP John Roebuck's motion for a committee of inquiry into the state of the Army before Sebastopol precipitated Aberdeen's resignation on 30 January after the previous day's vote of no confidence. Lord Palmerston succeeded him, and in Palmerston's new cabinet Sidney Herbert was briefly, for a few days, Colonial Secretary; he resigned, however, on 21 February, out of loyalty to Aberdeen, when Palmerston was unable to abide by his assurance that he would prevent the Roebuck inquiry. Herbert's examination before the inquiry in May impressed observers. Although, as Secretary of State at War (an office amalgamated with the Secretaryship of War in the new administration), Herbert was only responsible for financial control of the Medical Department, he had been well briefed about conditions at Scutari by the information contained in Florence's letters.

Lord Panmure, an irascible Scotsman, known as 'the Bison', who had served in the Cameron Highlanders for twelve years before entering Parliament in 1835, took Herbert's place. '. . . No one will do the work as you have done . . . ,' Florence wrote to Herbert, confessing that while she was very glad for his sake that he was 'out of the turmoil', she was sorry on her own behalf, and for the 5,000 'poor fellows' whose lives were at stake. In spite of her occasional asperity – to which, it should be noted, Herbert had never responded in kind – theirs was still a relationship founded on mutual respect. He had stood by her 'gallantly' in urging the reforms that they both considered essential, she told her mother, after her father, in the wake of the Stanley controversy, had grumbled that Herbert had failed to act supportively towards her; and he would stand by her as her protector in the future. 'Pray continue to write to me for anything you want, which you don't like to say to others,' Herbert told Florence at the beginning of March. 'I will do everything I can. I shall never forget how much I owe you for all you have done.' She would more than take him at his word.

Palmerston's government had been charged with bringing a new robustness to the management of the war, and among its first actions was the dispatch of a Sanitary Commission to the East, to carry out inspections and 'purify the hospitals . . . and exert all that science can do to save life where thousands are dying, not of their wounds, but of dysentery and diarrhea, the result of foul air and preventable mischiefs'. The idea for the Commission came from Lord Shaftesbury, Palmerston's son-in-law. With Palmerston's support, Shaftesbury won Panmure's approval and three commissioners were selected: Dr Hector Gavin (killed some weeks after his arrival in Constantinople when his brother accidentally discharged a pistol), Robert Rawlinson, a civil engineer under the General Board of Health, and Dr John Sutherland, the Commission's head, an inspector under the Board of Health, who had conducted several special inquiries, including one into the cholera epidemic of 1848-9. Although Florence's first impressions of Sutherland are not recorded, it was an auspicious meeting. Her friendship with Sutherland marks the true beginning of Florence's association with the sanitarian movement, which was to bulk large in so much of her subsequent work. While at Scutari, Sutherland acted as Florence's personal physician, and after the war, he was to serve for more than three decades as one of her most trusted advisers.

The Commission arrived at Scutari on 4 March, and began their work energetically. While the commissioners advised that the Barrack Hospital bore 'marks of much having been done to improve it', conditions there were, nevertheless, described as 'murderous' (by contrast, the General Hospital was described as scrupulously clean). The sewers beneath the building were clogged so that the hospital effectively sat on top of a large cesspool; the large pipe carrying water to other parts of the hospital was blocked by the decomposed carcass of a horse, one of more than twenty-five dead animals found at the site; and excrement from the prefabricated privies in the central courtyard was seeping out of the trench into the water tanks beside them. Orders were received to correct these evils and, on 16 March, Lord William Paulet, the Scutari commandant, confirmed that the work would be carried out to the best of his ability. Sewers were flushed out, openings made in the roof to improve air circulation, rotten floors torn out, walls and floors limewashed, and orderlies instructed to empty waste on a daily basis. On 18 March, Florence commented on progress: 'The Sanitary Commission is really doing something, & has set to work burying dead dogs & whitewashing walls, two prolific causes of fever . . . A Liverpool Inspector of Nuisances has been left us to do what we should have done long ago [the commissioners had been accompanied by three sanitary inspectors from Liverpool].'

The mortality rate at Scutari for March, down to 20 per cent of admissions from the previous month's peak of 52 per cent, has been taken as evidence of the success of the Commission's work. But the idea that such a striking decrease could be connected to improvements that had barely started two weeks earlier is, as John Shepherd, historian of the Crimean War medical services, once wrote, 'scarcely tenable' (and it's interesting to note that Florence's enthusiasm for the Commission was not shared by Charles Bracebridge, who complained that it was 'incompetent' and that 'these patchings are of little use'). Rather, the sharp decline in the number of deaths in the short term was almost certainly due to a reduction in overcrowding, owing to the fall in the number of admissions, as well as to the improved health of the medical cases arriving from the Crimea, partly as a consequence of the better weather with the onset of spring. A distant cousin of Florence's, William Woodward Shore (not to be confused with Aunt Mai's son Shore), visited the Barrack Hospital on 18 March and observed the work of the Commission. The kitchen had been 'turned inside out', and 'a large amount of scrubbing & white washing' was going on. But he also noted 'the greatly diminished numbers' in the wards, that cases of fever had 'died out', and that most of the invalids were 'generally convalescent'.

Florence believed that, in the long term, the Sanitary Commission saved the British Army. But neither this belief, nor the fact that she cooperated with the Commission's work once it reached Scutari, should be taken to mean that she personally drafted its terms of reference, or exerted special influence to have it sent out in the first place. A. W. Kinglake, who published his massive work *The Invasion of the Crimea* in eight volumes between 1863 and 1887 – and whom Florence regarded as 'utterly . . . in the dark' about the real causes of 'Crimean Mortality' – believed that the original brief given to the Commission, under Panmure's signature, 'had received impulsion from a woman's mind'; but nothing in the surviving Nightingale papers has ever emerged to confirm a theory that remains, as a consequence, purely speculative.

A not unrelated notion, prevalent among an older generation of historians, but still to be found in popular historical writing today, is that the dramatic decrease in mortality at Scutari in the first months of 1855 is directly attributable to Florence Nightingale herself. This was transparently not so. The only claim she made for her work, privately, in letters to the Herberts, but never publicly, was that 'We pulled this hospital through for 4 months & without us, it would have come to a stand-still.' In this conclusion, she was undoubtedly correct.

*

By the spring of 1855, the Bracebridges had hopes that Florence might soon be returning to England. They themselves were worn out, saddened by the recent death of Selina Bracebridge's favourite sister, and considering taking a few months' respite before returning to Scutari. They were encouraged by rumours that the military stalemate might shortly be over, and that summer would bring a decisive victory for the Allies, forcing Russia to sue for peace. 'I would wish you to consider,' Charles Bracebridge wrote conspiratorially to William Nightingale, 'supposing the battle over by then, if you could not get Florence herself safe away. I think the country will be of the opinion that she has done enough.'

No thoughts of this kind so much as entered Florence's mind. But improvements at Scutari, combined with the likelihood that the pressure in a future siege would be on the hospitals at Balaclava, had made her decide on a visit to the Crimea. This was in spite of the fact that her instructions appeared to give her no rights of jurisdiction there. Her visit was approved by the War Office, but only in the capacity of 'Almoner of Free Gifts in the British Hospitals in the Crimea', not as Superintendent of Nurses. The introduction of systematic arrangements at Scutari seemed as far off as ever – 'all our arrangements are of the Elizabethan era', Florence told Sidney Herbert at the end of February, as another purveying crisis took hold – but she trusted Mrs Bracebridge to oversee 'the bear-garden' while she was away. Mr Bracebridge would be accompanying Florence, along with the invaluable Mrs Roberts and three other nurses, Thomas, a twelve-year-old drummer boy, who called himself 'Miss Nightingale's man', an invalid soldier from the 68th Light Infantry who had been hired as a messenger, and two cooks, Alexis Soyer and his manservant. Soyer, the celebrated Reform Club chef and a flamboyant self-promoter, had arrived at Scutari in March, after offering the Government his services for free. In the Barrack Hospital kitchens he had cooked food that was nutritious and economically produced, and he was keen to make similar improvement to the kitchens at the hospitals in Balaclava.

On 2 May, the party set sail for 'Crim Tartary' on board the *Robert Lowe*, or the 'Robert Slow' as Florence impatiently nicknamed her. Florence hadn't been invited to the Crimea, and no one, certainly not Dr Hall, the Chief Medical Officer in the East, was expecting her. None the less, she had decided to lay claim to what she considered to be her rightful domain.

10. A Visible March to Heaven

On 24 February 1855, one of the most enduring and iconic images of the modern age – and of the nursing profession in particular – made its first appearance, when the depiction of Florence Nightingale as the Lady with the Lamp was published as an engraving in the *Illustrated London News*.* The newspaper, founded in 1842, had come of age during the Crimean War, its standards of pictorial journalism providing unrivalled coverage of Britain's most significant international military event since the Napoleonic Wars. The editor, Herbert Ingram, dispatched special artists to the fields of battle. Working to tight deadlines, these artists sent back to London their rapid sketches and quickfire pen and ink drawings, which were transferred, sometimes with a little editing, on to woodblocks. The effort behind this swift turnaround paid massive dividends. In November 1854, sales of the *Illustrated London News* already outstripped those of *The Times*; by the summer of 1855, the paper was selling 130,700 copies a week.

The *Illustrated London News* employed an assortment of marine artists, landscape painters and wood engravers. There is no signature or any mark of identification on the Lady with the Lamp image, though by a process of elimination it is possible to narrow down the authorship of the original sketch from which the engraving was produced to two men: J. A. Crowe, described by the paper as its 'correspondent' in the Crimea in 1855–6; or, a much more famous artist, the French Realist illustrator Constantin Guys. It has been suggested that Guys is the more likely candidate, as he was renowned for working from memory, which may be one explanation for the engraving's substitution of the type of lamp used at Scutari – an Arab pattern lantern – for a Grecian, or ceremonial genie lamp. Alternatively, it is just as possible that this alteration was

---

* The lamp later came to represent nurse education, following the foundation of the Nightingale Training School at St Thomas's Hospital.

made by the engraver in London as more in keeping with the picture's romantic, almost magical quality.

The portrayal of Florence with her lamp, on her night-time vigil in the wards at Scutari, rapidly became a part of her personal mythology, and a potent visual metaphor for the ideal of Christian womanhood she had come to represent. Aunt Patty was among those for whom the image in the *Illustrated London News* struck an immediate chord. It remained with her, insistently, she said, 'day & night for many weeks'. Visitors to Scutari in the months following the engraving's appearance kept an eye out for the lamp. One of them, an acquaintance of the Nightingales, had his hopes fulfilled when, 'called up accidentally at 3 in the morning', he found Florence 'about with her little lamp, ministering . . . as the men say themselves "like a guardian angel"'. During Aunt Mai's stay at the Barrack Hospital in the early autumn of 1855, assisting Florence with administrative duties, she wrote to her children, describing, with a strong degree of recognition, how she had been escorted home from the hospital by the light of 'the "little lamp"'. Printed reportage kept pace with pictorial representation in embracing the imagery of the lamp. John Macdonald, the *Times* fund manager, with whom Florence had worked closely in the purchase and distribution of stores, returned to England not long after the publication of the engraving and contributed this famous description to his newspaper:

She is a 'ministering angel' without any exaggeration in these hospitals, and as her slender form glides quietly along each corridor, every poor fellow's face softens with gratitude at the sight of her. When all the medical officers have retired for the night and sickness and darkness have settled down upon the miles of prostrate sick, she may be observed alone, with a little lamp in her hand, making her solitary rounds.

A poem in *Punch*, on 8 December 1855, took up the theme, clearly betraying as it did so its origins in Macdonald's account. 'Upon the darkness of the night how often, gliding late and lone,/Her little lamp, hope's beacon-light, to eyes with no hope else has shone!' By the time Fanny Taylor's memoir, *Eastern Hospitals and English Nurses*, appeared in 1857, reference to the famous lamp was seemingly obligatory. Taylor, one of Mary Stanley's ladies, who had served at Koulali as well as Scutari, remembered that 'A dim light burned here or there. Miss

Nightingale carried a lantern, which she would set down before she bent over her patients.'

The Christian connotations of this symbolic use of light were to become a commonplace in writing, especially verse writing, about Florence Nightingale and the widely perceived religious nature of her mission. The appeal of this sanctified imagery of light had found its strongest expression six months before the expedition to Scutari, in the spring of 1854, when William Holman Hunt's *The Light of the World* was exhibited at the Royal Academy in London to sensational effect. Hunt's painting, showing Christ knocking at a door overgrown with brambles, lantern in hand, possesses obvious visual parallels to the image of the Lady with the Lamp. Yet it's worth noting that the kind of lantern with which Florence would have been familiar at Scutari – a *fanoos*, similar to those that can still be bought in the Istanbul souk today – is distinctly Islamic in style, utilizing a simple ornamentation on its brass cover which reflects Islamic notions of divine unity. With her deep interest in oriental religion, and the spirit of latitudinarianism that pervaded her own faith, Florence would no doubt have appreciated this fact.

The *fanoos* may be hand held, set down on a flat surface, or suspended from a hook. A waxed linen concertina, slightly translucent in effect, protects the flame of a candle held in the circular brass or copper base. The metal cover has a shield, which may be moved aside to reveal the candle when the concertina is collapsed, and a handle with a hook from which the lantern can hang. There is no evidence that Florence placed any special significance on the means of lighting used by her at Scutari, and there are only two references in her surviving wartime correspondence, one in which she specifically refers to carrying a lantern while chasing rats (as one of the Bridgeman nuns noted, 'The rats of Scutari are something to be remembered'). Nor would she have used the same lantern all the time, which makes any identification of 'a Nightingale lantern', as has been sometimes attempted, a fruitless exercise. None the less, five Arab pattern lanterns with Crimean associations do survive, one of them, now in the National Army Museum in London, brought back to England by the Bracebridges as a souvenir. In 1913, a Bracebridge relation, Gwen Compton-Bracebridge, was turning out cupboards at Atherstone Hall when she made two discoveries. One was a bunch of grass – 'watered by men's blood' – picked by Florence at the site of the Battle of Inkerman in June 1856; the other was a lantern. 'This is like a round folding up Chinese lantern,' wrote Mrs Compton-Bracebridge to Margaret Stephen, Aunt Mai's granddaughter, unable to keep the hint of surprise out of her voice, 'with a tin socket for a candle & a parchment like outside . . . I think the general public would be very sceptical if they saw it, they are so imbued with the idea of the Grecian lamp.'

The publication, in 1857, of Henry Wadsworth Longfellow's poem 'Santa Filomena', in his collection *Birds of Passage*, finally elevated the image of Florence Nightingale as the Lady with the Lamp to the level of cultural icon. Early in the war, Florence had been compared to Longfellow's most famous heroine, Evangeline, who becomes a Sister of Mercy, and serves the sick, her presence falling 'on their hearts like a ray of sun on the walls of a prison'. In 'Santa Filomena', Longfellow, a friend of the Howes and of Arthur Clough, associates 'A Lady with a Lamp', going about her nightly rounds 'through the glimmering gloom', with a saint, Philomena, who was widely venerated in the mid-nineteenth century, and whose name means 'one who loves the moon'. Despite the poem's popularity, Longfellow himself expressed dissatisfaction with it. Sending a copy to Parthenope, he admitted to feeling 'how inadequate the verses are to the subject, and how the words, instead of outrunning the feeling, lag behind it'. Florence's only reported comment about the poem that spread her fame was both self-effacing and prosaic. Longfellow, she remarked to Clough, had simply failed to understand 'the true point' about the disasters of that first winter at Scutari.

Florence Nightingale's rise to secular sainthood, to 'a noble type of good/Heroic womanhood' in Longfellow's phrase, was assured, though not before matters relating to her femininity and religious beliefs had been paraded for inspection and approval in the pages of the national press. A letter signed by 'One Who Has Known Miss Nightingale' in *The Times* on 25 October 1854, four days after Florence left London, emphasized her acceptance of conventional womanly virtues, as well as the religious base of her mission, praising Florence for her charitable act of quitting 'the family circle which her taste and talents made her so fit to adorn', and for doing the healing work of 'our Saviour . . . in the spirit of the martyrs of old'. The emphasis on Florence's true domesticity was pushed further home in an article, 'Who is Mrs [sic] Nightingale?', initially appearing in *The Examiner* on 28 October, and subsequently reprinted in a number of other papers, including *The Times*. This underlines the fact that although Florence Nightingale is a well-educated woman with extraordinary ambitions, she is still 'feminine', and 'her happiest place is at home' where she lives – here the public rhetoric silently slides over the private struggle – 'in simplest obedience to her admiring parents'. Once again, the saintliness of her undertaking is described, a 'deliberate, sensitive, highly-endowed young lady . . . rendering the holiest of woman's charities to the sick, the dying, and the convalescent'. What is being offered here is an acceptable public counterpart to 'The Angel in the House', Coventry Patmore's portrayal of the perfect wife and mother, published for the first time that autumn: an 'Angel of Mercy' to validate a woman's sudden appearance at the scene of war. 'A sage few', the article concluded,

will no doubt condemn, sneer at, or pity an enthusiasm which to them seems eccentric or at best misplaced: but to the true heart of the country it will speak home, and be there felt, that there is not one of England's proudest and purest daughters who at this moment stands on so high a pinnacle as Florence Nightingale.

Those sneering voices were briefly heard before vanishing into the ether. A letter to *The Times* on 13 November, signed by 'Common Sense', offered grudging praise of Miss Nightingale and her 'reckless devotion', before proceeding to rehearse some of the arguments against the employment of women in military hospitals: that the work would be better done 'by 50 or 60 hospital orderlies', that women in such a situation might be difficult to control or discipline, and questioning the role of Nightingale herself as subordinate to the medical men but in charge of her nurses. Two days earlier, under the heading 'Nurses of Quality for the Crimea', *Punch* had pursued the subject in more satirical vein, in what purported to be a report of a meeting of women interested in nursing in the East. One of them, Dowager Lady Strongi'th'head, insists that it is the Government's business to provide nurses for military hospitals, 'and not to leave the duties of the soldier's nurse to be undertaken by ladies of rank and fashion, who knew not even as yet what it was to nurse a baby'. The activities of Florence Nightingale – the very reference in *Punch* to an individual woman, aside from the Queen, was itself a novelty – are described by the Dowager as a 'display of enthusiasm'.

While agreement that the Nightingale expedition to Scutari had been undertaken out of Christian duty was almost universal in the press, the religious composition of the original party swiftly became a matter of public controversy. A letter from an 'Anti-Puseyite'* in the *Daily News* on 28 October was characteristic of this feeling, deploring both that Florence had been chosen for the task of leading the nurses over Lady Maria Forester, who as the widow of an army officer was deemed more suitable, and that the nurses had been recruited 'from Miss Sellon's house and from a Romanist establishment'. Lady Maria herself wrote to Parthenope to express her concern at 'the peculiar favour' shown to the nuns by Government. '. . . I think I am no bigot but do feel . . . that . . . we who <u>have The Truth</u> must <u>keep it</u> pure & distant from <u>Error</u> . . .' A Dublin paper fanned the flames by printing that Florence was a Roman Catholic (leading the Dean of Salisbury to riposte that she was 'of that little sect of which we find scanty contributions from all churches – the good Samaritan sect'). In an effort to silence mounting fears of a Catholic conspiracy, Liz Herbert issued a statement that Florence was Low Church, but then regretted not having described her as Broad Church instead. Meanwhile, the variety of sectarian labels being pinned to Florence's name in different parts of the press – Unitarian, as well as Catholic and Low Church – left the *Standard* to conclude that this was 'pretty good proof that her creed is not very distinct'.

The question in these early months of whether the public figure of Florence Nightingale could be contained within mid-Victorian rhetoric about appropriate womanly behaviour and religious orthodoxy had a line neatly drawn under it, in the spring of 1855, with the publication of Sydney Godolphin Osborne's *Scutari and its Hospitals*. Osborne, who had returned from Scutari to give evidence before the Roebuck Committee, had been from the earliest stages one of Florence's firmest supporters. Yet the portrait he gives of her in his book is far from mere panegyric, and, moreover, explicitly confronts some of the problems connected to her personality and beliefs which had already been aired in print. Osborne's Florence is 'without the possession of positive beauty'.

* Edward Pusey and his supporters had become a contentious group in the early 1850s. Their Tractarian beliefs appeared to threaten both the spiritual and moral authority of the Anglican Church, by arguing that the Established Church was a divine institution and that its clergymen were direct descendants of the apostles, and supporting the wider employment of women within church and parish.

Instead, she has 'a manner and countenance' that betoken 'great self-possession'. Having disposed in this way of the issue of her femininity, Osborne moves on to the subject of Florence's reform of the hospitals. 'I can conceive her to be a strict disciplinarian,' he wrote; 'she throws herself into a work – as its head – as such she knows well how much success must depend upon literal obedience to her every order. She seems to understand business thoroughly, though to me she had the failure common to many "Heads", a too great love of management in the small details, which had better perhaps have been left to others.' As for Florence's religious views, Osborne silences the doubters. In 'her every word and action', he had found her 'a Christian'. 'I thought this quite enough ... Her work ought to answer for her faith.' Rarely, in the sentimental effusions that were to follow for the rest of the war, would anyone write or speak publicly about Florence Nightingale with such unflinching honesty and directness.

Inevitably, the Nightingales were caught up in the life of the family heroine. Aunt Mai and Shore, as we shall see, went to Scutari to assist Florence with her work. Uncle Sam, there more briefly in the summer of 1855, supervised her accounts, and was later involved in the setting up of the Nightingale Fund. Lothian Nicholson, sent to the Crimea in July 1855 in command of the 4th company, Royal Engineers – and soon to be mentioned in dispatches for his part in the demolition of the Sebastopol docks – paid a visit to Scutari, climbing the steep hill to the hospital to see his cousin and report back on her appearance and general health. Even Uncle Adams, one of Fanny Nightingale's younger siblings, went sightseeing near Varna in the summer of 1855, though it's unclear whether he met his famous niece in the course of his travels. There were demands on those left behind. Hilary Bonham Carter, who hoped at one stage, early in 1856, to take over from Aunt Mai at the Barrack Hospital, stayed in England and began work on a plaster figurine of Florence, not finally completed until 1862. Meanwhile, Aunt Patty, continuing her semi-invalid existence at Tenby, complained about 'the frequent calls at her door' from strangers wishing to obtain information about Florence Nightingale.

The impact of Florence's fame, naturally enough, fell most heavily on her parents and sister. They derived great pleasure from it – or at least Fanny and Parthenope did – while, at the same time, gently nurturing the image from which it sprang. Fanny, who attended closely to newspaper reports about her daughter, and interviewed Sidney Godolphin Osborne for 'an outpouring' of thirteen hours on his return from Scutari, took to the recognition as if it was something she had been dreaming about all her life. She lapped up personal tributes to 'the mother of so heroic a woman', and revelled in her heightened social status. An invitation came from Buckingham Palace, to watch the guards entering London from the privileged vantage point of the Palace forecourt. 'The Queen was on her Balcony just above us, with all the children', Fanny wrote, brimming with pride, '& the fine fellows, care worn & weary, in thin old Crimean clothes before us within a few feet. It was most touching to be in such close contact with some of those for whom she has been toiling . . .' In the spring of 1855, she and Parthenope 'ventured out' in London one evening, for the first time since Florence's departure, to a party given by Monckton Milnes. 'The ruck of people' inquiring about Florence, Fanny wrote afterwards, 'was formidable . . . All begin with [the words] "the only bright spot . . ."' Dickens, Bulwer Lytton and Thackeray asked to meet them. The only blight on the proceedings was that 'N', as Fanny referred to her husband, 'does not like celebrity', and refused to accompany them.

Indeed, the very idea of celebrity was anathema to William Nightingale. His daughter's 'apotheosis', he wrote, made him 'tremble for my own name'. Seeing it printed in a newspaper was 'simply an abomination', and he longed to hide himself away when he was recognized in the street or at his club. Lea Hurst and Embley no longer offered complete seclusion either. Trespassers, eager to see the Nightingale homes, had been apprehended on both estates. Hilary Bonham Carter proposed the simple expedient of putting up a 'No Entrance' sign on the gates at Lea Hurst. 'Surely it should be enough to go to some neighbouring hill from which Miss N's home may be pointed out, or even inspected thro' a telescope?' In the wood at Lea, one afternoon in May 1855, Mr Nightingale came upon an old soldier, walking in the company of some friends from nearby Lea Bridge. He described the encounter to Fanny:

They had just been up to Lea 'the Home of Miss Nightingale' & apologised for the intrusion. 'Well', said I, 'she has done her best I dare say.' He is now a recruiting serjeant for the Derbyshire Militia [&] therefore a man in authority, 'Yes . . . I have seen a good number of soldiers returned from Scutari – There she was with her dim lamp, in the night & there was not one who did not feel himself blessed by the sight of her. If she comes to London, she will be carried thro' the streets . . .'

'What next?', William Nightingale asked his wife, 'in wonder & in awe', but more than a little tongue in cheek. 'Will she call the dead to life?'

Florence's work was providing her sister with a true sense of purpose for the first time in her life. At root, Parthenope had transferred her obsessive feelings for Florence to a broader, more public canvas, becoming keeper of the flame; but her focus of love and admiration also widened to the point where Florence was now her 'inspiration'. Parthenope's workload on Florence's behalf was enormous, pursued with an intensity that never flagged: writing letters, endlessly copying and circulating any that touched on Florence's concerns to a large circle of family, friends and acquaintances, compiling vast albums of any scrap of material that so much as mentioned the Nightingale name, and acting generally as her younger sister's proxy in a multiplying number of situations. 'You . . . are becoming legendary as well,' Monckton Milnes wrote admiringly to her, as he contemplated the extent of her efforts. Parthenope was left with 'between 50 & 60 letters' to answer on Florence's departure, then swamped by another 300 from a 'cloud of applicants' for Scutari. Eventually the number settled at '12 or 13 letters per diem'. As Parthenope explained to her cousin Bertha Smith, '. . . the immense amount of writing which I have to do is incredible, in my sister's cause – I will tell you my day's work today. 2 presents to thank for, for what she has done in the East . . . 2 letters asking for advice [from] ladies who want to join her . . . 1 begging letter, 4 letters entreating for news of her, an Italian, an American & a German to answer, besides my own friends.' No wonder that Uncle Sam commiserated with her over her 'penworn fingers'. This one-woman secretariat didn't always operate smoothly. Confidential letters went astray before materializing in the press, while on at least one occasion Liz Herbert felt forced to refuse Parthenope a copy of one of Florence's letters to Sidney Herbert, on the grounds that it was '<u>strictly Private</u>'. In the matter of Florence's autograph – for instance, for the Bishop of Oxford, who was eager to procure one – it was Parthenope who turned down requests. 'Her writing is part of herself,' she wrote, '& I cannot bear to have her vulgarised.' Florence's hair was another matter, and Liz Herbert asked for, and received, a strand of it to wear in a locket around her neck.

In December 1854, when Queen Victoria requested, in a letter to Liz Herbert, that 'Miss Nightingale and the ladies would tell these poor, noble wounded and sick men, that *no one* takes a warmer interest or feels *more* for their sufferings or admires their courage and heroism *more* than their Queen', it was Parthenope who grasped the importance of this royal seal of approval, asking 'May we spread the Queen's letter a little?' At the same time, Florence arranged for Victoria's message to be read in the wards and posted on the walls of the hospitals, where it was received with tears by the men. In November 1855, the Queen would present Florence with a brooch – the recognition denied Mary Stanley – designed by the Prince Consort, with a St George's Cross in red enamel, and the royal cipher surmounted by a crown in diamonds. The inscription read 'Blessed are the Merciful'. Victoria's accompanying letter praised the 'Christian devotion' displayed by Florence 'during this great and bloody war', and looked forward to the prospect of making her acquaintance on her return to England.

The testimony of ordinary soldiers about their treatment at Scutari was assiduously collected by Parthenope. Stories abounded, and, exchanged and repeated by men at the front, or back home in England, they sometimes grew or were embellished at each retelling. 'Nothing can surpass the way in which the poor soldiers talk of her . . .,' noted Lothian Nicholson, citing the tale of the man, an ex-patient from Scutari, overheard in the trenches before Sebastopol telling his colleagues that they no longer need fear being wounded or falling sick as Florence Nightingale was there to care for them. Writing to his wife, Martha, and their friend Mrs Ivernay, from the Barrack Hospital, on 3 April 1855, Private John Swains responded to their inquiries about 'Miss Nightingale':

. . . if there is any Angels on Earth she is one how my Dear old friend Mrs Ivernay would glory to see her Delicate form gliding about Amongst hundreds of great ruff soldiers and to see the looks of love and gratitude that they cast on her beloved face it always does me good to see her it would be a brave man that dare insult her I would not give a peny for his Chance . . .

Soldiers' letters often emphasized Florence's feminine delicacy, or portrayed her as a substitute mother requiring manly protection ('. . . supposing a case in which <u>she</u> were in danger', were the reported remarks of one Private, '. . . he thought that of every 3 regiments 2 would fly to save her . . .'). Gifts from Miss Nightingale – a knapsack, a comb, or a handkerchief – might be mentioned, with the assurance that they would be treasured 'while life lasted', not, 'of course', for their value, but for remembrance. Personal descriptions of the lady might be vague, or perhaps the work of a romantic imagination. 'How did she look?' a soldier was asked. ' "Very small", was his reply – but surely she is very tall? Yes, but he meant thin.' Another man thought Florence had been wearing a veil, gold cross, blue slippers and 'a sort of brown' gown when he saw her.

'She's here, there, and everywhere,' wrote a former Scutari patient. 'You never lose sight of her.' And this power of omniscience was, indeed, part of the magical quality ascribed to Florence in some of the poetry she inspired, like, for example, John Davies's 1856 tribute to her, in which she is imagined as a goddess with a 'magic touch'. But, of course, in the crude light of reality, she possessed no such ability to be in several places at the same time, though it is entirely understandable that so many men rushed to claim that they had been personally nursed by her. The Reverend W. F. Hobson later took these claims to their logical conclusion in a memoir of his wife, Catharine (Kate) Hobson, née Anderson, who had been in the second party of nurses, at Koulali and Scutari. According to Hobson, Anderson bore a close resemblance to Florence Nightingale, and had been frequently mistaken for her. ' "Miss Nightingale",' Hobson concluded, not without a little justice, 'was to many a generic name to whom many things were assigned through mere ignorance and mistake.'

In the summer of 1855, Florence Nightingale mania, driven by the affection and esteem in which she was held by the British Army in the Crimea, was sweeping through Britain. 'The floating froth of public praise', as *Punch* called it, was to be found in scores of songs, with sentimental titles like 'The Shadow on the Pillow', 'The Star of the East' or, most popularly, 'The Nightingale in the East', with its refrain, 'So forward, my lads, may your hearts never fail,/You are cheer'd by the presence of a sweet Nightingale.' By the autumn of 1856, Parthenope calculated that the family was receiving copies of at least three new songs a week. Poetry and rhymed broadsheets, illustrated with rough woodcuts, poured from the presses in Seven Dials and Soho. Florence had become 'the heroine of the cottage, the workshop, and the alleys'. Tradesmen printed idealized likenesses and short lives of her, as well as 'the Nightingale pedigree', on their paper bags. There was a publication, 'the Florence Chronicle', and 'a Nightingale-coffee-house'. Ships were named after her. 'Did you see the account of the Iron Ship just launched at Hartlepool with her name, figure, bust,' Aunt Patty wrote excitedly to Fanny Nightingale in December 1855, 'built by Richardsons & Co for Mr Young of Wisbeach?' (This barque was followed two years later by a brigantine named in Florence's honour and, eventually, by a steamer, the *Florence Nightingale*, built in Sunderland in 1878.) Most unlikely of all, a racehorse called 'Florence Nightingale' won the Forest Plate Handicap. From Manchester, Mrs Gaskell informed Parthenope that 'Babies ad libitum are being christened Florence ... poor little factory babies, whose grimed stunted parents brighten up at the name ...' But it wasn't simply working-class parents who decided to associate their children with Florence in this way: George Eliot's future sister-in-law, for example, born in 1857, and baptized Florence Nightingale Cross, came from a middle-class banking family.*

'The mythical Florence is very, very curious,' Parthenope admitted. In the circles in which the Nightingales themselves moved, Florence was often compared to Joan of Arc. Lady Dunsany, a bit like Mrs Gaskell before her, had a bee in her bonnet that Florence was Joan of Arc 'come round again'. She possessed 'the same strange & sexless identity', Lady Dunsany wrote to Parthenope, expanding on her theory, 'which belonging ... neither to man nor woman seemed to ... combine the choicest results of both'. Mr Luck, a barrister, took up the theme in a series of public lectures on 'The Varieties of Heroine', including both Florence and Joan among his subjects, together with Miriam, Judith, Elizabeth I, Mary, Queen of Scots, and Charlotte Corday.

* There were plenty of more literal namesakes, too, of whom Florence Alma Nightingale, born in 1856, is perhaps the most memorable. On her return to England Florence became accustomed to contemplating her own death in the newspapers, 'always at the age of five', by which she meant the deaths in infancy of children named after her. In her own circle, children who were given her first name included Monckton Milnes's second daughter; Arthur and Blanche Clough's eldest child; the granddaughter of Sir John McNeill, leader of the Commissariat Commission in the Crimean War; and Florence Farr, daughter of Dr William Farr, Florence's collaborator in medical statistics, who was later actress-muse to both Shaw and Yeats. Florence Nightingale Shore (1865–1920), a distant cousin on William Nightingale's side, was also Florence's goddaughter, and became a nurse in emulation of her, serving with distinction in France during the First World War. She was murdered, with three heavy blows to the head, on the London to Hastings train in 1920. No one was ever arrested for her killing.

Florence Nightingale was projected by the middle classes as a symbol of efficient, effective, housewifely virtue to be set against the aristocratic – and masculine – mismanagement of the war. She was promoted by the Government itself as a heroine in a conflict that had signally failed to produce a figure of the stature of Nelson or Wellington, and as a useful diversionary tactic from the Government's own manifest failings of leadership (thus *Blackwood's Magazine*, reporting on Sidney Herbert's Commons speech of December 1854, in which he referred movingly to her work, portrayed Herbert as sheltering behind Miss Nightingale's skirts). Among women, however, views on Florence's significance as a standard-bearer for the future of her sex differed widely. Was she a suitable role model for other women? Ellen Tollet, an old family friend, was one of those who thought not. '. . . Let her be considered a great exception to general rules,' she suggested to Parthenope, 'as she is herself a great exception as to genius & character.' This idea, that Florence Nightingale was exceptional and could not be held up as an example for other refined and educated ladies, was one of the arguments developed in Emily Shirreff's *Intellectual Education and Its Influences on the Character and Happiness of Women*, a manual addressed to the women of the late 1850s, as Mrs Ellis had spoken to the generation before. For Elizabeth Barrett Browning, on the other hand, Florence Nightingale's career represented a retrograde step for her sex. While Mrs Browning expressed to Parthenope her admiration for 'your heroic sister', she privately thought that the portrayal of woman as a 'saintly nurse' was merely a revival of old virtues. By contrast, Caroline Bathurst, in a series of letters to Parthenope, was eloquent on the subject of the new ideal of woman embodied by Florence. She was convinced of the 'revolution' that Florence was working in English society – 'not with carnal, but (as woman must always work) with spiritual weapons' – and saw as evidence of this the wholesale change of opinion among those who, only a short time before, had ridiculed the idea of young ladies being made useful members of society, and who were now urging those who wished to devote themselves to nursing to obtain preparatory training in one of the London hospitals. 'Oh: Florence, Florence,' wrote Lady Bathurst, 'you will be the destruction of the "young lady class" in England – & with it, of how much suffering.' There were those in British society in Constantinople who thought that Florence's example might even influence the 'degraded womankind' of Turkey itself. It was regarded as a hopeful sign, at an Embassy ball in February 1856, that some Turkish women appeared without their faces veiled.

The essential precondition for this appropriation of Florence by different interests was that she herself, in line with the conventional expectations of her sex, should observe a rule of silence. This she resolutely did, establishing a pattern for the future, never defending herself publicly even when placed under the severest provocation. 'What a veiled & silent woman she has always been,' Caroline Bathurst commented approvingly, 'manifesting her Womanhood in deeds, not words, by the fulfilment of duties, not the assertion of rights' (and a concern with deeds not rights might be said to encapsulate Florence's later response to the growth of 'the Woman Question' in the course of the latter half of the century). Florence's reaction to the 'buz-fuz' surrounding her name tended to be generally dismissive. Her 'effigies & praises' were unwelcome, she told Parthenope in July 1855, not because she affected indifference towards 'real sympathy', but because she understood only too well 'the unmitigated harm' done to the enterprise by the 'vanity and frivolity' it had inspired. Such éclat, she believed, had lowered the standing of the nursing expedition in the eyes of the medical men, while attracting women to the hospitals who were 'desirous of notoriety' rather than the prospect of hard work. Nevertheless, one perhaps senses in Florence's repeated, somewhat over-emphatic insistence that she never so much as glanced at a newspaper to read about herself – despite Mary Stanley's assertion that the sofa in Florence's room at the Barrack Hospital was strewn with newspapers just come in by the post – a trace of the old struggle between her own small reputation and the will of God.

The demand for portraits of Florence, drawn from the imagination rather than life, seemed insatiable. An example turned up at Scutari in a box of stores from Embley. 'How unlike her!' said Selina Bracebridge, laughing it to scorn. Soldiers in the Crimea pasted them up in the mess. Back in Derbyshire, John Smedley, the Lea Mill owner, bought 'two pictures with the likeness of Miss Florence', and gave one to Fanny Wildgoose, the schoolmaster's wife, who proudly showed it off. On the Nightingale estates in nearby Pleasley, prints of Florence were distributed to every farmhouse and cottage.

Not everyone was happy about the proliferation of these fanciful images. Alfred Bonham Carter, a young cousin, marched into John Mabley's shop in the Strand in London, paid a shilling for 'the article so long the object of my contempt & hatred', an idealized portrait of Florence, and harangued the shopkeeper for selling it. Mabley's excuse was that he was meeting 'the wants of the poorer classes'. He had obtained the picture from a cheap market in Berlin, but would have preferred to sell something 'nearer to the truth'. Engravings of 'the Heroine of Scutari', like the one presented 'gratis', in May 1855, to subscribers of the *Weekly News*, generally showed a plump, dark-haired woman, not unlike Queen Victoria, dressed, if the print was in colour, in virginal blue, and holding a letter or a book. This rather bland facial template had a bizarre subsequent history, when it was used as an example to illustrate the fashionable science of physiognomy. In S. R. Wells's *New System of Physiognomy*, published in 1866, a drawing of Florence Nightingale's face is juxtaposed with one of 'Bridget McBruiser', an imaginary working-class woman, to represent class stereotypes and highlight the superiority of Nightingale's breeding as a pinnacle of British womanhood.

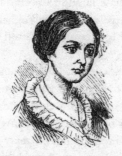 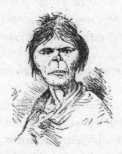

The porcelain figures produced by Staffordshire factories in 1855 took a further leap towards the imaginary in their depiction of Florence Nightingale. Interestingly, none of the three designs portrays her holding a lamp. In one she is veiled and standing beside a wounded Crimean soldier; in another, also veiled, she stands beside a pedestal, her hand resting on three books; in the third, she is bareheaded, dressed in a colourful jacket and skirt, and holding two drinking cups on a tray.

'Surely it would be charming to have a cheap likeness of Florence – really like,' wrote Aunt Patty in late 1855, 'done on stiff paper . . . to go in a pocket book.' In fact, two lithographs based on pre-Crimean portraits of Florence from life, one by Hilary Bonham Carter, the other, of Florence with Athena, by Parthenope, had been published by the Colnaghi Brothers, with the family's authorization, in the autumn of 1854. Small details from these, the flower in the hair, the check shawl, occasionally seep into the idealized pictures, but clearly, at a price of anywhere between 2s. 6d. and 7s. 6d., they were not for mass consumption. Fanny Nightingale sent copies to friends and wellwishers, and offered them for sale to benefit local charities like the Buxton Bath Bazaar.

Florence, however, continued to refuse sittings for a more up-to-date painting or photograph. She had a principled objection to having her likeness taken, later annotating her Bible, against Ecclesiastes, chapter 12, verse 8 ('Vanity of vanities ... all is vanity'), with the words: 'and the vanity of vanities – the idolatry of our fellow mortals'. She made an exception for two official requests after her return to England. One was to satisfy the Queen's wish for a photograph of her; the other was to sit for the sculptor Sir John Steell, and then only because the bust was made at the express wish of the British Army, and paid for out a fund raised from subscriptions from non-commissioned officers and men. Steell's bust, often declared by the Nightingale family to be the best artistic likeness of her, was visited in the artist's studio by 'soldiers, widows, orphans & sweethearts' who greeted it, according to Steell, 'with tears of gratitude'.

The artist Jerry Barrett, arriving at Scutari during Florence's closing weeks there, in the summer of 1856, to begin work on a group painting that would convey her 'mission of mercy', swiftly confronted Florence's refusal to sit for him. He wrote to her of the 'serious inconvenience' this caused him. His letter evidently stung her, but in replying to him, Florence referred again to the drawbacks created by publicity. She had determined 'in no way to forward the making a show of myself or of any ... thing connected with that work though I cannot always prevent them from being made a show of'. She hadn't counted, though, on Barrett's resourcefulness. On, or around, 27 July, the day before Florence's departure, he snatched a quick head and shoulders study, in profile, as she walked down by the harbour. Even so, this, together with a couple of earlier sketches, appears to have been inadequate for Barrett's purposes, and for the final painting he almost certainly relied on the photograph of Florence taken by Mayall for the Queen later that year. *The Mission of Mercy: Florence Nightingale Receiving the Wounded at*

Scutari – to give the painting its full title – was Barrett's second large-scale painting with a Crimean theme. *Queen Victoria's First Visit to Her Wounded Soldiers*, documenting the royal family's official inspection of Crimean invalids at the army hospital at Chatham, in the spring of 1855, had preceded it; and it was the success of this painting, with a renowned woman as its central protagonist, which had encouraged Barrett, who had been exhibiting at the Royal Academy since 1853, to choose Florence Nightingale for his next commission. Barrett's expenses for Scutari were met by Thomas Agnew, the Manchester art dealer, who was cornering the market in Crimean scenes. In the summer of 1857, Agnew would buy the finished work for £450, a sum which included the copyright of the picture, an essential feature of the transaction, as *The Mission of Mercy* was engraved in mixed media by Thomas Barlow, and published, with a key to the identity of the individuals depicted, in April 1858. This large edition of prints – over 1,000 engravings, in addition to the sale of hundreds of artist's proofs – pointed to the picture's impact on the Victorian public, and signalled its enormous popularity.

Barrett had a studio inside the Barrack Hospital (and may be glimpsed, in a self-portrait, through the window at the centre left of the painting), from where he must have made preliminary sketches of soldiers and some of the other participants, as well as capturing the view of the docks and minarets of Constantinople through the hospital gates as a stream of casualties arrived from the ships in the harbour beyond. However, the painting blends the real with the imaginary. Some of those represented, like the Bracebridges, and Mother Clare Moore, had already left Scutari by the time Barrett was working there, while the painting portrays three consecutive Commandants – Major Sillery, Lord William Paulet and Major-General Sir Harry Storks, the third commandant of the hospital, who succeeded Paulet in August 1855 – who were never all in residence at Scutari at the same time. In June 1857 Barrett was working in his London studio at 27 Gower Street, where Paulet, the Bracebridges and Miss Tebbutt, Superintendent of the General Hospital in 1855–6, were among those sitting for him. From Gower Street, Barrett wrote to Agnew, describing Fanny Nightingale's second visit to view the painting. She had sat for half an hour, 'looking at the picture and spoke in commendation of her daughter's portrait . . .' Florence herself never saw it.

Today, *The Mission of Mercy*, hanging in the National Portrait

Gallery, in London, is arguably the most famous, possibly the most frequently reproduced, portrait of Florence Nightingale, despite her efforts to deny Jerry Barrett a sitting. Yet it has only been on public display since 1993, when it was purchased by the Gallery (the preparatory oil sketch, with over thirty-four figures instead of the finished thirty-one, some of them in significantly different positions, has been in the Gallery's collection since 1963). Following its completion, the painting had been deposited at Buckingham Palace in June 1857 for royal inspection, and exhibited the following summer at Leggatt and Hayward, in Cornhill. In 1859, it was bought by Sir Edward Bates. Handed down through the Bates family, the painting effectively disappeared for more than 130 years, known to subsequent generations only through the medium of the engraved print.

Florence Nightingale stands at the centre of *The Mission of Mercy*, illuminated by a light that falls on her face and figure. At her feet lies a recumbent soldier, and her hand stretches out towards him – though without touching him – as if in a gesture of benediction, a clear echo of Raphael's cartoon of *Peter and John Healing the Lame Man at the Gate of the Temple*. The painting offers an implied reproach to those who have contributed to the neglect of the war's sick and wounded, while framing a new definition of the heroism of enterprising woman.

The first biography of Florence Nightingale, published in 1855 and entitled *The Only and Unabridged Edition of the Life of Miss Nightingale . . . The Heroine of European Philanthropy . . .* , was a slim sixteen-page book, costing a penny. Aside from its association of Florence's name with the idea of philanthropy, which she would certainly have loathed, the book rehearses aspects of her early life – the strong sympathy for the sick, the ministering to the needs of the poor, and the acts of self-denial despite her privileged background – that were already familiar from articles in the press. Florence was also asked to write a book about her Crimean experiences. One offer from a company in the United States, Childs & Petersen, anticipated sales in America alone of 50,000 copies and, hoping to tempt Florence, suggested that the profits might go towards funding a training hospital for nurses in the States. It goes almost without saying that she rejected any such request.

A handful of other women did capitalize on their time in the hospitals of the East by publishing memoirs of their experiences. The earliest was

the anonymous account that appeared in 1855, by a lady volunteer, of
the British hospital at Smyrna, though, staffed by nurses sent out by Lady
Canning, this never came under Florence's authority. The following year,
*Eastern Hospitals and English Nurses – a Narrative of Twelve Months'
Experience in the Hospitals of Koulali and Scutari* by Fanny Taylor, one
of Mary Stanley's ladies, was published. Neither of these found favour
in Florence's eyes. She had no time to read them anyway, she told Lady
Canning, but 'even had I, I would not', as she was unable to understand
why serving God and your country wasn't sufficient without having to
sit down and write a book about it. She did find the time, six years later,
to read the Sellonite Margaret Goodman's *Experiences of an English
Sister of Mercy*, and was appalled to discover the author's treachery:
not only in her discussion of Lydia Sellon's 'flannel shifts', but also
through her breach of privacy in mentioning those with whom she'd
served by name, with descriptions of 'all their peccadilloes'.

This kind of prose account generally made respectful obeisance to the
Nightingale name. One which certainly didn't was a book by Elizabeth
Davis, a vigorous Welsh woman in her late sixties, formerly a domestic
servant and nurse at Guy's, who came to Scutari as a member of the
Stanley party, but insisted on going on to Balaclava's General Hospital,
without Florence's blessing, after being accused of insubordination.
Davis's *Autobiography*, edited by Jane Williams from notes of conversations, was published in the summer of 1857, partly in order to
raise some badly needed cash (Davis died in poverty in 1860). Davis
announces her antagonism towards Florence from the outset. 'I did not
like the name of Nightingale. When I first hear a name I am very apt to
know by my feelings whether I shall like the person who bears it.' She
then proceeds to criticize Florence for her bureaucratic approach and
misuse of resources, claiming that while she and other nurses ate tough
old meat, Florence dined every day on the best French cooking (presumably Soyer's, though this is an unfounded allegation repeated by at least
one modern Nightingale biographer). Selina Bracebridge believed that
she detected a major motivation behind this 'odious lying Book'. Davis
was one of the supporters of Charlotte Salisbury, who had been dismissed from Scutari for dishonesty in her distribution of the Free Gifts
in the stores. Several of Davis's sentences were, in fact, the repetition of
phrases from Salisbury's own statement of defence.

These self-chroniclers are, however, the exception to the rule. Most of the women who nursed at Scutari or in the Crimea have left little mark on the early history of military nursing, beyond their names, and the brief – often nothing more than a few trifling words – résumé of their career in the surviving 'Register of Nurses Sent to Military Hospitals in the East'. This handwritten record, maintained by several people, including Mrs Bracebridge, Mary Stanley and Florence herself, contains the names of 229 women who left Britain in 1854–6 to nurse during the Crimean War. It is a vital historical resource, but one that is, nevertheless, demonstrably incomplete. Information about the later lives of most of these women depends on the vagaries of the census records; those who were unmarried or without permanent address are consequently lost to history. Often it is only the notorious that rise to the surface. Take Jane Gibson, for example. She had been sent home from Balaclava in disgrace, in June 1855, on the grounds of being intoxicated while treating a patient. Back in London, in the autumn of that year, she was accused of 'extensive robbery from the Hospitals at Scutari and Balaclava', and of having stolen items of clothing, linen and books. Later, after examinations at Southwark Police Court, and on the basis of evidence submitted by Mrs Polidori, the store keeper at Scutari, Gibson was acquitted, though the accusations were a stain on her record. Troublesome Emma Fagg, despite her dismissal for incompetence, has her own place in history. She returned to Kent to work as a private nurse, living out her old age in Thanet Union Workhouse, and dying, at the age of eighty-seven, in March 1913, the final survivor of Florence Nightingale's famous expedition of October 1854.

For the broader picture, we must rely on numbers and statistics. Of the 229 women, eleven died in the hospitals and were buried at Scutari, Balaclava and Smyrna, while only seventeen, including Florence herself, served for the duration of the war; forty-nine women were dismissed, eighteen of them for intoxication, while forty resigned. One analysis of these figures concludes that, in spite of the impression created by the high-profile cases of misconduct and disciplinable behaviour, as many as three-quarters of the women 'acquitted themselves in so satisfactory a manner that they were retained until no longer needed . . .'

In the course of his attempt to preserve the memory of his wife Catharine, who had nursed at Koulali and Scutari, the Reverend W. F. Hobson suggested that Florence Nightingale's reputation had overshadowed the other Crimean nurses, and effectively blotted them from history. The idea that she had received the credit due to other nurses was something that troubled Florence herself in her later years. 'I often think, or rather do not like to think,' she wrote to Aunt Mai in 1888, 'how all the people who were with me in the Crimea must feel how unjust it is that all the "Testimonial" went to me. I don't think Sister Bertha is without this feeling – how could she be? – though she never expresses it.' Her remarks were prompted by a visit from Bertha Turnbull, a Sellonite from the original party, whom Florence had singled out, years before, as among her most valued workers. One or two nurses, like Sarah Anne Terrot, who went to Balmoral in 1897 to be decorated with the Royal Red Cross by Queen Victoria, lived long enough to receive recognition. But the only woman to challenge Florence Nightingale's position as the archetypal Crimean nurse, in the popular imagination in recent years, has been the figure of the Jamaican-born Creole Mary Seacole.

'Have you read Mrs Seacole? She excites my sincere good will, & I hope F[lorence] thinks she deserves it.' This was Aunt Patty in a letter to Fanny Nightingale, in the summer of 1857, commenting on Mary Seacole's recently published autobiography, *Wonderful Adventures of Mrs Seacole in Many Lands*. This book, written to raise funds to compensate Seacole for the financial losses she had suffered at the end of the war, at her British Hotel on Spring Hill, two miles along the road from Balaclava, was a bestseller. Like Elizabeth Davis's memoir, Seacole's account of her travels, as 'a female Ulysses', on the Isthmus of Panama, and in the Crimea, where she had won a place in the hearts of many officers and men for her care of the sick and wounded, was probably dictated to an editor. It retains the energy and idiosyncrasies of her speech, and is as vivid and colourful as Seacole's favourite outfit, a canary-yellow dress and blue bonnet trimmed with red ribbons.

It is difficult not to be stirred by Mary Seacole's spirit of independence, her flamboyant sense of adventure, and the warm-heartedness that flows through her book's pages. The first two characteristics would be remarkable enough in any nineteenth-century woman, but for one of mixed race, regularly encountering prejudice on account of her colour – and negotiating complex strategies in her writing to associate herself with her predominantly British readership, while distancing herself from blacks – they are doubly impressive. Born Mary Jane Grant, in Kingston, Jamaica, in 1805, to a free Creole woman and a Scottish army officer, Seacole was technically a quadroon (of one mulatto and one white parent). From her mother, who kept a lodging-house for British army officers, she inherited her medical knowledge, including many Caribbean herbal treatments. After the death of her husband Edwin Horatio Seacole (a godson of Nelson's), in 1844, Seacole worked as a nurse and 'doctress' at the local military station at Newcastle before joining her brother in Panama in 1851. Over the next few years, while setting up a hotel and stores for gold prospectors, she gained invaluable experience of treating epidemics of cholera and yellow fever (she had already nursed in the cholera attack that swept Jamaica in 1850). She arrived in London in October 1854, just after the Battle of Alma, determined to offer herself as a nurse in the second party leaving for Scutari. However, in an interview at the Herberts' house in Belgrave Square, Seacole was rejected on the grounds that the full complement of nurses had been selected. Seacole believed that even if there had been a vacancy, prejudice against her colour would have prevented her from being allowed to fill it. Her surmise was probably correct. Records show that another applicant, Elizabeth Purcell, described as 'an exemplary character', was turned down for being 'too old and almost black'.

Mary Seacole wasn't to be thwarted, though, and set off under her own steam. As an hotelier on Spring Hill, she offered good food and hospitality – admittedly at heavy prices – earning praise from Alexis Soyer for 'her soups and dainties'. As a nurse and 'doctress', applying herbal remedies derived from Caribbean medicine, she successfully treated cases of diarrhoea, dysentery, even cholera. With a bag, containing lint, bandages, needles, thread and medicines, slung across her shoulder, she came under fire as she courageously navigated the fields of battle to tend to the injured and dying. In September 1855, Mary Seacole became the first woman to enter Sebastopol after the ending of the prolonged siege. The nicknames given her – 'Mother' or 'Aunty', or even 'the Creole with the Teacup' – testify to the enormous affection with which she was regarded by the British Army. When she fell on hard times, the military establishment organized a benefit in her honour. In *The Times*, one veteran had asked whether 'While the benevolent deeds of Florence Nightingale are being handed down to posterity with blessings and imperishable renown, are the humbler actions of Mrs Seacole to be entirely forgotten, and will none now substantially testify to the worth of those services of the late mistress of Spring Hill?' Seacole remained a celebrated figure among her contemporaries. When Anthony Trollope visited Jamaica in 1858, he was informed by Seacole's sister Louisa that Mary had wanted to go with the army to India during the Indian Mutiny, but that Queen Victoria would not let her because her life was 'too precious'. Mary Seacole's death in 1881 was commemorated by several newspapers, but by the beginning of the twentieth century, her name was beginning to be forgotten.

This neglect continued, to a large extent, until the 1980s. Then, twenty years ago, *Wonderful Adventures* was republished in Britain, and quickly became a rallying point in the teaching of multicultural history. Seacole was presented, justifiably, as a black woman whose achievements had been marginalized by white historians; a cottage industry developed around her exploits, her name was hitched to the bandwagon of political correctness, and she was dubbed in popular shorthand as 'the Black Nightingale'. The false comparisons between Mary Seacole and Florence Nightingale, which continue to this day, do not belong to the realm of serious history. Moreover, they fail to do justice to the significance of the Crimean work of either woman. There can be no doubt that, in terms of practical nursing expertise, Seacole far outdid Nightingale's experience of hands-on nursing. While Florence was on her visit to Kaiserswerth in the summer of 1850, for her brief, initial period of training, Mary Seacole was nursing victims of the Kingston cholera epidemic. Seacole's practice extended not simply to nursing, but also to the preparation of herbal and pharmaceutical medicines, to diagnosis, minor surgery, and even a postmortem (in *Wonderful Adventures* she describes carrying out her 'first and last' postmortem on a dead baby to learn more about the effects of cholera). Equally, though, the romantic myth surrounding Nightingale's name has often obscured her formidable organizing powers, and the reality that her primary responsibility during the war was not to nurse, but to administer the nascent military nursing service.

What were the women's impressions of each other? In her autobiography Mary Seacole recalls seeing Florence Nightingale – 'that English-woman whose name shall never die, but sound like music on the lips of men until the end of doom' – for the first time. Seacole was on her way to Balaclava, on her journey out, and stopped at Scutari, where she was found a bed for the night in the washerwomen's quarters. Introduced to

Florence through a letter of recommendation from one of the medical officers at the hospital, who had known her in Kingston, Seacole was ushered into her presence, where she was received in a 'gentle, but eminently practical and business-like way'. Florence is presented in deft strokes as standing in repose, while remaining 'keenly observant – the greatest sign of impatience . . . a slight, perhaps unwitting motion of the firmly planted right foot . . .'

Did Florence share Aunt Patty's feelings of 'sincere good will' towards Mary Seacole? The conclusions are mixed. On the one hand, Florence clearly respected all that Seacole had done for men at the front. In the account of his *Culinary Campaign* in the Crimea, Alexis Soyer quotes Florence as saying that she would like to see Mrs Seacole before she returned to England, 'as I hear she has done a great deal of good for the poor soldiers'; and recently discovered evidence reveals that Florence implicitly acknowledged this good work by contributing to Mary Seacole's Testimonial Fund, raised by wellwishers when Seacole faced bankruptcy in 1857.

But on the other hand, Florence remained wary of the reputation of the Seacole Hotel on Spring Hill for being a 'bad house', and was anxious that the good name of her own nursing establishment should not suffer by any association with it. She knew that Mrs Seacole encouraged drinking among her guests, turned a blind eye to immorality – and possibly even had an illegitimate teenage daughter of her own. Her prejudice against this 'woman of bad character', as she later called her, was unlikely to have been racially motivated. A more plausible, additional reason for any resentment she felt was that, at some stage during her time at Balaclava, Seacole won the protection of Florence's great adversary Dr John Hall, Inspector-General of Hospitals in the East, and received 'his sanction' to prescribe her own medicines. Seacole's nursing of, and hobnobbing with, high-ranking officers would not have found favour with Florence either. Florence's system of nursing concentrated on the ordinary ranks. Officers had servants to nurse them, or could pay for their nursing. She considered it no part of the main business of her work to attend to their needs.

Some of these feelings were to resurface in 1870, when Florence was asked for her view of Mary Seacole. 'She kept – I will not call it a "bad house" but something not very unlike it in the Crimean War. She was very kind to the men, &, what is more to the Officers – & did some

good & made many drunk ... I had the greatest difficulty in repelling
Mrs Seacole's advances, & in preventing associations between her & my
nurses (absolutely out of the question) when we established 2 hospitals
nursed by us between Kadikoi & the "Seacole Establishment" in the
Crimea.'

From poems in august journals and periodicals to doggerel verse printed
on paper bags, the poetry of the Crimean War captured the wave of
emotion surrounding Florence Nightingale's name, and presented her in
her most uncontroversial guise. A young mathematics don at Christ
Church, Oxford, Charles Dodgson, a decade away from becoming Lewis
Carroll, worked for many months on a poem celebrating her, completing
it soon after the bells that signalled the coming of peace rang out in
March 1856. 'The Path of Roses' reads like a Tennysonian parody,
employing the by now well-used imagery of a lamp lighting the 'creeping
gloom', and of fevered brows being cooled by the softest of touches.
'"Alas ... For what can Woman do?"' the Nightingale character asks
at the beginning of the poem. '"Her life is aimless, and her death
unknown:/Hemmed in by social forms she pines in vain./Man has his
work, but what can Woman do?"/And answer came there from the
creeping gloom ...'

   The answer, of course, lies in woman's acceptance of a religious-based
role, ministering to the sick and wounded in imitation of Christ. This
symbolism, of Florence Nightingale as 'the crown of Christian womanhood', is reflected in many poems, of variable quality, like Westland
Marston's 'At Scutari' (*Athenaeum*, 20 January 1855), for example,
or *Punch*'s anonymous contribution, 'Scutari', published the following
month. Martin Tupper's poem of that year, addressed to the eponymous
heroine, is filled with this religious theme, but goes further. To Tupper,
standing for a conservative, middle-class outlook, Florence Nightingale
is a 'calm dove of peace amid war's vulture woes', but also an image of
stability, and, most importantly, of consensus in an area where national
unity is difficult to achieve. It doesn't matter what Florence Nightingale
does, Tupper appears to suggest, so much as what she represents to the
public.

'... The people love you,' Parthenope had written to her sister, 'with
a ... passionate tenderness that goes to my heart.' Florence herself

experienced an unforgettable impression of the strength of this feeling, several days after her arrival at Balaclava, on 5 May 1855, when, accompanied by Soyer, Bracebridge, and other members of her entourage, she visited the trenches before Sebastopol. There was something sublime in the spectacle, she wrote afterwards. The men of the 39th 'turned out & gave Florence Nightingale three times three, as I rode away. There was nothing empty in that cheer nor in the heart which received it. I took it as a true expression of true sympathy – the sweetest I have ever had ... In all that has been said against & for me, no one soul has appreciated what I was really doing – none but the honest cheer of the brave 39th.'

On board the *Robert Lowe,* with the sound of gunfire in their ears, they had entered the harbour at Balaclava, filled with ships 'packed like herrings'. The decks of these surrounding vessels were crowded with spectators waiting to catch a glimpse of 'the Nightingale'. During the following week, Florence toured the regimental hospitals as well as two of the base hospitals: the General, established at an old stone house at the time of the invasion of the Crimea, in September 1854, and the Castle, a group of huts above Balaclava, in a scenic spot on the Genoese Heights, opened just weeks earlier. With Soyer's assistance, she made plans for extra diet kitchens at the General Hospital, and reorganized the Castle Hospital, where the cooking arrangements were wholly inadequate. She foresaw months of work ahead to introduce a semblance of the kind of order that now existed at Scutari. At Balaclava, the Army authorities seemed even more resistant to change. The Sanitary Commission had been obstructed in their work there, while, in a sign of difficulties to come, Florence was faced with instructions from David Fitzgerald, the Purveyor-in-Chief in the Crimea, and his patron Dr Hall, that all her requisitions should receive their personal sanction before being issued to her. Meanwhile, at her headquarters on board ship, she received Sir John McNeill and Colonel Alexander Tulloch, the two men heading an inquiry into the supply system. Florence reported that they had already worked wonders, ensuring fresh meat three times a week, and fresh bread from Constantinople on a regular basis. Sir John, another of her future allies, returned her admiration, having taken 'a wonderful fancy' to her, according to Charles Bracebridge.

She remained profoundly affected by this first contact with the troops in their wartime habitat. It seemed to reinforce her sense of special union with them. The camp was very striking – between 150,000 and 200,000 men in a space of twenty square miles – and it was impossible to be unmoved by the sight of soldiers, 'mustering & forming at sun-down' for their twenty-four-hour duty in the trenches. On horseback, Florence and Mr Bracebridge surveyed Sebastopol from the heights, as shells whizzed to the right and left of them. From ground 'ploughed with shot & shell', she picked some flowers, and a Minié bullet, to send home to Parthenope as a souvenir.

There was some cholera in the camp, which reignited concern for her health. But Florence remained as fearless as ever of the risk of illness. However, on 13 May, the day after her thirty-fifth birthday, she collapsed, suffering from weakness and exhaustion. Two days later, Colonel William Napier reported seeing her as she was carried in a litter by four guardsmen across to one of the huts at the Castle Hospital. The word passed rapidly through the camp. Florence Nightingale was close to death.

11. I Shall Never Forget

It was as bad a case of fever as any he had seen, said Dr Arthur Anderson, the Principal Medical Officer at Balaclava. For ten days, during the acute phase of her illness, Florence's condition oscillated wildly between satisfactory and critical. A sudden relapse in the morning was followed by recovery, and then another relapse in the evening. Her hair was cropped to stem the temperature from the brain, but at the height of her delirium she continued feverishly to write, producing strange figments of deceit and distrust from her imagination. In one letter, to Sir John McNeill, she described how a Persian phantom had appeared to her with the information that Mr Bracebridge had issued a draft on her account for £300,000. Could McNeill offer any advice? (At an early stage in his career, McNeill had been attached to the East India Company's legation in Persia, so there was some method in her madness.) The letter was returned. At Lord Raglan's orders, the telegram to her family containing news of her condition was delayed until the doctors could hold out the prospect of Florence's recovery.

On 22 May, she was pronounced better. The ninth day, 'which is called the crisis', had passed, Charles Bracebridge wrote to Sidney Herbert, though there was still the danger of a relapse. Florence had already communicated her intention of returning to her command, but Mr Bracebridge saw realistically that a long convalescence would be necessary. 'She was never a strong woman,' he wrote, and any recurrence of fever might well prove fatal. Three days later, Lord Panmure informed Herbert that Florence was out of danger, and a telegram from Bracebridge to Embley the following day reassured Florence's family that she was now 'convalescent'. The patient care of Mrs Roberts, nursing her as if she was her own child, Florence wrote afterwards, had saved her life. She remained unable to feed herself and was at first unable to speak above a whisper. On 28 May, Mr Bracebridge, who had been filling in time by riding over the line of the ill-fated Light Brigade charge, reported a definite improvement to Parthenope. 'She was able yesterday to talk a little, but lies with her head back & speaks very low. There is no disease left, but great prostration of strength.' Meanwhile, anxiety about Florence had been evident 'from one end of the Camp to the other'. Soldiers, who had wept openly at the possibility of Florence's imminent demise, wrote home to express their relief that she had been saved. Mrs Seacole's offer to 'quack' Florence with her special medicines was politely refused, while a call from Fanny Duberly, officer's wife and Camp busybody, was turned away. Admittance was also initially denied to Lord Raglan, when he paid a visit to Florence's hut on 24 May. Mrs Roberts, failing to recognize him, barred him from entering. When he persisted, she asked, 'And pray, who are you?' 'Only a soldier,' Raglan replied, 'but I have ridden a long way, and your patient knows me very well.' He was admitted. A month later, Raglan was dead, ostensibly from cholera, though Florence believed that he had died from a broken heart at the Army's unsuccessful assault on the Malakoff, which had been intended to precede the final attack on Sebastopol.

Friends and doctors hoped to persuade her to convalesce in Switzerland. She rejected the plan, insisting she would remain at Balaclava, and was only finally induced to return to Scutari as a compromise. Her best nurses were threatening to leave if she went, and there were too many 'jarring elements'. Without her presence as a central authority, she believed that everything would fall to pieces. On 5 June, she was escorted back across the Black Sea, Selina Bracebridge having arrived in time to accompany her. An odd tale of intrigue adheres to this return voyage. In a letter to Aunt Mai, several months later, Florence described how Dr Hadley, the Senior Medical Officer at the Castle Hospital, and a friend of Dr Hall's, had selected a transport ship, the *Jura*, for her journey, which was not calling at Scutari, but returning directly to England. At the last moment, Mr Bracebridge and Lord Ward had realized this, and transferred Florence to Ward's yacht instead. Are we to believe that Hall, in league with Hadley, would really have resorted to such underhand methods to rid himself of the interfering Lady Superintendent? Florence said that she was 'unconscious' while being taken off the ship; certainly she was so weak that she had to be carried on a stretcher. But no other evidence seems to exist to confirm the salient features of the accusation. Was it purely a product of her own fevered imagination, a version of events as she had been told them, or a paranoid interpretation based on her deteriorating relationship with Hall? It remains a mystery.

Back at Scutari, the Bracebridges had prepared a small house for her near the Barrack Hospital, which formed a base for her from now on (the house, a wooden construction on two floors of a kind common to the area, was probably swept away at the end of the 1860s when a horse-drawn tram service was introduced). At the beginning of July, Florence continued her convalescence at the Ambassador's summer residence at Therapia, still so weak that she was moved in the mode of transport to which she was becoming accustomed: a litter carried in relays by four guardsmen. 'F looks very nice indeed,' Selina Bracebridge wrote to Parthenope, in what was clearly an attempt to disguise the worst, 'her hair is quite short – she wears a black handkerchief, & in her white cap has that bright, innocent, almost childlike look which I remember of old . . .' Other accounts emphasized her emaciated appearance and how much older she looked, and that she was unable to stand for long without her legs giving out from under her. She busied herself writing letters, and was so anxious to resume her full workload that her mother felt forced to write to remind her that she should perfect the difficult lesson of learning how to wait. Gifts from home arrived to distract her. Sidney Herbert sent a terrier, Parthenope a short book, the 'Life and Death of Athena, an Owlet from the Parthenon', which she had written and illustrated. A lithographed version was later distributed among family, and friends like the Mohls and Lady Canning. 'You have done Athena's history very nicely, with great taste,' Fanny Allen told Parthenope, 'the silver thread, of part of its dear mistress's life running through it, makes it a valuable bit of biographical truth . . .' Athena had achieved posthumous fame. The drawing of her on a pedestal beside her mistress was in English shop windows that summer, and the troops at Scutari provided Florence with a replacement for her dead pet, though Athena's successor was similarly short-lived, eaten by rats early the following year.

The Bracebridges left for England on 28 July. Their return was long overdue, postponed by Florence's illness. Mrs Bracebridge was herself now failing, '& feeling so ill that she had to get away'. Florence paid fulsome tribute to them, while privately believing that she might get on better without Mr Bracebridge who, latterly, had been inclined to antagonize Army and medical officialdom. At Atherstone, their home town, the Bracebridges, accompanied by Parthenope, received a rousing welcome. Houses were decorated with flags and triumphal arches, and a celebratory rocket was launched from the railway station. 'We all know they have been as parents to her,' Sam Smith wrote a little tactlessly to his sister Fanny, '& without them she w[oul]d have been dead long ago.' Their place was taken by Aunt Mai, who arrived at Scutari in mid-September to supervise the Free Gifts store and assist with the accounts. Aunt Mai had delayed her decision about going, but had finally decided that she must not 'lose the chance of seeing dearest Flo', despite Florence's warning that their time together would be limited to '2 or 3 hours a day at my little house at Scutari where you would live'. The sight of her niece shocked Mai, but, like Mrs Bracebridge, she put a good face on it for the benefit of the family. 'She looks pretty well,' Mai wrote after being reunited with Florence, 'calm as usual, her hand & voice quite firm . . . tho she is altered, it is the firmness of her voice that comforts me. I feared I should see her shaken.'

The disease had far from run its course. At the beginning of October, on her return to the Crimea, Florence would be readmitted to hospital for a week with severe sciatica. In late November, she began to be plagued by earache, chronic laryngitis, dysentery, rheumatism and insomnia. As Dr Sutherland, Charles Bracebridge and Florence herself had recognized, she was suffering from 'Crimean Fever', but what precisely was this?

The report on the pathology of the diseases of the British Army in the Crimean War listed six forms of fever. Typhoid and typhus were the most common – and most fatal – followed in third place by a remittent fever, known popularly as 'Crimean Fever', but also under a bewildering number of alternative names, some (like Mediterranean or Malta fever) reflecting its geographical distribution, others (undulant fever) the marked tendency for the patient to relapse after a period of remission. The illness varies from a mild disorder to a severe affliction dominated by fever, shaking chills, and extreme physical and mental exhaustion (Florence had joked, back in June, that she was suffering from 'a compound fracture of the intellect'). It causes both acute and chronic symptoms, including generalized aches and pains, depression, loss of appetite, delusions (which might conceivably account for the *Jura* episode), insomnia, palpitations and breathlessness, and at its most serious,

sciatica, and the excruciatingly painful condition spondylitis, or inflammation of the spinal cord, which can lead to permanent disability.
Yet, despite all this, examination of patients often reveals only minor
physical abnormalities.

Medical understanding of the disease, under its generic name
brucellosis, kept pace with the remaining decades of Florence's life. The
first accurate description of the disorder was made by J. A. Marston, an
Assistant Surgeon in the Army Medical Department, in 1861, five years
after the end of the Crimean War. In 1887, David Bruce, a military
physician assigned to the Malta naval base, isolated the bacterium,
Brucella melitensis, responsible for the disease. The first monograph on
brucellosis followed ten years later. In 1906, the Mediterranean Fever
Commission identified the goat as the reservoir of the brucella infection,
and prohibited the use of goat's milk and its products in Government
establishments. The disease is transmitted to humans either through the
consumption of contaminated milk or cheese, or by direct contact with
infected animals or their environment. The incubation time of brucellosis
is between ten days and three weeks, which means that Florence was
certainly infected in April, in the Constantinople area, before her departure for the Crimea (Mrs Bracebridge had reported the high incidence
of fever at Scutari at this time).

Following her return to England, Florence was to suffer from a variety
of symptoms consistent with a particularly chronic form of brucellosis,
in a number of recurrent attacks, sometimes years apart, which were
also characteristic of the illness at its most virulent. Already, as she
picked up her work again at Scutari that August, she was exhibiting signs
of the depression and nervous irritability associated with the disease.
The intense heat hardly assisted matters. The atmosphere resembled a
steam-bath, and there were sudden tropical downpours. Florence shaved
her head and found it 'a great comfort'. But news of the unexpected
death at Balaclava, on 9 August, of Elizabeth Drake, a St John's nurse
from the original party, when it had been assumed that she was convalescing from fever, distressed Florence immoderately and plunged her
into gloom. Mrs Drake's body was brought back to Scutari, where
Florence arranged for a small marble cross to be erected over it in the
British cemetery. At the same time, her normally indefatigable manner
was exacerbated by a restlessness she seemed unable to control. Inevitable feelings of redundancy arising from the fact that the Scutari hos-

pitals were in good order (and the mortality rate down to 2 per cent in the three-month period ending in September 1855) only made her search for other areas requiring her improving touch, while she lashed out at those whom she perceived to be lacking in commitment or competence. 'When I lie down, which I never do, I think of all the things to be done & they start me up again.'

Writing at length to the Bracebridges, Florence ranged widely over a number of matters which she believed needed urgent attention: designs for new trench clothing to protect men from damp and frostbite, the need for huts at Balaclava to house troops before the onset of winter, and the perpetual worry about the proportion of Roman Catholics among the patients nursed by the Bridgeman nuns. Sometimes, she wrote, she felt like a figure in a Greek tragedy, 'where all is <u>fated</u> to ruin & struggle is useless'. She placed no faith in those around her. The support for reform of Dr McGrigor, Principal Medical Officer at Scutari, had once led Florence to urge for his promotion, feeding ill-natured gossip, designed to complicate her position, and given wide currency in the newspapers before she left for the Crimea, that she had married him. Now, however, she rejected McGrigor as 'incompetent'. Lord William Paulet was 'ignorant', while Robertson, the new Purveyor, of whom she had initially had high hopes, had come to her the worse for drink. As for her nurses, she had changed round all the wards 'to break off acquaintances' which 'were coming to bad'. She managed to brandish one minor triumph, though. Locking up the brandy in the kitchen closet, and holding on to the key, had kept Nurse Hawkins sober for 'two whole days'.

Her campaign to save the British soldier from idleness and drink provided an outlet for all this surplus energy. The Scutari hospitals were full of convalescents with time on their hands, who had nothing better to do than spend their pay on the highly intoxicating spirits manufactured by the Turks and the Greeks. In the face of some of their superiors who insisted that she was 'spoiling the brutes', Florence pursued a variety of initiatives which demonstrated the ordinary soldier's capacity for self-improvement. In the first week of August, although still scarcely able to stand, she attended the opening of the Inkerman Café in a house midway between the two hospitals, close to the shore of the Bosphorus. Working with Peter Pincoffs, one of the civilian doctors at Scutari, she provided supplies, advanced the cash, and sent them 'hams, butter, brandy, tea-urn, tent, prints, a band, newspapers etc' for the first day, when everything was free. Additionally, she established a scheme for reading-rooms and schools, which started at Scutari and later extended to the hospitals in the Crimea. Parthenope called this 'the education of the British Army', and the rounding up of gifts to equip the lectures, singing lessons and amateur theatricals became another of her duties. '. . . We have sent . . . 1000 copybooks,' Parthenope wrote in November, 'writing materials in proportion, Diagrams, Maps . . . *Macbeth* . . . to read 6 at a time . . . Chess, Footballs, other games, a magic Lanthern for Dissolving views, a Stereoscope (very fine!), plays for acting, music . . .' Despite Lord Panmure's assertion that the British soldier was not a remitting animal, Florence successfully continued the work that Sidney Godolphin Osborne had started, devoting each Saturday afternoon to receiving from the men money they wished to send home to their families, thereby diverting sums that might otherwise have been spent on alcohol. The Government, learning from this example, developed it into a system and, in January 1856, offices for money orders were established at a number of sites at Scutari and Balaclava.

Florence's influence on the men did indeed discourage many of them from drunkenness and ensured that others did not fall into debt. In turn her respect for the ordinary soldier grew, though she resisted the temptation to sentimentalize him. 'I have never been able to join the popular cry about the recklessness, sensuality, and helplessness of the soldiers . . . ,' she told her sister. 'Give them opportunity promptly and securely to send money home and they will use it. Give them schools and lectures and they will come to them. Give them books and games and amusements and they will leave off drinking. Give them suffering and they will bear it.' For years afterwards, she would sometimes go to extraordinary lengths to find employment for an ex-soldier, or treatment for one in poor health, often contributing to the doctors' fees herself. During the war, she was no less concerned for a soldier's wife and family, answering inquiries about the missing or the seriously ill, sending, for example, a grieving widow money with which to buy mourning clothes, and writing or dictating countless letters of condolence. This was perhaps the first time in any British war that such serious attention, from an official source, had been paid to the surviving relatives of the dead. From Scutari's General Hospital, in September 1855,

Florence wrote to Mrs Maria Hunt, in a letter typical of many others, with its concern for precise detail, and its respect for the feelings of a dead soldier's mother:

I grieve to be obliged to inform you that your son died in this Hospital on Sunday last . . . His complaint was Chronic Dysentery – he sank gradually from weakness, without much suffering. Everything was done that was possible to keep up his strength. He was fed every half hour with the most nourishing things he could take, & when there was anything he had a fancy for, it was taken to him immediately . . . [H]e spoke much of his Mother, & gave us the direction to you in his last moments . . . His great anxiety was that his Mother should receive the pay due to him, & should know that he had not received any since he had been Out . . . You may have the satisfaction of knowing that he had the most constant and careful attendance from the Doctors & the Nurses . . . He died very peacefully & sorrowful as this news is for his bereaved Mother, may she find comfort in thinking that his earthly sufferings were over, & in the hope that our Almighty Father will receive him into a better world . . .

Like an open sore, the question of Florence's jurisdiction in the Crimea, in the absence of any clarification of her orders, remained painfully unresolved. On 8 September 1855, Sebastopol finally fell after a siege of almost a year, and the Russians started their withdrawal. The end of the war was confidently in sight. But Florence's bitterest struggles to assert her authority over the nursing in the Crimean hospitals were only just beginning.

On her return to business, at the end of July, she had begun negotiations with Hall, testing the waters by proposing that she withdraw the nurses from the General Hospital at Balaclava, concentrating those who remained at the Castle Hospital, where her trusted lieutenant, Jane Shaw Stewart, was in charge. The overall number of patients in the hospitals in the Crimea, like those on the Bosphorus, had begun to fall, and Florence was acting on the likelihood that, at some point in the near future, the hospitals at Balaclava would be used merely as a short-term stopover for patients in transit to Scutari or England. She also badly wished to bring Margaret Wear, Superintendent of the General Hospital, to heel. Wear, who had long regarded herself as an independent agent, consistently flouting Florence's authority, had informed her that she, and the rest of her nurses, might be sent to the Monastery Hospital,

where patients were mainly ophthalmic and convalescent cases. Florence
sought Hall's assurance that this was not about to happen. She saw no
necessity for the introduction of nurses to another hospital at this stage
of the war, while remaining firmly of the view that nurses had no place
in a hospital for convalescents in the first place.

Hall's reply was curt. He had no intention of sending Miss Wear and
her nurses to the Monastery Hospital, but he seized the opportunity to
suggest that as he needed to retain two nurses at the General Hospital,
for the sake of 'convenience', he might obtain them elsewhere. Forced
to cling to what vestiges of authority she possessed in the Crimea, this
was, of course, something that Florence could not possibly allow. Miss
Wear and one other nurse were permitted to stay at the Balaclava
General Hospital, and for a short time an uneasy truce prevailed between
Florence and Hall. Within two months, however, Hall had reversed his
decision regarding Miss Wear. Under pressure from Wear herself, he
allowed her to abscond to the Monastery Hospital. This was a blatant
act of collusion on Hall's part in Wear's rebellion. But considerably
worse was to follow. By the late summer, the hospital at Koulali contained fewer than fifty patients, and was shortly to be handed over
for use by allied Sardinian troops. This presented Reverend Mother
Bridgeman, who had been working at Koulali with her sisters since
January, with a pressing dilemma. Since her superiors in Dublin were
anxious that the Kinsale nuns remained in the East for as long as
possible, and Bridgeman was adamant that she would not return to
Scutari to join her four nuns there and work under Nightingale, she
applied to Dr Hall, asking if she might instead transfer her sisters,
with reinforcements from Ireland, to work under him in the Crimea.
Addressing Hall through her intermediary, Father Woollett, a Jesuit
chaplain at the front, Bridgeman wrote that 'It may be well to add that
I would not undertake again to work with Miss Nightingale, as I learned
while I was at the Barrack Hospital, Scutari, how very DIFFERENT
from ours, are Miss Nightingale's views of nursing . . .' Hall leapt at the
chance to rid himself of 'Miss Nightingale'. In a nifty bit of deceit, he
invited Florence to recall her two nurses from the General Hospital at
Balaclava – but without informing her of his plan to restaff the hospital
with the Bridgeman nuns. Unaware of what had been going on behind
her back, Florence replied to Hall, on 21 September, pleased that they
were now of the same opinion about the withdrawal of 'the female

element' from the General Hospital, and hoping that she would have the pleasure of seeing him when she visited the Crimea in the near future. Hall left it to Bridgeman herself to deliver Florence the *coup de grâce* at the beginning of October. She was recalling her four sisters from Scutari, Bridgeman told her – even though the power to dispose of the nurses there remained officially Florence's – and hoping to sail for the Crimea, to start work at the General Hospital, 'at the beginning of next week'. Florence had been roundly tricked.

'Really, Dr Hall is so clever, it is almost a pleasure to contemplate such cleverness, even at one's own expense,' Florence commented later. Hall – or Sir John Hall as he had become in February 1855, decried by Florence as a 'Knight of the Crimean Burying-Grounds' – was, she acknowledged, able and efficient in many ways. Furthermore, he was responsible for overseeing a system of nursing that he had neither instituted nor been consulted about. None the less, she believed him vain on a Napoleonic scale, and as inclined to dirty tricks 'as that great ruffian'. She had no doubt that he intended to make her life as difficult as he could, and that ideally he would have liked to broil her slowly over the fires of one of her Crimean stoves. Twenty years earlier, Hall had expressed a favourable opinion about the use of female nurses in Army hospitals, but he scorned the Nightingale experiment for what he saw as its excessive refinement and extravagance, and took Florence's instructions at their word: that she had no control over the appointment and allocation of nurses outside Turkey.

How could she conduct the nursing establishment in a unified, disciplined manner while facing such intransigent opposition, and when arrangements for her nurses were continually made over her head? Florence appealed to Lord Stratford, the British Ambassador. He made sympathetic noises, but referred her to General Storks, who had succeeded Lord William Paulet as Commandant of the Turkish hospitals in August. In Storks, Florence discovered an ally. He advised her to accompany the Bridgeman nuns to the Crimea in order to maintain some semblance of her authority. On 8 October this ill-assorted party left Scutari, reaching Balaclava four days later. The voyage was grimly comic. 'Miss Nightingale appeared as sweet and amiable on board as if she was <u>charmed</u> at the idea of the "Sisters" going to Balaclava,' wrote Sister Joseph Croke, in one of the Crimean journals that the Bridgeman nuns were encouraged to keep. For the preservation of polite relations it was probably as well that both Florence and Bridgeman were forced to stay in their cabins on account of sea-sickness. The sight of Florence losing her footing as she rushed to get into the boat taking her ashore, to be sure that Bridgeman didn't enter the General Hospital before her, was recorded with spiteful glee by Sister Croke. The subduing of the Bridgeman nuns, with their 'papal aggression' or 'Irish-Catholic rebellion' as Florence intolerantly referred to it, had become a matter of principle for her. But Bridgeman was just as determined to maintain their independence, forging an alliance not only with Hall, but also with David Fitzgerald, the Purveyor, whose hostility towards Florence knew no bounds. Even Bridgeman found Fitzgerald 'most difficult to manage and most penitential to deal with'; but she persevered, realizing that he was 'one whom it was most essential we should win to work with us'. She was soon blessing God 'for winning this officer' who was prepared to risk his own career in defending their cause to the War Office.

Florence's six weeks in the Crimea were filled with minor harassments as she worked towards the opening of the Extra Diet Kitchen at the Castle Hospital, which would have been ready six months before had it not been for her illness. Fitzgerald continued to obstruct her requisitions, while Hall issued an official complaint when, for twenty-four hours during the installation of the new kitchen, it was impossible to make toast for the officers. Every day, until a bout of sciatica forced her to rest, Florence went to the General Hospital in an effort to impose her authority there. An attempt at a more conciliatory relationship with the Bridgeman group fell on stony ground. After the death from cholera of Sister Winifred, one of the sisters who had served at Scutari, Florence's offer to place a cross over her grave was ignored. 'She wishes to let it appear that she has control over us in life and death,' wrote Sister Croke. 'Mother Brickbat's conduct has been neither that of a Christian, a gentlewoman, or even a woman,' Florence observed.

Her frustration boiled over in a letter to Aunt Mai, who, back at Scutari, was at the receiving end of a constant stream of instructions about the daily running of the hospitals in her niece's absence. Marking the first anniversary of her appointment, Florence observed with typically dramatic overstatement that 'Christ was betrayed by one. But my cause has been betrayed by everyone – ruined, betrayed, destroyed by everyone alas! One may truly say excepting Mrs Roberts, Revd. Mother

[Moore], first, & Mrs Stewart . . . And Mrs Stewart is more than half mad. A cause which is supported by a mad woman & twenty fools must be a falling house.' Florence wasn't alone in considering Jane Shaw Stewart, for all her outstanding qualities as a nurse, more than a little eccentric. The Bridgeman nuns thought her very 'odd', while Assistant-Surgeon George Lawson agreed that Stewart was 'perfectly mad', observing that whenever she wanted to take a rest from nursing her patients, she simply lay on the ground wrapped in her cloak.

This sense of betrayal was intensified by the arrival at Balaclava, a week or so later, of a copy of The Times for 16 October, containing a report of a speech that Charles Bracebridge had made at Coventry. All the attention had gone to his head. Stirring up controversy, not for the first or last time in his life, Mr Bracebridge had made exaggerated claims for Florence's work at Scutari – on arrival there they had found 'neither kitchen, coals, nor candles', just 'naked walls' – while attacking the medical staff for failing to take advice from the French physicians about the treatment of various conditions, alleging that, as a result of their obstinacy, many of their patients had needlessly died. Bracebridge's remarks were widely reported and undermined Florence's position at exactly the time when she was under greatest pressure from Hall and his supporters. Hall poured scorn on the 'twaddling nonsense' spoken by 'the garrulous gentleman' who had talked about 'putting hospitals containing three or four thousand patients in order in a couple of days by means of the Times fund . . .' Florence was unjustly suspected of complicity in the attack, though she was as angry as the doctors themselves at Bracebridge's intervention, as it effectively undid all her hard work to win the support of the medical establishment at Scutari for her reforms. Bracebridge maintained that he had been misrepresented, but in fact his speech was consistent with arguments he had been putting forward for some time, that the public should be made aware that there was more to Florence Nightingale than her guise as 'a toady of Herbert's or a mere soft-hearted Nurse' would suggest. Florence's terse rejoinder to Bracebridge urged him to be an 'active friend' rather than a 'disagreeable enemy', and to avoid 'mere irresponsibility of opposition'.

In the third week of November, she was called back to Scutari (the Bridgeman nuns rejoiced and offered up a novena when they heard the news). A cholera epidemic had broken out, causing the mortality rate to rise again, to 15 per cent (among the victims were several doctors, including Alexander McGrigor, whose name had recently been linked with Florence's). The epidemic was rapidly brought under control, by sending those free from the disease to an encampment two miles away, and by nursing those suffering from cholera in segregated wards in the Barrack Hospital. As the disease burnt itself out, Florence allowed herself a rare respite from her duties by attending a Christmas party at Lord Stratford's residence on the other side of the Bosphorus. Here Emilia Hornby scrutinized 'her wasted figure, and the short brown hair combed over her forehead like a child's ... Her dress ... was black, its only ornament being a large enamelled brooch, which looked to me like the colours of a regiment ... She was still very weak, and could not join in the games, but she sat on a sofa, and looked on, laughing until the tears came into her eyes.'

There were no doubt tears of fury and indignation in her eyes that January, however, as she read a copy of the 'Confidential Report on the Nursing System, since its introduction to the Crimea on 23rd January 1855'. Prepared by Purveyor Fitzgerald, at the request of Colonel John Lefroy, Panmure's adviser on scientific matters, who had been in the Crimea at the end of the year interviewing Florence and other members of the nursing establishment, this report predictably lambasted Nightingale's nurses, for lax discipline, insubordination and drunkenness, while doling out praise to Bridgeman and her nuns. Many of Fitzgerald's statements were demonstrably inaccurate, and amounted to 'a malicious & scandalous libel' on the good names of those involved. Mrs Noble, for one, who, according to the report, had been dismissed for misbehaviour, had actually recently been recommended for an extra year's pay. Although he did not criticize Florence by name, Fitzgerald (described by Florence as like Dickens's character Squeers, 'only lower') questioned whether there had been sufficient number of nurses 'appropriate to the extent of Sickness', and disputed her claim to overall authority in the Crimea.

The report circulated in medical and army circles, while officially Florence was not provided with a copy. She had to rely on Lefroy, fast moving over to Florence's circle of admirers, leaking her one. Her denunciation of what she contemptuously called the 'Purveyor's Report' ran to more pages than the report itself, and ended by demanding that her position be clarified, once and for all. She rehearsed the point that whereas her instructions had placed her under the direction of the medical authorities, all matters relating to treatment of patients, the appointment, selection, and distribution of nurses 'were definitely committed to me'.

If the War Department desire me to continue to exercise these functions entrusted to me by themselves, I must request that they will support me . . . by notifying to the Inspector General of Hospitals that he is to second & not to oppose me in the performance of my duties. The incessant difficulties arising from the want of such support consume my time & strength to the impediment of the work.

But could she count on the support of the War Office? Junior officials seemed split along pro- and anti-Nightingale lines. 'I confess I think it is time that we curbed the pretensions of Miss Nightingale to unlimited & almost irresponsible command over the Nurses attached to the Army in the East,' was the view of one civil servant, scribbling on a departmental minute. In the end, it was Colonel Lefroy's influence with Panmure that proved decisive to Florence's cause. Without Florence's centralizing control, he argued, the whole – certainly the Protestant part of it – would dissolve into unconnected establishments and disappear. 'The medical men are jealous of it,' he wrote. 'Dr Hall would gladly upset it tomorrow, and he knows better than any one, that Miss Nightingale is its only anchor . . . If the Nightingale Institution is to bear any fruit to the Army she must be supported until it can do so.'

Florence, though, was by now feeling 'bruised & battered' after fifteen months of fighting against enemies 'who "strike below the knee" '. The governmental machine was moving too slowly, and she was beginning to think that the only solution was for a move to place all the relevant papers – her original instructions, the Confidential Report, and related correspondence from both herself and Hall – before the House of Commons. '. . . The War Office,' she wrote in a private letter to Sidney Herbert on 21 February, 'gives me tinsel & plenty of empty praise which I do not want – and does not give me the real business-like efficient standing which I do want.' If the English people knew of her treatment, she said, acknowledging the strength of her popular mandate, they would not stand to see her treated so. Herbert moved swiftly to advise her strongly against any notion of making the first move. As long as she was not publicly attacked, her standing would remain high; if, however, the papers she had mentioned were published, it would introduce doubt in the public mind about the value of nurses in the eyes of the

Army and medical establishments. With great wisdom, he warned her against her besetting sin, of writing with 'an irritation and vehemence' that only detracted from the strength of her case. He appreciated that she was 'overdone' with her 'long, anxious, harassing work', but she must try not to overrate the importance of 'onesided, unfair & unjust' reports of it.

The situation was finally reaching its resolution. On 25 February, Panmure wrote to Sir William Codrington, Raglan's replacement as Commander-in-Chief, censuring Dr Hall, and asking him to promulgate 'the rightful position of Miss Nightingale' in the General Orders. Hall's humiliation was complete. On 16 March 1856, Florence Nightingale became the first woman in the history of the British Army to find herself in General Orders. Her triumph came just in time. A fortnight later, the Treaty of Paris was signed, and the Crimean War was over.

It is strikingly ironic that just at the point when Florence's fortunes in the Crimea had sunk to their lowest ebb, her stock back in England had never been higher, as the public's affection for her found a new focus for its expression. In August 1855, plans had already been set in motion for a national appeal to recognize 'the noble exertions of Miss Nightingale in the hospitals of the East'. The Herberts, in consultation with the Nightingales, had assumed that Florence would refuse a personal tribute of the 'teapot and bracelet' variety, and put to her instead a scheme for raising a fund by public subscription that would enable her on her return home to establish a permanent training school for nurses, of the kind that she had had in mind in pre-war days.

Florence received the idea courteously, but without enthusiasm. In the midst of battling against Hall, Bridgeman, and bureaucratic red tape, exhausted and depressed by the possibility of failure, she was in no mood to consider the future. 'People seem to think I have nothing to do but to sit here and make plans,' she had responded irritably when Herbert requested an outline for the use of the proposed Nightingale Fund. Nevertheless, she did issue what she regarded as an essential proviso, one that she had learned from experience of using the *Times* fund at the Scutari hospitals: that she should be allowed full control of the money.

In the summer of 1855, a fund circular was sent out to 300 banking houses. A provisional committee of seventy distinguished names was appointed (Charles Dickens was one of only two refusals, excusing himself on the grounds that he was working in Paris, and unable therefore to take an active role). A lease was taken for a year on first-floor chambers at 5 Parliament Street. On 8 November, Sidney Herbert called a meeting of the committee to agree the resolutions for presentation to a public meeting. Among these were clauses decreeing that the subscription be opened to all classes, and that the sums collected would be used at Florence's discretion. '. . . Our only wish', Liz Herbert explained to Fanny Nightingale, 'is to direct the tide of popular feeling so as to be most acceptable (or least repulsive!) to Her . . .' Three weeks later, on 29 November, the Nightingale Fund was officially launched in London at Willis's Rooms, in King's Street, off St James's Square. The meeting was packed to overflowing, with 100 people on the platform, and as many as 1,250 in the body of the room. The Duke of Cambridge, the Army's Commander-in-Chief, took the chair, and resolutions were moved by, among others, the Duke of Argyll, Sydney Godolphin Osborne and ex-Prime Minister Lord Goderich. Sidney Herbert read out emotive letters from soldiers which described kissing Miss Nightingale's shadow as she passed through the wards. Trustees, including Herbert, Monckton Milnes and Charles Bracebridge, were confirmed (later, a finance committee was formed, with Edward Marjoribanks, who had been the treasurer at Upper Harley Street, as one of its members). To Mrs Nightingale, it was the most interesting day of a mother's life; even William Nightingale appeared overcome with joy at the 'universal oneness' of the meeting.

Only the recipient of the honour appeared wary of committing herself wholeheartedly to the venture. Early in the New Year, Florence responded formally to Herbert, expressing her gratitude for the 'sympathy and confidence' shown by the originators of the Fund, but also declaring her uncertainty as to when or whether she would ever be able to carry out the work she was asked to undertake. A private letter to him threw further light on her reasons for not wishing to be tied down. A correspondent in *The Times* had argued that she should provide 'a cut & dried Prospectus' of her plans before expecting people to subscribe money for them, which, she agreed, was all well and good. But it was simply impossible 'in the midst of one overpowering work to digest & concoct another', and even if she could, such a plan would only have subsequently to be altered or destroyed. To Selina Bracebridge, Florence went further: she would like to take the poorest and least organized hospital in London, put herself there, and not touch the Fund's money, perhaps for years, until experience had taught her how best it might be used. This, she announced to Bence Jones of London's St George's Hospital, one of four doctors appointed to the Fund's council of nine by Florence herself, 'is the only plan I have'.

The Nightingale Fund has been called the first national appeal in Britain aimed at all classes of society. Publicity was widespread. Twenty thousand circulars were sent out in the first month; W. H. Smith, the newsagent and politician, placed 1,000 leaflets about the Fund on his station bookstalls; *The Times* carried subscription lists and reports of meetings; and there was a spate of articles by various authors, including Sidney Herbert, in the journals and weeklies. In March, Jenny Lind, the world-famous soprano, gave a concert at the Strand's Exeter Hall, raising £1,872 for the Fund, as well as lending it a little glamour (one of *Punch*'s favoured nicknames for Florence was 'Jenny Lint', so the association seems apposite). Meanwhile, public meetings proliferated: Leeds, Manchester, Glasgow, Oxford, Bath and Brighton were among the initial venues. Mrs Gaskell attended her local Manchester meeting, in January 1856, and reported on its successful outcome to Parthenope. Mill workers, 'plenty of grimy hands', had attended to cheer and applaud their heroine – 'for they feel her as theirs, their brother's nurse, their dead friend's friend' – while a woman seated near her 'bowed her head down on her hands, and shook all over with her sobs'. The star turn was Monckton Milnes, who quite lost himself in nostalgic reverie about the young Florence Nightingale. 'His face grew quite pale, & you forgot the fat in the features – the eyes fixed on bye-gone scenes, not on all our poor upturned faces, – eyes & nostrils quite dilated . . .'

The Army was one major source of contributions, the Church another. Notice of the Fund was conveyed to the armed forces through General Orders, and it was suggested by General Codrington that donations should take the form of one day's pay. Clergymen, meanwhile, adapted their Sunday sermons to advertise the Fund, and collections were taken following the service. Inevitably, there was a renewed outburst of sectarian bickering in the press, associating Florence with Catholicism, as well as with Socinianism (the anti-Trinitarian sect), but this was silenced by an article in *The Times* denying that the Fund was connected to any particular religious group. Despite all the effort extended over a wide social field, the bulk of the total amount collected came from generous individual contributions from the upper and upper-middle classes, ranging from donations of £300 to £25 (while the Army contributed almost a quarter of the total). This outcome was scarcely surprising given the economic downturn being experienced by much of the industrial heartland in 1856. As Mrs Gaskell had observed of the Lancashire workers, there was 'a great deal of latent enthusiasm' surrounding the Nightingale name, but also 'so very much distress of all kinds' prevalent in the area at this time.

Nevertheless, when the Fund was wound up on 20 June 1856, it was revealed that £44,039 – more than £2 million in modern money – had been collected. A Deed of Trust was outlined, assigning Florence the power to direct the Fund as she saw fit. This was an extraordinary testament to the British public's faith in their heroine. But the ultimate disposal of the Fund was to hang like a millstone around Florence's neck in the years immediately ahead.

At Lea, in Derbyshire, celebrations to mark the end of the war were supervised by Aunt Julia. The centrepiece of a display was 'a figure as large as life of Miss Nightingale', dressed in a white shirt and blue jacket, with the words 'The Good Samaritan', made out in flowers above its head.

Peace made little difference to the daily lives of those encamped at Balaclava or working in the hospitals. Hostilities, after all, had ceased over six months earlier with the fall of Sebastopol. On 16 March, the day she appeared in General Orders, Florence, with a first detachment of nurses, had set sail for the Crimea. It was her third visit and, in some ways, the most arduous. One of her main tasks was to oversee the two hospitals of the newly formed Land Transport Corps at Karani, at the urgent request of their Principal Medical Officer, Dr George Taylor. Travel between these, and the other hospitals in the Crimea, was difficult. Distances were great, roads were practically non-existent, and the terrain rough. Florence had grown used to spending long days in the saddle in severe weather. Earlier experiments at transporting her in a cart drawn by a mule had failed after it overturned and threw her on to the track. For this latest trip, Colonel McMurdo of the Land Transport Corps presented Florence with a hooded baggage car, which had once belonged to a Prince Menschikoff, and she soon became a familiar sight driving about in it. It was 'a sort of luggage wagon', according to Aunt Mai, 'awning over head, latticed & curtained at the sides – drawn by 2 mules', with a 'padded behind'.

Florence returned to the Crimea, her authority confirmed. She was not, however, inclined to be generous in victory. Within days of her arrival, on 24 March, she was claiming to Herbert, and various members of her family, that the Purveyor Fitzgerald had attempted to starve her and her nurses by denying them rations, in what may have been a wily strategy to place him in the wrong. With Hall, who kept up a dignified front, despite describing himself in a letter to his wife as 'quite prostrate' at his humiliation in General Orders, she traded petty points and veered towards triumphalism. As for Bridgeman, Florence was intent on dissuading her and her eleven sisters from resigning their post, for fear that this might turn them into martyrs. In Bridgeman's account, Florence pressed her, to the point of 'rudeness', to stay. But Bridgeman insisted that they would be returning home at once. '. . . I cannot blame her after what is past . . .,' wrote Hall, who saw their departure as depriving the Army 'of the only real nurses we ever had'. On the day that the Bridgeman nuns vacated the General Hospital, 11 April, Florence demanded that the keys be handed over to her. Fitzgerald, determined to keep her out, refused. Waiting until Fitzgerald was at dinner, Florence inveigled them from one of the doctors. Vilification of Bridgeman's nursing subsequently poured from her pen. 'Your pig sty is cleaner than our Quarters or than the wards of the Hospital, as left by Mrs Bridgeman,' she told Uncle Sam. 'The patients were grimed with dirt, infected with vermin, with bed sores like Lazarus (Mrs Bridgeman, I suppose thought it holy).' Two years later, after the gist of these remarks was incorporated into the Royal Commission's findings on the health of the Army, Bridgeman made her defence in a private letter to Hall. It was true, she said, that one patient had had bed sores on his back, but these were dressed twice a day by the doctor responsible until the patient became so exhausted and miserable at being moved that latterly he was dressed only once a day. '. . . This is one of the many cases,' wrote Bridgeman, 'in which a truth may be forced to the work of a falsehood.'

The contrast with Florence's attitude to the Superior of the Bermondsey Sisters, Reverend Mother Mary Clare Moore, who returned to

England from Scutari in May, suffering from dysentery, could not have been greater. Florence's farewell letter to her was filled – 'gratefully, lovingly, overflowingly' – with endearments, and the admission that Moore had been far better suited than her, in both worldly talents and spiritual qualities, to the superintendence of the military hospitals. Soon afterwards, Florence's own health faltered, a reminder that she was still under constant threat from vestiges of the disease. Writing to the Nightingales, Aunt Mai warned them gently about the change in Florence that might not be immediately apparent when they saw her again. '. . . She has a spirit within that works upon her appearance without,' she told them, following Florence's return to Scutari at the end of June. 'To judge how her health & spirits really are, one must live with her closely for months – I see her at times when she seems hardly able to walk across the room from fatigue & deeply depressed in spirits.'

The nagging question for her parents, understandably enough, was when exactly would they see her again? The only answer she could obtain, Mai advised them, was that just as the Army came home by degrees, 'so must their Nurses', and Florence must come home 'last of all'. Proposals that her mother, father and sister might meet her at Aix, or at some continental watering place, were pushed aside. Florence intended to leave the date and time of her return undefined for as long as possible, as doing so would increase the chances of her getting home 'privately'. Dr Sutherland alarmed her one day by saying it would be impossible to avoid some public notice when she reached England. 'I can't tell you the dislike she expresses to anything of the kind & she is bent on avoiding it,' wrote Aunt Mai, '& as she is very clever at accomplishing what she wishes, I think it possible she will in this instance.' Parthenope was instructed to pour cold water on any mass demonstrations of affection. 'I think we have extinguished the Mayors,' she reported in July, '& . . . the proposal of the 3 bands', of the Coldstreams, Grenadiers and Fusiliers.

'The curtain begins to fall on this scene,' Aunt Mai wrote to her brother William on 18 June. Three days later, only five nurses remained at Scutari, as the redoubtable Mrs Clarke prepared to leave. Florence still had accounts to complete, records of requisitions to check, and character references for each nurse to write. She began to send home her 'spoils of war': William Jones, a 'fine spirited' young sailor, who had lost a leg; Thomas, the twelve-year-old drummer boy; and Peter

Grillage, a Russian orphan, also twelve, later to become footman at Embley. All three, Florence said, were to be sent to school until she came home. She also dispatched 'a "Rooshan" trophy', a rare breed of puppy given to her by some soldiers, whose 'mama is about as big as a calf'.

On 17 July, she wrote to her family to say that she was working as hard as possible to get home and that, when the time came, she intended to travel incognito as Miss Smith, her mother's maiden name. 'A "nom de guerre", naturally,' joked Monckton Milnes. Eleven days later, Florence and Aunt Mai embarked at Constantinople for the voyage to Marseilles. At Paris, the two women separated, Florence spending the night at the Mohls in the rue du Bac. 'I have many things to say,' Florence told her aunt as they parted, 'but I cannot speak . . .'

———

Two groups emerged from the Crimean War with their status dramatically enhanced. The British Army had been shown that ordinary soldiers were no longer to be regarded as blackguards, but were deserving of respect as 'Christian men'. At the same time, perception of nurses had also changed. The Nightingale mission of mercy had given a powerful boost to a new and positive image. There was hope that, with proper training, nursing might provide a suitable occupation for respectable, middle-class women.

By the end of the war, the Scutari hospitals had been transformed into efficiently organized, smooth-running operations. The mortality rates from illness in all the hospitals of the East were no higher than those of a comparable civilian population in an industrial city like Manchester. The hospitals of the French Army, with their Sisters of Charity, once the object of such admiration, were now suffering from death rates that significantly outran those experienced by the British at the height of the terrible winter of 1854–5.

In all these improvements, Florence Nightingale may be said to have played a significant, even a decisive, role. Yet she returned to England, obsessed by failure, and burdened by an increasing sense of identification with the memory of the Crimean dead. 'Oh my poor men who endured so patiently,' ran a private note, 'I feel I have been such a bad mother to you, to come home and leave you lying in your Crimean graves, 73 per cent in eight regiments during six months from disease alone.' Despite her efforts, nothing, she believed, had fundamentally changed.

The Army had settled into a new routine, but still lacked the kind of system that could only come about through root and branch reform. Everything in the Army, she informed Sidney Herbert in April 1856, 'is just where it was eighteen months ago. The only difference is that we are now rolling in stores. But indeed we were so then – only most of them were at Varna.' Moreover, no one in England 'has yet <u>realized</u> the graves of Scutari or the Crimea – or their causes'.

She was the obvious person to spearhead reform, besides which, her allies in the Government and the Army needed her standing and popularity to counter the conservative elements of rank and privilege. Her wartime correspondence, even at times of crisis, seethes with new ideas, for an army medical school, for instance, close to the seat of war, or for the introduction of proper statistical methods in the records of mortality and sickness in the Army hospitals. In all, she calculated, she had fifteen points to make, 'five pertaining to Army reform, ten to Army and medical reform mixed'. But did she have the stomach for it? She, like many people, viewed with disgust the fate of the McNeill-Tulloch report's findings on the issue of supplies. This far-reaching attempt to deal with the breakdown of the Commissariat had been overthrown in a whitewashing exercise by seven generals on the Chelsea Board, who exonerated all the senior officers named in the report. It made her feel that all such work was hopeless. Would it not be better for everyone if she buried herself away in some small, remote hospital, pursuing her original objective of training women as nurses? She shrank from the prospect of 'the laudation of friends & abuse of enemies' that would inevitably accompany the enterprise. Furthermore, she had serious doubts that her health would hold out long enough for the work to be completed.

Within weeks of coming home, however, Florence would commit herself to reform. She was haunted by thoughts of the 'living skeletons' of that dreadful first winter; men, ulcerated and covered with vermin, who wrapped their heads in their blankets, and died without uttering a word. Overwhelming herself with work might at least keep these memories at bay. Almost a decade after the war, she was to look back, and shudder at the memory of the 'slaughter houses' of Scutari. It was like 'a horrid spectre' that she was afraid of conjuring up from the dark corners of her mind, where it was ever present, waiting to spring out on her.

She had long ago resolved to be a 'saviour', and she was not afraid of self-sacrifice. 'I stand at the Altar of the murdered men and while I live I fight their cause,' she vowed. Her deepest feelings, for the foreseeable future, lay not with the living, but with the dead.

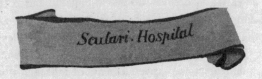

Part Three
Mother of the Army
1856–71

It would be a noble beginning of the new order of things, to use hygiene as the handmaid of civilization.

FN, *Notes on Matters Affecting the Health, Efficiency, and Hospital Administration of the British Army* ... (1858)

... I have thought that I could work better for others off the stage than on it.

FN to J. S. Mill, 11 August 1867

Oh dear Papa, my soul is sometimes exceedingly sorrowful, even unto death.

FN to William Nightingale, *c.* 1867

12. A Turbulent Fellow

Florence Nightingale's home for much of the five years following her return to England in the summer of 1856 would be London's Burlington Hotel. Established in the mid-1820s, the Burlington consisted of a collection of houses situated between Cork Street and Old Burlington Street, at the heart of the city's fashionable West End. At number 30 Old Burlington Street, where she took a suite of rooms at the beginning of November, Florence would oversee the reforms for improvement of the health of the British Army, becoming the driving force behind the campaign, and earning the house its nickname of the 'Little War Office'. Here, too, she would write *Notes on Hospitals* and *Notes on Nursing*, probably the most influential of her books. In 1913, Edward Cook, Nightingale's official biographer, described the Burlington as possessing the strongest associations with Florence Nightingale's public work of any location in Britain, and envisaged a time when a memorial tablet might be affixed to number 30. These associations – let alone the architectural distinction of the building as a fine eighteenth-century town house designed by Lord Burlington himself – should have ensured its survival. Nevertheless, in the autumn of 1935, the entire Burlington Hotel was demolished to make way for a block of service flats. A sliver of the wall of number 30 still clings to the building next door, while the outstanding feature of the interior, its great neo-Palladian staircase, found a new home at Buxted Park in Sussex.

Florence had first stayed at the Burlington in 1842, when it became the hotel most often frequented by the Nightingales during the London season. Her overall opinion of the Burlington had never been high, despite the rich decoration of its principal rooms, and she had once referred to it in a letter to her cousin Hilary as 'dingy'. But, while expensive, it was central, convenient and discreet, advantages that led her to prefer it to the apartment in Kensington Palace offered to her by Queen Victoria at the beginning of the 1860s. As she embarked on her

work in the autumn of 1856, in such secrecy that even close members
of her family were unaware of the nature of the task she had set herself, the Burlington also served another useful purpose. Casual acquaintances were likely to be deterred from calling, as the hotel address encouraged the impression that Florence was merely on a fleeting visit to
London.

The Burlington Hotel comprised three houses besides number 30,
which Florence called the 'private' house, 'composed mainly of family
suites of rooms'. Its chief entrance was at 19 Cork Street, where staff
prepared evening meals for guests in the private suites. Behind this,
buried within the hotel, and suffering from progressive architectural
maltreatment, lay numbers 29 and 30 Old Burlington Street, the former
built in the 1720s to another famous design by Burlington, for his client
General Wade. A further house, not far away at 22 Albemarle Street,
served as a hotel annexe, and it was to a 'light lofty two windowed front
room' at this address that Florence occasionally moved in the course of
1857, during the intensive bursts of writing, for instance, that accompanied the preparation of her own detailed account of her Crimean
experiences and recommendations for army welfare, *Notes on Matters
Affecting the Health, Efficiency and Hospital Administration of the
British Army* ... (Today, as the only significant surviving London
building once occupied by Florence Nightingale, 22 Albemarle Street,
currently part of the rear of Asprey's the Jewellers, certainly merits a
commemorative plaque.)

Florence's status as a distinguished, long-term occupant of the Burlington did not save her from being subjected to the inefficiency of the
staff and management. She despaired of its servants, who ignored the
basic sanitary precepts of fresh air, open windows and cleanliness that
she so fervently espoused, and was pleased when her description of these
failings, in the first edition of *Notes on Nursing,* was identified with the
Burlington '& very much injured' the hotel. In the winter of 1860–61,
she was once again disgusted 'at the carelessness of the Burlington
people' when, with a loud bang, the cistern above her bedroom burst
and emptied its contents over her head. By that time, Atkinson Morley,
her landlord and the original proprietor, had partly redeemed himself
and his hotel, having died and bequeathed £150,000 for the building of
a new hospital.

Florence's homecoming was more muted than she could have hoped for. Only a young girl presenting some flowers to her, as she made her way from London to Derbyshire on the afternoon of 7 August, after spending the morning at the Sisters of Mercy Convent in Bermondsey in prayer and meditation with Mother Clare Moore and her community, must have briefly revived fears of wider recognition. Faced with her 'noiseless' reappearance in England, Florence's expectant public had to make do with the return of her Crimean carriage, which rolled off the steamer at Southampton ten days later, exciting a great deal of interest. Rescued by Alexis Soyer, who had discovered it among some discarded wagons and carts waiting to be auctioned, the carriage was eventually returned to Embley, where it was shut away from public view.

On the early evening of the seventh, Florence arrived at Whatstandwell station. In fading light and still unrecognized, she walked the one-and-a-half miles across the fields, through the garden gate at the back of Lea Hurst. Her astonished parents and sister suddenly saw her from the windows of the drawing room. 'She came in like a bird,' wrote Parthenope, '. . . so quietly that no one found her out.' The next day the local churches rang their bells, and prayers of thanksgiving were offered at the Methodist Chapel at Lea.

Twenty-one months had passed since Florence's departure. During that time she had endured anxiety, strain and hardship, become a national heroine, and sailed perilously close to death. For her family at first there was the simple relief of hearing Florence's voice and seeing her face again, 'a blessing', as Fanny wrote, 'for which we cannot be too thankful'. They understood her need, after such an arduous ordeal, for a breathing space, for the time to restore her to the strength she would need for work in the future, and tiptoed round her, trying to be as unobtrusive as possible, keeping other wellwishers at bay. But they rapidly became concerned at the profound exhaustion, continuing insomnia, breathlessness and severe nausea at the merest sight of food from which she was suffering. Rest was difficult when 'heaps' of letters, some with vague addresses like 'Miss N at her home England', arrived by every post. There were begging letters, like one from a costermonger requiring 'a donkey & cart by return of post'; or another, from a young lady requesting a correspondence with Florence 'because I admire you so. I hope you will answer me by Tuesday.' Parthenope dealt with most of these 'effusions', but acknowledgement of gifts, like the large clasped

Bible inscribed by the female tenantry of the Nightingale estate at Pleasley, or the set of Sheffield cutlery donated by the city's artisans, required a personal response. Additionally, there was still an enormous backlog of correspondence relating to individual nurses and their claims to be answered, and the money given by the Sultan of Turkey to the nursing parties in recognition of their service to be distributed. Assisted by Uncle Sam and the Bracebridges, Florence also had to balance her own accounts and begin work on the breakdown, which she eventually published, of all the various voluntary contributions made to the hospitals in the East. Not surprisingly, the end of August found Parthenope anxiously writing to Liz Herbert that the improvement in Florence's health was not as marked as they might have wished. On an optimistic note, Florence was beginning to talk about her experiences, in a vein of self-abnegation that constantly amazed Parthenope, and contributed to the picture of her sister's saintliness that she was intent on impressing on her audience of fascinated correspondents. '. . . She is so calm, so holy – I can use no other word. In telling of all the horrors she has gone through . . . it is as if she dwelt in another atmosphere of peace & trust in God where nothing wicked can touch her. The physical horrors we cannot get her to tell us of, & she speaks of the mental ones, which are so far worse to bear, the indifference, ignorance, bigotry and cruelty as one fancies they must be looked upon in Heaven . . .'

As Florence regained something of her strength, the calm evaporated with her growing frustration. August was hardly the ideal month to start agitating the Government about reform of the health administration of the British Army. She wrote to Panmure at the War Office, soon after her return, proposing to report to him personally, but his reply recommended that she rest, and denied that there was any urgency for them to meet. Meanwhile, he was off to Scotland to shoot grouse. Her obvious ally, Sidney Herbert, was fishing salmon in Ireland. He told his wife that accounts of Florence's condition were 'disturbing', but agreed with Charles Bracebridge that with a mind 'constituted as hers is', complete rest from 'active business' would be a greater trial than a life of moderate occupation. Nevertheless, when Florence and he were reunited at the Bracebridges' home at Atherstone Hall, at the end of the first week of September, she came away disappointed at what she considered to be only a lukewarm interest in her ideas. By then, though, she had received an invitation that went a long way to lifting her spirits. Sir James Clark, the Queen's physician who had treated Parthenope at the time of her breakdown four years earlier, had written from Osborne on 23 August, asking Florence to stay at his house, Birk Hall, near Ballater, that September. The court would be in residence nearby at Balmoral, providing Queen Victoria, who had sanctioned the plan, with the opportunity to have an informal talk with her, and to hear at first hand her account of her experiences. Florence immediately sought advice from other advocates of reform about how best to take advantage of such a meeting. Dr Sutherland suggested that she should stick to facts when talking to the Queen. 'Facts are always facts; while advice may be returned without thanks . . .' Colonel Lefroy urged her to propose a Royal Commission to inquire into the state of the barracks, hospitals, and the Army's Medical Department. Both men left her in no doubt that while it would be comparatively straightforward to remedy 'the scientific defects' in the living conditions of the private soldier in peace and war, the wholesale reform of the Army Medical Department, which necessitated a strike at the root of the Army's system, would be a mammoth task that would face obstruction not only from the conservative elements of the ruling Horse Guards clique, but also from the forces of the Treasury, War Office, and senior medical staff combined.

Accompanied by her father, Florence set off for the Highlands in mid-September, stopping off in Edinburgh for several days to confer with Sir John McNeill and Colonel Tulloch, and to sift through some of the evidence that they had collected in the course of preparing their report into the failings of the Army supply system. At Balmoral, on 21 September, she was introduced to the Queen and the Prince Consort by Sir James Clark and, as Victoria noted in her Journal, 'talked principally of the want of system and organization which had existed and been the cause of so much suffering and misery'. The next evening she attended the first of a series of court balls. 'Flo says the Balls are dull affairs & the Queen ought not to dance,' reported Blanche Clough. 'When she is quiet her manner is just what it ought to be . . . but she looks very undignified . . . [dancing a] Sir Roger de Coverley.' Four days later, Florence had another, more informal talk with the Queen over tea at Birk Hall, and it was agreed – by 'command' – that she would extend her stay with the Clarks to await the arrival of Panmure at Balmoral. The Queen believed that with royal backing, Panmure might be convinced of the case for reform. 'I don't,' wrote Florence. 'But I am obliged to succumb.'

'I wish we had her at the War Office.' The Queen's famous remark about Florence (from a letter to her cousin, the Duke of Cambridge, who had recently become the Army's general commander-in-chief) has often been quoted as evidence of Victoria's unquestioning support for Florence's point of view. But it obscures the much more complex state of affairs surrounding the struggle between the Army's High Command and the Government for control of Her Majesty's Army. Certainly Victoria and Albert were both impressed by Florence's modesty, cleverness and lucidity. The Queen had been expecting 'a rather cold, stiff, reserved person', and was pleasantly surprised to find an altogether more engaging and much less intimidating 'ladylike' individual, dressed simply in black, with cropped hair. It also flattered Victoria to be told how much her own interest in the soldiers' welfare had been appreciated by the men themselves. However, the Queen's notion of reform, as Florence would come to realize, did not extend to the overhaul of a system, merely to the shuffling of personnel at the top. Neither she, nor the Prince Consort, whom Florence already suspected of being predisposed to the Horse Guards, would be likely to countenance yet another commission arising from the war that would once again air the deficiencies of the Army's top brass in public as the McNeill-Tulloch report so recently had. In any case, although the monarch might possess the desire to influence her ministers' decisions, constitutionally she was not invested with the power to act. That power rested with Palmerston's government, and the War Office led by Lord Panmure. Florence's insights into the royal couple show how acute her judgement of individuals could be. The Queen she was later to describe as 'the least self-reliant person she had ever known'. If Victoria was left alone with someone for ten minutes, she would send for Prince Albert to begin the conversation. Albert himself, so intelligent and well-informed, with his faith in a world that could be managed 'by prizes and exhibitions and good intentions', seemed oppressed by his situation, and 'was like a person who wanted to die'.

The Times reported Miss Nightingale's continuing stay in Scotland for the benefit of her health. Meanwhile, Florence attended church with the royal family, and talked metaphysics and religion with Prince Albert. On 5 October she at last met Panmure at Balmoral, and repeated the case that she had already laid before the Queen. A further meeting was arranged at Birk Hall. 'Panmure comes here today to eat his lunch &

me,' she wrote on 8 October to her father, who had retreated home with
a bad cold. 'He is civil, shrewd, impracticable & inert, good at parrying,
bad at acting . . .' The results of this second encounter must then have
agreeably surprised her. Not only did Panmure acquiesce in principle to
the appointment of a Royal Commission, he also, at Palmerston's urging,
requested that Florence commit her observations and recommendations based on her experiences into a formal and confidential report.
One other matter, which was to prove a considerable headache for some
time ahead, was thrown in for her consideration. The plans for the
country's first general military hospital at Netley on Southampton Water
were nearing completion, and Florence's opinion of them was eagerly
sought.

She felt the flush of success as she journeyed south from Aberdeen
after almost a month away. '. . . For the next three or four months,' she
warned her family, 'I shall have business . . . which will require hard
work & time spent in London & elsewhere to see men & Institutions
whom & which I must see to get up my Précis, demanded of me by Pan.'
At Lea Hurst, Parthenope marvelled at Florence's 'great mind' as she
began to assemble her materials. It was 'so wonderful', Parthenope told
her friend Ellen Tollet, just to sit by and watch her at work, even though
much that went on was behind closed doors after she was in bed.
And she confessed to feeling no longer any bitterness, or more than a
moment's regret, that Florence 'is not my sister any more, but the Mother
of a great army . . .'

Moving to the Burlington on 1 November, Florence drew up her list for
membership of the Commission. She had cut her teeth on the cunning
management of her committee at Upper Harley Street before the war,
but this time, in selecting commissioners, she tried to ensure that candidates of her own frame of mind were well to the fore. Her ten-man
selection balanced civilian and military representation equally and, most
vitally, was heavily packed with her former Crimean allies. During a
three-hour interview with Panmure on 16 November, she fought hard
for her nominees, bargaining man for man, revelling afterwards in her
triumphs, especially when she believed that she had pulled the wool over
the War Secretary's eyes, and finally ceding four names in favour of
Panmure's alternatives. Only one of these, Dr Andrew Smith, shortly to
retire as Director-General of the Army Medical Department, was a

member of the old regime, and Florence won a substantial victory over her old enemy Sir John Hall in persuading Panmure not to appoint Hall as Smith's successor. She had failed to secure the inclusion of Colonel Lefroy or Dr William Farr, the pioneering statistician she had met at Colonel Tulloch's house in Edinburgh earlier that autumn; but Lefroy had his own instructions, confirmed by Panmure, to draw up a scheme for an Army Medical School, while Farr was to act as her essential co-worker in assisting her investigations into the comparative mortality rates of army and civilian populations and, furthermore, would appear as an expert witness before the commission. Among her personal choices as commission members were Dr Sutherland, as a leading sanitary authority, Dr Thomas Alexander, an outstanding staff-surgeon in the Crimea of rare organizational ability, and General Storks, who as the final serving commandant at Scutari had been one of her most committed supporters, and had joined her in promoting various Army welfare schemes. Florence's estimate of Sir James Clark was not high, but his place on the commission was intended to act as a sop to Queen Victoria. Most importantly, Sidney Herbert would be chairman. He had severe reservations about taking the post, besides which his health was not good. His faith in commissions, he admitted, was 'rather shaken'. On the one hand, a commission might draw out the truth, and strengthen the hand of the executive to take action; on the other, it might postpone the necessity for immediate remedies until public feeling, which had been roused to unprecedented heights in support of the Army rank and file, had died away. Over the next few years, Florence would steel his resolve, as together they put pressure on the War Office to grant the commission the liberty to pursue active change.

The Commission's instructions, she recorded triumphantly after Panmure had gone, 'were general and comprehensive, comprising the whole Army Medical Department, and the health of the Army, at home and abroad . . .' This, according to her interpretation, encompassed not only hospital and barrack design with their respective sanitary arrangements, the introduction of a new system of pay, promotion and education for Army doctors – including the 'absolute necessity of a Practical Army Medical School at home' – but a welter of other points dealing with everything from the supply and transport arrangements, to the diet of the ordinary soldier, the collection of accurate statistics and, low down the list, the introduction of male and female nurses to military hospitals.

'You must drag it through,' she reminded herself at the end of her personal memorandum on the interview. 'If not you no one else.'

Her elation, though, swiftly vanished. Almost another six months were to pass before Panmure issued the Royal Warrant for the Royal Commission, while she seethed at his indolence, and at what she considered as the unnecessary delay. 'Gout is a very <u>handy</u> thing,' she complained to Sir John McNeill, who had begged her not to be discouraged, '& Lord Panmure always has it in his <u>hands</u> whenever he is called upon to do something.' Waiting for him to act was nothing less than torture. The idea that men were playing 'the game of party politics over the graves of our brave men, & trying to prevent us learning the terrible lesson which our colossal calamity should have taught us' was utterly abhorrent to her. In her mind it reawakened the idea that only she truly cared, that she alone appreciated the urgency of the situation, and that she was 'a bad mother' because she had failed to achieve more for her dead sons. 'You will say, who is this woman who thinks she can do what our great men don't?' she asked herself rhetorically, before declaring that in the last resort she might take her appeal to the country in the manner of Cobden and the Anti-Corn Law League.

But was Florence doing Panmure an injustice? It has been plausibly argued that far from sitting on his gouty hands, the War Secretary was actively engaged in raising support for the commission in Parliament. He knew that without it, and in the face of certain Army opposition, a commission of such wide-ranging scope and independence would stand no chance of survival. Panmure had, moreover, a personal motive in ensuring that an inquiry into the Army's health was not shelved in the way that the McNeill-Tulloch report had been: his own brother had died in the outbreak of cholera that had overwhelmed the British troops at Varna in the summer of 1854. Florence knew that Panmure had some trick in his head, but she couldn't see exactly what. In February 1857, she did receive his letter formally authorizing her own confidential report. She was already busy inspecting public and military institutions, and compiling data and statistics on sickness and mortality in the Crimean War. She visited the military base at Chatham at the end of 1856, where she was besieged by 'crowds of students and medicals'. In the New Year, she went over the naval hospital at Haslar at the request of Sir John Liddell, Director-General of the Navy's Medical Department. In March, she spent five hours at St Mary's, Paddington, accompanied by Hilary Bonham Carter, who mounted a guard over the entrance to the wards to protect her against unwanted onlookers.

In the preparation of her report, Florence leaned heavily on the intellectual support of two men, John Sutherland and William Farr. Sutherland was her master in sanitary administration and practice. He was in his late forties, had studied medicine at Edinburgh, and had a decade of experience of working in public health. He had headed an investigation into the law and practice of burial, and had brought into operation the act for abolishing intramural interments, before heading out to Turkey and the Crimea as head of the Sanitary Commission. 'The Sanitary reformers are quite accustomed to that sort of thing,' he wrote to Florence in December 1856, receiving her into the sanitarian fold, after she had told him of her problems in convincing Panmure that the designs for the new hospital at Netley were defective, as they were based on the old corridor system, and therefore encouraged overcrowding and poor ventilation. '. . . All we can often do is to state the truth and leave it.' She depended on Sutherland's technical advice and expertise, and his cool-headed analysis of any given situation, so much so that it is sometimes difficult to draw a distinguishing line between her original material and the points at which she has incorporated his briefing notes into her drafts, though generally she was inclined to liven up his somewhat colourless prose.

Their close collaboration across three decades – and the fact that Sutherland's growing deafness, despite her attempts to get him to use an ear trumpet, encouraged them to communicate by written notes though they worked in adjoining rooms – has left behind an extraordinary trail of paper: eight volumes of letters and notes in the British Library, which vividly convey the impatience, stubbornness, sheer fatigue ('You must think because I cannot', she writes at one especially exhausting moment), but rarely the personal affection, that was present on both sides in their unique working relationship. They were an oddly matched couple. As time wore on, Florence was unable to work effectively without Sutherland, but found working with him increasingly exasperating. At worst he became her pet aversion. She complained incessantly about his untidiness and unpunctuality, his flippancy and, in later years, his reluctance to be constantly at her beck and call when he would rather be tending his garden. Browbeaten, Sutherland referred to himself as 'one of your wives', but it was his own spouse, Sarah, who

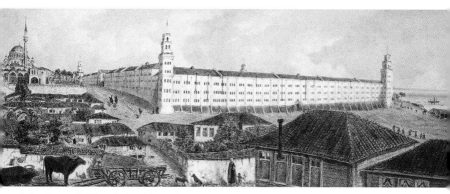

22. The Barrack Hospital at Scutari.

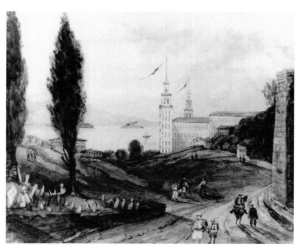

23. A view of the cemetery at Scutari, with the Nurses' Tower in the background.

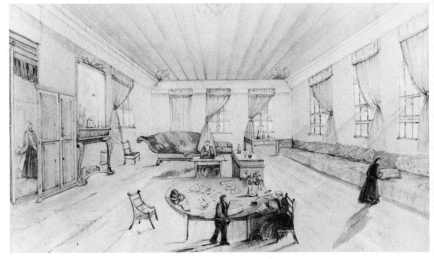

24. Florence's room in the Nurses' Tower at Scutari. One of a number of sketches by the Scutari matron, Anne Morton, this gives a misleading impression of the size of the room, which, in reality, was much smaller and more cramped.

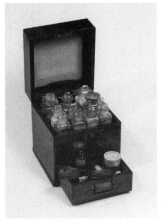

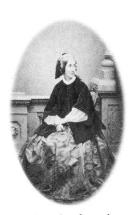

25. Mary Stanley, who led the second party of nurses sent to Scutari in December 1854. In Florence's eyes, Stanley assumed the role of the disciple who had betrayed her mistress.

26. The medicine chest, consisting of thirteen bottles, two pill boxes, and scales and measures, which Florence took with her to Scutari. It contains a range of medicines, such as carbonate of magnesia and carbonate of soda, as well as herbal remedies like powdered rhubarb.

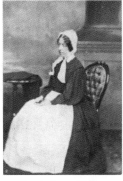

27. Sarah Anne Terrot, one of the Sellonite Sisters who formed part of the first expedition to Scutari.

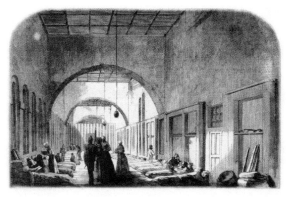

28. A sick ward at Scutari.

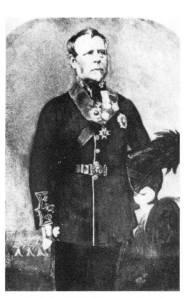

29. Sir John Hall, Florence's major adversary in the Crimea.

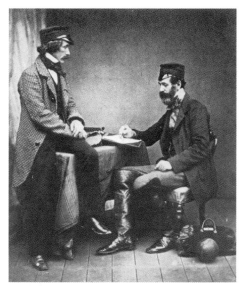

30. Roger Fenton's photograph of Dr John Sutherland (*left*) and Robert Rawlinson, two members of the Sanitary Commission sent out to Scutari and the Crimea. Sutherland was to be Florence's chief adviser for three decades following the Crimean War.

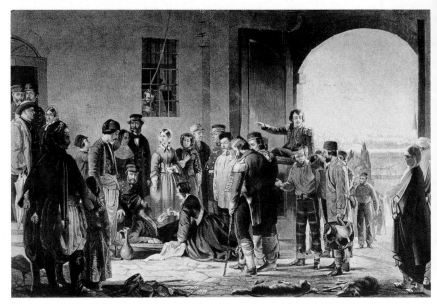

31. An engraving from 1861 of Jerry Barrett's painting *The Mission of Mercy* (1857). Mary Clare Moore, dressed in her habit, is to the left of Florence, Mrs Bracebridge stands to the right of her. Eliza Roberts, who nursed Florence during her dangerous illness in May 1855, kneels at her feet, attending to a wounded soldier.

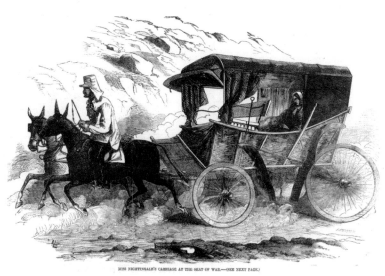

MISS NIGHTINGALE'S CARRIAGE AT THE SEAT OF WAR.—(SEE NEXT PAGE.)

32. An engraving from the *Illustrated London News* of Florence's carriage, used to drive her around the Crimea. In later years, when it was put on display, Florence referred to the carriage as 'that wretched Russian car'.

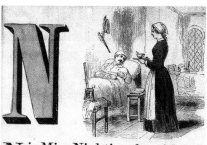

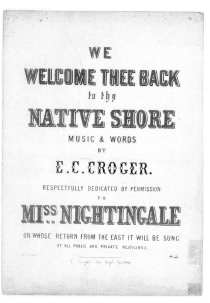

N is Miss Nightingale, with her
   fair band,
Who solaced our sick in a far distant land.

33. A poem celebrating Florence
from *The Panorama of Peace* (1856). At
the height of Florence Nightingale
mania during the Crimean War, the
Nightingales received three new songs
or poems about her every week.

34. The title page of a popular song
about Florence Nightingale.

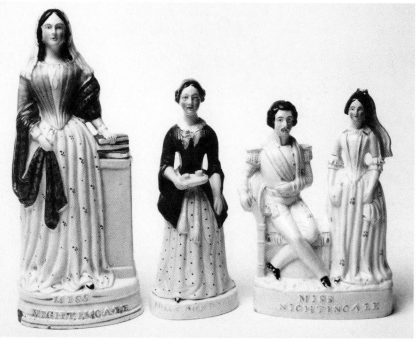

35. Staffordshire figurines of Florence Nightingale. Interestingly none of them
portrays her with the famous lamp.

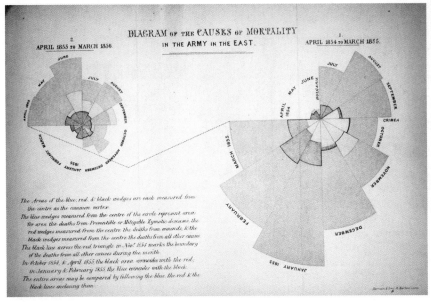

DIAGRAM OF THE CAUSES OF MORTALITY
IN THE ARMY IN THE EAST.

2.
APRIL 1855 to MARCH 1856

1.
APRIL 1854 to MARCH 1855.

The Areas of the blue, red, & black wedges are each measured from the centre as the common vertex.

The blue wedges measured from the centre of the circle represent area for area the deaths from Preventible or Mitigable Zymotic diseases, the red wedges measured from the centre the deaths from wounds, & the black wedges measured from the centre the deaths from all other causes.

The black line across the red triangle in Nov.r 1854 marks the boundary of the deaths from all other causes during the month.

In October 1854, & April 1855, the black area coincides with the red, in January & February 1855, the blue coincides with the black.

The entire areas may be compared by following the blue, the red & the black lines enclosing them.

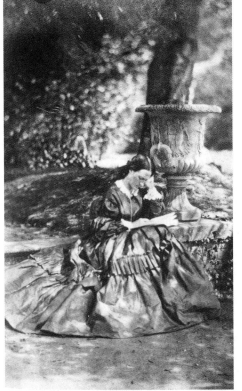

36. A detail from Florence's 'coxcomb', the coloured statistical diagrams designed by her to demonstrate the causes of mortality in the army in the east. The largest category presents visual data for deaths from infectious diseases, including cholera and dysentery.

37. Florence in May 1858, during her last visit to Embley for eight years. This photograph, which came to light in 2006, belonged to William Slater, the local chemist in Church Street, Romsey, and was probably taken by his assistant William Frost.

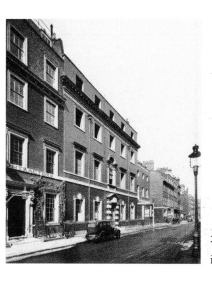

38. The Burlington Hotel, Florence's 'Little War Office', photographed shortly before its demolition in 1935.

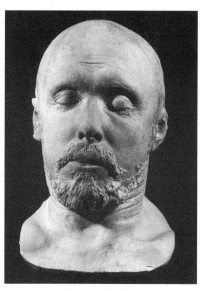

39. A cast of the head of Arthur Hugh Clough, taken in the hours following his death in Florence in November 1861.

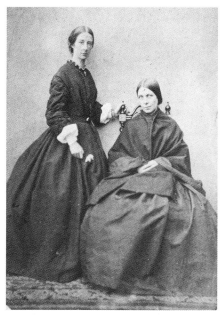

40. Florence's cousins, Bertha Smith (*left*) and her sister Blanche Clough, *c.* 1861. Bertha's resemblance to Florence is striking.

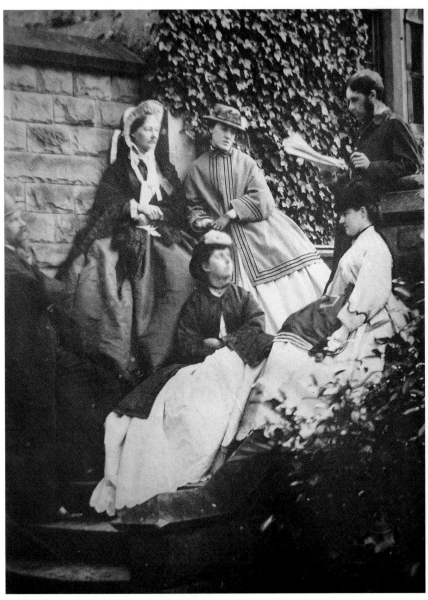

41. Parthenope as Lady Verney of Claydon House, *c.* 1865, with her step-daughter Emily, Miss Trevelyan, George Trevelyan, and Miss Storey.

evoked Florence's stronger feelings as her 'Dearest, kindest friend'. Mrs Sutherland was just as devoted to Florence, offering practical help, and at one time viewing forty-one houses on her behalf before settling on the best temporary lodgings for her. Suspecting that Sutherland was domineering towards his wife, and that he was something of a male chauvinist at home (he once 'went off about the "rights of man"' after objecting to the notion of women having the responsibility of filling out statistical forms for hospitals), Florence plotted to out-manoeuvre him by arranging for Mrs Sutherland to be offered the honorary secretaryship of the Ladies' Sanitary Association.

Florence's relationship with Farr, her 'Patron Saint' as she called him, was quite another matter, characterized as it was by a spirit of deference. She felt like a small boy writing to Aristotle when she sought his advice on statistics, she told him after they had been working together for more than a decade. On at least one occasion during 1857, she ordered her carriage to drive to the other side of Regent's Park so that she could visit Farr at his home in St John's Wood, and 'sit at his feet' to consult him about some pressing matter. By this time, Farr possessed a considerable reputation as an authority on vital statistics and epidemiology, in particular for his statistical nosology for tabulating reported deaths. Born in 1807, the child of a farm labourer, Farr had trained as a doctor after becoming apprenticed to a local patron who recognized his promise, provided him with some education, and offered him a route out of the poverty of his background and into the professional class. In 1837, Farr joined the General Register Office to help in the organization of the flood of data arising from the new registration of births, deaths and marriages. He was later appointed compiler of abstracts, and eventually, superintendent of the statistical department. For almost forty years Farr was to use his position to collate and interpret, with ever more ingenious methodology, statistical information on the condition of public health in England and Wales. In his *First Annual Report*, for example, he pointed to the increases in mortality that occurred whenever population density increased.

'It has been held that the world is governed by numbers . . .,' Farr wrote to Florence, quoting Goethe, in the summer of 1857; 'this I know . . . Numbers teach us whether the world is <u>well or ill governed</u>.' He, like her, was a passionate statistician (though possibly a less gifted mathematician); an admirer of Quetelet (the Belgian author of *Physique*

Sociale, whom Florence had venerated since pre-war days for his guidance in discovering the laws of God, and whom, with girlish enthusiasm, she met in mid-1860 when the great man breakfasted in her rooms at the Burlington, during the International Statistical Congress organized by Farr); and he was prepared to place not only his knowledge, but also unpublished records and the services of his trained clerks at her disposal. In return he asked for her assistance 'in the attempts that are now being made to improve the Health of the civil population'.

Farr's emphasis on the significance of mortality tables at their very first meeting had encouraged Florence to compare the mortality among civilians to that among soldiers. The results were shocking. In peacetime, soldiers in England between the ages of twenty and thirty-five – so-called 'picked lives', as they had passed a medical examination at the time they were recruited – had a mortality rate nearly twice that of civilians. Moreover, in the Crimean War, the death rate from sickness and disease among British soldiers in Turkey was 'not much more' than it was among healthy soldiers at home. Even more startlingly, the mortality for all British troops in the Crimea was just two-thirds of what it was 'among our troops at home'. The inference was clear. It was just as criminal, Florence wrote later with typically hard-hitting pungency, 'to have a mortality of 17, 19, and 20 per thousand in the Line, Artillery and Guards in England, when that of Civil life is only 11 per 1,000, as it would be to take 1,100 men per annum out upon Salisbury Plain and shoot them'.

But how best to grab the public's attention and bring these dramatic conclusions home to them? Figures were impressive, but the employment of diagrams was a more arresting means of presenting the material. Florence's 'coxcomb', later appended to the Royal Commission's report as well as to her confidential précis, was a series of circular diagrams, like a piechart, designed 'to affect thro' the Eyes what we may fail to convey to the brains of the public through their word-proof ears' (she also employed '<u>line to line</u>' diagrams, but preferred the area ones 'as being mathematically more correct'). Farr oversaw the design of the coxcombs, as well as rigorously checking the figures that were fed into them. He remained, however, suspicious of this resort to pictorial material, and her evident flair for popularizing statistical findings. Statistics, he advised her, should be as dry as possible – 'the dryer the better'.

Florence's groundwork for the investigation into the health of the

Army demonstrates what were to be some of the hallmarks of her working style in years to come: the careful marshalling of the most accurate raw data and, if this was unavailable or inadequate, the dispatch of questionnaires to obtain it, together with the enlistment of the finest expertise to help understand it and formulate solutions. She was above all a brilliant assimilator, with the ability to state a case with clarity and unrelenting force. 'How she collects the honey out of each man's information & sense,' noted Parthenope, '& binds it up into the whole that is to carry on the work.' Almost as extraordinary perhaps was her capacity to retain the loyalty down the years of so many of the doctors, cabinet ministers, and other officials who worked with her. Of paramount importance, of course, was the fact that, for the most part, these co-workers shared her vision. In respect of Army health reform, feelings of outrage at the neglect of the rank and file during the war remained high until the late 1850s, and the urgent necessity of securing the Army's future health was a burning issue. Nor should it be overlooked that for men like Sutherland and Farr there were considerable advantages in an association with Florence Nightingale which could ensure that their ideas reached well beyond the boundaries of their natural audience to the attention of the politically influential.

There can be no doubt, though, of the significant role played by the attraction of such men to the steadying strength of Florence's moral certainty, and to the energy she put into drawing them as individuals into an irresistible ongoing drama. As a woman, her position was unprecedented. She could not herself be included as a member of an official inquiry, nor appear publicly in its support, yet she was to remain throughout the mainspring of the operation. She might complain of the problems that attached to a woman 'in official life' – that her word tended not to be taken as evidence because 'a Lady' could not be contradicted, that, on the one hand, she could be used as a scapegoat for failure and, on the other, be denied any credit for success – but only a woman could have got away with the mix of cajolery, bullying, flattery of susceptible male egos and plain scolding that she employed to such demonstrable effect. 'My dear Lady, do not be unreasonable,' Sutherland wrote pleadingly after he had missed an appointment with her. 'I fear that your sex is much given to being so. I would have been with you yesterday, had I been able, but alas! My will was stronger than my legs.' In a moment of levity, Sutherland might compare Florence to an Amazon

Queen, and Panmure describe her as a 'turbulent fellow' (a description to which Florence responded by calling herself 'a bothering woman'), but it was Sidney Herbert who appealed to her femininity with a flutter of light flirtatiousness. Returning 'a batch' of Florence's letters to her at one stage, at her request, he cast himself for a moment in the role of a disappointed suitor, mourning a broken engagement. Florence's failing health, as she worked herself to the point of exhaustion in the cause of reform, was regarded by her male collaborators not as indicative of the weakness of her sex, but rather, in Dr Sutherland's words, as illustrative of a woman's preparedness to 'suffer knowingly where men would shrink'. While her illness aroused the protective instincts of those men in regular contact with her, the example of her 'self devotion' also presented them with something of a challenge to spur them on to greater efforts of their own.

Florence's status as a national heroine remained the most significant weapon in her personal armoury, and the source of what in time would become known as 'Nightingale Power'. Since returning to England, she had held firm to her resolve to resist any publicity as likely to have only harmful consequences for her future work, but the threat that she might have to resort to an appeal to the country, above the heads of its government, was kept in readiness, in the event of it being needed. In February 1857, her patience finally snapped. 'I have been home six months . . .,' she told Sutherland. 'And Lord Panmure has amused himself with our suffering.' On 12 February, she sent Herbert a formal warning: 'three months from this day I publish my experience of the Crimea campaign, and my suggestions for improvement, unless there has been a fair and tangible pledge by that time for reform.' Despite her continuing pessimism, there were signs that the political climate was changing. In March, the McNeill-Tulloch report was at last vindicated when a Commons motion to honour its two authors was carried without division. On 5 May, Panmure issued the Royal Warrant, and a week later the Royal Commission on the Health of the Army finally began its sittings.

A draft of Florence's *Notes on Matters Affecting the Health, Efficiency, and Hospital Administration of the British Army* . . . was nearing completion as the Royal Commission was appointed. Its relationship to the main report, written by Sidney Herbert later that summer, was mutually beneficial. In fact, the two fed off one another. As Chairman, Herbert depended on Florence's findings, and the voluminous materials she had assembled, to enable the Commission to move more rapidly over similar ground than it otherwise would have done; for her part, the *Notes* incorporated a mass of official correspondence unearthed by the Commission, throwing new light on defects in the Army medical system, and included at the last minute so that the pagination of her 830-page text had to be hastily, and somewhat erratically, amended. Its length may have stretched to breaking point conventional definition of the term 'précis', but in its combination of argumentative rigour, caustic analysis and well-directed sarcasm, this remarkable document was as far removed from the dry, dusty tone of the Blue Books as it was possible to conceive. It is at once a passionate elegy for the British soldier as well as a plea for his more humane treatment in the future.

The *Notes* begin with the descriptive, and a devastating collection of facts, letters and statistics to tell 'the whole history of the frightful Scutari calamity', subsequently moving on to the prescriptive, and a detailed blueprint for the thorough overhaul of the soldier's living conditions in peacetime and at war. Every element in this administrative programme for change is outlined with rhetorical skill as well as statistical precision: the need for general hospitals in addition to the regimental ones; a new educational and career path for the Army's medical officers to attract better men to the service; the introduction of sanitary officers ultimately answerable to the War Office; the establishment of a proper method of statistical accounting to combat slipshod practices during the war, when, to take one example, the chief medical officer's record for the last quarter of 1854 showed 400 fewer deaths than the adjutant's listing of burials; and the construction of hospitals and barracks with proper ventilation and adequate sanitation. Netley, the country's first general military hospital, she wrote, 'will not answer the purpose'. What was required in its place was a design to aid the constant movement of air: 'separate pavilions, placed side by side or line by line'. Along with these broad schemes were a host of smaller recommendations, relating to soldiers' pay and stoppages, soldiers' wives, washing and canteens, and dietary provisions (including a recipe for 'Cheap Plain Rice Pudding for Campaigning'), deriving directly from Florence's experiences at Scutari.

The angry scorn she reserves for individuals like Andrew Smith, the

Director-General, and John Hall, the Principal Medical Officer, who placed the reputation of the Army's medical department before the welfare of the men, is inescapable. Scrutinizing Smith's correspondence, she constantly ridicules his refusal to accept any notion of accountability as he turns a blind eye to deep-rooted systemic problems, and takes false comfort from the misleading interpretation of statistics. 'The administrative principle of the Horse Guards,' she observes, 'is an admirable plan for shifting all responsibility till it is not known where it lies. If you treat your Director-General like a school-boy, you will have a school-boy for your Director-General.' Rarely does she allow her own emotion to get the better of her and divert her from the presentation of her case – except at one point, when 'the tears come into my eyes as I think how, amidst scenes of horrible filth, of loathsome disease and death, there arose above it all the innate dignity, gentleness, and chivalry of the men . . .'

The final printed version of Florence's *Notes*, restricted under its confidential heading, reflected her conversion to the belief that it had been the disastrous sanitary arrangements in the hospitals at Scutari, rather than the inadequate food and supplies she had originally believed responsible, that were the primary cause of so many deaths. While admitting that there was 'still some difference of opinion' on the subject, she appears to have reached this conclusion herself only after Farr had convinced her of the differences in mortality between the front-line hospitals in the Crimea and the base hospitals at Scutari. Exactly when this conversion took place, it is impossible to say. But by May 1857, just as the commission was beginning its proceedings, she was able to write to Sir John McNeill about Scutari as 'a historical instance of sufficient importance to furnish us with much absolute knowledge, no longer within the domain of hypothesis'. What this absolute knowledge was, she went on to explain:

It is true that the Sanitary arrangements adopted [with the arrival of the Sanitary Commission in March 1855] brought the mortality down to 1.8 per cent in the latter year of the war. But in what condition? That of not allowing above 1000 patients in a building 700 feet square, three floors in height. Had this building been differently distributed as to its construction, it might easily have accommodated 3000 patients with good recovery conditions . . . The question is to find a construction which will accommodate the greatest number of Patients upon a given area with the greatest facilities for recovery.

I do not hesitate to say that the causes of the great catastrophe at Scutari were want of ventilation, want of draining, want of cleanliness (too disgusting to detail further) ... frightful overcrowding. However good the construction and ventilation of the corridors, if you fill them with patients, it is the same as building two hospitals back to back ...

If it is objected that the condition of the men sent down from the Crimea during the first winter was such that they could not have recovered under <u>any</u> circumstances, I answer that the Land Transport Corps sent down men in exactly the same condition the second winter, and that under different circumstances they did recover. Witness our rates of mortality – 1.8 per cent.

She had, of course, been fully aware since the spring of 1855, when the Sanitary Commission started its investigations, that the Barrack Hospital had been built over a cesspool. What must have come as a considerable shock to her was the discovery that the death rate at her own hospital was far higher than at any other, higher even than the General Hospital at Balaclava, which she had previously believed to be the worst. There is no evidence to suggest that this discovery was a factor in the ensuing breakdown of her health later that summer (a plausible connection between the two would require Florence to have accepted responsibility for the original choice of the Barrack Hospital site, when clearly she had had nothing to do with it). However, the shocking truth about Scutari did drive her to an unsuccessful attempt to make the facts about the high mortality rate at her hospital one of the major constituents of the Commission's public report. Herbert refused. He didn't want to taint the Nightingale legend; nor perhaps did he wish to embroil his report in the kind of public attention that had surrounded the last major sanitary controversy: the dismissal in 1854 (by the government of which he had been a member) of Edwin Chadwick, leading sanitary reformer, and member of the first national board of public health. But the significance of the discovery would not be lost on Florence. From now on, 'the sanitary question' would be the touchstone of her working life.

She had put to one side the writing of her *Notes* to concentrate on priming Herbert for his appearances as Chairman of the Commission. Like a solicitor issuing instructions for the case, she advised him on witnesses, and the order in which to call them, and then set about coaching him on how to present his materials and what questions to ask, often preparing the briefs for cross-examination as well as examination. 'Dear Miss Nightingale, I should very much like to have a Cabinet council with you today,' Herbert would write, signalling that they were to meet to decide on a course of action. He was a quick learner, and she a relentless taskmaster, impatiently pushing him on at the merest sign of any slackening of pace. She coached Sutherland too, up at his house in Highgate, but worried incessantly that he didn't carry the weight on the Commission that his brains ought to have given him. His lack of 'pith' preoccupied her in the middle of June as the Commission prepared to examine her old adversary, Sir John Hall. She agreed that the Commission shouldn't 'badger the old man . . . which would do us no good and him harm', though the memory of his 'incredible apathy' soon reasserted itself. In the event, though, Sutherland was not present at this particular sitting, and Hall's evidence 'broke down utterly from want of truthfulness and perpetual doubling'. Florence claimed not to be without sympathy for Hall as a victim of a system 'of which he could know nothing until the results appeared'. Hall crept away, retired on half-pay, and died in Pisa in 1866.

More problematic was the question of Florence's own evidence. Calling a woman as a witness in a public inquiry was not entirely without precedent (Caroline Chisholm had appeared before a House of Lords committee looking at Australian settlement in 1847). But Florence's poor physical condition, coupled with the inevitable furore that would result were she to appear in public, even behind closed doors, seemed to rule it out, as did the potential for political damage to Herbert himself should it become known that, both during his time as Secretary at War and subsequently, he had been receiving information from Florence through unofficial channels. He shared Sir John McNeill's 'repugnance' at the idea of her being examined 'viva voce', Herbert told Florence on 8 July, but considered that her evidence would 'fortify our proceedings, and hasten the adoption of our recommendations'. He suggested that she submit extracts from her *Notes*, 'or otherwise in writing', but then tried to restrict her evidence to the area of hospital construction. She resisted his move. It would be 'treachery to the memory of her dead' were she to leave 'untouched the great matters which will affect (& have affected) the mortality of our sick more than mere Architecture could do . . .' The evidence she did finally submit occupied thirty-three closely printed pages of Herbert's published report, and covered a wide variety of subjects, including sanitation. But the most controversial section of her *Notes*, the data on the higher mortality at Scutari, was omitted. It was to remain buried for several generations.

In the summer heat, the rooms at the Burlington were unbearably hot and stuffy. If the windows were shut, the atmosphere became 'pestilential'; if they were open, the noise made it impossible for anyone to hear themselves speak. The constant presence of Florence's mother and sister was another persistent source of irritation. 'Your ceaseless watchfulness to ease and help me in the time we have been together can never be forgotten by me,' Florence had assured her mother six months earlier after they had spent a few days together at Embley. Several weeks closeted in her hotel suite with Fanny and Parthenope that summer was enough to change her mind on that score. The Burlington was completely booked on their arrival. This forced Florence to spend her nights at the Albermarle Street annexe, and to work during the day in the small parlour at number 30, while her mother and sister occupied the main drawing room, receiving visitors and welcoming friends. Fanny, who was to become increasingly resentful of the cost of maintaining 'a public servant' in London, quibbled about unnecessary expense. Florence, meanwhile, accused her mother of engendering financial confusion by attempting to smuggle her own expenses, like 'contraband', into Florence's accounts.

It must have seemed all too reminiscent of being a daughter at home again, back in the drawing room at Embley. Her resentment against her family – never far from the surface – spilled over into several angry pages of private notes on the subject of Fanny and Parthenope's hypocrisy. She could not forget the way in which they had for so many years, 'inexorably' and 'overbearingly', opposed her work.

What have my mother & sister ever done for me? They like my glory . . . Is there anything else they like in me? I was the same person who went to Harley St & who went to the Crimea. There was nothing different except my popularity. Yet the person who went to Harley St was to be cursed & the other was to be blessed . . . this false popularity, based on ignorance, has made all the difference in the feeling of my 'family' towards me. There has been nothing really learnt by them from experience. But the world thinks of me differently – i.e. I have won, but by an accident . . .

Florence's attitude was understandable. The pressure on her was intense, her physical condition failing, and the last thing she needed was unnecessary interruptions from her mother and sister. But her frustration also led her to overlook the ways in which Fanny and Parthenope were attempting to make amends for all the misunderstandings of the past. In a letter written well over a decade later, Florence would portray the two women at the Burlington, in the summer of 1857, as lazy and self-indulgent, lounging about on their sofas, and complaining of their own fatigue, while she slaved away for the report. This isn't entirely fair. During this same period, Parthenope was continuing to work tirelessly on her sister's behalf, writing and copying letters, fielding requests and receiving the odd imperious demand from Florence when she got some detail wrong. For her part Fanny – who saw Florence's work for the Army as being on a par with the campaign her father had once waged for the abolition of slavery – took pride whenever she was 'allowed to lift a finger' to help her daughter 'with her burthen', describing to her husband, on one occasion, her assistance with the practical arrangements for Florence's briefing of the commissioners, and often relaying her excitement, as the Commission got under way, when its members returned to the Burlington 'quite elated with their success'.

Both mother and sister were alarmed by Florence's deteriorating health, but powerless to persuade her do anything to conserve her strength. 'The irritable desire of perfection grows upon her,' Parthenope observed, and 'She will not let one even write a note if she can help it.' Bratby, the Nightingales' steward, went daily to the Herberts in Belgrave Square for supplies of chicken, 'soup, beef tea & Jelly' for members of the 'Little War Office', but Florence, according to her mother, 'so entirely forgets herself that she would not eat at all unless the food were put before her'. Herbert went fishing in the second week of August, having outlined the gist of their findings to Panmure, as well as putting before him an active programme of reform which he had agreed with Florence. Before leaving London, he wrote to tell Florence how much he owed her 'for all your help during the last three months', and tried to persuade her to take some rest. She showed no sign of heeding his advice. 'Last night,' Fanny told William Nightingale on 17 August, 'I looked out at 1½ to see if the light was still burning in her room & there it was & when I remonstrate, she says "when I have work to do which must be finished by a certain time I work . . . sometimes twenty hours out of the 24."' By this point, Florence's lips were 'quite blue with exhaustion', and she was barely able to stand. Some time in the third week of August she collapsed with an attack of severe palpitations. Her overwhelming desire to complete her task had kept her going, but now nature was taking its course.

13. Thorn in the Flesh

Florence Nightingale has become one of history's most famous invalids. The image we have of her, tirelessly continuing to work while confined to bed, or reclining on a sofa, has become a dominant impression in many people's minds, second only to the popular notion of the Lady with the Lamp. Yet for decades, biographers and historians speculated about the true nature of the illness that afflicted her after her return from the Crimean War, which, at its height, left her bedridden for years, and convinced that she was going to die. Most, if not all, of these commentators questioned whether she had suffered from an organic illness at all, arguing instead that her symptoms had been the product of neuroses. Cook attributed Florence's condition to 'dilation of the heart' and 'neurasthenia' (a catch-all term favoured by the nineteenth and early twentieth centuries for unexplained psychosomatic symptoms). Subsequent writers saw her illness as a product of stress brought on by her struggles with officialdom over the Royal Commission, or produced by her unresolved conflict with her mother and sister, though what neither of these theories could explain was why the anxiety produced by both these conditions should have caused no disturbance whatever to her intellectual powers. In more recent years, there has been a tendency towards less charitable explanations. She feigned illness and lied about her health in order to protect herself from people she didn't want to see, particularly Fanny and Parthenope, was the conclusion of the most damaging account. By the early 1990s, the growing body of research about Nightingale appeared to have reached agreement that, at best, Florence Nightingale was a malingerer, and, at worst, her illness was a pretence that she used to her own ends.

Posthumous diagnoses are rarely successful in establishing with any degree of certainty the nature of an illness experienced by an individual long dead. In 1995, however, David Young, a former principal scientist at the Wellcome Institute in London, put forward a compelling case for

Florence as a sufferer from chronic brucellosis, which, as we have seen, originated in the Crimean fever that had caused her collapse in May 1856. Florence's attack in August 1857 was similar in many ways to the one she had suffered in the Crimea: palpitations, tachycardia (abnormally rapid heart action), accompanied by depression, insomnia and nausea at the sight of food. Two years later, in the summer of 1859, she suffered her second severe attack, adding shortness of breath, weakness, syncope (temporary loss of consciousness from a fall in blood pressure), indigestion and flushing of the face and hands to her growing list of complaints. The form of chronic brucellosis of these episodes, and the three further instances of serious illness that Florence was to experience in the course of 1861, are difficult to distinguish from neurosis because of their non-distinctive symptoms. But the attack Florence suffered in December 1861, when she developed spinal pain so severe that she was unable to walk, and had to be carried to and from her bed, showed distinctive symptoms that can accurately be ascribed to what is known, in modern medical parlance, as the specific form of the disease. This spinal pain, almost certainly due to spondylitis, together with shortness of breath and muscle spasms, afflicted her at various periods throughout the 1860s. The effect could be devastating. Spondylitis has been described as 'one of the most incapacitating and painful maladies that can affect man'.

The ramifications of the disease for Florence's way of life and work took effect instantaneously. Before her collapse in August 1857, she had visited institutions, paid personal calls and attended dinner parties given by friends and associates, while continuing to shun public attention. From the autumn of that year, and for much of the next few decades, she would impose a rule of strict seclusion upon herself. This meant concentrating her limited strength on the work in hand, and keeping visitors, even members of her immediate family, to the absolute minimum, receiving them at her invitation, generally one at a time and with the appointment specified to the nearest half-hour. In one significant respect, Florence's illness served her work. It gave it urgency. 'She always talks as if her time were short,' Dr Sutherland reported to Aunt Mai, '. . . so that the work must be done now or never.' Later, Sutherland would change his mind to a more optimistic long-term prognosis for Florence's life expectancy, arguing that individuals with 'afflictions of the heart' – which, since he consistently denied the presence of 'organic disease', is what he believed Florence to be suffering from – often lived on for years. Her family, though, was in little doubt, in these first years of illness, that her time was running out. 'I fear Florence's power of work & therefore hold of life is disappearing from month to month,' her father wrote at the end of 1857. 'I see no possible continuance for long – she might have lived a comparatively long life ... but this was inconsistent with Greater Events.' Florence shared his conviction of this gloomy scenario. Her feelings were encouraged by the crippling depression that was such a pronounced feature of her brucellosis, and she met each episode of virulent illness in the late 1850s, and at the start of the new decade, with preparations for her own death: making and remaking her will, drafting final letters, deciding to leave her body to science (because, as she flippantly told a friend, she wanted to 'go down to posterity in a bottle of spirits'), or conceiving the romantic idea of burial in the Crimea. There were periods of respite from her more serious symptoms, some lasting for months, which may have left some visitors wondering why she was committed to her regime of enforced invalidism when to all appearances she seemed calm and well. Aunt Julia, for one, thought that Florence's face was 'deceptive', and might make 'unin-formed people' suppose her 'to be much less suffering' than she was. (Florence underlined the contrast between herself and Mrs McLeay, another resident of the Burlington, who was 'one of the gayest & most flighty hypochondriacs in London – in bed one day & at a ball the next'.) Florence may have been surprised by her continuing survival, but the threat of another, possibly fatal, attack remained always present. As Harriet Martineau, another professional invalid who had defeated medical prognostications, wrote to her in 1858: '... Every stroke of work is more likely than not to be the last. Yet I may go on, as I <u>have</u> gone on, – much longer than could be expected.' Florence responded in agreement. '... I too have "no future" & must do what I can without delay.' By the time that Florence's symptoms began to subside, at the beginning of the 1880s, her invalidism formed part of the grain of her everyday working life, and the descriptions of herself in her letters as an incurable, or as 'entirely a prisoner to my bed', had become her constant mantra to the outside world.

In August 1857 Florence returned to Malvern, and to Dr Johnson, who had treated her at Umberslade, and had subsequently set up an establishment at Malvern's Bury House. She had set her heart on being 'quite alone' at the water-cure. Her greatest sacrifice over the past four years, she said, had been to give up the longing for silence and solitude once so vital to her. While there Florence underwent a ten-day course of hydrotherapy, followed by several weeks of recuperation. '. . . I was told that my life was not worth 24 hours purchase – and I knew it too,' she recalled later. She tried to relax, in spite of her racing pulse, and sent to Parthenope for a bottle of cologne and a novel; but her privacy was threatened when a Worcester newspaper reported that she was staying at Malvern, and her mother annoyed her by attempting to obtain details of her condition in writing from Dr Johnson. She was determined that as far as possible news of her illness should not leak out. Sutherland, alarmed by the sight of her as she left London – 'it appeared as if all your blood wanted renewing' – wrote, anxiously counselling her not to think, but to eat, drink and rest. She replied with a 'long scold of a letter'. If she had lost the Report, 'what would the health I should have saved have "profited" me? Or what would ten years of life have advantaged me, exchanged for the ten weeks this summer? Yes, but, you say, you might have walked or driven or eaten meat. Well . . . let me tell you, O Doctor, that after any walk or drive I sat up all night with palpitation. And the sight of animal food increased the sickness.' She had recently dreamed of Athena, her pet owl, lying dead and being pecked at by Sutherland's canary. '. . . You', she wrote accusingly, 'all peck at me.' Although still weak and confined to her room for most of the day, she was nevertheless unable to resist the pull of work when it unexpectedly presented itself. At the beginning of September, a hospital expert, passing through Malvern, contacted her about the plans for Netley. Florence was at once fired with interest, and insisted on seeing him.

Sutherland inadvisably proposed that she return to the 'bosom of your family' for a couple of months to convalesce. He could then join her at Lea Hurst so that they could continue their work together. She was having none of it. Instead, she called upon her old ally Aunt Mai to absent herself from her husband and children, and move into the Burlington to help manage her domestic and business affairs. Aunt Mai's fervent response suggests that this was just the invitation she had been waiting for. 'You know my heart too well – my child, my friend, my guide & uplifter, my dearest on earth & in heaven . . .' On 1 October, Florence and Aunt Mai, who had gone to Malvern to accompany her niece back to London, arrived at Euston Square station where they were met by Arthur Clough, Mai's son-in-law. Clough placed Florence in a brougham with her aunt, who dosed her with sal volatile, and then followed in a cab with the luggage. At the Burlington, Florence was given twenty drops of henbane to help her sleep. 'She is extremely calm as ever,' Mai wrote to the Nightingales the next day, '. . . but she did say that her state of nerves makes her hear sounds at a distance quite beyond hearing when she is well, & that when a cart went along at Malvern . . . it was the feeling of an earthquake'. Everything possible was done to prevent Florence from becoming agitated, though the rapid breathing caused by her palpitations much distressed her. No more than one person at a time sat with her in her room, and she disliked anyone being present unnecessarily. Logan, a trusted former surgical nurse, was hired as a general help, and 'to spare her opening a box or drawer'. Arthur Clough came twice a day, on the way to and from his work at the Education Office in Downing Street. He was proving a godsend in the complicated process of assembling Florence's *Notes* for printing, and was keen for 'any more commissions'. Dr Sutherland sat in an adjoining room to Florence's, the messages between them delivered by Aunt Mai. As the other members of the 'Little War Office' returned to the Burlington, Florence would see members of the Commission in the parlour for half an hour. By the end of the year, as the regulations for the implementation of the report were being drawn up, she was attending more intensive meetings in the morning and afternoon, lying down in her bedroom in between to muster her strength. Her input was considered vital because she had 'both the smallest details at her fingers' ends and the great general views of the whole . . .'

Aunt Mai was the key to the success of this operation. Her devotion to Florence, living out the life of a 'porter's wife' for her, was plain. For Fanny and Parthenope, on the other hand, Mai was the dragon at the gate, keeping them at bay, issuing lengthy, almost daily, bulletins on Florence's condition, her general spirits, and appetite, but restricting their access to her with resolute authority. 'I am afraid of any drop of excitement we can help . . .,' Mai wrote to them about one of their visits to London, discouraging their stay at the Burlington, and strongly urging that they try an alternative hotel. 'If you were in Cork St[reet] I am sure she would be uneasy <u>not</u> to have you with her & <u>not</u> to have you in these rooms . . . It seems to me it would be best for her to see each of you on separate days . . .' Mai proved her point a little later, when Fanny booked into the Burlington, 'after sending to 2 or 3 other hotels in vain', and attempted to conceal her stay from Florence. Florence heard her mother's voice, '& saw her at her open window – & all Saturday she was feverish & restless whilst too hard at work to be able to see her mother before Sunday'. Both Fanny and Parthenope were sufficiently disturbed by Florence's appearance to keep their distance when pressed to do so, though on one occasion, after Mai had become exasperated by their 'selfishness & thick skinnedness', she turned to Arthur Clough to back her up. Clough was sympathetic to their position, but brutally frank and to the point. 'These things are more cruel upon you than upon any others,' he wrote to Parthenope. 'But they are the more necessary – You are the nearest to her & must make the most severe sacrifices. Sutherland & Dr Farr & I may see her safely – when you must tremble & stay away.'

Undoubtedly, it suited Florence to be able to control her mother and sister's visits, with all their potential for unwarranted interruption and upset, and in that sense she did exploit her ill-health to protect herself from them. The inordinate fuss that ensued, on at least one occasion in the late 1850s, when Mary Bratby, the steward's wife, gave Parthenope the impression that Florence was well enough to see her – in spite of Aunt Mai's insistence to the contrary – shows that she was probably wise to do so. But the situation regarding her family wasn't generally as calculated as this makes it sound. Florence was genuinely ill and anxious to conserve her time for her work, something she repeatedly emphasized to her family. 'If I could give companionship or receive it,' she wrote affectionately to her mother in January 1858, 'I would beg you to come and share it with me.' Often, over the next couple of decades, she was to refuse to receive many other visitors, some of whom, like her old friends Madame Mohl and Louisa Ashburton, she was eager to see. Sophia, the liberal intellectual Queen of the Netherlands, General Gordon, whose work Florence considered unique, and William Rathbone, the Liverpool philanthropist with whom she collaborated on workhouse nursing, were all, at some point, turned away. Gladstone twice made 'an unnecessary call' at her door. The first time she had to put him off because of another appointment; on the second occasion, in 1884, when he was Prime Minister, she could not see him, despite her longing to discuss Indian policy, as she was ill in bed 'with inflammation of the eyes'.

Other aspects of her life were deliberately curtailed. Florence gave

up church attendance for good in 1857, though, given her dislike of
the Church of England, it is unlikely that she much regretted the loss.
She continued to practise her observance in private, and to receive the
sacrament in her room. Music, one of the great pleasures of her youth,
was a greater sacrifice. The singer Clara Novello came to sing privately
for her in 1860, which was 'a treat', but she found listening to piano music,
even her beloved Mendelssohn, especially nerve-racking. She rarely ventured out. Five minutes on the pavement outside the Burlington after 'a
hard day' often sufficed. Occasional drives in invalid carriages, designed
to protect the passenger from being thrown about on uneven road surfaces, left her 'much fatigued' and 'panting for breath'. In May 1858 she
went home to Embley, her final visit for eight years. She didn't return to
Lea Hurst until 1867. At the end of 1857, she went back to Malvern for
the water-cure, and returned in the summer and autumn of 1858, and
again in early 1859, but then not subsequently until 1867.

In the absence of knowledge about her condition, Florence's doctors
were able to prescribe little more for her than bed rest, and it was to her
bed that she increasingly retreated to work, unable to find a sofa that
would allow her, as she put it, 'to do something' other than simply
lolling about ('Stuffing not springy but too much stuffed – throws the
Patient up upon a hillock,' she noted critically of one sofa recommended
by Parthenope). With the onset of severe spinal pain in 1861, Florence
was seen in consultation by Dr Charles Edouard Brown-Sequard, the
leading spine specialist of the day, who diagnosed 'congestion of the
spine', caused by constant worry. But again, all he could advise was rest,
together with a moratorium on her incessant letter-writing, which was
obviously out of the question. When the pain became so intolerable that
she was unable to work, Florence accepted the temporary relief afforded
by subcutaneous opium, though she complained that it muddled her
brain and made it difficult for her to concentrate.*

---

* She made the same complaint of the spirit chloroform that she sometimes took in the
1880s, and of the bromide which she was prescribed during the same period. In the course
of earlier attacks she had sometimes relied on morphia to induce sleep. A letter written by
Florence to Dr Lauder Brunton, in December 1887, thanking him for arranging her 'first
séance from your Swedish Masseuse', and mentioning the bromide prescription, provoked
sensational headlines like 'Sexy Florence and mystery masseuse' when it surfaced in Britain
in 1996. These headlines conveniently overlooked the fact that the masseuse was employed
to alleviate Florence's back pain, and that in the nineteenth century bromide was often taken
as a sedative, quite apart from its use as a drug to curb the sexual libido.

One inevitable consequence of Florence's lack of exercise was the loss of her slim figure. Mary Mohl, visiting her for the first time for three years, in the autumn of 1861, was surprised to find that she had grown 'fat, which is I believe no good sign, in so abstemious a person'. Five years later, in a portrait by the artist G. F. Watts, Florence was shockingly unrecognizable, her face puffy and swollen, with a look of searing pain written across her features. Watts hoped to include Florence in his series of portraits of famous contemporaries, which he had begun sporadically to paint, and made his approach through Parthenope. Reluctant as Florence was to sit for him, she caved in under pressure from her sister, though she appears to have given Watts at most only two sittings, leaving him eventually to abandon the study as unfinished.

Her personality was being transformed as surely as the contours of her face. As a young woman, so later family opinion went, Florence had been 'touching'. This left unspoken the implied sequel that in middle age she had become increasingly querulous, demanding and difficult. Already, in the autumn of 1857, Aunt Mai observed that Florence's manner was 'often cold & dry, some might say cross', though she also expressed her amazement that, in the circumstances, there was not 'more revulsion & irritation'. Whether this change was a product of Florence's general incarceration and social isolation, or of the chronic form of brucellosis from which she was suffering, which often brings irritability and depression in its wake, and can have serious repercussions on the personality – or a result of both these factors – it's impossible to say. Florence herself later remarked that '. . . the main part of the suffering of a long illness is the morbid mind of a person who has no variety, no amusement, no gratification or change of any kind'.

Conversations with her father, on his rare visits to London, were a pleasure she did not forgo. Florence 'was only too full of talk for a good hour by the clock', William Nightingale wrote after one of their meetings, confessing that he had been unable to resist staying, 'so interesting was her general review of many subjects', though he feared that she probably suffered for the exertion afterwards. He noticed how Florence's solitude 'tells upon her more & more', and that she was also 'maledicting Sutherland rather more (if possible) than usual'. At the sight of her 'weak footsteps', he fought hard to disguise his grief. 'Who shall write the epitaph of a woman working in silent majesty,' he wondered aloud, early in 1859, 'without a soul to mark her bravery in death

or life, without stimulant, without reward, expectant only of still harder
work . . . in the wide fields of God's vast creations?'

———

The scope of that work, relentlessly pursued, with manifold projects
always being tackled simultaneously, is one of the most remarkable
aspects of the second half of Florence Nightingale's life, made all the
more extraordinary by the fact that such a workload would have
defeated most able-bodied individuals, let alone, one would have
thought, someone suffering the effects of a chronic and debilitating
illness. Her reforming mission was to encompass a wide range of issues
across the public health spectrum, including Army and civilian health
in Britain and India, hospital design, as well as nursing reform. Underlying them all is a single unifying theme: a personal worldview of
disease, centring on its relationship to the individual, and on his or her
moral responsibility for dealing with the threat that disease poses to
human life.

This worldview was of dual origin. Fundamental to it was a belief in
the primary role of the atmosphere in causing disease. Florence adhered
to a miasmatic theory of transmission, according to which certain airborne poisons, or miasmata, when inhaled into the lungs caused disease.
There was much that remained mysterious about the process, but
Thomas Southwood Smith, miasmatist and leading sanitarian of the
early Victorian period, offered one compact explanation: 'The immediate, or exciting cause of fever, is a poison formed by the corruption or
the decomposition of organic matter. Vegetable and animal matter,
during the process of putrefaction, give off a principle, or give origin to
a new compound, which, when applied to the human body, produces
the phenomena constituting fever.' For Florence this belief went hand-in-
hand with a commitment to the type of policies of public hygiene that
had dominated Britain in the 1840s, through which Edwin Chadwick's
programme of removing filth, reducing overcrowding, and promoting
cleanliness would be transferred from its urban and industrial environment to a new setting of urban hospitals and their patients. Florence
had studied Chadwick's famous report linking unsanitary living to the
prevalence of disease among the poor when it first appeared in 1842
(interestingly around the time that Chadwick himself became a member
of the Nightingales' London circle). She had even introduced new openings for light and air in certain rooms at Embley in the early 1850s,

as a minor domestic response to the sanitarians' insistence on proper ventilation. But ultimately it took the calamity at Scutari to convince her of the crucial importance of sanitary doctrines, and of the deadly consequences of overlooking or ignoring them. After the war, Florence and Chadwick began to correspond. She sought statistical data from him for the army report, and recruited his services for publicizing its findings, while remaining wary of Chadwick's tendency to aggravate situations through his antagonism to those who did not share his opinions. He encouraged her, as 'the great national nurse', to use her standing to promote sanitary measures for the prevention of disease.

Aside from perceptions about its effectiveness in combating disease, sanitary reform was bound to appeal to Florence on an additional level. Put simply, it offered the individual an opening for personal action in a way that by definition contagionism, and later, germ theory, simply could not. Contagion, assumed at mid-century to involve the transmission of disease by touch, seemed alarmingly random, and embodied a threat to a programme of pragmatic reform intent on pursuing a link between sickness and contamination of the environment by poisonous gases. The implications of contagion for treatment, by quarantining infected patients, specifically denied the role of personal responsibility in the prevention of disease. 'Were "contagion" a fact,' Florence asserted, 'what would be its lesson? To isolate and fly from the fever and cholera patient, and leave him to die; to kill the cattle; instead of improving the conditions of either.' Miasmatism, on the other hand, entailed practical lessons consistent with Florence's belief that mankind is called to discover the workings of God's laws, thereby actively encouraging the promotion of vigorous measures to remove conditions of dirt, overcrowding, and 'foulness of every kind'. 'Do you believe that God's word is not "pray" but "work",' she asked her father in March 1857. 'Do you believe that He stops the fever, in answer not to "from plague, pestilence and famine, good Lord, deliver us," but to His word and thought being carried out in a drain, a pipe tile, a wash house?'

From this it followed that Florence was resistant to the claims, advanced increasingly as the laboratory replaced the hospital as the major source of medical knowledge, that diseases had specific causes, and could therefore be subjected to standardized treatments. She believed, for instance, that even smallpox, long regarded atypically as a contagious disease, could be bred in the stagnant air of a closed room.

It was wrong, she said, to look upon diseases as separate things, like cats and dogs. Rather, we should consider them 'as conditions, like a dirty and clean condition, and just as much under our control'. Like Chadwick before her, Florence emphasized that sanitary knowledge was not a part of medicine. On the contrary, it was knowledge that everyone ought to have, 'distinct from medical knowledge, which only a profession can have'. She was in any case generally critical of the medical profession for treating diseases that had already developed rather than seeking to prevent illness arising in the first place. 'Medicine does not cure,' she once wrote. 'It is only Nature that cures.' Here the nurse stepped in to play her vital role in the scheme, ensuring that patients were in the best possible condition for nature's cure to take effect, through the proper use of fresh air, light, and cleanliness, and the introduction of a good diet. This was a system in which disease existed not as a separate entity, but as a state of disequilibrium, with the human body as a dynamic organism constantly interacting with its environment.

Florence's ideas were practical, not scientific, as she often said, almost revelling in the distinction. Essentially, she was unconcerned with the finer points of medical theory. In common with other sanitarians, offering guidance to the public and campaigning against official policies like quarantine for fear that they might reverse sanitary advances in public health, she relied on rhetoric and clearly stated advice of a practical bent – 'All foul smell indicates disease' being one notable example – to press her message home. Men with theories, she dismissed as 'mere weeds occupying the ground and preventing useful vegetation . . .' The more scientifically inclined in her circle, like William Farr, sometimes despaired of this attitude. While unwavering in his commitment to sanitary reform, Farr refused to 'fanaticize' about it, and had for some years assigned a large role to contagionism in the causation of disease. Discussing quarantine with Florence, in a letter of 1859, he asked her not to 'Chadwickize', and to try to be scientific. She displayed not a trace of moderation in her response: '. . . I do not venture to argue with you – because, as you say, I am not scientific . . . I only modestly & really humbly say, I never saw a fact adduced in favour of contagion which would bear scientific enquiry. And I could name to you men whom you would acknowledge as scientific who would place "contagion" on the same footing as witch-craft & other superstitions.'

It is hardly surprising then to find that Florence opposed the new germ theory – or perhaps one should say 'germ theories', given the bewildering number of views about what disease-germs were that proliferated in the period following the pioneering work of Pasteur, Lister and others in the 1860s. This opposition, or at least position of serious doubt, was shared by many of Florence's medical contemporaries. In 1864, the *British Medical Journal* observed that the great majority of doctors still believed that 'sundry disease poisons' were spontaneously generated 'by the material conditions which surround us'. It was, after all, to be another fifteen years before Robert Koch's landmark paper, 'The Etiology of Traumatic Infectious Diseases', appeared, in 1879, finally confirming that germs cause disease. Evidence, in the form of a chapter that Florence wrote in the late 1870s for *Quain's Medical Dictionary*, first published in 1882, in which she urges nurses to use antiseptic precautions (the use of chemicals against germs), suggests that it was at about this time that she came to accept germ theory. She continued, though, to worry about the complacency that germ theory might induce, and advocated that public health authorities should emphasize the impact of bad sanitation in causing the different strains of bacteria.

Without recourse to the correct theory, many of Florence's practical suggestions about hygiene and cleanliness had, of course, eliminated germs in the course of removing 'filth'. Her methods, therefore, must have often proved effective, though they were rooted in what would come to be seen as an outdated framework.

One decisive victory for the sanitarians, and for Florence in particular, lay in the field of hospital design. She lost the battle over the new military hospital at Netley, despite strenuous efforts to get the building halted, including the orchestration of a major press campaign against it, in the summer of 1858. The massive frontage, and vast central hall and dome, merely disguised the fact that Netley was a traditional corridor hospital with all the sanitary defects common to structures of its kind. Its many small rooms, leading off a single continuous corridor, with windows on one side only, the placing of bath and WCs in between rooms, and its marshy site, with ten square miles of mud, were all condemned; while the report on the health of the Army concluded that the small size of the wards would result in it costing as much money to nurse the sick efficiently in them as had already been spent on the site and the works.

Netley, Lord Palmerston said, exemplified a hospital where the care of the patient had been sacrificed to the vanity of the architect, who had designed a building intended to cut a dash when looked at from Southampton Water. None the less, although Palmerston intervened over Panmure's head, recommending that Netley should be pulled down and rebuilt, financial rectitude finally asserted itself after Panmure protested that the abandonment of the plan would cost over £70,000. Florence was given the opportunity to suggest ways of correcting defects by widening corridors and increasing the number of windows, and the 1,000-bed hospital opened in 1863 (its administrators, meanwhile, answered critics by saying that, in peacetime at any rate, Netley would be largely a convalescent hospital, with a large proportion of its patients out of bed for most of the time).

In the eyes of Florence and other protesters, the opportunity to build a large-scale military hospital, on up-to-date sanitary lines, had been squandered. But the principle of hospitals designed according to the pavilion style, with separate wings to prevent the spread of infection, and the positioning of windows on opposite sides of the ward to permit natural cross-ventilation, was established. It was enshrined in the report of the Royal Commission, and carried by Florence and her collaborators, with the ringing fervency of a new gospel, into the hearts of the medical and architectural professions. The military hospital which began construction at Woolwich in 1859, later known as the Herbert Military Hospital, was the first large-scale pavilion hospital to be completed in England. This drew its inspiration from the Lariboisière Hospital in Paris, opened in 1854, and often commended by Florence as one of the best hospitals in existence. However, whereas the Lariboisière had an artificial heating and ventilation system imposed on it at a late stage, causing serious problems of airborne cross-infection, the Herbert depended on a natural supply of air. For Florence, supervising the hospital's design, the issue of ventilation was paramount. Ideally a provision of at least 2,500 cubic feet of fresh air per bed was to be allowed 'to keep the wards perfectly sweet'. She was unable to forget the lesson of the Barrack Hospital at Scutari, before the arrival of the Sanitary Commission, when scarcely anything had been done about the flow of air, 'not even as much as breaking a pane of glass in the privies'.

The Herbert rapidly evolved into the model for civil as well as military hospitals, proclaiming the pavilion principle throughout the world, and

ensuring its dominance in British hospital design until well into the
twentieth century. Florence's influence in making the pavilion plan the
icon of all new hospital design was bolstered by the support of two other
leading campaigners, George Godwin and John Roberton. Godwin,
editor of *The Builder*, seized the chance to popularize its principles in
the pages of his professional journal of the architectural and building
world, while Roberton, a Manchester obstetrician and old ally of Chadwick's, also contributed articles on the application of sanitary science
to medical institutions. Florence's own initial contributions to the subject
appeared anonymously in this 'discreet little paper', as she called it,
'which always puts me in'. In October 1858, two papers by her on
hospital construction were presented at a meeting of the National Association for the Promotion of Social Science in Liverpool. She made Uncle
Sam read one of the papers out loud in a trial run beforehand. 'It was
longer than the <u>sacred</u> time [twenty minutes],' she told Chadwick, who
was presenting both her papers and his own, rather prolix effort, to the
Association. 'So I remodelled it and cut it in two – <u>You</u> should cut yours
in three.'

These papers, together with Florence's evidence before the Royal
Commission, and three articles by her from *The Builder*, were published
in 1859 as *Notes on Hospitals*. A second edition followed later the
same year, and a third, enlarged and substantially rewritten, in 1863.
Concentrating on the fresh air, light and ample space she considered
essential for a reformed hospital, she contrasted the pavilion model with
the defective arrangements in existing hospitals. Pre-reform hospitals
were often built on retentive clay subsoils, which impeded drainage.
Their wards were overcrowded by as much as three or four times
Florence's stated maximum of thirty-two beds, with beds placed along
'dead' walls, so that no light or air supply could reach them. The floors,
walls and ceilings were made of non-absorbent materials and, as a result,
streamed with damp and fungus. Florence's first enunciated principle of
hospital construction was the division of the sick among separate pavilions, each with its own nurses' rooms, ward sculleries, and lavatories
and baths (sometimes incorporated into 'sanitary towers' at the end of
the wards), and unconnected to the administrative offices except by
'light airy passages or corridors'. Advice for interior design reflected
the overriding concern with sanitation. Parian cement for walls was
recommended for a smooth, impervious surface, and oak, waxed,

polished, and closely fitted, for the floors. Large spacious wards supplied another prerequisite of hospital order: the absence of 'skulking' places. Nurses and ward attendants should be able to see their patients at a glance. Hospitals were still to be regarded as places in which nefarious deeds might run riot without the imposition of surveillance and discipline. Florence was therefore later to insist that morally contaminating venereal patients required 'a head nurse of the utmost strength of character . . . to prevent assignations for further vice by these wicked women under her very nose'.

On its first, abbreviated, appearance in book form, *Notes on Hospitals* was immediately greeted by George Godwin as essential reading for architects, who were advised to 'obtain the volume and master it'. Publication brought Florence a stream of requests from architects, hospitals and local authorities consulting her about hospital construction, and one from the King of Portugal, who wanted to build a hospital in Lisbon, in memory of his wife. They received her views, she observed, 'as from the mouth of an oracle'. William Butterfield, the architect chosen to design the Royal Hampshire County Hospital at Winchester, was among those who approached her. She thought that he had planned 'a model hospital', but offered some criticisms. For instance, she did not like his small day room for nurses, which she felt resembled 'the parlour of a discreditable public house', and, in line with her resistance to theory, made it clear that she did not support the idea of a room for one Winchester doctor to pursue his 'microscopic investigations'. Gilbert Scott's designs for Leeds General Infirmary were the first application of the pavilion principle to a large-scale voluntary general hospital. Florence surveyed his proposals and issued instructions for thirty patients per ward, and a ward height of sixteen to eighteen feet. Unfortunately, her estimate of costs was wildly out. She had suggested a likely cost of £100 per bed. It turned out to be closer to £400. On a smaller scale, she was also involved in the designs for the Buckinghamshire General Infirmary, in Aylesbury, which, with its 'in-line', two-storey configuration of blocks, formed an early model for the small pavilion hospital.

Notes on Hospitals' 'terse phrases', according to the *Lancet*, provided a welcome change from the 'brown-suited dullness' of other books on the subject. The 1863 edition carried a preface with an opening couple of sentences that instantly arrest the reader's attention: 'It may seem a strange principle to enunciate as the very first requirement in a hospital that it should do the sick no harm. It is quite necessary, nevertheless, to lay down such a principle, because the actual mortality *in* hospitals, especially in those of large cities, is very much higher than any calculation founded on the mortality of the same class of diseases among patients treated *out* of hospital would lead us to expect.' Those calculations, however, based on Florence's inclusion in the third edition of the mortality rates in 106 English hospitals, derived from the tabulated results of forms specially designed by her, provoked controversy among the medical and surgical staffs of the London hospitals. They denied that metropolitan hospitals could be fairly compared with the provincial variety, dealing as they did with more serious cases, and serving a population in poorer general health.

More damaging was the critical reaction to Florence's dogmatic anti-contagionism in the later version of *Notes on Hospitals*. The idea of isolating infectious patients in smaller wards, especially the separation of surgical and general wards, continued to be resisted by her. Patients, she maintained, preferred 'a full large ward and think it "so cheerful"', and accidents and operations were better nursed in a single ward. If such views hadn't been promulgated by a lady, said the *Medical Times*, they would have required 'rough treatment'; while the *Lancet* compared Florence to a brave soldier who refused to think about, and even scorned, the dangers that he had passed unharmed.

———

'In England we ferret out abuses & leave them in the blue book.' This, William Nightingale had feared, might be the fate of the Royal Commission on the Health of the Army. Back in the late summer and early autumn of 1857, Panmure had procrastinated. He was torn between committing the Government to immediate reform in anticipation of the Report's publication – which might help appease public reaction to it – and giving in to reactionary elements within the War Office who were gearing up to fight every recommendation tooth and nail. One thing was certain. With post-Crimean feeling about the suffering of British troops continuing to run high, the Report, and especially its major contention that mortality in the Army was considerably greater than that of the civilian male population of the same age, possessed the power to provoke outrage and inflict incalculable damage on Palmerston's Government. Sidney Herbert urged Panmure to publish the Report, and the details of the proposed reforms derived from it, simultaneously. Florence, returning to a frenetic pace of work after her time in Malvern, once more railed against Panmure's 'unmanly & stupid indifference', and drafted – and then redrafted – the regulations for the four sub-commissions which were awaiting final approval. These sub-commissions were to put the Army barracks in sanitary order; establish a statistical department for the Army; institute an Army Medical School; and restructure the Army Medical Department, revise the hospital regulations, and draw up a warrant for the promotion of medical officers. This last, and most far-reaching of the four, known as the 'Wiping Commission', not surprisingly caused the most soul-searching at the War Office as Panmure first revoked, and then reinstated it at Herbert's insistence. By December 1857, everything was set, and each of the four sub-commissions granted. All that was necessary now, Florence told Sir John McNeill, was 'to keep Mr Herbert up to the point'. The strength of his character, she declared, lay in its 'simplicity and candour' and 'extreme quickness of perception'. But she faulted him on his 'excessive eclecticism', and complained that 'Ten years have I been endeavouring to obtain an expression of opinion from him & have never succeeded yet.'

As expected, the publication of the Report, at the beginning of February 1858, produced widespread press interest in its findings. *The Times* accused the Horse Guards of a neglect 'which could hardly be exceeded under any Government, however indifferent to human life'. There was little doubt 'that the chief cause of the evil is the deficient accommodation and the consequent overcrowding in barracks . . . the closeness, the dirt, the indecency spoken of remind one of a slave-ship more than of a place for English soldiers to inhabit . . .' Less than a fortnight later, Palmerston's unexpected resignation following his Government's defeat over the Conspiracy Bill placed a momentary question mark over the future for reform. Panmure was gone, just when he was most needed, and as part of Lord Derby's incoming administration, General Jonathan Peel (another brother of the former Prime Minister) was appointed to succeed him as Secretary for War. In spite of this, it proved a smooth transition. In the Commons, on 10 May, Herbert defended the Derby Government against the charge of having 'fooled' away money on barracks and hospitals, and demonstrated how great an economy could be achieved by keeping the soldier in good health. Two days later, Lord Ebrington, a supporter of Chadwick's and a former secretary to the

THORN IN THE FLESH

Poor Law Board, especially selected for the task by Herbert and Florence, moved resolutions based on the Army Report, calling attention to the high mortality in the barracks caused by their poor sanitary condition. His remarks were resoundingly cheered.

This was very encouraging, and Florence allowed herself some cautious optimism. But as the sub-commissions pressed ahead with their work, she mounted a second line of attack, this time in the pages of the quarterlies and reviews. 'Not because it signifies a farthing now . . .,' she had explained to Herbert in March, but because it was essential to maintaining momentum for reform in the future. She earmarked J. T. Howell to summarize the Commission's findings in the *Edinburgh Review* (the editor, Henry Reeve, was the widower of her old friend Hope Richardson), and for the *Quarterly* hoped to retain the services of Chadwick himself (though, in the end, it was Andrew Wynter, a popular essayist on medical topics, who contributed the article on 'The Lodging, Food, and Dress of Soldiers'). For the *Westminster Review*, the flagship of radical freethinking, she turned to Herbert himself, though, thinking him somewhat dilatory, she felt forced to chivvy him to finish his piece. Herbert's article, 'The Sanitary Reform of the British Army', published, in a departure from usual practice, with his initials, appeared in January 1859, and bears the clear impress of Florence's mind. After replying to the statistician, G. P. Nelson, who had challenged the Report by arguing against overcrowding as explanation for high mortality, substituting 'want of exercise' in its place, Herbert concluded that any further delay in implementing its findings would be not just a loss, but a sin.

Florence remained steadfastly in the background. She was the engine driving the machine forward, but her anonymity remained as important to her as ever. 'I had much rather that you had no chivalrous ideas about what is "due" to me,' she wrote to Herbert after he had proposed mentioning her efforts for Army health in plans he was drawing up for the distribution of the Nightingale Fund. '. . . Whatever of information your own judgement has accepted from me will come with far greater force from yourself . . . I had much rather therefore that any mention of my late occupations were left out – not from any modesty or candour, but simply from a feeling of what is best for the troops.' Her personal contributions to driving the campaign home included her *Mortality of the British Army*, a pamphlet compiled from her diagrams and statistical data reproduced in the Report, 2,000 copies of which were printed and circulated to the Queen, other members of the royal family, ministers, MPs, and medical and commanding officers in Britain, India and the colonies. She also dusted off her *Notes . . . on the British Army*, lying unread in its lilac binding since its printing in the final months of 1857, and distributed it among a corresponding range of public figures. Harriet Martineau, who had not met Florence since the latter was a child, but with whom there was 'a tie' through Aunt Julia and Hilary Bonham Carter, was among the influential recipients of this 'confidential' report, which she described as 'one of the most remarkable political or social productions ever seen'. Martineau drew on it for a series of leaders in the *Daily News* at the beginning of 1859; and then, later the same year, used it with Florence's approval as the basis for her book, *England and Her Soldiers*, a popular account of the Commission's results, which reproduced Florence's pioneering 'coxcombs'. Once held in reserve as a weapon to brandish against the delaying tactics of Government ministers, the *Notes*, in Martineau's treatment, would reach a wide readership. However, there could be no question of betraying the work's confidentiality. The pretence agreed between the two women was that Martineau's book was based on extracts from public documents, even though material from the *Notes* had been used for background information. 'The book is to be mine, as to form, style, & responsibility in every literary sense,' Martineau told Henry Reeve, 'but F.N. is (at my request) to see the whole, in order to preclude mistakes of fact, & to keep me informed of the latest movements.' Florence supplemented Martineau's meagre payment from her publishers, Smith, Elder, partially offset expenses by providing Martineau with the printer's blocks so that they could be reused, advised on the price and quantity of books printed, and paid to have copies of the book placed in soldiers' reading rooms across the country. How great a hand she had in the final text, it is difficult to say. It is probably no coincidence, however, that the Florence Nightingale of *England and Her Soldiers* is light years removed from the sentimental individual of popular myth. Indeed, at times she appears as a helpless participant in the ongoing drama rather than its ministering angel. Moreover, unlike the Royal Commission's Report, Martineau's résumé of the catastrophe makes no bones about the fact that Florence's own Barrack Hospital at Scutari had been the worst ventilated of any British hospital in Turkey or the Crimea.

While not formally a member of any of the four sub-commissions, Florence participated in the day-to-day work of all of them, and 'the cabal' continued to congregate regularly at the Burlington. '. . . We could have a Barrack meeting in the morning and a Statistical one if Farr's papers are ready in the afternoon,' Herbert wrote to her in March 1858. A significant early triumph was the appointment in June of that year of one of their number, Dr Thomas Alexander, to the position of Director-General of the Army Medical Department in succession to Andrew Smith (the sense of victory would be short-lived, as Alexander died suddenly in early 1860). In June 1859, the return of Palmerston to power brought Herbert himself back to the Government as Secretary for War. This was 'a great national benefit', Florence wrote to Liz Herbert, while wondering whether she should really offer congratulations as 'I am afraid he has inefficient servants, a disorganized department and a silly commander-in-chief [the Duke of Cambridge, who had insisted that the British soldier hadn't been neglected in the past, but was simply more appreciated by the present].' She was right that the War Office was cumbrous, weighed down by bureaucratic convention and overly concerned with pettifogging detail. She viewed Sir Benjamin Hawes, Permanent Under-Secretary to the department, as the chief culprit of official opposition to reform, in particular to changes in the Army Medical Department, and, as usual when she had someone in her sights, there was a vein of exaggeration in her pronouncements. Hawes may not have been quite the blinkered reactionary of Florence's portrayal. He had, after all, been responsible for commissioning his brother-in-law, Isambard Kingdom Brunel, to design the war hospital at Renkioi, which, in its adherence to sanitary principles, was a precursor of the later pavilion model. Hawes was as anxious as Florence to wrest domination of the Army away from the Horse Guards clique. Equally, though, he was unprepared to see control of Army medicine handed over in its place to a cabal outside Government centring on the Lady-in-Chief, as Florence was known, and members of the Royal Commission.

As far as the health of the Army was concerned, Herbert's tenure of office produced mixed results in the period leading up to his presentation before Parliament of the reports of the four sub-commissions in April 1861. One unquestioned achievement was the reorganization of Army medical statistics, which had struck Florence forcibly as an important objective since Crimean days. With Farr as one of its three-man team, this sub-commission oversaw the setting up of a statistical branch of the Army Medical Department. Within a short time British medical statistics had become the most reliable of any in Europe. The situation regarding barrack and hospital improvement was less clear-cut (as we have already seen in the arguments over Netley). Between 1858 and 1861 this sub-commission, later reconstituted on a permanent basis as the Army Sanitary Committee, visited every barrack and army hospital in Britain, reporting on structural improvements to ventilation, sewage disposal, water supplies and washing facilities. Its findings revealed the scale of the task that confronted them, from the provision of the minimum 600 cubic feet of space per man in barracks and guardrooms, to arrangements for separate marital accommodation, and the removal of urine tubs from barrack rooms. Expenditure upon construction, enlargement and repair of barracks, which had expanded six-fold to £726,841 by 1859–60, shows the commitment with which these problems were tackled. Even so, by 1861, following its inspection of 108 barracks and fifty-eight hospitals, 30 per cent of barracks and 10 per cent of hospitals remained without adequate ventilation. These figures reflect the fact that, for all the pressure exerted by the reformers, the sense of urgency had been lost within just a few years, as other priorities supervened. As Secretary of State, Herbert ensured that works were carried out according to the principles laid down by the Royal Commission, but he could do little to overcome the Treasury's resistance to sustained financing of barrack improvements. '. . . A cry for economy has become audible,' Gladstone, the Chancellor of the Exchequer, told Herbert in January 1861, and in the course of the next decade, expenditure on barracks began to be run down significantly. Interest in barrack reform only revived in the late 1870s, when a serious outbreak of enteric fever at Dublin's Royal Barracks once again provoked questions about the conditions under which troops were housed in Britain.

One of the members of the barrack sub-commission was Douglas Galton, a leading Royal Engineer, who was the Army's expert on matters as diverse as the application of iron to railway structures, the laying of underwater telegraph cables, and sanitary engineering in the construction of barracks and hospitals (he designed the Herbert Hospital at Woolwich). Galton also happened to be married to Florence's cousin, Marianne. Marriage had improved Marianne, though she was still capable on occasion of 'a nasty little sneer' at 'the mysterious proceedings of the lady Flo' (the Galtons' London home in Chester Street, rather oddly, had a room set aside for prints of Florence portrayed in heroic mould, nursing the wounded at Scutari, and surveying Sebastopol from Cathcart's Heights). Beginning in the spring of 1858, and stretching across the next four decades, Douglas Galton was in regular contact with Florence, absorbed into her circle as he advised on innumerable subjects connected with the War Office, hospitals and sanitary improvements. Florence became godmother to the Galtons' daughter Gwendolen, scribbled messages of 'best love' to Marianne at the foot of letters to her husband, but otherwise kept this, perhaps unwelcome, reminder of the past at a firm distance.

The two remaining sub-commissions accomplished reform with varying degrees of success. An Army Medical School was founded at Chatham in 1858 to provide four months' instruction for all Army doctors in the treatment of gunshot wounds, tropical diseases, and other subjects relating to military hygiene and sanitation, though the first students arriving there discovered that the War Office had failed to authorize payment for their instruments. It was later moved to Netley, in the face of Florence's stringent opposition, where it established a European reputation (she did ensure that Edmund Parkes, a former supporter of hers from Renkioi, was appointed Professor of Military Hygiene). Nevertheless, in 1876 the War Office proposed the school's abolition in order to make money available for an increase in the pay of Army doctors, and only canvassing by Florence and Sutherland of the then Secretary of State, Gathorne Hardy, managed to avert its closure. The Army Medical Department was reorganized and a new warrant issued for Army medical officers, but Florence's hopes of attracting better doctors to the service stumbled on problems of pay and professional status which did not match those accorded combatant officers. As a result, recruitment dropped sharply.

By the end of the century, despite these setbacks, an extraordinary improvement had taken place in the health of the British Army. The comparison between civilian and Army mortality was now reversed, to the detriment of civilian health. Examining the statistics in the annual reports of the Army Medical Department, which she had worked so hard to establish, Florence would have observed an almost continuous steady decline, in the decades after 1857, in the rate of mortality from accident and disease throughout the entire service. A decade before her death, mortality in the ranks had declined to a rate of four or five men per 1,000 each year.

Sidney Herbert, Florence later wrote, should be remembered 'as the first War Minister who ever seriously set himself the task of saving life . . .' Her own part in securing the health of the Army was no less crucial. In 1860, prayers 'on behalf of Florence Nightingale, now dangerously ill', were offered in all the garrison chapels in England. Most ordinary soldiers must have thought they were praying for a lady with a lamp whose memory was already growing as dim and distant as the shadow that had once flickered on the walls of the Barrack Hospital. They were unlikely to have been aware of the far-reaching consequences of her role in instituting reform.

In the summer of 1857, as the sheets of Florence's *Notes . . . on the British Army* passed through the press, news reached London of the 'lamentable occurrences' taking place in India: the eruption of the Great Revolt, or Indian Mutiny, challenging British rule in India. As accounts emerged of the horrifying casualties from the defence of Lucknow, '4 Ladies' were reported as having gone to India to nurse, following 'the example of Miss Nightingale'. That autumn, as Florence struggled to regain her health at Malvern, she wrote to Lady Canning, now Vicereine of India, saying she would come out to India, at twenty-four hours' notice, if there was 'anything for her to do in her "line of business"'. She was quickly dissuaded from pursuing the idea further. For a start, she was clearly in too weak a state for such a major undertaking, while Sidney Herbert and Sir John McNeill pointed out how much the Royal Commission would suffer without her presence in London.

But the seed of a new idea, and a new commission to inquire into the conditions of the British Army in India, had been planted, and was starting to expand in her mind. For 'a great deal may be done to diminish the disease & mortality in a large army of occupation by which we must hereafter hold our Indian Empire . . .,' she wrote in the postscript to her *Notes*. The problems connected to the health of a whole sub-continent were slowly opening before her.

14. Dying by Inches

In the latter half of 1857, a tall, spindly man in his mid-fifties became a persistent caller at the Burlington Hotel, asking to see Florence Nightingale. Sir Harry Verney of Claydon House, in Buckinghamshire, was the respected Liberal MP for Buckingham, and a widower with a large family. His wife Eliza had died earlier that year, and he was anxious to fulfil one of her final wishes, that their daughter should become personally acquainted with the heroine of the age. This was impossible. 'Poor F.,' noted Fanny Nightingale, 'has no time for the education of young ladies.' Sir Harry's visits to the Burlington were usually politely declined; Miss Nightingale was invariably not well enough to see him, and on the one occasion he was admitted to her quarters, he was able to observe for himself Florence's 'overwrought, careworn look of mental exertion'. Instead, he gravitated towards her parents and sister, whom he had met in the past at the home of the Bunsens. By the end of the year he was a regular guest at Embley, his presence there encouraged by his 'hot pursuit' of Parthenope. 'He woos like a soldier in haste as if he was just setting off for the wars,' her mother wrote, 'which rather alarms her.'

This military style of engagement was a product of his early background. In 1819, the year of Parthenope's birth, Harry Calvert, as he then was, had been in training as one of the first cadets at the Royal Military College, Sandhurst. He had resigned his commission with the Grenadier Guards at the age of twenty-three, and succeeded to the Calvert baronetcy on his father's death in 1826. The following year, he inherited the Verney estates at Claydon from his first cousin Catherine Wright, and changed his name to Verney under royal licence. Before settling down to the management of his inheritance, Sir Harry Verney embarked on a series of adventurous travels in South America, making a perilous journey across the Andes, and narrowly escaping death while helping to put down an insurrection at Santiago. Returning to England, he was elected, in 1832, to the Buckingham seat he was to hold, with two short interruptions, for the next half-century. His marriage, in 1836, to Eliza Hope produced four surviving children: Edmund, George, Emily and Frederick.

Harry Verney's intimacy with Parthenope began, innocently enough, when they read a passage from the Book of Isaiah together. Her health, he recognized, was delicate, but in other respects – 'her character, pursuits & education' – Parthenope reminded him of his late wife; moreover, he believed that she was the kind of woman his wife would have chosen as her successor. On her side, Parthenope liked Sir Harry's Liberal politics, shared his interest in the new biblical criticism, and was grateful for the reports on Florence's health that he prised from Aunt Mai and Dr Sutherland on trips to London. But she did not see herself as his future wife. At Christmas 1857 Sir Harry wore down her resistance, and had gone so far as to announce the news of her acceptance of his proposal to his brother and eldest son when, in the spring, Parthenope suddenly retracted her agreement and rejected him. She hadn't the feelings for him 'that would make it safe' for her to become his wife. Pressed further, she admitted fearing that Sir Harry's Evangelical beliefs might come between them. Unlike him, she could not believe in the doctrine of eternal punishment, and needed the freedom to worship God in her own way, otherwise she would feel 'like a bird in a cage'. He begged her not to give him up. 'Don't think of it,' he wrote, confessing that he had 'lost his heart' to her. Sir Harry's desperation, and the likelihood that he would make himself ill, began to sway her. In late April, or early May, Parthenope finally agreed to marry him.

Their marriage plans demanded a major readjustment on Parthenope's part. At thirty-nine, an age when most women had either long since married or accepted spinsterhood, she was to acquire what her father acknowledged was an 'independent existence', as mistress of her own home. The separation from her parents represented 'a sore struggle', as much on Mr Nightingale's part as her own, for, in the five years since Florence had left home, Parthenope had become his 'constant & much loved companion'. Even more disorienting was the recognition that becoming Sir Harry's wife implied a definitive break in her relationship with Florence. 'I never thought to marry any one but F,' she wrote to Mrs Gaskell, informing her of the engagement, 'but life has cut me off from her. I cannot help her now.' Mrs Gaskell's kindhearted response showed that Parthenope had been right to choose her as the recipient of her confidence. She had often wondered, she said, what future there would hold for one, 'whose life has been so long absorbed in care & thought for others', and expressed her relief that Parthenope was 'going to be loved & sympathized with', as someone's 'principal object'.

Before the engagement, Florence had unkindly dismissed Sir Harry as 'a pompous princess', but she soon had cause to revise her judgement, especially after she discovered that he had long been an enthusiastic participant in hospital reform, as a fundraiser for the county hospital established in his constituency at Aylesbury. In late 1857 she apologized for not being able to meet his daughter Emily, as she only saw people 'on business', but shared with him her views on the pavilion principle. By February 1858, when he visited her at Malvern to discuss hospital engineering, she told Sidney Herbert that he was 'ignorant but agog'. Soon, though, she began to find his judgement invaluable on numerous matters connected with the issues of reform in which she was interested, and declared that a search of all England might not find another man so worthy to be loved.

As a husband for Parthenope, one of Sir Harry's advantages in Florence's eyes was that he came with a ready-made family. Some of those Verney children, however, regarded their prospective stepmother with suspicion. Fifteen-year-old Emily seems initially to have been most hostile, though her father claimed that Parthenope mistook Emily's shyness for dislike. Edmund, the eldest, who, at nineteen, was pursuing a naval career, had seen action in the Crimean War, and was currently serving in India in the aftermath of the Mutiny, was more open about his fears concerning his father's second marriage. Supposing, he asked, Parthenope's 'mental qualities' turned out to resemble those of her sister? 'I have always suspected that Miss Florence Nightingale possesses, in addition to her kind and benevolent disposition, a strong and imperious mind,' Edmund warned his father; 'that under a gentle exterior, she is very self-willed, and also susceptible to strong prejudices.' Furthermore, he had heard differing reports of her religious opinions. A gentleman at Constantinople had confidently assured him that she was an atheist, while Mr Hill of Athens, with whom Florence had stayed in 1850, had given him 'an account of her diametrically opposed to this'. Emily Fremantle, Sir Harry's sister, who was married to the Vicar of Claydon, was alarmed about the Nightingales' Unitarian leanings, but was relieved to note that her future sister-in-law went to church, took communion, and 'agreed with us on the main points'.

In time Edmund would take to Parthenope 'as if he had known me all his life'. He was unable to reach home in time for the wedding, which took place at Claydon on 22 June 1858. It was a distinctly muted affair, 'befitting a pair of respectables of mature age': 'no honeymoon – trousseau – no wedding cake . . . no breakfast or splash of any description'. Florence, too unwell to make a journey outside London, sent a message of goodwill to her sister. 'God bless you, my dear Pop – and take my blessing and my best thoughts with you on your marriage day.' Sir Harry, having changed his name once in his lifetime, now considered a further alteration, that of adding Nightingale to Verney. The name would, of course, have to be 'Nightingale Verney rather than Verney Nightingale', he told Parthenope, pulling rank, the Verneys 'having owned my estate for 4 centuries & other lands in Derbyshire long before' (Sir Harry, of course, had no direct blood link to this earlier Verney line). Sensibly, Parthenope persuaded her husband to drop the idea.

The Verneys may have possessed a long pedigree, dating back to the 1460s when they first owned property in the village of Middle Claydon, but their house and lands had been subject to a period of long neglect. The house itself, the family seat since 1620, which had been substantially remodelled in the second half of the eighteenth century, was dilapidated and sparsely furnished. When Sir Harry arrived there in the 1820s, he had found family portraits by Lely and Van Dyck stacked in outhouses, with one painting fastened over a hole to keep out rats. Florence had described Sir Harry as rich, but in fact he was badly in need of funds to restore the house and continue with his programme of building and repairing cottages and farms on his estate. A thorough restoration of the house alone was estimated at £20,000, to which Parthenope's marriage settlement made a healthy contribution. Parthenope immediately started improvements to the part of the house occupied by the family, rescuing and identifying the portraits, and supervising the construction of a new library. She created 'a very delightful drawing room', her mother reported admiringly, 'by bunging into it sofas & chairs & tables & books innumerable'. And in the long gallery, at the top of the house, she started to examine the great mass of family papers, dating back to the fourteenth century. Among them, the seventeenth-century correspondence, the largest continuous private collection of the period in the world, would one day form the basis of Parthenope's classic study of the Verneys during the English Civil War.

With her marriage, as Fanny Nightingale observed, Parthenope's 'difficulties' were 'wonderfully cleared away'. She did indeed blossom. Her time was consumed by the management of a large household, and by Sir Harry's 'constant demand for her sympathy in all his pursuits', as well as by the beginnings of a writing career that would eventually encompass five novels, several historical works, and a number of articles on the social and religious questions of the day. It may have been during these early years of married life that Parthenope started to write a memoir of her younger sister. Certainly there are letters from this period, from various friends and acquaintances, urging her to write 'A life of your dear one', even though it must have been obvious that no such biography could appear in Florence's lifetime. The draft that survives today breaks off at the start of the Crimean War, but scattered notes of conversations with Florence about Scutari, and other research material, suggests that she intended to continue with it. Given the precarious state of Florence's health at the time, Parthenope may have conceived of it ultimately being published as a literary memorial to her sister. In a different sense, the memoir represents Parthenope's own farewell to a way of life that had been unhealthily centred on her sister's existence, whether as obstructive elder sibling, or devoted keeper of the flame. There appears to be recognition of this in Parthenope's opening sentence: 'I have lived too passionately in her life to get far enough off to make her picture.' It is unlikely that Florence would have approved of such a venture. 'Those female ink-bottles', as she called them, intent on collecting material for her biography, were her 'dread and despair'.

There was another way in which Parthenope believed she could memorialize Florence in the event of her sister's premature death, and that was by giving birth to a daughter to 'fill the void'. In the final months of 1858, Parthenope discovered that she was pregnant, but at the beginning of December, in the pregnancy's early stages, she suffered a miscarriage. The hope, which both she and Sir Harry had nurtured, of producing 'that little Flo', would never be fulfilled.

At the Burlington, Florence's seclusion continued. Hilary Bonham Carter was now often in attendance, allowing Aunt Mai an occasional opportunity to slip off to see her family, while Arthur Clough had become the equivalent of Florence's secretary and general factotum in his spare time from the Education Department. Introducing Hilary to their working routine, he recommended her to fit in a number of hours each day 'during which you will be understood to be occupied with your own affairs so that unless [Florence] sends for you during that time, she is not to expect to see you'. Aunt Mai remained strict on the point of admitting no visitors to the hotel suite unless they were specifically invited on business, so that even Hilary had to obtain special dispensation for her younger sister Elinor to pay her a visit. It was considered vital, in moving from her sitting room to her bedroom, that Florence shouldn't run the risk of coming upon some unexpected individual who might 'take off her feeling of quiet & necessity'.

From the spring of 1859, Florence's existence became more peripatetic. The Burlington was still her base, but a series of houses in Highgate and Hampstead provided a respite, often for weeks at a time, from the bustle of the city and tedium of hotel life. She would return to the Burlington for meetings, or, sometimes, Sidney Herbert, Sutherland and the others would ride out to see her. Florence took a short lease of West Hill Lodge in Highgate Rise, the first of these houses (belonging to the writers Mary and William Howitt) for April and May 1859; in the autumn of 1859, she resided at Montague Grove in Hampstead; in the winter of 1859–60, and again in the summer of 1861, she was at Oak Hill House, part of a new development, at 7 Oak Hill Park, in Frognal; and in the final months of 1860, she settled again in Hampstead, this time at 3 Upper Terrace. The scanty furnishings, the taste 'of the dust of centuries', and, in particular, the poor natural light, were constant sources of dissatisfaction, and Florence became convinced that this area of north London, damp, cold, and built on clay, was too unhealthy for a permanent home. One of its minor attractions, though, was that the donkey rides on Hampstead Heath offered amusement for younger visitors like Gwendoline Galton, who came to see Florence with her father, Douglas, and later, for Arthur and Blanche Clough's small children.

Fanny Nightingale, invited to Oak Hill Park to spend a day with her daughter for the first time in over six months, found Hilary downstairs sketching 'a striking woman', while upstairs, Florence was lying in bed with the window open and a fire blazing. Fanny was touched that '3 or 4 times when I got up to go', Florence 'put her hand upon me & made me sit down again, & when I did go, she insisted upon my coming again . . .' Florence's parents protested when they heard nothing of her for months, though not generally to any avail. Meanwhile, Fanny dispatched a stream of gifts, of pheasant, fruit and flowers to London, and responded dutifully whenever Florence asked her to provide hospitality at Lea Hurst or Embley for a co-worker or valued servant. A former housemaid of the Cloughs, for example, suffering from a prolapse of the womb, stayed five weeks with the Nightingale household in order that she might be treated by a Romsey doctor; while Robert Rawlinson, a member of the wartime sanitary commission whom Florence was consulting on barrack and hospital reform, spent a night at the Hurst on his way to a meeting in Liverpool. 'Pray forgive him for murdering the Queen's English,' Florence told her father, in anticipation of Rawlinson's arrival. 'I think it is so creditable to him; he was the son of a private soldier.' Realizing that her parents might deduce from her description that Rawlinson was 'a kind of foreman & that you would not know where he was to dine or sleep', she had to write hurriedly the next day to explain that 'He is just as much a gentleman as you or I.'

It was inevitable that, in her deepest troughs of depression, Florence should strike out verbally at those closest to her. She once accused her family of denying her 'one word of feeling . . . though I am sure they have never seen anyone strained to the utmost pitch of endurance and mind as I am', and another time wrote that Aunt Mai was 'unfeeling and unmanageable', despite the fact that it was Florence who deliberately kept their daily contact to a minimum. Arthur Clough was different. His help and sympathy appeared to admit no bounds. But then, Florence reflected, Clough was an angel, not a man. No task was regarded by Clough as too mundane, or as being beneath him. Settling bills, acting as a courier, checking train timetables and arranging transport from Malvern in an invalid carriage with 'noiseless wheels', changing her newspaper from the *Daily News* to *The Times* – everything was carried out with a dedicated efficiency. On one occasion at least his efforts on Florence's behalf went far beyond the call of duty. When Blanche was within days of giving birth to their second child, a daughter later named in Florence's honour, Clough was prepared to leave his wife's side, go down to Malvern, spend the night there, and return with Florence the next day, excusing himself from home on the grounds that there was 'no apparent reason to expect the event in our household just yet'. Such behaviour seems all the more extraordinary when considered in the light of Blanche's loss of their first baby, three years earlier.

Clough's willing enslavement to Florence Nightingale provoked posterity's ridicule in the earlier part of the twentieth century. In Lytton Strachey's *Eminent Victorians*, he was mocked for it, and famously portrayed tying up her brown paper parcels (a job he may not literally have undertaken, but which was well in keeping with the more ordinary of his occupations on Florence's behalf). Florence herself later confessed to the 'blundering harasses which were the uses to which we put him', and compared Clough to 'a race-horse harnessed to a coal-truck'. However, she offered no further clues to his underlying motivation beyond the observation that here was a man of rare mind and temper who gladly undertook 'plain work'. The most implausible hypothesis, offered by one of Clough's modern biographers, is that he must have found Florence sexually attractive. There is no evidence of this, and certainly nothing in their correspondence to suggest that their relationship was characterized by anything other than a formal, and very unromantic, propriety. It is more likely that Clough interpreted his role as being in some way a fulfilment of a personal ideal of service. But in the act of committing himself to that ideal, Clough was driven by a compulsion of his own, one that called on not so much a sense of duty, as an almost masochistic desire for self-punishment. His old friend Matthew Arnold sensed Clough wearing himself out by becoming 'ordinary and different from what he was'. He seemed to have turned his back on writing poetry in the years since his marriage, and to be searching for what he had referred to in one of his earliest poems as 'Some poor mechanic task . . . to play the drudge.'

Working like a drudge for Florence was not without its compensations. She was unusually forthcoming in her gratitude, showed her faith in Clough by agreeing to his later appointment as Secretary of the Nightingale Fund, which carried a small salary, and was generous in arranging for him to receive other payments to supplement his meagre income. In the summer of 1858, Florence gave him £500, the equivalent of a whole year's salary, to help with the purchase of the Cloughs' new home. '. . . If I could give him £10,000 a year,' she told Uncle Sam, responsible for handling her financial affairs, 'it would be a poor acknowledgement of what he has done for us.' The following April, when Florence was staying at West Hill Lodge, 'suffering from severe illness' and believing her death to be imminent, he witnessed changes to her will, including a note bequeathing him all that would otherwise have come to her on her parents' deaths.

Clough showed himself of service in another way. Intimations of her mortality had encouraged Florence to resume work on what she called her 'Stuff', the 'Science of Theology', dedicated to the artisans of England, which she had put to one side before leaving for Paris to work with the Sisters of Charity in 1853. Clough's own rejection of Anglican orthodoxy, and his enthusiasm for the project, made him the perfect sounding-board for her ideas. One Sunday evening at West Hill Lodge, he and Hilary sat with Florence before dinner as she inveighed against the message on a scroll pinned to the wall in her room, 'Wait on the Lord – Wait patiently on him.' 'If I did not believe that God was working out a scheme in which I was taking part,' she declares in Clough's notes of her remarks, 'I could give up working altogether.' Later, she turned to another theme that was to figure prominently in the revision of her 'Stuff', '. . . the mischief of Christianity as reflected in parents' treatment of their children'. Parents, Florence told Clough and Hilary, to whom her words were particularly relevant as she was constantly at her own family's beck and call, believed that their children belonged to them. This belief was paralleled in Christianity, where God was placed in the position of the parent. 'But we are not meant for servants, to look after so many pairs of sheets,' she concluded, 'but for something much higher.'

Outwardly, at least, Clough's life began to prosper. In 1859 he was promoted at the Education Office as private secretary to Robert Lowe, and moved with his family to a larger house in Campden Hill Road, Kensington, where, at the end of that year, a son, Arthur, joined their one-year-old daughter. At this point, the pressure of work began to tell on his health and nerves. His constitution had always been robust, but at Christmas 1859 a bad attack of scarlatina weakened him, and his recovery wasn't helped by his insistence on going back to work too soon. From there it was a downward spiral, as further illness, and a recurrence of the depression that had been a feature of his troubled Oxford days, took hold of him. Clough suffered from lameness in one of his legs, and then crushed a toe, while the death of his mother from a paralytic stroke contributed to his depressive state. He went to Malvern for the water cure for two months in 1860, but remained poorly despite some improvement in his condition. Florence showed concern about his illness, arranging a consultation for him with William Bowman when his symptoms after the accident with his toe began to resemble tetanus. She was anxious about him going home late at night, and in all weathers, and pressed him to stay at Hampstead, saying she would not see him at all unless he'd agree to sleep there. To make things easier, she suggested that Blanche and the children accompany him.

There was never any question, though, of Clough forsaking Florence altogether. Clearly he had no wish to, while the departure of Aunt Mai from her role as Florence's protector and helpmate, in the early summer of 1860, made Clough's support more essential to her than ever. Uncle Sam had been making tentative approaches for the best part of a year to Fanny and Parthenope, anxious for their influence in what he regarded as the long overdue return of his wife to her family and home. He was grateful for their 'very kind & soothing' support, acknowledging that the 'one great impediment' to the plan was Mai's own reluctance 'to leave Flo'. Mai's age (she was over sixty), her rheumatism, combined with Sam's persuasive powers, finally made her reconsider where her priorities lay. The gap left by Aunt Mai was filled by Hilary, supplemented with an occasional round of duty by Beatrice, Mai's youngest daughter. Uncle Sam continued to appear at the Burlington every Wednesday to consult with Florence about business; and Clough, as far as his health permitted, was still on hand to do her bidding.

This was not enough for Florence. She interpreted Aunt Mai's departure as nothing less than an act of gross personal betrayal, seeing it as a desertion not just of herself as an individual, but of her work, which, in happier times, Mai had been proud to admit Florence had undertaken 'for each & all of us'. The sudden withdrawal of sympathy from the woman who had always doted on her with the concentrated feelings of a surrogate mother for a surrogate child was a devastating blow, leaving Florence unwilling even to conceive of the possibility of another perspective on what swiftly became a bitter estrangement. 'Do what I will, my mind is always hanging on my Aunt and all those grievances,' Florence told Madame Mohl, three years after the break. 'I do what I can to chase it away, but it will come back.' The situation was a sad product of Florence's isolation, and an example of what Clarkey saw as her intensity verging on madness. Aunt Mai's greatest sin, in Florence's eyes, was that she had chosen to leave her in order to return to the bosom of her family. Once back at home, Florence predicted scornfully, Mai would devour her children, and be devoured by them.

The sick, particularly the bedridden, think of painful things more than pleasant ones. '. . . The very walls of their sickrooms seem hung with their cares' and 'the ghosts of their troubles haunt their beds . . .' This was one of the insights developed in a chapter of Florence's *Notes on Nursing: What It Is and What It Is Not*, the most popular and enduring of her books. Published in Britain by Harrison and Sons, in the first week of January 1860, it sold 15,000 copies within two months, and went on being steadily reprinted for the rest of Victoria's reign and beyond. As Florence warned in her preface, *Notes on Nursing* was not intended as a manual to teach nurses how to nurse, but offered instead 'hints for thought to women who have personal charge of the health of others'; to help them, in other words, to teach themselves. In language of wit and incisiveness, it blends everyday sanitary knowledge – 'how to put the constitution in such a state as that it will have no disease' – with observations based on Florence's own experience both as a nurse and as a patient. Above all, the book encourages the notion that good nursing stems from an ability to engage in imaginative sympathy with someone else's feelings, feelings that by definition you yourself can never have felt. Florence's physiology may be limited, her understanding of disease as a reparative process based on a rationale that makes no sense to the modern reader; but her ideas about how a nurse can bring about healing are still resonant. 'If a patient is cold, if a patient is feverish, if a patient is faint, if he is sick after taking food, if he has a bed-sore, it is generally the fault not of the disease, but of the nursing.'

The idea for *Notes on Nursing* had originated with Edwin Chadwick, at the end of 1858. He wanted Florence to reach a wider audience than she had through her work on hospital construction, and suggested at first that she provide practical instructions for her 'hundred thousand children' in the Army on how to treat wounds and look after themselves when medical care was unavailable. What caught her attention, however, was his alternative suggestion, that she offer advice to nursing or young mothers on sanitary matters 'before the arrival of the physician'. Among the subjects Chadwick outlined for inclusion were advice on temperature, air, light and food, along with practical hints for the treatment of a cold, a furred tongue, headaches and skin eruptions. All these were to be found in the finished work, but in the writing its scope broadened as *Notes on Nursing* attempted to focus the public's attention on care for its own health, enshrining a principle of prevention rather than cure.

Already, by early February 1859, Florence had prepared an outline for Dr Sutherland's perusal. After reading it, he urged her to be 'more preceptive and less doctrinal', and recommended that she soften her critical remarks against the medical profession. He also reminded her that her primary audience was the class from whom nurses were taken, among them the domestic servants whose duties included nursing and caring for young children within the home, and that she should therefore write in simple sentences which appealed to common sense. She did precisely that, in a punchy, epigrammatic style: 'A nurse who rustles . . . is the horror of a patient'; 'Feverishness is generally supposed to be a symptom of fever; in nine cases out of ten, it is a symptom of bedding;' 'it is . . . certain that there is nothing yet discovered which is a substitute to the English patient for his cup of tea – he can take it when he can take nothing else, and he often can't take anything else if he has it not.'

In December, Chadwick received his complimentary copy of the finished work, a slim charcoal-coloured volume of seventy-six pages, priced at two shillings. Six months later, noting the continuing demand for *Notes on Nursing*, he prophesied to Florence that more good would arise from it than from her labours for Army reform, 'great as those have been'. The critics had been united in their praise. 'We never read any book on any subject in which so much is said, and said so well, in shorter space,' ran the review in *The Times*, while the *Lancet* concluded that if the book produced 'one-half the good which it ought to effect, Florence Nightingale will have conferred a greater benefit on her kind, and have achieved a higher claim to their gratitude, than any woman of her time'. In the *Quarterly Review*, Harriet Martineau described it as 'a work of genius' – while squeezing in a piece of blatant self-advertisement by referring, under the veil of anonymity, to her own book, *Life in the Sick-Room*, published sixteen years earlier. *Notes on Nursing* was in homes everywhere, Martineau told Florence in a letter in June, and everyone was talking about it. As the first book written by Florence for the general reading public, this was only to be expected. The Crimean heroine, assumed by many to have retreated into private life following the end of war, now reappeared before the public eye again. And here and there in the book were subtle touches of autobiography to remind the reader of the Lady with the Lamp: Florence's acknowledgement of her 'sadly large experience of death-beds' for instance, or her memory, in the chapter 'Variety', of her attack of fever at Balaclava and 'the acute suffering produced from the patient (in a hut) not being able to see out of the window'.

Characteristically, despite this success, Florence could not rest on her laurels. She was dissatisfied with the poor standard of printing and the host of minor errors that had crept into the text as a result of its hasty preparation. She had no formal agreement with Harrison, the publisher – an oversight she later attributed to the poor health that both she and Clough were suffering from at the time the manuscript was submitted to him – and saw evidence of 'roguery' in the publisher's reluctance to provide a proper accounting of copies sold, and his unwillingness to countenance a cheaper edition while sales of the first remained strong. In the end, Florence sold the copyright of *Notes on Nursing* to Harrison's for 500 guineas (a comparative bargain for them), and negotiated the appearance, within sixteen months, of two further, heavily revised, editions of the book, each addressed to a different audience. As she explained to Sutherland, she saw the necessity of both 'a cheap Manual for the uneducated and a Library Standard book for the educated', to produce 'a real permanent effect'. In July 1860, 2,000 copies of a library standard edition were published at five shillings each. This new version redirected Florence's nursing hints towards professional hospital nurses – it was no coincidence that the Nightingale Training School at St Thomas's, as we shall see, was admitting its first probationers that month – and in so doing doubled the book's length. Some of the vigorous rhythms of the original were lost as Florence tinkered with the punctuation, and allowed herself space for the development of new ideas. A supplementary chapter, 'What Is a Nurse?', defined 'the very alphabet' of a nurse as the ability to read every change that comes over a patient's face 'without causing him the exertion of saying what he feels', and emphasized the essential quality of good nursing as deriving from the nurse's constant observation of her patient's condition: 'the state of the pulse, the effect of the diet, of sleep, whether it has been disturbed ... the state of expectoration ... the state of secretions ... whether the motions are costive or relaxed, and what is their colour' – and so on. '... We are often told that a nurse needs only to be "devoted and obedient" ,' Florence wrote in a memorable passage. 'This definition would do just as well for a porter. It might even do for a horse. It would not do for a policeman.'

A third, sixpenny, edition, geared to popular use in working-class households, appeared in April 1861 under a new title, *Notes on Nursing for the Labouring Classes*. Revising the book with the inhabitants of country cottages in mind, and specifically those in the neighbourhood of Lea Hurst, Florence simplified the vocabulary (so, for instance, 'pyemia' becomes simply 'sickness'), eliminating technical language and learned allusions as far as she could. 'Minding Baby', an additional chapter addressed directly to young girls 'nursing mother's baby at home', was, she thought, the best thing she'd ever written (the chapter title, unlike the others in the book, is placed in quotation marks in accordance with labouring-class usage). It was included at the suggestion of a Peckham schoolmaster, Mr Shields, who had referred her to the part played by his female pupils in removing dung-heaps from their parents' doorways and ensuring that windows were kept open at night. Reaching out to this younger readership, Florence attempts to win their attention by first expressing her respect for them: 'Do you know that one-half of all the nurses in service are girls of from five to twenty years old? You see you are very important little people.'

Harriet Martineau was more enthusiastic than ever about this latest version. Writing from her home in Ambleside, she told Florence that she had ordered a new batch of copies, and that 'the parson, the Arnolds [Matthew Arnold and his family, who lived nearby] and I shall soon see that everybody here has it who can profit by it'. Chadwick's teenage daughter Marion, meanwhile, ordered 300 copies for her schoolmates. Yet even at this stage, Florence was not done with *Notes on Nursing*, and continued to prepare new material for inclusion. In a further edition of 1868, she added three substantial passages, on purifying village wells, on telling patients the truth about their illnesses, and on the risk of death by fire to women wearing crinolines. This last was the subject of an inquiry to Dr Farr at the General Register Office. 'What would be a safe statement,' Florence asked him, 'as to Death from clothes catching fire in women at the "fashionable" ages to put in my text?' Farr replied that the returns didn't necessarily distinguish 'deaths by Clothes-taking-fire', but he was inclined to believe that nearly all the women burnt to death, particularly those over sixty who were asleep when they caught fire, were burnt in their clothes. '. . . The account to be laid at the door of women's clothes is cruel indeed!' Florence concluded in the augmented *Notes on Nursing*, calculating from the returns of 1863–4 that 'If the crinoline age begins after ten and continues onwards, then 277 lives are known to have been sacrificed by fire during two years only to this absurd and hideous custom.'

Another edition was prepared in 1875, but remained unpublished. In it, Florence discussed the relationship between disease and the air from sewers, and warned of the sale of substandard milk. She also wished to examine the habits, especially among factory workers, of smoking and drinking, which 'make our race degenerate'. If she had been alive in the second half of the twentieth century, there is little doubt that Florence Nightingale would have been in the vanguard of anti-smoking protest.

———

Translations of *Notes on Nursing* almost immediately sprang up abroad, in France, Denmark and Sweden. The book was translated into German by one of the Bunsen daughters, while an Italian translation appeared simultaneously in Turin, Florence and Nice. In the United States, where British copyright laws did not apply, there were two separate editions in 1860, one in New York, the other in Boston. The New York pirated version, in its cheap format, quickly became a bestseller, and was frequently reprinted. American readers were also able to read *Notes on Nursing* as part of a popular compendium of *Domestic Medicine*, published in 1863.

A copy of the book reached Dorothea Dix, the New England reformer best known for her work on behalf of the mentally ill. She had spent much of the 1840s travelling throughout the United States, surveying the shocking conditions of the country's mental asylums, and successfully agitating for the design and building of better facilities for the indigent insane. Americans had been comparing Dix to Florence Nightingale ever since the Crimean War. A popular journal, *Godey's Lady's Book*, which reprinted portions of *Notes on Nursing*, advising 'every lady' to study its recommendations, placed an illustration of benevolent womanhood on the cover of its issue of January 1861, depicting Dix and Nightingale, together with Elizabeth Fry, Grace Darling and Mary DuBois (founder of the New York Nursery and Child Hospital). This association with Nightingale was one that Dix was more than happy to accept. She had followed Florence's career with intense interest, encouraged by their mutual friend Samuel Howe, with whom Dix had worked on various reform initiatives and, to her disappointment, had narrowly missed meeting her on two occasions. In the spring of 1856, Dix had arrived at Scutari only to discover that Florence was at Balaclava; later that year, following Florence's return to England, Dix had been all set to join her, at the Bracebridges' invitation, at Atherstone Hall, when Florence was suddenly called away to Scotland for her momentous interview with Queen Victoria.

The American Civil War cemented the parallels between the two women when, in June 1861, the Secretary of War, Simon Cameron, appointed Dorothea Dix as Superintendent of Women Nurses for the Union forces. At the outset, Dix appeared to possess a number of advantages in her new role in comparison to her British predecessor's situation during the Crimean War, six years earlier, not least that she had the example of Florence's experience to learn from. There was widespread debate in the press about the appropriate treatment of the sick and wounded soldier, and the Federal Government's determination not to let its forces suffer the fate of the British and French armies in the earlier war, by falling victim to preventable disease, was signalled by President Lincoln's agreement to the appointment of a United States Sanitary Commission, in imitation of its British counterpart. Furthermore, Dix was vested by the Government with broader administrative powers than Florence had received from Sidney Herbert in 1854. Dix's jurisdiction extended across the country. She had the right to visit every military hospital, and her powers of 'diligent oversight' extended to all nurses. Mindful of Florence's problems in disciplining her nursing staff, 'Dragon Dix', as she was known, required nurses to be over thirty (she herself was fifty-nine), plain-looking, and to wear dresses of brown or black, 'with no bows, no curls, no jewellery, and no hoop-skirts'.

She quickly met with challenges to her authority. In New York, Elizabeth Blackwell, Florence's old friend and a founder of the volunteer Women's Central Association of Relief, called Dix the 'meddler general', and complained that she had no system or any practical knowledge of nursing. Public criticism of Dix swelled to a climax when a journalist called Jane Grey Swisshelm visited Army hospitals in Washington in the wake of the Union defeat at Chancellorsville, in the spring of 1863, and reported that Dix had refused to give a patient something more flavoursome than water to drink because she was unprepared to act against the rules imposed by the doctors. Swisshelm appealed to the country for the distribution of lemonade to hospitalized soldiers, and labelled Dix a 'self-sealing can of horror tied up with red tape'. This was an entirely different reception from the one that had greeted Florence Nightingale. Whereas Florence's role as purveyor to her wartime hospitals had allowed her to be seen as a free agent in her battles against the restrictions of red tape, Dix was well on her way to becoming the personification of needless bureaucracy. 'This is not the work I would have my life judged by!' Dix exclaimed as she faced personal humiliation. Louisa M. Alcott, briefly one of Dix's nurses, offered a more sympathetic picture of the Superintendent, in her portrayal of Dix's solicitude for her fictional alter ego, Nurse Periwinkle. 'Daily our Florence Nightingale climbed the stairs, stealing a moment from her busy life, to watch over the stranger, of whom she was as thoughtfully tender as any mother.'

'All our women are Florence Nightingales,' declared the *New York Herald*. If the American Civil War was a woman's war, as contemporary commentators claimed it was, because of the significant involvement for the first time in a major conflict of women in aid schemes at home, and in nursing at the front, then Florence Nightingale was the female exemplar that most American women looked to for their inspiration. Indeed her wartime popularity amounted at times to a cult. Not only was her name synonymous with nursing, her insistence that a woman's skill in 'sanitary domestic economy, and more particularly in cleanliness and tidiness' was superior to a man's made her an apostle of cleanliness to women in both the Northern and Southern states.* Louisa M. Alcott was one among many who read *Notes on Nursing*, and felt that as a consequence she was well versed in 'the canons of the profession'.

For the United States Sanitary Commission, wrapping 'cleanliness and order in the mantle of patriotism and victory', the Nightingale emphasis on preventative sanitary measures for the Army's benefit was a role model. Through Harriet Martineau, who had requested detailed information that could be sent to the Union army about hospital management and treatment of the sick and wounded, Florence provided a collection

---

* Women in the South had their Florence Nightingales too, like the Confederate nurse Fannie Beers, who served as chief matron in hospitals in Virginia, Alabama and Georgia during the Civil War. However, the Confederates were never to possess any equivalent of the Union Government's Sanitary Commission.

of official guidelines, including a copy of the 1858 report on the Health of the Army. Led by Frederick Law Olmsted, its chief executive, and with Samuel Howe as one of its board members, the United States Sanitary Commission investigated the conditions of camp sites, promoting hygiene and providing instruction about the relationship of dirt to disease, and authorizing the building of pavilion-style military hospitals. Thanks to these measures, the Commission was able to report, after two years of war, that the Union army had suffered far lower rates of disease than European armies earlier in the century.

In the spring of 1864, Emanuel Leutze, America's leading history painter, exhibited a painting of *Florence Nightingale at Scutari* at a New York Sanitary Fair organized to raise money for the Commission. Leutze's most famous historical subject was his painting of *Washington Crossing the Delaware*, which was also placed on show in New York. But for his depiction of Nightingale, Leutze eschewed a heroic theme. No attempt is made at an authentic representation, while the only concession to popular myth is the shadow of Nightingale's profile, cast on the wall above a soldier's bed. In Leutze's painting, Florence Nightingale is imagined as a kind of American Everywoman: a golden-haired nurse, leaning wearily on a table, fatigued by the exigencies of war.

———

At the end of the 1850s, the Nightingale Fund, the £44,039 donated by a grateful nation to permit Florence to establish a training programme for nurses, was lying idle in the bank. Florence had not asked for the money, as she sometimes rather bitterly reminded correspondents, but was expected nevertheless to direct and manage its disposal. Preoccupied with Army medical reform, and struggling with ill-health, she had appealed to Sidney Herbert, the Fund's Chairman, in the spring of 1858, to be released from the responsibility. He advised against taking such a step, and asked her to reconsider her decision. The public was growing restless at the absence of any news about the school, and without Florence as its figurehead the success of the scheme could hardly be guaranteed.

Florence's wariness about the Fund arose from more than simply a lack of time to devote to the development of a training school, or from her unwillingness to make it a priority. She was also deeply ambivalent about the lines along which nursing training should develop, and recognized that success might only be achieved after years of trial and experiment. Then there was the question of who should instruct the trainees. Florence's idea of nursing as a distinct branch of knowledge from medicine, and her definition of the reformed nurse as, above all, a missionary spreading sanitary doctrines, made her suspicious of participation by the medical profession in any training programme she might devise. But, in that case, where were the educated women, free of contamination from medical knowledge, who would be available to teach the less educated probationers? And what precisely were these probationers to be taught? From its beginnings, the Nightingale School, as eventually founded at St Thomas's Hospital, would grapple with the central problem that has been at the heart of the debate about nursing education ever since. Was the training to be theory or practice based? In Florence's eyes, examinations were little more than a test of memory, and could not test performance on the ward; nor were they able to offer any clue as to the development of a nurse's personal and moral character, which Florence considered to be the main object of nurse training. A nurse's technical ability was dependent on her moral powers and, in particular, on her moral responsibility in taking action to ensure that her patients didn't succumb to illness or disease.

Florence had already taken some tentative steps towards clarifying her approach to nursing in yet another confidential report written at Panmure's request, which she had subsequently expanded into *Subsidiary Notes as to the Introduction of Female Nursing into Military Hospitals in Peace and War*. Privately printed in 1858, the *Subsidiary Notes* formed a much shorter, more anecdotal complement to Florence's *Notes ... on the British Army*, and was consumed eagerly by Mrs Gaskell in a single long sitting. Unknown to Gaskell and other early readers, the book amounted to a work of dual authorship. Three of its chapters were drawn from a memorandum prepared by Jane Shaw Stewart, Florence's trusted lieutenant, who had served with her at Balaclava's Castle Hospital, and who, since the end of the war, had been receiving instruction in surgical nursing at St Thomas's. Its tone is guarded, for despite – or perhaps one should say, because of – the Crimean experience, it was far from a foregone conclusion that women would be employed in military nursing in the future. Just a week before Florence sent the initial report to Panmure on which the book was based, Woolwich Artillery Hospital had removed all but two of its female nurses. None the less, while it contains no hint of how nurses should be

trained, the book does enunciate several principles that would resonate
in the scheme later adopted and financed by the Nightingale Fund for
the civil hospital. There is the draconian ward routine, the allocation of
cleaning, sweeping and bedmaking tasks; the military terms – 'on' or
'off duty', 'absent on sick leave', for example – that would seep into
civilian nursing usage; and most importantly, the defining innovation of
the Nightingale model of nursing, that the Lady Superintendent – or
Matron – should exercise complete authority over her nurses. Only the
Matron would have the power to hire or discipline a nurse and, under
this system, any doctor with a problem relating to an individual nurse
was required to apply to her.

Herbert, anxious to get things moving, had suggested that the Fund be
used to finance training at King's College Hospital, where the St John's
sisterhood under Mary Jones had been in charge of nursing since 1856.
Florence disagreed. She recalled the problems she had experienced with
the St John's nurses at Scutari. Furthermore, she wanted any school she
established – 'if I can when I can' – to be non-denominational and free
from the risk of sectarian strife. Other hospitals were considered, the
Middlesex, University College Hospital, and the Royal Free. But in the
end there was only one serious contender, St Thomas's, still at that
time in crumbling, dilapidated buildings in Borough High Street in
Southwark, on a site that it had occupied for the past 600 years. Florence
had met the Matron there, Sarah Elizabeth Wardroper, before setting
off for Scutari. Wardroper, a forty-two-year-old widow and mother of
four who had been Matron since 1854, and was to hold the post until
1887, had won a reputation for good management (she wasn't herself
a nurse) and for her efforts at recruiting better-quality nurses. One
outstanding member of her staff was Mrs Roberts, who had nursed
Florence so devotedly at Balaclava in 1855. Also familiar to Florence
was St Thomas's Resident Medical Officer, Richard Whitfield, who
supplemented his income by instructing nursing students.

Further, more complex, considerations, though, underlay the decision
to choose St Thomas's. In 1858, the South Eastern Railway Company
suddenly gave notice of their intention to extend the line from London
Bridge to Charing Cross through part of St Thomas's garden. Most of
the hospital's governors were in favour of rebuilding St Thomas's at a
new location, provided the rail company could be convinced to purchase
the entire hospital site. Richard Whitfield, an advocate of sanitary reform

who had read Florence's articles in *The Builder*, sought Florence's support for rebuilding the hospital in the suburbs, a plan resisted by many of the medical staff on the grounds that it restricted access for patients. She didn't need much persuasion. Hospitals should never be built 'among dense unhealthy populations', and she had a wealth of statistics to prove it. If St Thomas's was moved to a healthy location, Florence told Whitfield in February 1859, the opportunity would exist 'to build the finest hospital in the world'. She thought Blackheath would be ideal. A casualty department could be built in Southwark, and patients transported by rail, 'like the war wounded'.

She mobilized opinion in the press, attempted to influence Prince Albert, one of the hospital governors, and enlisted the help of Sir Harry Verney, persuading him to raise the matter in Parliament. As a quid pro quo, Whitfield smoothed the path of the Nightingale Training School at St Thomas's. He appreciated that the state of Florence's health made it unlikely that she would ever be able personally to superintend the school, but made it clear that her prime candidate for the job, Elizabeth Blackwell, would not, as a woman doctor, be acceptable to St Thomas's (Blackwell had in any case declined the offer, preferring to continue with her career as a doctor). Whitfield imposed a further condition, that St Thomas's own Matron, Mrs Wardroper, should act as superintendent of the new school. 'It is not the <u>best conceivable</u> way of beginning,' Florence admitted to Herbert in May 1859. 'But it seems to me the <u>best possible</u>. It will be a beginning in a very humble way. But at all events it will not be beginning with a failure, i.e. the possibility of upsetting a large hospital – for she is a <u>tried</u> matron.'

It was indeed a solution of reduced expectations, shaped by compromise, and out of Florence's reluctance at the time to be either actively or regularly involved. The Fund appointed a committee of four to negotiate with St Thomas's, comprising Sir John McNeill, Sir James Clark, William Bowman and Sir Joshua Jebb, three doctors and a prison reformer; and Clough was named as secretary. The Matron was given the power to select probationers and to dismiss them. She was also expected to recommend sisters who would provide instruction to the probationers, while Whitfield would give whatever medical instruction was considered necessary. Probationers would acquire fundamental nursing skills, including the application of dressings and leeches, the administering of enemas, the making and applying of bandages; and, naturally, every nurse would be taught to ensure the constant flow of a clean air supply. No syllabus was issued, and no thought apparently given to who would vet and oversee the ability of the sisters selected to teach. Despite Mrs Wardroper's assumption of absolute power, she appears not to have been interviewed by the Fund officials, and to have had just one meeting with Florence when negotiations had already reached a late stage. The first fifteen probationers, it was calculated, would cost the Fund about £800 a year, including their board and lodging and an annual £10 wage for each probationer. Meanwhile, the Fund's payments to Mrs Wardroper and Whitfield inflated their salaries to the extent that they were among the highest paid men and women of their day.

The three-year contract offered to probationers was designed to attract respectable young women from the lower classes, between the ages of twenty-five and thirty-five, though in practice the standard of literacy among these women sometimes fell short, so that instructors in reading and writing had to be employed. Five years into the School's history, a dual system of 'Specials' would be introduced, of lady volunteers who paid for their training. There would be considerable criticism of this idea of ladies training with nurses but, as Florence said, 'the lady must be educated with her cook'; she would then become a Superintendent not simply by virtue of her education and station in life, but because she had done the same training, and knew what was involved. Applicants responding to the advertisements that began to appear in May 1860 were expected to be 'sober, honest, truthful, trustworthy, punctual, quiet and orderly, clean and neat', and Florence drew up a printed sheet to record their monthly assessments. The Nightingale School of Nursing opened on 24 June 1860. For the first time, women with a vocation could learn nursing skills outside a religious environment. 'It is true *we* make no vows,' Florence wrote later, though she left no one in any doubt about the sanctity of the calling.

A fortnight later, the first group of probationers began to arrive in their brown dresses and 'snowy caps and aprons', looking, as one observer fondly imagined, 'like bits of extra light'. They were to live in a series of partitioned cubicles at the top of one of St Thomas's newer wings – but not for long. Within two years, with the battle for the hospital's suburban site still raging, St Thomas's would move to a temporary home in what had once been the Surrey pleasure gardens in Newington, with its music hall and zoo. Here, space was cramped. The former Giraffe House was used as the cholera ward, while the Elephant House served as the dissecting room. The bed quota was reduced, and consequently the number of probationers fell to ten. It was a humble beginning, and one that stored up plenty of trouble for the future.

Florence had resumed the writing and revision of her religious and philosophical work. From the summer of 1858, and throughout the following year, she returned to it in intervals from other business, assisted by Clough and, before her departure, by Aunt Mai, who had originally played such an important role in encouraging her niece's speculations about religion. 'She _is_ working at the winding up of her "Stuff" . . .,' Hilary told her Uncle Nightingale in early 1859. 'The first thick portion (half of the whole)' had been sent, in great secrecy, to Julius Mohl in Paris, who pronounced it 'very noble & beautiful', but insisted on reading it all 'before venturing remarks'. In the summer of 1860, six copies of the three-volume work, under the title _Suggestions for Thought to the Searchers after Truth among the Artizans of England_, were privately printed with wide margins for readers' annotations, and circulated for comment.*

The chosen recipients were William Nightingale, Sam Smith, Richard Monckton Milnes, Sir John McNeill, John Stuart Mill and Benjamin Jowett. Jowett, Regius Professor of Greek at Oxford and a Fellow of Balliol, had been a college contemporary of Clough's, while the approach to Mill, the philosopher whose _System of Logic_ had been a formative influence on Florence's 'Stuff', was made through Edwin Chadwick. Chadwick had forwarded a copy of _Notes on Nursing_ to Mill, recommending that he consult them for nursing his own 'neglected & weakly body'. Mill's response was terse. He didn't need the _Notes_ for himself, but shared the universal high regard for Miss Nightingale, and indicated her 'right to write to him, or any person else without any introduction'. Florence responded to Mill almost immediately, as one of his 'most "faithful" adherents', initially sending him only volume one of _Suggestions_, and admitting as she did so that there were two other ' "devils" (I mean volumes) "worse than the first" ' to come. The copy sent to Uncle Sam was intended for Aunt Mai. In the wake of Mai's

---

* A further, unknown number of copies, presumably very few, were also printed, 'in a tidy octavo form', without the margins. Florence's own copy of this edition, bequeathed to her cousin Rosalind Vaughan Nash, is now in the Florence Nightingale Museum in London.

return to her family, a source of such bitter resentment for Florence, all direct communication between the two women had ceased. Yet, in spite of this ill-feeling, Mai dedicated herself immediately to further work on the 'Stuff', rising early each morning to answer Jowett's queries about the sections on free will, and feeling depressed when she was unable to come to any satisfactory conclusions. Observing his wife's sadness, Sam Smith made a pathetic plea to Florence on Mai's behalf. 'No one can have known her as I have, without being sure that she has the good will to work on this, or in any other good cause, if she did but see the way.'

In the first volume of *Suggestions for Thought*, Florence introduced the main outline of her creed, the idea of 'Law, as the basis of a New Theology'. The second, 'Practical Deductions', embodied criticism of the religious and social life of the day, including a long critique of the institution of the family, especially in its relationship to the lives of women. Appended rather awkwardly to this volume is a revision of the 'Daughter at Home' novel, in its final recension in essay form as 'Cassandra' (one of the work's organizational flaws is that there is considerable overlap, in subject matter and expression, between this and Florence's comments on the plight of daughters earlier in the same volume). The third part is a summary, restating the ideas expounded in the earlier volumes. The title of the second and third volumes was shortened to *Suggestions for Thought to Searchers after Truth*. The social criticism of 'Practical Deductions', which breaks in abruptly on the religious and philosophical discussion, was palpably irrelevant to the audience of artisans that Florence had hoped to reach.

'God's scheme for us was not that He should give us what we asked for,' Florence wrote, announcing her major theme, 'but that mankind should obtain it for mankind.' The laws of God are discoverable by experience, research and analysis, and not least by careful statistical inquiry. Attempting to resolve the age-old philosophical conundrum of the conflict between the idea of God as Law and the individual's capacity for freedom of action, Florence conceives of 'a Being who, willing only good, leaves evil in the world solely in order to stimulate human faculties by an unremitting struggle against every form of it'. Mankind is not therefore powerless to bring about its own salvation, but is able to discover the laws of God, and thereby move towards a state of perfection. Truth, Florence insists, does not come to us by way of a 'miraculous light', but only through hard work, suffering, and human error.

Many of the radical ideas discussed in *Suggestions for Thought* – the book's questioning of the authenticity of miracles, its call for critical evaluation of the Bible, its rejection of the doctrine of eternal damnation – allied it strongly with beliefs being expressed by liberal Anglicans, members of the so-called Broad Church movement within the Established Church. The publication of *Essays and Reviews* by seven of these thinkers, united by their desire for a free spirit of inquiry in matters of doctrine and scripture, just months before Florence distributed the specimen copies of her 'Stuff', had caused an outcry in the Church, and had led to the conviction of two of the essayists for heresy in the ecclesiastical courts. A third, Benjamin Jowett, who had contributed the essay 'On the Interpretation of Scripture', was denied an increase in his college stipend at Balliol, and saw his appointment to the Mastership of the college blocked for the next decade. It was not surprising then that Jowett found himself in sympathy with much of the content of *Suggestions for Thought*. To Clough, who had sent him his copy without at first revealing the identity of its author, he wrote that he felt as if he had received the impress of a new mind. Later, after he began a correspondence with Florence herself, Jowett commended her larger purpose, the brave attempt 'to unite science & religion'. In the world of 1860, rocked by not only the parochial controversy of *Essays and Reviews*, but also, a short time before, by the revolutionary theory of natural selection outlined by Darwin in *The Origin of Species*, Jowett had no doubt that 'Many sparks' would 'blaze up in people's minds' if they were permitted to read Florence's work.

But, stimulated though he was, Jowett could not ignore the book's deficiencies: its repetitiveness, endless digressions, and the angry tone that pervades its reflections on the family. Florence subsequently admitted that she could not bear to read the book herself, and anyone today seeking a short-cut to the ideas it contains would be well advised to read the two articles that Florence published, in May and July 1873, in *Fraser's Magazine*, which cover some of the same ground and share the larger work's concern with the loss of religion among ordinary people. Jowett, laboriously annotating his copy, urged Florence to edit the book extensively before seeking publication. J. S. Mill similarly acknowledged that *Suggestions for Thought* would benefit from editing because of its 'want of arrangement', but praised the substance of the book. While he could not agree that 'all of the arrangements of Nature' had necessarily to emanate from a divine will, he would not regret 'the adoption of the same creed by anyone to whose intellect and feelings it may be able to recommend itself'.

Suggestions for Thought, however, remained unpublished, and so never found its wider readership. Five years after her initial approach, Florence asked Jowett to edit her 'Stuff', but he reiterated that it needed to be recast entirely, and that in effect it was the materials for a book rather than the book itself. Florence had neither the time, nor did she show any inclination, to do the recasting herself. There was a sense in which *Suggestions for Thought* had achieved its purpose for her, allowing her to formulate the personal philosophy that her life's work depended upon. It was also true that literary creation held no appeal for her. Writing was a means to action; literary craftsmanship could be dismissed as 'mere artistry'.

Something of that prejudice against writing as anything other than a means to an end filters through the extensive revisions that Florence made to 'Cassandra' before it became part of volume two of *Suggestions for Thought*, transforming it from the drafts of the autobiographical novel she had written at the beginning of the 1850s to a more generalized, third-person essay. The surviving manuscript twists and weaves a path around a large proportion of passages that are heavily scored through and cancelled; many other paragraphs are littered with minor excisions and interpolations, altering pronouns and changing the tenses of verbs. Speeches made by the heroine Nofriani are removed from their quotation marks, and the 'I' of her first-person narration is changed to the first-person plural, 'we', or the third-person plural, 'they'. At the end of this protracted editorial process, 'Cassandra' is no longer an account of the personal suffering from which Florence had managed to liberate herself, but an anonymously narrated commentary on the lives of women of her class in mid-nineteenth-century Britain. These are women who can find no outlet in 'a cold and oppressive conventional atmosphere' to satisfy their 'Passion, intellect' and 'moral activity'. They are 'never supposed to have any occupation of sufficient importance *not* to be interrupted', and so fritter away their days in looking at prints, doing worsted work, reading out loud, and taking drives in the carriage. At night they pay the price for their inactivity: 'the accumulation of nervous energy . . . makes them feel . . . when they go to bed, as if they were going mad.'

In preparing 'Cassandra' for publication, Florence was undoubtedly hoping to effect change for women by highlighting the destructive influence of the family on their lives. Her own memories of 'The prison which is called a family' remained searing. When her father had suggested sending her some furnishings for her 'drawing room' at the Burlington, she had replied indignantly that she had no drawing room; a thing that was 'the destruction of so many women's lives'. Refashioning her novel in the form of an impersonal tract allowed Florence to present her arguments more objectively. It also enabled her to disguise the autobiographical origins of the piece. Most importantly, by eliminating the fantasy elements of the novel, and its mysteriously exotic setting, she could distance herself from the world of dreaming, which had once provided her with such an important escape valve from the humdrum concerns of family routine, while commenting on the problem of consuming daydreams for women in society as a whole. As a woman of power, working invisibly behind the scenes, the need to cloak herself in anonymity was paramount.

It was no wonder therefore that Florence baulked at Jowett's identification of herself with the subject of her essay. She must have been further disheartened by his suggestion – a 'rather impertinent thing', as he admitted – that she should not throw away her advantage of writing as a woman, as well as by Sir John McNeill's observation that she was more likely to reach a mass audience through a work of the imagination than through one of reason. For both these male critics there was something profoundly disagreeable about the prevailing tone of 'Cassandra'. Almost seventy years later, Virginia Woolf put her finger on what troubled them when she described 'Cassandra' as more like screaming than writing. The removal of fictional devices only emphasized the autobiographical roots of the original. Deprived of these framing mechanisms, the naked force of Florence's account of women's imprisonment within the confines of society struck early male readers like Jowett and McNeill as resembling nothing less than a case of indecent exposure.

J. S. Mill was not so much interested in the emotional temperature of the piece as he was in its relevance to his own theories about the condition of women. He was particularly drawn to its depiction of the family as an instrument of tyranny. 'Cassandra' provided valuable first-hand testimony to back up his own indictment of the family in the book he was working on in the winter of 1860–61. In *The Subjection of Women*, unpublished until 1869, Mill argued that women's subordination to domestic life was one means of ensuring that they did not make themselves 'remarkable', and of thus denying them equality with men. The influence of 'Cassandra' is strongest in Mill's depiction of the way in which a lifestyle of conventional idleness – 'the dinner parties, concerts, evening parties, morning visits, letter writing, and all that goes with them' – prevents women from pursuing any opportunity of useful work. At one point, his observation that only illness in the family, or some other extraordinary development, enabled women to devote attention to their own affairs is almost a paraphrase of Florence's report of a married woman who 'was heard to wish that she could break a limb that she might have a little time to herself'. Acknowledging his debt to Florence, Mill wrote that 'a celebrated woman, in a work which I hope will some day be published, remarks truly that everything a woman does is done at odd times'.

Mill had crossed swords with Florence on the subject of women's rights in an exchange of letters in the autumn of 1860. He had objected to several paragraphs in the second edition of *Notes on Nursing* in which Florence had advised her 'sisters' to avoid the two kinds of jargon she saw as prevalent. The first was 'the rights of women which urges women to do all men do, including the medical and other professions, merely because men do it, and without regard to whether this *is* the best women can do'. The second was the jargon that urged women to avoid everything men did

merely because they are women, and should be 'recalled to a sense of their duty,' and because 'this is women's work,' and 'that is men's' and 'there are things which women should not do . . .' Surely any woman should bring the best she has, *whatever* that is, to the work of God's world, without attending to either of these cries.

Mill told Chadwick that he would have preferred Florence to have omitted this lecture. By including it, he feared that she had lent the prestige of her name to those who wished peremptorily to exclude women from everything without first giving them the opportunity to test their suitability for different kinds of work. Learning of Mill's criticism, Florence wrote to him that he had misunderstood her. He replied that he was glad that this was so, and added that advocates of women's rights already made 'what appear to me far too great con-

cessions as to the comparative unfitness of women for some occupations', but that he did not believe that they could fairly be accused of
jargon. Florence's response made it clear who she considered the chief
perpetrators of this jargon were: the American contingent of doctors led
by Elizabeth Blackwell, the first British woman to practise medicine,
who had been in London giving a series of lectures, advocating the entry
of women into the medical profession. Evidently still smarting from
Blackwell's rejection of the job of superintendent at the new nursing
school at St Thomas's, Florence told Mill that Dr Blackwell was 'a dear
& intimate & valued' friend. But, she went on, Blackwell talked a
jargon, '& a very mischievous one' at that. Women doctors had 'tried
to be "men"', but had only succeeded in being 'third-rate men', able to
earn their livelihood, while at the same time failing to introduce overdue
improvements to medical practice. Florence was far from alone in her
negative view of the medical profession, which had only recently become
self-regulating, though the need for reform was not in itself a reason to
prevent women from becoming doctors. What her words to Mill did
not convey was her concern that the diversion of educated women into
medicine was likely to cause a shortfall in the number of good candidates
applying to train as nurses or midwives; or that women might regard
nursing training, not as part of a distinct profession in its own right, but
as a short-cut to medicine.

In time, Florence's attitude to woman doctors would soften, and
she would become a public supporter of women's entry to medicine
(Florence's own last two doctors would be women, Caroline Keith and
May Thorne). Yet she continued to maintain her ambivalent stance
both towards women's rights, and towards those who campaigned for
them, whom she contemptuously referred to as 'Women's Missionaries'.
Fundamentally, the language of rights was not a part of Florence's
vocabulary, and she relied instead on more traditional concepts like
duty, the desire to serve and the idea of a calling. She was, however, a
signatory to the three petitions on women's suffrage presented to Parliament by J. S. Mill, in 1866, in 1867 and 1868, together with other
prominent names, including Mary Somerville, Harriet Martineau and
Josephine Butler. She remained unconvinced, though, by the case for
votes for women, arguing that women's suffrage would take many years
to obtain, and that in the meantime there were evils, pressing 'much
more hardly' on women – such as the law's prohibition of a married

woman's right to own property, or the absence of equal pay among ordinary women workers – which could be swept away by the legislature as it stood.

Writing, in 1867, to solicit Florence's support for the London National Society for Women's Suffrage, Mill emphasized that until women exercised power openly and directly, these evils would never be satisfactorily dealt with. Florence's reply – 'if you will not think me egotistical' – underlined the difference in their respective approaches. She had never felt the want of a vote. Indeed, if she had been 'a borough returning two members to Parliament, I should have had less administrative influence. And I have thought that I could work better for others off the stage than on it.' Mill disagreed. He understood that it was possible to get a great deal of work done swiftly, 'and apparently effectually', by working through others. But he was certain that it would have a salutary effect on the world to know 'how much of all its important work is and always has been done by women . . .', and that the disabilities that blighted many women's lives would only be removed by giving them an equal voice in their own affairs.

Florence was almost certainly correct in her assumption that she was able to wield greater influence by working through men behind the scenes than if she had pursued legally constituted power of her own. Nevertheless, her absence of understanding of women far less exceptional than herself, unable to breach the barriers that she had broken through, partly by virtue of her prestige, and her apparent refusal to perceive how truly unique her position was, are at times impossible to ignore. If she, as 'a woman of very ordinary ability', as she on one occasion disingenuously described herself, could break through, why couldn't others of her sex follow her example and do the same?

But then her view of women was not generally high – though there were obvious exceptions like Mary Clare Moore – and in characterizing herself as 'a man of business' called 'to a man's work', she sometimes appears to be making an attempt to distance herself from the rest of her sex. 'Women have no sympathy,' Florence declared to Mary Mohl in 1861. '. . . Women crave for being loved, not for loving. They scream out at you for sympathy all day long, they are incapable of giving any in return, for they cannot remember your affairs long enough to do so.' Conveniently overlooking the fact that Mrs Bracebridge and Aunt Mai had both made considerable sacrifices on her behalf, Florence claimed

that she had never found one woman prepared to alter her life 'one iota
for me or my opinions'. She could only contrast this with her experience of men. Arthur Clough, 'a poet born if there ever was one', had
taken to nursing administration for her. Sidney Herbert had remodelled
his entire political life for her, learning 'a science . . . by writing dry
regulations in a London room by my sofa with me'.

Tragically, though, Sidney Herbert, author of her destiny and the man
who, more than any other, had given her access to that influence, was
dying at the age of fifty. Early in December 1860, Bence Jones of
St George's diagnosed Herbert with diabetes and renal sclerosis, a hardening of the kidney tissue then commonly known as Bright's disease.
Florence's reaction to the news was one of shock, a refusal to admit the
gravity of the situation, accompanied by the immediate realization of
what it might mean for the future of the Army reforms they were engaged
upon together. 'You know I don't believe in fatal diseases,' she wrote to
Uncle Sam, 'but fatal to his work I believe this will be.'
  Signs of the decline in Herbert's health had been evident for a couple
of years. At the beginning of 1858, he had complained of suffering from
a 'neuralgic headache and tic in the temple and jaw'. Florence 'was very
sorry' to hear of it, and worried that Herbert's inspections of barracks
in cold weather would do nothing to alleviate his complaint. She suggested he try the water cure at Malvern. Instead he experimented with
a concoction called 'Christchurch Remedy', a mixture of camphor and
chloroform inhaled through the nostril, followed by several glasses of
brandy. A couple of months later, he admitted to her that he was 'heartily
ashamed' of having idled away two days in bed 'instead of minding my
business in London'; but then, sensing her concern, he wrote again to
reassure her that 'I really am not ill . . .'
  As an invalid herself, Florence wasn't exactly unsympathetic to the
state of Herbert's health, though habitual disregard of her own ailments
tended to make her dismissive of the illnesses of others. She failed,
though, to understand fully enough that the renewed strains of Herbert's
political life from the summer of 1859 when he became Secretary for
War, along with his family responsibilities at Wilton, did not allow him
the freedom from distraction and opportunity to conserve his energy
that her own lifestyle provided. In the space of just one year at the War
Office, Herbert's attention had been diverted on many fronts, in addition

to the sanitary programme. He had overseen the development of the volunteer movement, a war against China, the transfer of the Indian Army to the crown, the reorganization of the national defences, and had been embroiled in a wounding battle with the Chancellor, his old Oxford friend Gladstone, over increased expenditure on the Army. In the parliamentary session that opened 1860, Herbert estimated that he had spoken in the Commons nearly 200 times. Every speech, he later told his wife, had shortened his life.

And now Florence was bent on directing him towards one last push, the greatest of all, the reform of the War Office itself. Without such reform, the permanence of the Army reforms already achieved could not be guaranteed. The War Office, she had told Herbert in November 1859, was not only a very slow and expensive department, it was also one in which the Minister's intentions could be overturned 'by all his sub-departments and those of each of the sub-departments by every other'. Lord de Grey, Herbert's Under-Secretary, drafted one scheme for re-organization; with Sutherland's assistance, Florence drew up another, abolishing divided responsibility, defining clearly the duties of departmental heads and making them directly responsible to the Secretary of State. The scale of the task, and the entrenched opposition it was likely to encounter from the Horse Guards, and from Sir Benjamin Hawes, the Permanent Under-Secretary, would have defeated an individual of sound body. It was utterly beyond a man facing an incurable illness, whose strength and stamina were in steady decline. Yet Florence, reluctant to accept the seriousness of his condition, disguised her fear by alternately hounding and chiding Herbert, while keeping up a regular barrage of complaint about his deficiencies to others. 'Sidney Herbert is very forgetful,' she confided to Douglas Galton, adding that while she appreciated Herbert's 'great qualities . . . no one feels more the defect in him of all administrative capacity in details'. To her father, she complained of Herbert's 'increasing sleeplessness & consequent unfitness for work'. And, in a letter to Harriet Martineau, she wrote that Herbert was 'no statesman' and had 'no organizing capacity', but that he possessed 'great persuasiveness' which would 'carry the Estimates . . . [and] the reorganization of the War Office'.

Following his consultation with Bence Jones, at the beginning of December 1860, Herbert called on Florence and placed three alternatives before her: he could retire from public life altogether; he could retire from office and keep his seat in the House of Commons; or he could keep the Secretaryship of War, leave the Commons and go to the House of Lords. She urged him, with the support of Liz Herbert, to accept the third option, despite his own reservations about taking it. She now realized it as imperative, she told Liz, that Herbert leave the Commons. However, in opposition to Bence Jones's opinion, she was convinced that retiring from political life altogether was more likely to kill than cure him. On 8 December, Florence wrote to Herbert to make certain that he wasn't retreating on the decision. '. . . I do hope you won't have any vain ideas that you can be spared out of the W[ar] O[ffice],' she warned him, before indulging in an unpleasant bit of emotional blackmail, that he wouldn't be sacrificing himself 'to the "good of the cabinet" ' by resigning office, but the lives of 'hundreds of thousands of men'.

She saw death written on Herbert's face, but out of sheer desperation pressed on, endlessly dispensing advice to the dying man and his wife, as 'an old Nurse', while decrying the efforts of his doctors. Herbert must eat beef and beer – 'not sauces or acids' – because 'that makes blood'. He should wear a flannel belt around his body, not go out at night ('One night's party is worth ten days' disease to him'), sleep out of London where the air was better, and take plenty of exercise. He was to beware of another danger, namely 'that doctors often produce the very disease they prescribe for'. She was encouraged by tests showing the presence of protein in his urine, which might be a sign of nature working out its healing course by 'getting rid of something which ought not to be there'. In lifting the spirits of the Herberts, Florence was clearly also trying to raise her own. For who, 'after you', she confessed to Liz, 'has such a stake in his life as I have?' Common sense told her never 'to interfere between a physician and his patient', but writing to Bence Jones, who saw Herbert weekly, she begged him to recommend an additional doctor who would be able to keep an eye on the patient on a more frequent basis. 'Pray, pray, pray,' she ended her letter, 'think of what I say.'

It was all quite hopeless. Meanwhile, Arthur Clough, who was in no better health, had been advised to take extended leave from his duties at the Education Office, and from his other work. Florence agreed that a long convalescence was necessary, of 'travelling, amusement, want of thought'. It looked at first as if any travel plans might have to be postponed. Blanche was pregnant again. However, interfering on this

occasion between husband and wife, Florence was insistent that difficulties caused by Blanche's condition 'should be got over'. After a spell
with his family and the Tennysons at Freshwater on the Isle of Wight,
Clough set off for Athens at the end of April. He returned briefly to
England in June, and left the following month for a tour of the Auvergne
and the Pyrenees.

By the end of May, Sidney Herbert's weakness and thinness, his
trembling and breathlessness, were evident to everyone who saw him.
But Florence had convinced herself that he was no worse, and even that
he was getting better, which only increased her angry resentment at his
inaction on War Office reform. 'There is an "uneasiness" between me
& Lord Herbert,' she admitted to Uncle Sam. 'I am sure that he does
not at all realize what I feel about his failure – but thinks I do not see
him or write to him because of my own health.' At the beginning of
June, Herbert collapsed, and the game was up. 'There is an end of the
War Office for me,' he wrote to Florence. 'I feel that I am not now doing
justice to it or myself.' Most mornings he spent on a sofa, gulping down
brandy until he was 'fit to crank down to the office'. He hoped to remain
at his post until the end of the year, as there were various matters he
wished to complete. But War Office reorganization wasn't one of them.
'The real truth,' he told her, 'is I do not understand it. I have not the
bump of system in me. I believe more in good men than in good systems.'
Florence's tight-lipped reply left him in no doubt as to her displeasure.
'I consider your letter as quite final about the reorganization of the
W.O. . . . Hawes has won. If you will not think me profane I will say
"Hell hath gotten the victory".' In a draft letter, which may or may not
have been sent to him, she summed up her feelings with a devastating
directness: 'I am disappointed in you.'

One of Herbert's final actions as Secretary of State was to confirm
Jane Shaw Stewart, who had been initially reluctant to accept the
appointment, as Superintendent of the first female nursing establishment
at the new general military hospital at Woolwich, soon to be named in
his memory. On 9 July, he went to take his leave of Florence before
departing for the continent for the water-cure at Spa. He was by now so
weak that he had to be assisted climbing the stairs to her rooms at the
Burlington. She received him coolly. Later, in the only note of regret she
ever expressed on the subject, she admitted that she had been too hard
on him, but that his 'angelic temper' bore everything she had to say

without rebuke. With the words, 'No man in my day has thrown away so noble a game with all the winning cards in his hands,' ringing in his ears, Herbert left her. It was their last meeting. As he waited at the station later that evening, a train transporting a hearse passed by on the opposite track. Pointing at it, he said, 'That's the only carriage I shall ever want.'

Sidney Herbert died, surrounded by his wife and five children, on the morning of 2 August, after a hurried return to England so that he could see his beloved Wilton once more. A telegram informing Florence of the news arrived that night at the house at Oak Hill Park, in Hampstead, where she was staying. Aunt Mai and Uncle Sam came the next day to comfort her. Florence 'seemed very overpowered and cried, but quite in a natural way', Blanche reported to her husband, far away in the Pyrenees. Dr Sutherland stoutly defended Florence from any imputation that she had contributed to Herbert's death by suddenly declaring that she had only done herself what she had given him to do. There had been no reconciliation between Florence and her aunt, but Mai could only feel 'the deepest grief' for her niece. After a year apart, Mai thought Florence looked 'very much worse, her face & hands so swollen . . .'

The funeral was held in the little church at Wilton. Florence did not attend – although she composed 'some particulars' to be used at the service – but such was her association with Herbert in the public mind that newspapers automatically assumed she had been there. 'Many men were weeping,' Gladstone wrote to her afterwards. Already Florence was sustained by a report from Herbert's widow that some of the dying man's last words – a description soon to be amended to 'His last articulate words' in Florence's litany of grieving – had been addressed to her. 'He said more than once,' she wrote to Parthenope, embroidering them still further, on 7 August, ' "Poor Florence and our unfinished work".' In the same letter, she took her place as 'Sidney Herbert's constant mourner'. '. . . No one understood & knew him but me. No one loved & served him like me.'

The obituaries were grudging. Some blamed Sidney Herbert for the breakdown in military administration at the beginning of the Crimean War. Few mentioned his part in the reforms of more recent years. At Gladstone's instigation, Florence attempted to vindicate Herbert in a memorandum on his work as an Army reformer. In draft after draft she made endless revisions to the precise wording of the piece, apparently

struggling with the degree of public recognition due to her own contribution to their unique partnership. In letters to the outside world, she
continued to portray herself as the pupil and Sidney Herbert as her
'dear master'. In private documents, she presented the truth about the
relationship as having been something closer to the reverse. Herbert had
possessed 'a most rapid power of perception'. Yet 'even after he actually
begun his famous Report . . . he was totally ignorant of the real causes
of the loss of that Army'.

By the second half of August, Arthur Clough was in the foothills of the
Pyrenees, walking solitarily, or tagging along after the Tennyson family,
who were also on holiday in the area. In an atmosphere of contentment,
he had started to write poetry again. 'Mari Magno' ('On the Open Sea')
is a sequence of tales on the theme of marriage, some little more than
doggerel, others of a darker hue, narrated by a group of transatlantic
voyagers. Clough and Blanche's third child, a daughter called Blanche
Athena – after Florence had attempted unsuccessfully to have 'Sidney'
incorporated into her name – had been born on 5 August; and in
September, Blanche travelled to France to join her husband. By train
and diligence they crossed the Swiss border into Italy, reaching Florence,
after several stops, on 10 October. Here they managed only a couple of
days of sightseeing before Clough collapsed, having suffered the first in
a series of strokes. He died on 12 November. As his body was prepared
for burial in the city's Protestant cemetery, a cast of his head – 'the
features came out so beautifully after death' – was taken.

For his widow, there was immediate remorse for what might have
been. If only Clough had given up 'all the money-making and working
for F. Nightingale which had worn him out', and gone to rest by the
seaside, to 'follow his heart' by writing more poetry. Her misery was at
times greater than she could bear. '. . . If grief could kill . . .,' Blanche
wrote at the end of November, 'I ought to have died before this.'

15. Philomela

At Hampstead, Sidney Herbert's death had left Florence also nursing an inconsolable grief. She was Herbert's 'true widow', she lamented, for her work, the object of her life, and the means to do it, had all disappeared with him. Although gripped by many of the familiar symptoms of her illness – weakness, fainting fits and nausea – she nevertheless moved in October to stay at the Verneys' town house at 32 South Street, off Park Lane. She was determined to be in reach of developments at the War Office, where, to her dismay, Sir George Lewis, whom she labelled a 'muff', had been appointed Herbert's successor as Secretary for War. Florence was at South Street when she learned of Clough's death. She had known of his collapse, but the news still hit her hard, provoking further reflections about the dead, heavily laden with self-pity. 'He was my <u>support</u> in life, as my dear master was my <u>object</u> in life,' she told Liz Herbert. Clough had been a man 'of the highest and tenderest of spirit it has ever been my lot to meet, of uncommon genius, worn and fretted by the necessity of working at hard and uncongenial matters for daily bread'.

Florence requested that particulars of Clough's end be sent to her. None were at first forthcoming. In fact, from Italy, Blanche had specifically instructed Aunt Mai not to send any, and it was only after Florence 'vehemently insisted' that she was allowed a few sparse details of Clough's last days. Blanche's ill-will towards Florence, founded on her belief that she bore some measure of responsibility for her husband's death, ran deep. Others had come to the same conclusion. 'I hardly know whether it lessens the pang of his loss, to be told, (as I <u>have</u> been told) that the fatal weakness of the brain was induced by overwork in the cause of Florence Nightingale and her benign plans,' Francis Newman, the classicist and younger brother of John Henry, wrote to her. 'Alas, we cannot be satisfied that one martyrdom should thus entail another.' Rumours about Florence working Clough to death joined those already circulating about her part in Sidney Herbert's demise. People were labouring 'under such strange & hurtful mistakes about me . . .', Florence wrote as stories reached her ears. In December 1861, Elizabeth Blackwell blithely remarked in passing to Barbara Bodichon, Florence's cousin, that had she accepted the superintendency of the Nightingale Nursing School, she too would probably have found herself worked to death.

It may have been awareness of malicious gossip that prevented Florence from writing sooner to Blanche with her condolences. When she finally did so, she asked her to accept that, although silent, she had deeply felt the extent of Blanche's loss, 'at every waking hour'. Blanche's response was terse and grimly ironic. 'I know that his loss has been to you what it could hardly be to any one, & I have truly grieved for you in your great suffering . . .'

A sea-change had transformed the attitude of Aunt Mai, Blanche, and Blanche's sister Beatrice, who sometimes attended on Florence, towards the niece and cousin who had once been the object of so much of their 'reverence & affection'. Clough's death had certainly stirred up family ill-feeling against her. But while Blanche's hostility was understandable, it was unfair that so much of the blame for Clough's final illness was laid at Florence's door. Florence may have been indirectly responsible for some degree of the strain that Clough had been under at the end of his life; but it was Clough who had seemed determined to overload himself with work. More to the point, Florence's continuing rejection of her aunt was viewed as cruel and vindictive, and of a piece with her strangely 'overwrought' state of mind. According to Aunt Mai, those who spent prolonged periods of time with Florence felt forced continually to weigh up what she said, and to distinguish what was exaggerated, and what entirely fanciful. And yet, as Mai acknowledged, 'It does not do to disregard what she says, for at times there appears an extraordinary power & penetration.'

Ten days after Clough's death, Mai reflected sadly on her relationship with Florence in a letter to Blanche, remembering how they had previously cared for her 'in love, in veneration, in sorrow':

There were times when a doubt came over me about some of the things she said & did but I never spoke of it to anyone. I believed in her till what she said became so preposterous that I could not. Now I look on her quite differently. Imagination

& Pride. These words applied to her explain much. I believe her not capable of
... human tenderness or gratitude more than the blind can see. Beatrice has no
devotion to her, finds being with her painful ... There are good reasons against
giving her up. One is that there is not any other person about her whom she can
take pleasure in. Hilary clings to her, is ready to fly & serve as ever, but I think
her more wearisome & unnatural than ever. Flo lets her go a good deal to South
St, but not stay. Dr & Mrs Sutherland go to her faithfully & admiringly, but
finding fault very freely when they speak of her. Her maid is a capable woman
who it is hoped will stay, but there will never be fond devotion there. As to
myself, she will not harm me except from wounds already given. We have not
the slightest intercourse ... no kind word concerning what has befallen us ...
No longer wanting me, not only she drops me, but [her] imagination has been at
work, abusing me.

Mai hoped that it was some consolation to her daughter that her husband
had been sacrificed to a worthwhile cause.

We cannot doubt that the cause was good & much good done. She may truly
[be] said to have worked for an idea with a strength & persistence that could not
but draw a good & capable mind to work for her ... since the idea was true &
good & noble like himself.

There were no such recriminations from the Herbert family, not least
because Liz Herbert had been at one with Florence in demands that
her husband remain at the War Office when he was already fatally ill.
The relationship between the two women remained close for the next
few years, though Florence was disappointed by Liz's conversion to
Roman Catholicism at the beginning of 1865, a step which almost cost
Liz the custody of her children when the Herbert family threatened to
make them wards of chancery. They habitually wrote or sent flowers
to each other on the anniversary of Sidney Herbert's death; and, in
1862, Liz sought Florence's intervention when the Parliamentary Fine
Arts Committee – or 'No Arts Committee' as Florence called them,
'for the pictures they have admitted you would put into your cellar' –
turned down the proposal to place a statue of Herbert within the pre-
cincts of the Houses of Parliament. In 1867, a bronze statue of Herbert
by J. H. Foley was erected outside the War Office in Pall Mall. Three
years earlier, J. B. Phillip's marble effigy of Herbert had been unveiled
at Wilton Church. Among the bas-reliefs of scenes from the Crimean

War, below the recumbent figure, is one of Florence Nightingale at Scutari.

An urgent appeal to Florence from the War Office, a fortnight after Clough's death, rescued her temporarily from her all-consuming grief. She felt as if she was back in harness again, 'working just as I did in the time of Sidney Herbert'. It appeared that Britain and the United States might be on the brink of war. At the beginning of November, a Union naval frigate had stopped the neutral British ship *Trent,* and had abducted two commissioners from the southern states, who were seeking the support of Britain and France for the Confederate cause. Lord Palmerston's Government was outraged, sending the Union an ultimatum, and demanding an apology and the release of the commissioners. While negotiations were taking place, and in order to strengthen their hand, the British Government decided to send reinforcements to Canada to bolster the garrisons there in the event of war breaking out. Lord de Grey, the Under-Secretary for War, consulted Florence about sanitary arrangements for these troops. She complied with his request by drafting instructions about clothing and supplies for soldiers, and comforts for the sick, along with observations about more general dangers that might confront an army facing the winter cold. All her suggestions were adopted, though the conflict itself was averted. 'The War Office,' she explained to Clarkey, 'were so terrified at the idea of the national indignation if they lost another army, that they have consented to everything.' Once again, Florence demonstrated that there were no limits on the lengths to which she would go to serve her soldiers. The extent of her preparation, and the way in which, from the confines of her room, she was able to envisage the scene of operations, are astonishing. She calculated the distances which might have to be covered by sledges, and compared the relative weights and warming capacities of blankets and buffalo robes.

There could be no doubt of Florence's continuing usefulness to the Army, even though she despaired of Sir George Lewis's suitability for his new position at the War Office, and believed that with the beginning of 'the reign of muffishness', the days of her own influence were over. She and Lewis had encountered each other in 1860 when he was Home Secretary. There had been a sharp disagreement between them over questions Florence wanted added to the 1861 Census, which she hoped would provide information about the number of sick people in each house, and the diseases they were suffering from. Lewis had dismissed the idea as 'too indeterminate', arguing that any results obtained in this way would be inaccurate. As the new Secretary for War, and a noted classical scholar, Lewis tried to make amends by sending Florence first some of his Latin squibs – including a translation of the nursery rhyme 'Hey diddle diddle' – and then a copy of his book on early Roman history (in which he attacked Niebuhr, a historian she admired). She was not impressed. Why was the War Secretary wasting his time with such 'trash' instead of reforming his department? She enjoyed an easier relationship with Lewis's Under-Secretary, Lord de Grey, a more self-conscious reformer in the Herbert mould, and when Lewis died suddenly in the spring of 1863, Florence successfully petitioned Palmerston to appoint de Grey in Lewis's place ('Agitate, agitate, for Lord de Grey to succeed Sir George Lewis', Florence telegraphed Harriet Martineau). The death of her old adversary Sir Benjamin Hawes, in the first half of 1862, had renewed Florence's hopes of root and branch reform of the War Office, but it was once again to prove elusive. Instead, with Douglas Galton as Assistant Under-Secretary in charge of the health and sanitary administration of the army, another important ally was in place.

Wholesale reform would have to wait, but, together, Lord de Grey and Galton ensured the continuance of sound sanitary principles. While Florence would never again experience the kind of close working relationship she had enjoyed with Herbert, her position, for much of the rest of the decade, acting as a kind of 'Advisory Council to the War Office', was unparalleled. She was consulted on any problem relating to the health of the Army. The War Office Abstracts list the matters in which she was involved in one year: a new *Warrant for Apothecaries*, *Proposals for Equipment of Military Hospitals,* a scheme for the *Organisation of Hospitals for Soldiers' Wives*, *Proposals for the Revision of Army Rations, Warrant and Instructions for Staff Surgeons, Instructions for the Treatment of Yellow Fever, Proposals for Appointments at Netley and Chatham, Instructions for Treatment of Cholera.* In 1947, the Select Committee on Estimates would report favourably on the cost-accounting system used by the Army Medical Services, which eighty years after its introduction was still in use, and which worked more effectively than those introduced by other departments in more recent times. With

considerable surprise, the Committee learned that the originator of this
system was none other than Florence Nightingale.

As 1861, 'this fatal year', drew to its close, however, Florence was more
despondent than ever about the future. An attack of illness on Christmas
Eve, the severest since 1857, with a new torture, intense spinal pain, left
her again preparing for death. In January, she moved from South Street
to Peary's Hotel at 31 Dover Street, off Piccadilly, freeing the Verneys'
London home for Sir Harry and Parthenope to return. Here Florence
revised her will, bequeathing mementoes from every stage of her life –
including her shells, her 'unique collection' of the rules of French
religious orders, 'the memorials of My Roman Stay and Egyptian and
Greek journey', her prints from Upper Harley Street and 'the Crimean
remains' – to her father, and organizing the dispersal of her papers. She
would not return to the Burlington. Since Herbert's death, she 'could
not bear even to look down Burlington St where I had seen him so often'.
At the beginning of March, thanks to Mr Nightingale's generosity, she
moved again, to 'a fashionable old maid's house' at 9 Chesterfield Street,
in Mayfair. She had hoped that her new home, rented from the widow of
the politician Robert Plumer Ward, would open 'a new and independent
course in my broken old age', but soon took to calling the house 'The
Pigsty' on account of the squalid condition of its furnishings and bedding. Workmen were called, and carried away 'Two VANS FULL' of
stinking materials. 'Dr Sutherland said, if I had not persisted, we should
have had typhus . . .' It could be no coincidence that this was the disease
that had killed Mrs Plumer Ward's husband – 'through her dirt'. In the
autumn, Florence returned with relief to Oak Hill Park.

She was lonely, her pain acute. 'Sometimes I wonder that I should be
so impatient for death,' Florence wrote to her mother in March. 'Had I
only to stand and wait I think it would be nothing, though the pain is
so great that I wonder how anybody can dread an operation. If Paget
[the surgeon, Sir James Paget] could amputate my left forequarter I am
sure I would have sent for him in half an hour . . . I think what I have
felt most (during my last three months of extreme weakness) is not
having one single person to give me one inspiring word or even one
correct fact. I am glad to end a day which never can come back, gladder
to end a night, gladdest to end a month.' She compared herself to Queen
Victoria, in mourning for Prince Albert, who had died in December,

and half-mad with grief. 'She is never able to see but one person at a time ... Lord Palmerston says she is half the size she was.' People who said that time healed the deepest griefs were wrong. 'Time makes us feel what <u>are</u> the deepest griefs every day only the more by showing of the blank ...'

And having lost Aunt Mai and Clough, she had also deprived herself of Hilary Bonham Carter as a live-in companion. Hilary still visited her, but in 1861 Florence had sent her back home, convinced that Hilary was wasting her life and artistic talent as her cousin's housekeeper and amanuensis. 'Few things, I believe I may say nothing, weigh now so much on my mind,' Florence had written to her, 'as that I should have authorised, i.e. by its being done in my service, an expenditure of life to avoid which I left home.' In her redrafted will, Florence left Hilary £1,000 in the hope that she might provide herself with an atelier, or some other means of pursuing her art. Hilary was passionate about Florence, but her art lacked fire. In 1862, the plaster statuette of Florence, over which she had laboured for so long and with a growing sense of dissatisfaction, was exhibited at the Royal Academy in London (twenty or so small copies in porcelain, around fifteen inches high, were presented to friends and institutions). Fanny Nightingale was 'shocked at the poor little finnikin minnikin', and confided to Parthenope that she would like to 'annihilate' all the copies. Meanwhile, as one member of the Bonham Carter family departed, another was drawn into Florence's service. Hilary's younger brother Henry Bonham Carter, a thirty-four-year-old barrister, had been persuaded to take over Clough's position as Secretary of the Nightingale Fund. He was to remain in the job for more than half a century.

In the two years since he had begun to comment on *Suggestions for Thought*, Benjamin Jowett had kept up an irregular correspondence with Florence, sympathizing with her in her ill-health, sharing reminiscences of Clough from their Balliol student days, and offering professorial assistance in the 'sewing' together of her 'Stuff'. They had yet to meet, and when, at the beginning of October 1862, Florence asked him to come to Oak Hill Park to give her the sacrament, Jowett accepted the invitation with pleasure. He requested permission from the Bishop of London, Archibald Tait (as he was performing a private service in someone else's parish), assuring the Bishop that he would not mention the occasion to anyone, for fear that newspapers might get hold of the information. 'I do not think she is near her end,' Jowett reported to Tait, after the service had taken place on 19 October. 'I imagine she may live for many years though she does not think this herself. It is possible also that she may be taken at any moment. Her sufferings are very great and continual. Her mind appears to be as clear and as strong as ever. The illness affects her character more than her intellect.' This was the beginning of a remarkable friendship that would extend over the next thirty years. Once a month on a Sunday, he visited Florence to take communion with her, and any other members of her family, and friends like Mrs Bracebridge, who were present; while apart, they exchanged long confiding letters (many of Jowett's have survived, but he appears to have obeyed Florence's wishes about the destruction of hers, which only occasionally survive, and generally as drafts or copies). It would be a relationship founded on common interests – particularly in religion, and a variety of social problems – mutual respect of each other's intellectual gifts, and the need of both of them for an intimate friend. Interestingly, long before he had had any personal contact with her, Jowett had idealized Florence. In his contribution to *Essays and Reviews*, he had seen her as an example of an individual following the true religion of Christ: 'a tender and delicate woman . . . who feels that she has a divine vocation to fulfil the most repulsive offices towards . . . the soldier perishing in a foreign land'. Following their meeting, though, it was Florence's 'patient, solitary, unknown toil', rather than her legendary exploits as the Lady with a Lamp, which appealed to him as more extraordinary.

At forty-five, Benjamin Jowett was three years Florence's senior; 'a soft smooth round man', as the poet and diarist William Allingham described him, 'with fat soft hands'. Jowett's high-pitched voice was remembered by many former Oxford undergraduates, and according to his twentieth-century biographer, he spoke 'something like a eunuch' as a result of an inherited glandular complaint. He knew about the 'unhappiness of families', Jowett told Florence early on, finding common cause with her, for his own relations with his parents and siblings were strained and distant. Born in Peckham, the third of nine children, his father was a literary-minded furrier, author of a metrical translation of the Psalms, who failed to earn a living adequate enough to keep his large family. Benjamin's upbringing was marked by increasingly straitened circumstances, and by his growing reputation as a precocious young

classical scholar. Awarded a scholarship to Balliol College in 1836, he
was elected to a fellowship while still an undergraduate, appointed a
Tutor in 1842, and ordained in the Church of England three years later.
Balliol, and the wider University, which he hoped to rescue from narrow
ecclesiasticism, became the focus of his life, and the task of educating
bright young men, shaping character and sending them out into the
world equipped for future careers, his central challenge. Classics, even
the study of his beloved Plato, was not to be regarded as a work of
narrow scholarship; on the contrary, the wisdom of the ancients was
needed to teach us how to live. Yet Jowett's relationship with Balliol in
the early years of his friendship with Florence was ridden with strife, and
he once compared his problems at the hands of the College authorities to
hers with War Office officials. His heretical views had blocked his
advancement, creating an atmosphere of friction with the Fellows who
opposed his opinions. Jowett withdrew from high table and took his
meals in his lodgings in Broad Street. Not until 1870, after internal
politics ensured a majority in his favour at College meetings, would
Jowett become Master of Balliol. He then set about making it the college
of his dreams, 'a sort of heaven on earth'.

   Among Jowett's acknowledged characteristics was his power of pro-
jecting himself into the lives of others and of 'finding the better part' of
those he associated with. Soon after their first meeting, he wrote to
Florence about the distress she unknowingly caused family and friends
by isolating herself from them: 'Forgive me: I am not finding fault – I
am aware that difficulties of character & nervous states are very great;
also that your public duties leave no time for gossip and friendships.'
Nevertheless, Jowett possessed enough sensitivity to realize the damage
that was being done to Florence's balance of mind by estrangement
from old friends. He successfully interceded with Blanche Clough on
Florence's behalf, and soon the little Cloughs, including young Arthur,
whose gentleness reminded everyone of his father, were once more
paying her calls. He may also have played a part in reconciling Florence
with Aunt Mai. Certainly, by the autumn of 1863, the two women were
on friendly terms again. They could never resume their former closeness,
but their shared passion for religious inquiry revived in subsequent
letters between them. Jowett became a friend of the Nightingales, visiting
William and Fanny at both their country homes and, once Parthenope's
in-laws, the Fremantles, had adopted a more relaxed attitude to Jowett's

heresy, staying at Claydon with the Verneys too. Touchingly, while in Derbyshire, he would go to many of Florence's favourite spots near Lea Hurst so that he could describe them to her on subsequent visits to London.

By the spring of 1865, Jowett could write to Florence that he was sure that he was 'the better & happier always for coming to see you'. She told him that it also did her good 'to know that you are in the world'. As they became more familiar, he felt free to offer constructive criticism (though he once wrote that reproving Florence was like pouring cold water on a red hot iron, and producing a 'terrible hissing'). 'Bodily affliction,' he recognized, 'at times clouds your mind – and takes away self control.' He advised her never to forfeit the power afforded by her incognito, and to avoid personal controversy at all times. It was a vain hope, but he recommended that she shouldn't personalize her political dislikes so much. She felt things too intensely, and this meant that she was 'always getting scalded & hurt'. After all, Sir George Lewis, whatever his faults, wasn't really Ahriman, the principle of evil perpetually at war with the god of light in the Zoroastrian system, as Florence had said he was. Jowett saw that one of the barriers to any peace of mind for her was that she expected her ideals to be put into practice immediately and was too quickly disillusioned, as some other of her correspondents, like Sir John McNeill, had noted, by the slightest delay. She confessed, at one point in the mid-1860s, with a frankness she rarely revealed to anyone else, that he was right about her impatience:

I mar the work of God by my impatience & discontent. I will try to take your advice. I have tried. But I am afraid it is too late. I lost my serenity some years ago then I lost clearness of perception, so that sometimes I did not know whether I was doing right or wrong for two minutes together – the horrible loneliness – but I don't mean to waste your time. Only I would say that my life having been a fever, not even a fitful one, is not my own fault. Neck or nothing, has been all my public life. It has never been in my power to arrange my work. No more than I could help having to receive & provide for 4000 patients in 17 days (in the Crimean War, and how easy that was compared with what has happened since!).

Florence was held in high esteem by Jowett as the most important critic of his work. He sent her drafts of his sermons for comment, and later received her help with selections for a *School and Children's Bible* he was assembling. In May 1865, Jowett gave her some of his translations of Plato's *Dialogues* to read, the work that preoccupied him for a large part of his academic career. 'Hardly anything important about law or religion which has ever been said may not be found in Plato,' he told her, a conclusion with which Florence tended to agree, finding much in Plato to confirm her belief in God as the creator of laws, which are used to bring mankind to perfection. It was twenty years since Florence had floored a visitor to Embley with her Greek, but her detailed remarks on Jowett's work showed that her critical perception of the language was as fresh as ever. What she found exasperating were her unsuccessful efforts to persuade Jowett, as he endlessly polished his translations, to write his own theodicy, and reveal to educated Victorians the nature of God and the manner of his working in the world. 'Mr Jowett put as much of his genius into Plato as Plato did into Mr Jowett,' she wrote with a sense of the missed opportunity after the 'Dear (tho' Perfidious) Professor' was dead.

Jowett's affection for Florence was at its peak between 1863 and 1866. During this time, the relationship has been described as offering him 'the excitement of gallantry' from a distance. While he was enduring snubs from his colleagues at Oxford, it must have been curiously thrilling to have been on such close terms with so famous a woman. As he was drawn back into College affairs in the latter part of the decade, his affection for her remained strong, but some of the intensity waned. All the same, if the rumours, circulating strongly before Jowett's death, that he once proposed marriage to Florence have any basis in fact, it is to the second decade of their friendship – the 1870s – that such a proposal must belong. Until 1870, it would have been impossible for Jowett to marry and retain his Fellowship. As Master of a College, he was permitted to do so. There was one Balliol Fellowship that was compatible with matrimony, and when paying court, in 1862, to the Dean of Bristol's daughter, Margaret Elliot, Jowett may have applied for it. But the Fellowship went elsewhere, and Jowett seems to have accepted that he would remain married to his College instead, while bitterly regretting that he would never enjoy the support and companionship of a wife. However, did his thoughts of marriage revive when he became Master? And is it possible that he asked Florence Nightingale to marry him?

Jowett's editors and biographers have havered over this issue. Yet the evidence, although limited and far from decisive, none the less supports the idea that Jowett wished at some stage to marry Florence. Cornelia

Sorabji, later India's first female barrister, was up at Somerville studying law at the beginning of the 1890s and found herself taken under the Master of Balliol's wing. In her memoir, *India Calling*, published in 1934, Sorabji remembered a visit to Florence, by then in her early seventies, which had been arranged through an introduction from Jowett. Lunching with him afterwards to report on the meeting, Sorabji was 'struck dumb' when he suddenly pointed at the picture of Florence hanging on his study wall, a print of Parthenope's portrait of her sister with Athena the owl, and exclaimed, 'When she was like that, I asked her to marry me.' (Jowett later bequeathed the picture to Somerville, where it hangs today in the Senior Common Room.)

Either Sorabji's memory was hazy, or the Master's chronology unreliable, as the drawing of Florence and Athena belongs to Florence's early thirties, not to her middle age, when the friendship with Jowett began. But Sorabji produced a further piece of evidence to back up her story. When Cook's *Life* was published, one of Florence's cousins, probably Rosalind Vaughan Nash, showed Sorabji a one-line entry from Florence's diary, which Sorabji believed referred to this episode. It said simply, 'Benjamin Jowett came to see me. Disastrous!' This diary appears to be no longer extant. It may have formed part of the material which Rosalind Vaughan Nash, together with Florence's other executors, destroyed following the publication of Cook's biography. Only one diary (as opposed to diary notes) from this period does survive, for a single year, 1877. It is written in a small 'Gentleman's Pocket Daily Companion', with room only for a very concise description of each day's events.*

Jowett may then have seriously nurtured hopes of making Florence his wife, though the mind rather boggles at how he imagined marriage with a woman who was not only an invalid, but also insisted on living as a recluse, would have worked in practice (in this context, though, it's interesting to note how often he argued that Florence's closeted lifestyle was not beneficial for her health, while bearing in mind that the 1870s were the decade when the worst of the symptoms of her illness began to

---

* One should perhaps take with a pinch of salt the story told by Margot Asquith in the first volume of her amusing but unreliable *Autobiography* (1920). As Margot Tennant, before her marriage, she was befriended by Jowett, and having heard that he had been in love only once – with Florence Nightingale – she asked him what his 'lady-love' had been like. 'Violent . . . very violent,' was his 'disconcerting' reply.

recede). It is perhaps a temptation too far to make a connection between Florence's refusal of Jowett and the breakdown he suffered in 1873, when he became seriously ill, and made an agreement with her not to work more than three hours a day, and never more than an hour at a time. All that can be said with certainty is that Jowett went to his grave lamenting his unmarried state. In 1880 he wrote, with an air of finality, that 'The great want of life can never be supplied, and I must do without it.'

India created another common bond between Florence and Jowett. Two of Jowett's brothers, William and Alfred, one an officer, the other a surgeon, had served in the Indian Army. Both had died of disease in India in the 1850s, leaving Jowett to criticize the poor conditions of the barracks in Calcutta, and to wonder whether 'the natives themselves' might not be 'educated to cleanliness & health by the enforcement of sanitary regulations in the large towns . . .' Florence had turned her attention to India following the Mutiny in May 1857. Almost immediately she had started to press for another Royal Commission, this time to investigate the health of the British Army in India. In May 1859 the warrant for a second Royal Commission had been signed, and Sidney Herbert appointed as its Chairman. Herbert's ill-health, however, led to him resigning the post, and to Lord Stanley taking his place. By the autumn of 1861, the collection of data from the 200 largest military stations in India was well under way. For Florence it was the beginning of one of the great undertakings of her life: four decades of work to improve public health in India. Initially her focus was on the British soldiers serving there; but increasingly, flattering, coercing and cajoling five successive Viceroys, she would adapt to the 'noble task' of 'creating India anew', by devoting herself to the health and welfare of Indians themselves, earning Jowett's sobriquet, 'Governess of the Governors of India'.

In 1892, a Calcutta newspaper reported that Florence Nightingale had once visited India. While there, she realized that if the country 'needed anything it was village sanitation'. Consequently, she had collected 'masses of facts and has since been agitating in England'. Despite this confident assertion, Florence had in fact never visited India. There was 'really nothing', she told J. Pattison Walker, Secretary to the Bengal Sanitary Commission, in 1865, that she longed to do so much, 'this side

of the grave', as to go there, but her health was never to permit it. The
Calcutta correspondent's mistake was understandable enough. After
years of study, Florence's knowledge of the country – of its water and
drainage systems, for example, its experience of famine and urgent
need for irrigation schemes as a preventative measure, and of the lives
of the *ryots*, the Indian peasantry, and their suffering at the hands
of unscrupulous *zemindars*, the revenue collectors who challenged the
peasants' rights to occupancy of their land – was invariably so profound
that it was natural to make the assumption that she must have observed
these conditions at first hand. Yet all this knowledge had been assimilated from her home in London. Florence had gathered her facts from
reports, Blue Books and other official records, requesting information
by letter and in person from Governors-General, administrators in
Britain and India, and from both ordinary citizens and experts in various
fields. If she had ever gone to India, she once said, it would have been
like going home rather than visiting a strange country.

The idea for a Royal Commission to inquire into the Sanitary State
of the Army in India appears a relatively uncontentious one when compared with the difficulties that had been faced by the original commission
pressing for reforms to the health of the Army at home. The Mutiny
had come as a rude awakening for British rule in India, and there was
general acceptance of the view that reform of the Army was an essential
prerequisite for holding the Empire in the future. In the aftermath of the
rebellion, the Army had been reorganized in the three presidencies,
Bengal, Bombay and Madras, with fewer Indian and more British
soldiers. The health of these British troops was seen as a vital component
in transforming the Indian Army into an efficient fighting machine and
occupying force. It had already been reported that sanitary problems
had affected the campaign to subdue mutineers and rebels, and it was
clear, once again, that health conditions were killing more troops than
war itself. The statistics of the Indian Sanitary Commission were later
to reveal that, since 1817, the annual death rate of British soldiers in
India had reached sixty-nine per 1,000, three times higher than the death
rate of troops at home *before* the 1857–61 reforms. Florence's analysis
would show that nine per 1,000 had died of natural causes, sixty per
1,000 from causes relating to poor sanitation. In stark human terms,
British control of India was being maintained at a cost of the sacrifice
of one company per regiment every twenty months.

Reforms to the Indian Army in the wake of the Mutiny were part of a much wider programme of change by the British Government. In August 1858, Parliament had passed the India Act. This marked the end of rule by the East India Company and the beginning of the British Raj. The Act created a Secretary of State for India, with a consultative body, the Council of India. The Secretary of State operated from the India Office, situated at first in the Westminster Palace Hotel, and from 1867 in a new building adjacent to the Foreign Office in Whitehall. Meanwhile, thousands of miles away in Calcutta, the Viceroy, or Governor-General, presided over the largest imperial bureaucracy in the world. Although the Viceroy reported to the India Office in London, the civil servants under them, controlling the individual districts, enjoyed a large degree of autonomy. Florence communicated directly with the Secretaries of State (until 1866 the office was held by Sir Charles Wood, followed by Sir Stafford Northcote). To lobby effectively, she relied on establishing good personal relations with each Viceroy, and counted on finding allies for reform among Governors of individual provinces, like Sir Charles Trevelyan, the Governor of Madras, a family friend who had been Assistant Secretary to the Treasury during the Crimean War, and his successor, Lord Napier.

The Sanitary Commission for India included members of Florence's circle: Farr, this time actually sitting on the Commission, rather than merely advising it, Sutherland, Dr Thomas Arnold, and Dr Ranald Martin, an authority on tropical medicine. Additionally there were two members of the India Council, Sir Robert Vivian and Sir Proby Cautley, and 'a Queen's officer with acknowledged Indian experience', Colonel Edward Greathed. There was talk of including J. S. Mill, but his former employment with the East India Company eventually ruled him out. Florence had believed that the 'sanitary salvation' of India depended on Sidney Herbert heading the Commission, and regarded Lord Stanley very much as second best. Stanley, a Conservative with liberal tendencies, still only in his thirties, who had spoken at the 1855 meeting for the creation of the Nightingale Fund, was well qualified to deal with Indian affairs, having served for a short time, prior to the fall of Lord Derby's Government, as Secretary for State for India. But although, in the long run, he established a good working relationship with Florence, the fact that he wasn't Herbert counted against him, and she soon damned him with faint praise – or worse. He was 'a deal better than nothing', she wrote;

or, on another occasion, 'If we could have put Hamlet's ghost into the chair . . . he would have served us better!'

With the assistance of Farr and Sutherland, Florence designed a *Circular of Enquiry* to be sent to the barracks and Army stations in India, incorporating 'the most minute statistics' from the Government reports in East India House. As before, she suggested witnesses for examination before the Commission. Reviewing the evidence as it began to emerge, she was struck immediately by two factors that were contributing to the prevalence of disease in the Indian Army. The first was the belief that the climate of India alone was responsible for ill-health among the troops, when the reality of the situation was that the climatic condition of the country intensified the major causes of disease, bad water and drainage, overcrowding and lack of ventilation; the second was the tendency in the replies from stations to use the 'caste system', and the supposed Indian apathy towards sanitation, as an excuse for their failure to introduce up-to-date sanitary measures. How far, she asked herself, was 'caste' merely an excuse for the Europeans' own 'laziness & want of judgement?' She was appalled by some of the replies that mentioned the sepoys, the native troops. 'We look upon the native troops . . . much as Virginians look upon slaves,' she told Dr Farr. She was fast coming to the conclusion that without reforming the health of the Indian community as a whole, the sanitary conditions of the Army could stand no chance of long-term improvement.

Throughout the first half of 1862, the massive Commission Report was being assembled. Florence, as she reported to her mother in March, had now written 'the biggest part' of it. She was also writing her *Observations*, a ninety-two-page summary of the Commission's findings to accompany the Report, relayed in an accessible and, at times, agreeably sarcastic style. Drawing attention to the Indian *bheestiewallas*, who carried water in an animal skin to deliver it to the barracks, she jokingly referred to one man as the 'beginning' of a water pipe and to another as the 'end', commenting that these water pipes had a will of their own. Describing the practice of using cow dung to polish barrack-room floors, she remarked: 'At some stations, the floors are of earth, varnished over periodically with cow dung a practice borrowed from the natives. Like Mahomet and the mountain, if men won't go to the dunghill, the dunghill, it appears, comes to them.' The *Observations*, like the Report itself, conclude that the main obstacles to soldiers' health are 'camp disease', bad living conditions and neglect of sanitary measures, as well as 'liver disease', due to over-drinking, exacerbated by over-eating and lack of physical exercise. According to Florence, a soldier's routine day consisted of the following:

bed till day break;
drill for an hour;
breakfast served to him by native servants;
bed;
dinner served to him by native servants;
bed;
tea served to him by native servants;
drink;
bed – and da capo [repeat from the beginning].

In September, Florence commissioned Hilary to provide some illustrations for the *Observations*, to enliven the text further. They were for woodcuts, 'so the less picturesque, the fewer lines, the less laborious the better'. Florence added, 'I do think this is a more useful thing to do, for you. So I make no apology.' Hilary happily complied.

The Report was published in early July 1863. Florence did not under-estimate the importance of disseminating its findings widely to fight parliamentary complacency about Indian affairs (Stanley noted the empty chambers whenever India had been discussed in the past two years). She rallied Chadwick and Martineau to publicize the cause. 'By dint of sending three times a day to the printers and almost every half hour to the lithographer, I have got a few copies of our Indian Army Sanitary Report, before it is issued,' she wrote to Chadwick. 'Can you do anything for us in the way of publicizing it? And, if so, where shall I send you a copy?' She had a number of copies of her *Observations* produced for private use through the printer William Spottiswoode, and distributed them among friends, and anyone else who might be influential (she sent one to the Queen, who replied by sending her a copy of Prince Albert's speeches). Her arrangements for review coverage ensured that there were notices in most of the leading journals and newspapers. But she was almost stymied by the incompetence of the clerical staff of the House of Commons, who, in cutting down the enormous Blue Book to fit a small edition, had scrapped the *Observations*, the abstracts and the entire second volume of station questionnaires, and then submitted this abridged version to Parliament. Circumventing these difficulties imposed a further workload. Florence was told that the mistakes could not be rectified, as the typeface had been broken up. She requested that an unabridged copy be kept in the Hansard Office and, with Sir Harry Verney's assistance, wrote to all the MPs she was acquainted with, asking them to go and see the full report to make sure it had been placed there. For the first time, there was a run on a Blue Book. As a further corrective, the *Observations* were reprinted as a separate book in a red binding. Known as 'the little red book', the *Observations* were widely reviewed. Years later, when asked what had set the sanitary crusade in motion in India, Sir Bartle Frere, one of India's leading statesmen, replied that it was 'a certain little red book of hers . . . which made some of us very savage at the time, but did us all immense good'.

There were indeed some very savage critics of the Report in the wake of its publication. British officials in India, whose criticism Florence referred to as like 'thunder', were indignant that the Royal Commission seemed to ignore their own attempts at sanitary improvements (part of the problem here was that much of the data had been collected in 1859–60, four years before the Report reached India, and in the intervening period some of the evils had been remedied). Close to home, Colonel Baker at the India Office was a formidable opponent. He wrote to Stanley, impugning the Report's statistics, which he said exaggerated the facts and figures of soldiers' deaths. Florence was swift, though, to pour scorn on one of his arguments, that the highest death rates resulted from the war years, and that peace, therefore, and not sanitary measures, was the solution. 'The suggestion that, to reduce the mortality of the army, the sole course is to avoid war,' she remarked witheringly in a paper written in response to the criticisms, 'requires no discussion.' Most damaging were the attacks made by Dr Leith, the Chairman of the Bombay Sanitary Commission, who, again, was incensed by the lack of recognition given to the medical establishment in India, and questioned the statistics used. Florence's reply to Leith was 'moderate in tone, and conclusive in argument', though from a historical perspec- tive it's possible to conclude that doctors in India were denied the credit that they deserved for making sanitary reform, leading them to be portrayed in some quarters 'as obstructive, obscurantist, and woefully out-of-touch'. But, no doubt, the publicity given to the Royal Com- mission's Report allowed those same doctors to press their arguments for change more effectively on an administration that had previously been largely indifferent to reform.

A meeting of the National Social Science Association, in Edinburgh, in October 1863, gave Florence the opportunity to restate the Commission's case in terms that were addressed directly to the British public. Her paper, *How People May Live and Not Die in India*, was delivered on her behalf by Dr Scoresby Jackson. In it she emphasized her paternalist view that the British were not in India simply to rule; they were there to plant the seeds of a higher civilization, with hygiene as its handmaid. And she signposted the fundamental direction of her own work for the country in the future. 'The time has gone past when India was considered a mere appanage of British commerce. In holding India we must be able to show the moral right of our tenure.'

However, reports were not self-executive, as she always reminded herself. Sir Charles Wood had granted the appointment of three Sanitary Commissions in each of the presidencies, Bengal, Madras and Bombay, to implement the recommendations, and these began their work early in 1864. But Florence, as ever, recognized the importance of mobilizing individuals to combat inertia at the War and India Offices, and there could be no greater ally than the new Viceroy himself, Sir John Lawrence. '. . . There is no more fervent joy, there are no stronger good wishes, than those of one of the humblest of your servants,' Florence wrote to Lawrence at news of his appointment in the autumn of 1863, ending her letter with the plea, '. . . In the midst of your pressure pray think of us, and of our sanitary things on which such millions of lives and health depend.' On 4 December, before his departure for India, Lawrence called on her, leaving Florence elated by the determination he had expressed to expedite improvements to the health of the Army.

Lawrence was in his early fifties, a former Chief Commissioner of the Punjab, and possessed of a deeply held Evangelical faith (he was descended from John Knox on his mother's side). He had returned to Britain in 1859, a hero of the Mutiny for his part in preventing the spread of the rebellion to the Punjab. Florence had met him in 1860 when Lawrence was serving on the Council of India, and he had given evidence before the Royal Commission. Towards the end of her life, Florence claimed to have played a decisive role in the appointment of Lawrence as Viceroy when Lord Elgin, Lawrence's predecessor, was suddenly taken ill. Sidney Herbert had been a chivalrous medieval knight

– the 'Cid' as Florence had called him – but she saw Lawrence as more of a Homeric hero (though she would sometimes criticize him for his 'Caesarism'). Somewhat improbably, for he had a rough manner and was described by one of his adversaries as behaving more like a navvy than a gentleman, Florence was struck by Lawrence's blue eyes, which, she said, had the expression of a girl of sixteen. In later years, a photograph of Watts's portrait of Lawrence always hung in her room.

At the outset of the new Viceroyalty, there were the usual frustrating problems of surmounting the bureaucratic delays of Government departments. Florence, with Farr, Sutherland and Robert Rawlinson, had prepared a comprehensive list of *Suggestions* for improvements to be carried out in the Indian barracks, but six months after its completion the document was still waiting to be dispatched to India. 'Our great want is your standard plans and rules,' Lawrence wrote to Florence in May 1864, from his summer residence at Simla, 'without which we are quite at sea, and so far from doing better than formerly I shall be in danger of doing worse.' In August, the *Suggestions* finally arrived, though only after Florence had resorted to sending out private copies herself. Although Lawrence found fault with some of the Commission's figures, and supported the arguments that the Report failed to recognize the good work that had already been carried out to improve the soldiers' health and welfare, his Government speedily set to work on an expansive programme of barrack building, over a period of four or five years, at a cost estimated at £10 million. This kind of reform played to Lawrence's strength – he was better at implementing plans than at making policy – but Florence wasn't slow to lavish praise on him. He was 'the greatest figure in history', she told him, undertaking 'the greatest work in history, in modern times'. Lawrence modestly demurred from such enthusiasm. 'All that I really do is to try and help you where I think that your plans & propositions are feasible. Few things are more difficult to accomplish in India than real sanitary improvements, & their expense is very large, & almost beyond our means. We must therefore of necessity progress but slowly.' Nevertheless, in early 1867 Lawrence was able to report to Florence that the death rate among British troops had fallen to 20.11 per 1,000; by 1911, the death rate had dropped to five per 1,000.

Naturally they had their disagreements. The most serious of these centred on the subject of the introduction of female military nursing to India. There was general agreement among Indian medical authorities of the need to replace the ward coolies who served Army hospitals with properly trained nurses and orderlies. In 1864 Dr Pattison Walker of the Bengal Sanitary Commission, which had recommended that female nurses be introduced to all large hospitals in India, including regimental hospitals, approached Florence and asked for her advice about the organization of such a plan. Florence understood the necessity for a 'seed' of trained nurses and matrons to be sent to India to recruit and train women of English or Anglo-Indian parentage (upper- and middle-class native women could not be considered, as they were in purdah). In collaboration with Sir John McNeill, she produced a comprehensive survey of the requirements, recommending, in accordance with her common method, that female nursing should be tried first in a single hospital in Calcutta under 'the fostering care of the Governor-General'. In the meantime Florence was visited by Mary Carpenter, the Unitarian educationist and penal reformer, who attempted to persuade her to send nurses to India, describing the terrible conditions in Bombay and Madras hospitals, and arguing that if the Indian Government did not take the initiative by training nurses for hospitals, 'the Natives' themselves would, without reference to proper procedures. Florence was reluctant to involve herself in anything that lacked Government authorization, but after three years of waiting 'long & anxiously for some movement', she wrote to Lawrence to inquire about progress. His reply could not have been more discouraging. Instead of following her advice of beginning female nursing on a small scale, Lawrence and his Council had 'constructed an immense scheme' upon hers, which had subsequently been abandoned on the grounds that it was too expensive.

Financial constraints were responsible for other setbacks. In 1866, Lawrence, who had consistently maintained that the Sanitary Commission was too costly, restructured it, and reduced the Commission in the three presidencies to two members from the original five. Increasingly, Florence complained about the lack of administrative organization to secure the permanence of reforms at the end of Lawrence's term of office, while bemoaning the snail's pace of change itself. There were too many memoranda and dispatches produced by officials – a large proportion of them sent to Florence until 1906, four years before her death – busy theorizing instead of taking action. 'Any foolscap is sent all over India to see how many fools' heads it will fit. Of course it fits a good many,' she wrote to McNeill. Furthermore, the old argument about the apathy of Indians as an obstacle to sanitary progress had resurfaced with a vengeance, and was now applied to the question of how a comprehensive system of civil sanitation could be introduced throughout the country. Indians didn't want it, she was told. In Calcutta, where most of the Europeans lived, or Bombay, sanitary schemes were in operation. But in the villages, the Government showed little evidence of an appetite for progress. In vain, Florence informed Lawrence that it was a mistake 'to suppose that Natives take little interest or would object to pay for improvements', only to face a rigid colonial attitude which declared that she was wrong, and that it was preferable to reduce expenditure rather than increase taxation.

In 1870, the year after Lawrence retired as Viceroy – to be replaced by Lord Mayo – Florence published a paper on *The Sanitary Progress in India*. The new barracks, built at such great expense, without paying full attention to proper drainage or clean drinking water, were still too close to 'unhealthy native towns and bazaars'. The Government had failed to apply the sanitary engineering advances of the West to the wants of the civil population, who, it was now clear, lived 'under social and domestic conditions quite other than paradisiacal'. In the second phase of her work for India, Florence would reach out to Indians themselves, attempting to make them more socially aware and concentrating on their overwhelming need for education. By doing so, she would be attempting to find an answer to a question that she posed herself: 'For many ages the people of India were more civilized and more clean than almost any nations of Europe. Why has this condition of things been in later days reversed?'

One contentious issue that divided Florence and Jowett was the Contagious Diseases legislation of the 1860s. These Acts, passed in 1864, 1866 and 1869, sought to control the spread of venereal disease in the Army and Navy by the forcible registration and internal examination of women, in garrison towns and naval ports, who were suspected of being prostitutes. Those found to be diseased, following a painful and degrading process, were detained for periods of up to nine months. To their opponents, the Contagious Diseases Acts were tantamount to state-regulated vice for the armed forces, protecting men from 'unclean women'. As Josephine Butler, the Anglican clergyman's wife who spearheaded the campaign to repeal the Acts, pointed out, if these women were unclean they had not become so by themselves. They were being declared to exist for the gratification of men's sexual urges, and in the process were being treated with vicious cruelty which denied a woman her inalienable personal rights.

In 1870, as the repeal movement gathered momentum, Jowett expressed his hope that Florence would have nothing to do with 'Mrs Butler & Co.', who were 'getting excited' about the Contagious Diseases Acts, 'for they are not wise people, & are, I think, on a wrong tack'. However, by that time Florence's interest in the subject, and her opposition to the introduction of a system of compulsory inspection and treatment of prostitutes, modelled on the one that existed in France, extended back over almost a decade. She possessed no illusions about the seriousness of the problem. '. . . The dreadful sin & amount of syphilis in our army is not be denied,' she had written, in 1861, to Sidney Herbert, who favoured Britain's adoption of the continental model. Statistical data suggested that as much as one half of all sickness in the Army at home was caused by sexually transmitted disease. But Florence's study of the available evidence also showed that rates of venereal disease among troops abroad was not lower where the 'protection' of legislation existed, so that 'you actually have the demoralization of that licensing of vice, <u>without</u> the diminution of disease'. In 1862, in an attempt to influence Lord de Grey at the War Office against the implementation of the French method of state regulation of prostitution, Florence had gathered together her figures, and the conclusions drawn from them, in a privately circulated 'Note on the Supposed Protection Afforded against Venereal Disease, by Recognizing Prostitution and Putting It under Police Regulation'. He was apparently shaken by the strength of her evidence, though a similar approach to Gladstone, well known for his work in the reclamation of prostitutes, met with an unrewarding response.

A major plank of Florence's argument centred on her unshakeable faith in the ordinary soldier. 'The great men in office always look upon the soldier as an animal, whom nothing can check,' but she argued that he should be treated as a moral agent, given practical encouragement to enable him to marry early, and provided with comfortable barracks, day rooms and reading rooms, which would occupy his time and prevent him from wishing to go out. In this way the authorities would prevent prostitution 'more than by reclaiming ten prostitutes', and she advanced the case of the 5th Dragoon Guards, who were equipped with these kind of amusements and consequently had a minimum number of instances of disease. The alternative was legislation which actually supported the idea of prostitution – so long as it was healthy. What this amounted to, she informed Parthenope, was a law that effectively told an individual, ' "You may murder as much as you please, provided you give no pain to the victim & do not hurt your own hand. If you do, we will put you into hospital to cure your hand, so that you may be able to murder someone else & learn to do it without giving him pain" . . . This is exactly what they want to do about prostitution in the War Office, & what the *Times*, *Saturday Review* & Mr Jowett advocate . . .'

Despite her efforts, the first Contagious Diseases Act became law in the summer of 1864 with the overwhelming support of the Commons, 'placing the whole female populations of the towns', as Florence told Sir Harry, '. . . at the mercy of the inspector of police, & with nothing but a pecuniary compensation for a mistake!!!' Florence was drawn into the national campaign for repeal as a second and then a third Act was adopted, extending the area of application of the original legislation; and at the end of December 1869, she joined Harriet Martineau and Josephine Butler as a signatory to a petition for repeal, published in the *Daily News*. The full rigour of Florence's invective against those in favour of the Acts was reserved for two letters which she published in the *Pall Mall Gazette*, in the spring of 1870, unusually for her, under a pseudonym, 'Justina'. Elizabeth Garrett, the first woman to qualify as a doctor in Britain, who had written in the journal about the success of the legislation, was the unhappy recipient of her scorn, in particular when it came to the undermining of Garrett's own statistical evidence. '. . . I must say,' comments 'Justina', 'she [Garrett] has shown great skill in weaving the few scattered threads of advantage into a substantial-looking piece of stuff, with which she has succeeded in hiding from the eyes of a large number of your readers how really naked of good results the act is.'

It may have been Josephine Butler's own slipshod way with facts and figures, as well as what Florence termed 'the doctrinaire, not to say amateur mode, of action' of the association which Butler headed, that caused Florence to decline the offer of the Vice-Presidency of 'the Anti-C.D. Acts Society'. Nevertheless, she responded positively, in 1877, when Butler asked for her support for a congress in Geneva on the repeal of contagious diseases legislation internationally. Repeal in Britain finally came nine years later, in 1886. The 'legal recognition of prostitution as an indispensable national institution', which had so perturbed Florence, was over.

Her formidable mass of papers, especially those relating to India, made moving an expensive business. And Florence was constantly on the move in the first half of the 1860s, often spending part of the summer in Hampstead, but the rest of the year in a series of rented houses and lodgings. At the beginning of 1863 she was at 4 Cleveland Row, in the vicinity of St James's Palace; back at 32 South Street again at the beginning of 1864, and then at 115 Park Street, a house belonging to the Grosvenor Hotel, throughout the rest of that year; from November 1864 to May 1865 she was at 27 Norfolk Street, also in Mayfair; and then it was back to South Street, this time to number 34. The effort of finding a suitable house, getting into it, and making it comfortable was extremely wearing for everyone involved, but once settled, Florence lived on one floor, as stairs were difficult for her to manage, and mainly confined herself to her bedroom.

In April 1864, while she was at Park Street, Florence agreed to receive Garibaldi, the Italian patriot and hero of the Risorgimento, who was on a visit to England. Garibaldi hysteria was rife. He had been welcomed by a crowd of over 100,000 at Charing Cross station, and entertained in all the great houses of London (though not at Buckingham Palace). Florence had twice refused to see him. Although she had contributed to the fund for the rising in Naples, she had been disappointed by Garibaldi's tactics in attempting to march on Rome in 1862. She was finally persuaded to see him only after friends like Jowett insisted that it was her duty to use her influence to prevent Garibaldi stirring up future disturbance in Italy, which would threaten Austrian intervention. Garibaldi drew up at Park Street in Sir Harry Verney's carriage, supposedly in secrecy, though 'the whole world' seemed to have heard about the meeting. In the course of a long interview, for which she had carefully prepared, Florence was struck by Garibaldi's 'utter impracticality'. He looked flushed, very ill and worn, talked of caring, not for 'repubblica' or 'monarchia', but only for 'the right'. He had a heart of gold, she told Hilary, but the head of a schoolboy. What is more, he had departed before Florence had succeeded in securing his support for sanitary reform.

The burden of the expenditure on his daughter's temporary accommodation finally became too much for William Nightingale. Not only was
he required to pay as much as £500 a year for a Mayfair town house,
with the added expense of Florence's sojourns in Hampstead, he also
had to cover the cost of making good the decoration and furnishings both
before her arrival and following her departure at any rented property. In
1865, Fanny and Parthenope convinced Mr Nightingale of the necessity
of providing Florence with a permanent home in London. His offer of
£7,000 for 35 South Street was accepted, but as there were some months
to run on Florence's lease of number 34, Florence urged her father to
offer a short let of number 35 to Dr Sutherland and his wife. She was
worried that the Sutherlands' proposed move from Finchley to Norwood
might impede Sutherland's daily visits to her, and inconvenience their
work. '. . . The anxiety it would save me to have him next door for
business all the autumn and winter (our busiest time),' Florence
explained to her mother; '. . . People little know the way Dr S. treats me.
One little instance, I will give. He told me he was "dying" . . . and could
not come to me, and went to Epsom for the Derby. Now, if he were
next door, these insane tricks would not agitate me . . .' Dr Sutherland
clearly did not relish the idea of being so close at hand, choosing a house
in south London instead. In November, Florence moved to 35 South
Street, which was to be her home for the rest of her life.*

Before she went, there came news of the death, on 6 September, of
Hilary Bonham Carter, her close friend from childhood. Hilary was
forty-four and had been ill with cancer for some months. In May, Jowett
had visited her at Florence's request, and had written afterwards that
Hilary seemed to be at peace, though he was unable to forget her 'pale,
broken face'. Her own suffering, Hilary told him, had made her think
of all that Florence must have gone through. It was a characteristically
selfless remark from a woman who seemed incapable of putting her
own concerns before those of others. As Madame Mohl said, Hilary's
'beautiful softness' did her harm because she possessed not the smallest

---

* In 1878 the houses in South Street were renumbered and 35 became number 10. On
Florence's death in 1910, so many petitions were received by the London County Council,
requesting that a plaque be placed on the building to commemorate her residence there, that
the rule that an individual had to be dead for twenty years before a memorial could be
considered was waived, and, in July 1912, the Duke of Westminster unveiled a plaque. In
1929, 10 South Street was demolished, and in 1955 a new plaque to Florence Nightingale
was unveiled by the Princess Royal at the apartment block which stands on the site.

element of self-preservation. For a time Florence was distraught. Hilary had been slowly murdered by her family, with their incessant demands on her, as surely as if they had taken a knife to her throat, and she berated herself for having failed to rescue her cousin from the self-sacrifice that had swallowed up her life. The only saving grace was that Hilary was now at peace, for her end had been lingering and painful. 'The golden bowl is broken,' Florence wrote to Clarkey, '& it was the purest gold – and the most unworked gold – I have ever known.'

Number 35 South Street was 'truly a beautiful house', Florence wrote appreciatively of her father's generosity. There was enough glass, china and kitchen utensils, she reported sardonically after the move, 'to enable me to give the largest dinner parties, and the largest of my evening routs'. The principal rooms were at the back, and from the windows of her second-storey bedroom Florence had a fine view of Hyde Park across the grounds of palatial Dorchester House. The front of the property offered a less attractive prospect. Regularly there were 'disgraceful' scenes – 'and, after hours' – of 'drunken bad women' falling out of the pub opposite and rolling about in the mud in the street (it isn't clear whether Florence ever realized that, from 1872, one of the houses opposite was the home of the courtesan Catherine Walters, known as 'Skittles').

In the late 1870s, when number 35 was plagued with sanitary problems, Florence sought Douglas Galton's expertise. Her cook had a bad case of diphtheria, which Florence naturally attributed to a defect in the house's drainage. A recommended sanitary engineer called, inspected the situation 'most vigorously', and set about removing the upstairs WC and installing new soil pipes. The other major problem connected with the house arose in 1885 when the initial rent increase proposed by the Duke of Westminster, following the expiry of Florence's lease, almost compelled her to move. The Duke's kindness in reducing the rent enabled her to avoid this course of action, though she joked that she would have to leave if the Duke ever succeeded in his intention of renaming South Street 'Florence Nightingale Street'. One further disadvantage of living there was that Florence was practically on her sister's doorstep, and Parthenope had to be dissuaded from dropping in whenever it suited her. 'It is very good of you to offer to come tomorrow,' Florence wrote to Parthenope in the mid-1860s, 'but I could not see anyone, not if it were to save my life. I thought you knew that I worked every day from

7.30 to 5.30, & that <u>before</u> 1.00 I could not see anyone <u>except</u> to save the Indian Empire.'

Florence's bedroom was simply furnished, and decorated in white with no blinds or curtains. Visitors were struck by the light streaming through the windows, and by the lack of clutter, which formed a marked contrast to prevailing fashions of the period. Several pictures hung on the walls: a watercolour of an Egyptian sunset, an unframed copy of Guercino's *Ecce Homo*, and a chromolithograph of *The Ground above Sebastopol*; and on the mantelpiece facing the bed was a framed text, 'It is I. Be not afraid.' A long shelf was placed behind the bed for books and papers. Flowers were sent every week by Louisa Ashburton, Florence's friend from girlhood, who begged to be allowed to see her, 'through the keyhole' if necessary. Dr Sutherland had once accused Florence of being 'a vain thing' for having decorated her room. 'There are some people,' she riposted, 'who always say the wrong thing.' The drawing room was even more sparsely furnished. On the walls were engravings of the Sistine Chapel, but the room's predominant feature was the bookcases, mostly full of Blue Books.

Florence's household at South Street generally consisted of four or five servants: a cook and kitchen maid, one or two housemaids, and Florence's personal maid, a position filled for several years by Temperance Hatcher (Florence also employed the services of a messenger called, aptly, Messenger). Temperance had been born at Sherfield, near Embley, where she had entered service. Later she married Peter Grillage – the Russian orphan from Balaclava whom Florence had sent to England where he became her parents' footman – and they moved to Plymouth. Florence considered Temperance to be one of the more trustworthy of the servants she employed. The Dowding sisters – Jane (or Jenny), Ann and Fanny – born in Hampshire and similarly put through their paces by Fanny Nightingale before entering Florence's service in London, were also above average, and Fanny Dowding, like Temperance Hatcher, would be remembered in Florence's will. But more often than not, maids and cooks were found wanting, and Florence's correspondence bridles with terms of abuse about them – 'half-witted', 'slattern', 'drunk', 'flirt', 'cheat'. Even by the lofty standards of her mother and sister, Florence was an exacting mistress, especially when it came to hygiene. Delany, one 'feeble, incapable creature', who was always doing her own hair in Florence's presence, was described as being deficient 'in common decency,

tidiness, cleanliness', and accused of putting Florence's cap on a chair '&
the po [chamber pot] atop of it'. It's hardly surprising, therefore, to find
Florence throughout the 1860s in a 'perennial state of hunt' for good
maids. Number 35 South Street, she admitted, was 'a very strict place
owing to my invalid life'. Some prospective employees baulked at the
rules. A maid refused to take a job as it involved her taking her mistress's
meals up several flights of stairs; and a cook resented having to take her
orders through a maid, in the absence of a housekeeper.

There is no surviving testimony from the servants themselves to tell
us what it was like to be in Florence's service. To her credit, she paid
them generous wages (though, in a competitive market, this was one
way of ensuring their loyalty): £14 a year in the early 1860s, plus 1s.
6d. a week beer money and 1s. 6d. a week washing money, 'and everything else found'. In later years she rewarded faithful retainers with
contributions to savings bank accounts. She made sure that her younger
maids were carefully instructed for their first communion, and was
assiduous in caring for their health, writing personally to doctors about
the smallest complaint, or addressing a 'Hair-cutter' in Oxford Street
about a kitchen maid's hair, which was alive with lice. Her attitude to
her staff was summed up in a remark she once made about one of her
cooks, Mrs Neild. 'As Mrs N. to me, so have I been to God.'

Food was one creature comfort that Florence enjoyed whenever she
was well enough. In 1861 she was the inspiration for 'Rice à la Sœur
Nightingale', a recipe concocted by Francatelli, formerly chef at the
Reform Club, which, appropriately, was a kedgeree, an English form of
an Indian dish. Having expended considerable energy on the question
of nutritive diets for patients, Florence was no less concerned when it
came to her own diet as an invalid. There are recipes in her own hand
for her favourite meals, boiled mutton and turnips among them, along
with instructions about the best means of digesting food, drawn up for
Jowett when he was ill ('the main thing is to roll the food well about in
the mouth till it excites the saliva and so becomes a pulp'). A disappointing meal might result in a pointed query directed at the kitchen
staff: 'Why was the glue pot used for the lamb cutlets?' Alcohol was
welcomed in moderation, ginger and port wine being especial favourites.
Florence thought soldiers should drink less, nuns more, and she sent a
gift of brandy to Bermondsey when Mother Mary Clare Moore was
recovering from illness in 1864.

From the late 1860s, boxes of produce – containing fruit, game, chicken and cake – were regularly sent up to Florence at South Street from the kitchen at Embley. This was an expedient designed to save her household from paying the exorbitant London food prices of the time, though there was a charge of £150 a year for the service. Retrenchment became Florence's watchword. By the beginning of the 1870s, her father had increased her allowance from its 1853 figure of £500 a year to more than double that amount, paid quarterly in advance. On top of this, Mr Nightingale was also responsible for Florence's rates and ground rent. But income sometimes fell short of her expenditure, and she was forced to request an advance from Uncle Sam. Her enormous printing bill often accounted for her overspending, but so also did her generosity to worthy causes. She showed fierce loyalty to the villagers of Lea Hurst, and donated generously to the annual medical bill for the village's old and sick.

A succession of cats formed an important part of the household at 35 South Street, providing Florence with much solace, companionship and amusement. 'Dumb beasts observe you so much more than talking beings,' she wrote while mourning Sidney Herbert, 'and know so much better, what you are thinking of.' A story did the rounds in the 1870s that she kept seventeen cats, with a nurse to attend to each, and that the cats were periodically sent to the country for a change of air. Apart from the bit about the nurses, this isn't so far from the truth. Cats figure largely in her correspondence, especially in letters to fellow ailurophiles like her mother and Madame Mohl, and sometimes literally stalk through her papers, leaving a trail of inky paw prints. Mr Bismark [sic] was a large white, 'the most sensitively affectionate of cats, very gentle and really a lady', who moved to South Street in 1867. A little earlier, Tom and Topsy had taken up residence on Florence's bed, 'greatly to the horror of big Pussie, who does nothing but snarl at them'. Through the years, cats come and go: a large Persian called Gladstone, Mr Darky, Tib, Mrs Tit, and poor old Mr Muff who ended up being shot by a gamekeeper while out taking a stroll at Embley. Mr Bismark was especi-ally prized for being a 'very clean cat' who 'never makes a mistake'. He was rewarded with a precise regime to serve his needs. A newspaper was spread like a tablecloth on the floor for his meals, 'which he eats like a gentleman out of a plate', and he was particularly partial to a little rice pudding with his five o'clock tea. In keeping with her emphasis on hygiene, Florence had little patience with messy cats, like Fluffy and Jubilee, who lived at Claydon, and instructed the housekeeper there that, 'If cats cannot be taught to be clean, they must be destroyed.' The ignorance of vets was on a par with the failings of the medical profession. One London vet was responsible for the deaths of two Nightingale cats, a mother and her kitten. Much to Florence's distress, a patent treatment intended to destroy parasites turned out to be an extract of tar, resulting in a cruel death for both pets. She vowed to save future animals from veterinary surgeons.

Temporarily losing a roaming cat was a regular occurrence: '. . . I have had quite too much of policemen, and printing handbills, and offering rewards and paying them, for lost or stolen tomcats in London.' In 1869 Tib strayed into the house of Florence's neighbour, Lord Lucan, ignominious leader of the Charge of the Light Brigade, from where he was hastily retrieved. Joseph and Pickle, two other toms who went missing, were not so fortunate, and were never found. Florence mated her cats carefully and distributed their litters to specially selected homes, for instance, sending a kitten to Parthenope's stepson Frederick Verney when he was at school at Harrow. But over the breeding of cats she could exercise only limited control. 'My present Pussie has been married twice and no signs of little cats,' she complained in 1862. Even worse was a 'mesalliance'. Repeatedly Florence chose husbands of high extraction as mates, only to find that her cats preferred to take up with low toms from the local mews.

Relaxation was rare, but when Florence did spare time for herself, reading was a suitably sedentary occupation, although no novel possessed the excitement for her of a solid work of statistics (in 1857 she had told Sidney Herbert that Dr Balfour, the head of the Army Statistical Department, was putting together some returns of disease in India as a Christmas present for her). Books were borrowed and loaned (Jowett sent Florence books that she was having difficulty in obtaining from the Oxford Union library). Devotional works, increasingly mystical writings sometimes lent to her by Mary Clare Moore, were carefully annotated. Thomas à Kempis's *Imitation of Christ* was turned to by Florence at critical junctures in her life, for example, during her estrangement from Aunt Mai, when she writes of being 'altogether without any human fellowship' in the margins of one chapter. In the wider secular canon of literature, Florence had a profound admiration for Aeschylus. She loved Homer and thought that his stories of Andromache and Antigone were 'worth all the women in the Old Testament put together, nay almost all the women in the Bible'. She was well versed in Shakespeare, sometimes quoting passages from the plays and poetry in her letters, though she complained that Shakespeare didn't portray heroic women. *Henry V* was used to describe Crimean heroes; Constance's speech in *King John* on the death of her child – 'Grief fills the room up of my absent child' – was paraphrased to describe Florence's own grief at the death of Sidney Herbert; and *Hamlet* was often referred to, though, as can be imagined, she had no time for his indecision. Milton was a favourite poet for all the Nightingales, and in her mother's old age Florence shared his sonnets with her. Florence's estimate of Jane Austen's novels was common to many Victorians: 'not striking, like Walter Scott's, but of which one feels the truth to be like that of a Dutch picture so characteristically is it painted'.

Among contemporary writers, she was conversant with the works of popular novelists like Bulwer Lytton, and enjoyed Mrs Gaskell's *Sylvia's Lovers* and the political novels of Trollope. Florence supported her sister's career as a writer by buying copies of her novels and distributing them to friends (this may have been welcomed, as George Smith of Smith, Elder, who published the early ones, commiserated with Parthenope that her public was not a large one). The first of Parthenope's five novels was *Avonhoe*, published in 1867 (and criticized by Florence for including the death of a fictional cat). They are all solid family sagas, mostly set in parts of the country – Derbyshire, Hampshire, the Midlands – that Parthenope knew well, and with little to recommend them to a modern readership aside from a fact of incidental interest, that the heroine of *Stone Edge* (1868) is called Cassandra.

Florence was an avid reader of George Eliot's fiction. She was especially interested in *Romola* for its portrayal of Savonarola, the fifteenth-century Dominican who ruled Florence in the 1490s and attempted to reform the Roman Catholic Church from within by appeals to mysticism. Savonarola was one of Florence's personal heroes. He was the only religious leader, she wrote, who recognized the duty, 'as a religious duty and claim, of every citizen to aid in forming a free government' (whereas most English people thought of God as 'an old woman', who didn't understand politics, and had nothing to do with the House of Commons). While acclaiming *Middlemarch*, on its appearance in 1873, as a 'novel of genius', Florence took Eliot severely to task for finding no better fate for Dorothea, that latter-day Teresa of Avila, than a marriage to 'an elderly sort of literary imposter, and quick after him, his relation, a baby sort of Cluricaune [a type of Irish fairy that has a taste for alcohol]'. Why couldn't Dorothea have been made to follow the example of someone like Octavia Hill, the housing reformer (who was related to George Eliot by marriage)? Or, better still, why couldn't she have been a nurse?

Novels about nurses touched another sore point. Florence admired Charles Kingsley, not least for his work for the sanitarian cause. But she strongly disapproved of his novel *Two Years Ago* (1857), because Kingsley had had the temerity to give his heroine, Grace Harvey, a nurse in the Crimean War, a romance plot in which she searches for the doctor she loves and finally marries him. The 'doctrine', Florence declared, that disappointment in love was the quality of a good nurse, did incalculable 'mischief'. In the first edition of *Notes on Nursing* she had singled out for criticism novelists who depicted 'ladies disappointed in love or fresh out of the drawing room turning into the war-hospitals to find their wounded loves'. One such example of this genre, which she had read, and been appalled by, was *Sword and Gown*, a melodrama of the Crimean War by George Alfred Lawrence, which was serialized in *Fraser's Magazine* in 1859 and subsequently published in book form. Lawrence portrays a death-bed scene between Royston Keene, a wounded soldier, and Cecil Tresilyan, an old flame now nursing with the Sisters of Charity. However, Cecil is praised by the novelist for her 'defiance of conventionality' when she abandons her duties to spend the night in Royston's bed: 'no one came in to molest them; there was work enough and to spare, that night, for all in Scutari.'

In the early 1860s, Florence recalled the occasion at Lea Hurst, a decade before the war, when Richard Monckton Milnes had read out loud from the newly published poems of the Brontë sisters. A poem by Emily Brontë had particularly appealed to her, and she asked Milnes if he could lend her the book. She thought that the poem in question was called 'The Captive'. In fact its title is 'The Prisoner' – though the poem's heroine is referred to as 'The captive' – and one can immediately see how apposite it must have appeared to Florence, both as an expression of her confinement as an invalid, and as a description in lyric terms of a mystic experience of overwhelming power. 'The captive' suffers, but, she tells her jailer, his 'bolts and irons strong;/And were they forged in steel they could not hold me long'. However, 'A messenger of hope comes every night to me, and offers, for short life, eternal liberty.'

> He comes with western winds, with evening's wandering airs,
> With that clear dusk of heaven that brings the thickest stars;
> Winds take a pensive tone, and stars a tender fire,
> And visions rise, and change, that kill me with desire.

16. A Crying Evil

On Christmas Eve 1864, a letter in *The Times* drew attention to a shocking case of workhouse neglect. Timothy Daly, a twenty-eight-year-old pauper and former Irish labourer, had died at the Holborn Workhouse in London from conditions of filthiness caused by inadequate nursing. Less than a week later, as public outcry at Daly's treatment continued unabated, Florence wrote to C. P. Villiers, the President of the Poor Law Board. Daly's tragic end, she told him, had highlighted the fact that there was no nursing worthy of the name in any workhouse in England. She was well aware of the difficulties of the Poor Law guardians in steering an effective course between pauperism and real want. But, she went on, a cardinal distinction in Poor Law relief as it operated in the workhouse system badly needed asserting: from the moment a pauper becomes sick, 'he ceases to be a pauper & becomes brother to the best of us & as a brother he should be cared for'.

Florence was no stranger to workhouse infirmaries. In the 1840s she had been a 'lady visitor' at the St Marylebone Workhouse; and, in 1847, she had also visited a workhouse outside London with Selina Bracebridge, probably in Warwickshire, near the Bracebridges' home. The experience, she wrote later, had been enough to break her heart. Significantly, in an exchange of letters with Henry Bence Jones during the Crimean War, Florence had discussed the appalling state of workhouse infirmaries, and had informed him that her only plan for the future was to bring trained nursing to 'the poorest and most neglected institution' she could find. By the mid-1860s, the visible improvement in the standards of care of the sick poor in the voluntary hospitals – where the poor were supported by charitable subscriptions – formed a shocking contrast to the provision made for sick paupers in the workhouses, which now held five patients for every one in an ordinary hospital. Over one-third of workhouse inmates were sick, and in the Metropolitan workhouses the figure for the adult able-bodied was as low as 10 per cent. The workhouse infirmaries had become the 'great state hospitals of the metropolis', commented a *Lancet* commission in 1866. Yet there were no trained nurses for these workhouse patients, only pauper nurses, women inmates who were not themselves ill, and who were notorious for drunkenness, and for stealing the food and gin of their patients.* The majority of workhouse infirmaries exhibited only a superficial veneer of cleanliness. Ventilation was poor, there was a deficiency of toilet and washing facilities (at Kensington and Paddington some of the sick washed in their chamber pots), beds were made up in dirty linen which was sometimes left unchanged for weeks, and overcrowding was prevalent. Medical attendance was occasional and, as few of the pauper nurses were able to read, the distribution of medicines invariably haphazard and irregular.

The Poor Law Amendment Act of 1834 had established some 650 Poor Law unions administered by boards of locally elected guardians under the supervision of the Poor Law Commissioners in London. Outdoor relief for the able-bodied unemployed, instituted under the Elizabethan Act of 1601, had been abolished, and the principle of 'less eligibility' introduced. From now on, anyone seeking public aid would enter a residential workhouse where they would receive food and shelter in return for performing menial tasks. Conditions in the workhouse were deliberately harsh and austere so that only the most destitute and desperate would apply. Within a decade, however, the high level of unemployment had fallen, and the workhouses had become homes for sick adults, children, the elderly and incurable, in addition to the jobless poor, even though, as Florence later remarked, the revised Poor Law legislation had never made express provision for medical or nursing care.

Florence was always a staunch critic of the Poor Law reforms of the 1830s, especially in arguments with her father, who had once been a member of his local board of guardians in Derbyshire and, latterly, in discussions with Jowett, who shared her sense of urgency about the need for change. The Poor Law was rotten at the heart, she once said, and wanted cutting down to the root. The 'workhouse test', far from reducing pauperism, had actually increased it. The punishment doled out to 'these pitiable paupers', by giving them unproductive labour at unre-

---

* In 1866, in the forty London workhouses, it was recorded that there were 142 non-pauper paid nurses attending on 21,500 sick and infirm patients. However, these women, usually scrubbers or laundresses who had been given promotion, possessed no hospital training.

munerative prices, had proved itself of no avail, 'for the workhouses are overflowing and the people are starving', and instead of helping the able-bodied to self-dependence the Poor Law had simply perpetuated the problems. The result was that the ratepayer was burdened with the cost, and society denied the benefit of its citizens' full productiveness.

Florence's plan of introducing trained nursing to the workhouse infirmaries was part of a broader scheme to reform the entire workhouse system, which envisaged the eventual dismantling of its punitive element, except for cases of the wilfully unemployed. From mid-century, many individuals had actively involved themselves in attempts to eliminate abuses in workhouses. In 1853 Louisa Twining started reporting on the hardship and neglect she had uncovered at the Strand Workhouse. Five years later she founded the Workhouse Visiting Society with the intention of infiltrating lady visitors into a number of Metropolitan workhouses. The medical profession had formed an association for the improvement of London workhouses; while in the wake of Timothy Daly's death, and another death in similar circumstances shortly afterwards at St Giles's Workhouse, the new owner of the *Lancet*, James Wakley, commissioned three doctors to visit the London workhouses and publish the results of their inquiry. The conclusion of their 'soberly sensational' reports was that only far-reaching reform would bring an end to 'scandal' and 'reproach'. This was precisely what Florence, working in conjunction with Dr Sutherland, would prescribe, that the care for the sick poor offered by the workhouse infirmaries should be of the same quality as that provided by the best civil hospitals in the country.

Coincidentally, at the time the Daly scandal emerged, Florence was already supervising a small-scale experiment designed to test the introduction of skilled nursing into workhouses. In January 1864 she was overwhelmed with other work, but unable to ignore an approach from William Rathbone, the philanthropist and member of the Liverpool shipping family, offering to fund a 'lady visitor' at the Brownlow Hill Workhouse infirmary in Liverpool, and asking for Florence's assistance. William Rathbone was the sixth of that name, the latest in the line of a high-minded dynasty that prided itself on having become the conscience of its home city. Rathbone was impetuous: he was once compared to someone driving his railway engine at full speed without bothering first to lay down the track. His and Florence's paths had crossed at the start of the decade when he had consulted her about his plans for the training school for nurses opened by him in Liverpool in 1862. His interest in nursing arose from the skilful care that his first wife had received as she was dying. The difference this comfort had made to her final hours had turned his thoughts to the suffering of the poor, who were unable to afford such aid. Florence's reaction to his proposal regarding the Liverpool workhouse infirmary was to recommend that he guarantee the cost of a superintendent and team of nurses for a time rather than a visitor, 'who sees how much could be done and cannot do it'. Rathbone wholeheartedly agreed. Twelve nurses, together with a Lady Superintendent, would be selected from St Thomas's. The approval of the Vestry, the governing body of the infirmary, to which Rathbone belonged, was sought and won, with Florence herself writing to George Carr, the Governor, smoothing the way and encouraging him to believe that he would personally receive the kudos for the scheme. There was a chance, she told Rathbone, that the Vestry might eventually take all the cost on themselves once they saw the advantages and economy of good nursing. 'A good wise matron' might save many of her patients from pauperism by first nursing them well, 'and then rousing them to exertion and helping them to employment'. As the project steamed ahead in the first half of 1864, one overriding question remained: who would fill the post of wise matron?

The field of potential candidates was limited. Since opening its doors in 1860, sixty trainees had been accepted by the Nightingale Training School, and only twenty-five of these were still working. One woman stood out above the rest. Agnes Jones was thirty-one years old, the upper-middle-class daughter of an Irish family, and had completed the year's training at St Thomas's. Her father, who was dead, had reached the rank of lieutenant-colonel in the British Army. Her uncle was Sir John Lawrence, the Viceroy of India. It is difficult to know what kind of person Agnes Jones really was, as our impression of her has been muddied by the hagiographical accounts of her life and character produced shortly after her death both by Florence, and by Agnes's family. Superficially she fitted the Nightingale mould exactly. As a girl in Dublin, Agnes had taught at the local ragged school and visited the sick. In 1853, while on a continental holiday with her family, she had spent a week at Kaiserswerth. Inspired by Florence Nightingale's Crimean example, Agnes subsequently determined to become a nurse, though some years passed before she could overcome her mother's opposition. In 1860 she returned to Kaiserswerth for eight months' training, and, after leaving St Thomas's in 1863 with sterling references from Mrs Wardroper, worked as a sister at the Great Northern Hospital in London.

After Agnes Jones's early death, Florence was to remark on her prettiness and wit, writing that she resembled a Louis XIV shepherdess, while also recalling how quickly her face had become lined with care. But her early encounters with Agnes, during which she became aware of the younger woman's strident religious fervour, gave her cause for concern. Agnes's aggressive evangelical beliefs were a characteristic that William Rathbone had come across two years earlier, when he was considering her as first superintendent of his new training school. 'Is its foundation and cornerstone to be Christ and Him crucified, the only Saviour?' she had asked him, after he sent her the ground plan. '. . . I shall not embark in any work whose great aim is not obedience to the command: "Preach the gospel to every creature." ' Florence believed that Agnes Jones hid a complete lack of religious modesty behind her religious zeal. She thought her 'impertinent', and had advised Agnes 'to work for twenty years for the Lord' before ascending to the pulpit. Agnes's health was a concern, in particular her partial deafness in both ears, a condition possibly of nervous origin. She was also subject to bouts of serious depression, though once Agnes had embarked on her grim task at the Liverpool Workhouse it was scarcely surprising that she was at times prone to low spirits. In her diary Agnes recorded her sense of 'dreariness . . . loneliness' and isolation, though Florence later maintained that these entries were generally written late at night when she was overtired.

Despite these reservations, Agnes Jones was selected. After a holiday in Ireland to recuperate and prepare for her coming ordeal, Agnes made a preliminary visit to Liverpool in August 1864. She arrived alone at the great black gates of the Brownlow Hill Workhouse, where the porter quibbled about admitting her, and experienced strong feelings of imprisonment as the gates closed around her. The following April, awaiting the arrival of the main party of twelve trained nurses and fifteen probationers, Agnes wrote that 'It almost seems as if over so many of these beds NO HOPE must be written . . .' All the available evidence suggests that conditions in Liverpool's workhouse infirmary, one of the largest in England, were somewhat better than in those in other parts of the country – not least because of Rathbone's humane influence on the committee – but Agnes Jones's initial impression of the wards was that they resembled Dante's *Inferno*. There were roughly 1,200 inmates, divided between three hospitals housing male, female and fever patients (Agnes's brief was to begin with the male and fever wards). The thirty-seven pauper nurses she found on arrival there were to be trained to an acceptable standard, but in practice they offered unsatisfactory material, were inclined to spend their wages on drink, and many were eventually dismissed. From London, Florence sent alternately chivvying and encouraging messages as Agnes assumed command as 'an apostle of good order'. It was Scutari all over again, Florence wrote, the same kind of filth and immorality, but Agnes must never forget that she was doing great work in the midst of considerable difficulties. The eyes and expectations of half the kingdom were fixed on her, Florence told her in August 1865, in a note dictated to Sutherland, and if she succeeded, 'your workhouse will become the centre of one of the greatest reforms of the age'.

However, there was 'unhappiness, and tears'. That first autumn the new system almost broke down in a dispute between Governor Carr and Miss Jones on the thorny problem of who could claim authority over the nurses. This was a significant stumbling point. Carr refused 'to require' the pauper nurses to be subordinate to the Lady Superintendent; not only that, but he subordinated the trained nurses to himself 'as if they were paupers'. 'Hibernian rows', according to Dr Sutherland, ensued between the Irish Agnes Jones and Carr. Florence was sympathetic to Agnes's predicament. As the disagreement simmered on into 1866, Florence confessed to Rathbone that it was difficult to know how Agnes Jones 'can get on for a single day' with the government of the infirmary divided against itself. She feared that the experiment was doomed, along with the whole future of nursing in workhouses. '. . . I feel that none but a woman, and a woman who has gone through the same kind of thing, for herself, and for others . . . can tell men the absolute necessity of giving a proper position to the matron, on the obvious ground that, unless this is done, it is impossible . . . to do anything really important.' Privately she thought that Agnes Jones should resign.

It did not come to that. Concerted efforts on all sides were made at reconciliation, and although the problem remained unresolved, and the control of the sick wards continued to rest with the workhouse master, in the short term a modus vivendi was reached. In March 1867, nearly two years after Agnes Jones and her team had started their work in Liverpool, the Workhouse Vestry presented a favourable report on the trained nurses project, so favourable that the Vestry considered placing all the wards under their management. Yet the statistical evaluation of the new system of nursing appeared to produce mixed results. The mortality rates for 1866 and 1867 were not lower in the wards with trained nurses as had been expected. It was left to Florence to point out that proper controls in the analysis of data had not been observed. The worst cases might have been assigned to the wards with trained nurses, leaving patients with better prognoses to the pauper nurses in other parts of the infirmary.

Agnes Jones was praised for her 'indefatigable exertion' in 'a most difficult and arduous post'. Governor Carr commended her zeal and devotion to duty. Both wards and patients were cleaner, discipline and obedience were being maintained, and medical instructions followed assiduously. A report by one of the infirmary doctors suggested that Agnes's success could not be easily measured, but would be 'inscribed in the hearts and memories of grateful recipients, of the convalescent, the suffering, the dying'. To read, though, in Agnes's diary of her reaction to the children's death-beds she attended, and to remember as one does so the importance that she attached to saving their souls, cannot but leave a rather chilling impression. '. . . A great many children die,' runs an entry for 1867, 'and I can scarcely be sorry when I think of what might be; but it is often sad to see them dying. They look so pretty in their little coffins, and we lay them out so nicely.'

Meanwhile, the death of the unfortunate Timothy Daly in Holborn Workhouse had been used by Florence as a pretext to push for the extension of trained nursing to the Metropolitan workhouses. The Liverpool experiment, which was still months away from being implemented when details of Daly's treatment came to light, was to stand as a model of what might be achieved on a wider basis, first in London, then throughout the country. Florence's initial approach to Villiers, President of the Poor Law Board (a cabinet office), at the end of 1864, was deliberately confined to the provision of trained nursing under the Nightingale Fund, though in fact she suffered no illusion that anything less than a sweeping overhaul of the system of Poor Law finance and administration was likely to effect lasting change. Her moderation worked and Villiers was hooked. '. . . I shall be happy to communicate with you personally at any time most convenient to yourself,' he wrote to her.

Charles Villiers had been a liberal Tory in the 1820s, and had developed increasingly radical views during the following decade as he entered Parliament, opposed the Corn Laws, and became a firm supporter of the new Poor Law. Greville, the Whig diarist, found him 'always sensible, unprejudiced and the most satisfactory person to talk to', a view with which Florence would not necessarily have disagreed. In January 1865 Villiers called on her, demonstrated that he was open to persuasion, and a process of collaboration was set in motion. When he was unable to attend an appointment on a subsequent occasion – he was overseeing a major reform to the Poor Law, the important change in the unit of financial responsibility from parish to union – he sent the Poor Law Inspector for the Metropolitan district, Henry Farnall, in his place. Farnall was less cautious than his master, and quickly became a vital ally for Florence in her programme for drastic reform. Farnall shared her 'divine impatience', and there was no one in the Poor Law office, Florence told Harry Verney, 'who can hold a candle to him in powers of administration'. Maintaining the pressure on Villiers, who informed the Commons in May that he was hopeful of great improvements in nursing in the workhouses, Florence joined forces with the Association for Improving Workhouse Infirmaries, a new pressure group with a committee of distinguished figures including Dickens, Mill and the Archbishop of York. They had been sending earls, archbishops and MPs, she wrote to Harriet Martineau, to storm Villiers in his den.

But Villiers's first attempt at framing an amended Bill fell far short of what had been expected when a clause which would have enabled the Poor Law Board to compel guardians to improve their workhouses was struck out. Disheartened, Florence turned to the Prime Minister, Palmerston, who promised his support for a fuller measure of reform in the next parliamentary session. Farnall agreed that they must work even harder so that they could taste 'next year's ripened fruit'; and with his and Sutherland's help, Florence drew up a new scheme for Villiers's agreement. Her 'ABC of Workhouse Reform' enshrined three guiding principles. The first, and most fundamental of these, was that the sick, insane, incurable – 'and, above all, the children' – should be separated from the rest of the population of the workhouse. 'The care and government of the <u>sick</u> poor is a thing totally different from the government of paupers.' Secondly, a central administration should be introduced for economy and efficiency. Finally, this administration should be supported by a general rate levied throughout the Metropolitan area. This was the most radical idea of all. The entire medical treatment of Londoners in this plan would come under one central management. This management would possess the power to allocate vacant beds, 'and be able so to distribute the Sick . . . as to use all the establishments in the most economical way'.

Villiers gave his assent to this outline, and matters began to look hopeful again. Then disaster struck. On 18 October 1865, Palmerston died. Florence had lost a friend as well as a 'powerful protector'. He was the only man, she told William Farr, who could have dragged 'a too-liberal bill, especially in the Poor Law, through the Cabinet'. The Whig Government, with its precarious majority, limped on until it was toppled the following summer. Villiers was out, though he continued to advise the reformers from behind the scenes. Lord Derby's incoming minority Government, led by Disraeli in the Commons, introduced a politician of a very different character and calibre into the post of President of the Poor Law Board. Gathorne Hardy, a hunting, fishing, shooting gentleman, was a Tory of the traditional type and a strong opponent of radicalism (including the extension of the franchise being proposed by Derby and Disraeli). Not wishing to waste a moment, Florence immediately sent Hardy a letter, offering her assistance 'in the great work you are about to enter', and signing off with a bid for sympathy, that she could do this only in so far as her 'feeble health' permitted. His reply gave small encouragement. Hardy respectfully acknowledged that Florence had 'earned no common title to advise and suggest upon anything which affects the treatment of the sick' – advice of which he would 'in all probability' avail himself – but stated that he was currently unavailable on other business. Soon afterwards, he removed Farnall from his Whitehall post, and banished him to the Yorkshire Poor Law district.

Yet even diehard conservatives like Gathorne Hardy recognized that some show of reform would be necessary to satisfy popular clamour. In the autumn of 1866 he appointed a committee to determine the cubic space requirement in workhouse infirmaries. The committee was largely made up of doctors, while Douglas Galton, Florence's cousin by marriage, contributed his sanitary expertise. The chairman, Sir Thomas Watson, the President of the Royal College of Physicians, knew Florence from her Upper Harley Street days, and invited her to make a submission on nurse training. She regarded the question of cubic space as the least of the prevalent evils – indeed, as she joked with black humour to Galton, it might be a very good thing 'to suffocate the "pauper sick" out of their misery' – but she dealt comprehensively with the structural arrangements in hospitals she considered essential for good nursing, at the same time reiterating her belief that there was no place for pauper nursing in the workhouse infirmaries, and drawing attention to the 'great experiment' in operation in Liverpool.

She was in the dark about what use Hardy was going to make of the committee's findings, believing that he probably intended to do nothing. In the event, she must have been surprised that he made as much of it as he did, though she was savagely critical of the Bill that he unveiled in the Commons in February 1867, arguing that it went nowhere near far enough, and asking Sir Harry Verney to raise objections and put forward amendments. For a start, Hardy proposed taking no direct action on workhouse nursing reform. This meant that the introduction of trained nurses would have to be fought for workhouse by workhouse. On the other hand, the new legislation did make specific improvements. Separate infirmaries were formed for fever cases and lunatics, set up under a Metropolitan Asylums Board with the power to build and run such hospitals from a Common Fund, similar to the one of Florence's devising. The non-infectious sick presented a different problem. If they had been removed, the guardians would have been left with just 11 per cent of their inmates, and the principle of 'less eligibility' would have been considerably undermined. The Bill therefore encouraged the building of separate infirmaries for the non-infectious sick without actually compelling the Poor Law Unions to comply.

The Metropolitan Poor Act became law in March 1867. During the second reading of the Bill, recognition of Florence's influence in making the new legislation possible was made in speeches in both the Lords and Commons. It was, as she herself said when the uproar surrounding the debates had died down, a beginning: the first explicit acknowledgement, as it has since been called, of the duty of the state to provide hospitals for the poor. Eighty years later, the idea would come to fruition with the foundation of Britain's National Health Service.

The woman to whom Florence turned most often in these years as a professional colleague was Mary Jones – no relation of Agnes – the Superintendent of the St John's House nursing sisterhood. She regularly consulted Mary Jones on all manner of nursing issues, not least over matters in Liverpool. At a time when the training of nurses for ordinary hospitals was not a priority for her, Florence constantly deferred to the older woman's greater practical experience. Out of this a personal friendship had been forged. Their differences during the Crimean War, when Florence had criticized the behaviour of St John's nurses sent to Scutari, were long forgotten. Mary Jones was her 'Very dearest friend', Florence, Jones's 'Dearest Mistress'. Mary Jones was among the few permitted to disturb Florence's seclusion. They shared spiritual interests and prayed together, though Mary was High Church (unlike her sister-hood, which was a Broad Church foundation). Gifts of 'a brace of grouse in their mountain heather', honey, pictures and books – even a bedstead when she complained of back pain – were sent to Mary Jones from Embley; and when Mary was in ill-health, as she often was, she was invited to sleep at South Street, or take holidays at the Nightingale homes in the country. 'A drive in an open carriage occasionally is all she is fit for & to be sent to bed at 9 o'clock', were Florence's instructions to her mother in advance of one of these visits. Mary required complete rest of body and mind. 'Hers is such a valuable life.'

Mary Jones is a largely overlooked pioneer of modern nursing. Born in 1812, she was the daughter of a cabinet-maker. She demonstrated early gifts as a nurse, entering St John's House following its formation in 1848, and becoming its second Lady Superintendent in 1853. The St John's sisters took no vows, and observed no monastic rule. The only religious requirement was that they should be members of the Church of England. They could be married or single, were able to live at home, and had the choice of working full- or part-time. Members of the community, sisters and probationers, pursued an apprenticeship in nurs-ing, at the end of which they received a certificate of excellence. As important an inspiration as the Protestant deaconesses at Kaiserswerth in providing a model for St John's were the training schools for school teachers being established in the first half of the century.

The officers of St John's House consisted of four individuals, the Master, the Lady Superintendent and two doctors, governed by a council of twenty-four men presided over by the Bishop of London. Like Florence, Mary Jones subscribed fully to the position that the Lady Superintendent should have complete control of the female staff in her hospital. In 1856, under Jones's supervision, the St John's sisterhood assumed responsibility for the nursing at the recently rebuilt King's College Hospital. Here, as an autonomous community within the hospital, St John's House established a reputation for their leading system of modern nursing. It was a system studied closely by Florence. In general she was prejudiced against the role of nursing sisterhoods – a hangover in part from her dealings with the Bridgeman nuns in the Crimea – and believed that better nursing arose from a spiritual commitment to patients carried out in a secular context. But she made an exception for Jones's sisters, incorporating a host of details from the St John's House experience of nurse training into her own plans for St Thomas's. At the end of 1860, the year that had seen the arrival of the Nightingale School's first probationers, Florence credited Mary Jones with having accomplished '(quietly and sensibly) the greatest work in hospital nursing which has been done'.

It was in response to a suggestion from Jones that Florence used the income that remained from the Nightingale Fund, following the foundation of the School, to support the training of midwives at King's by St John's House nurses. From October 1861, the Fund furnished and maintained ten lying-in beds in a 'capacious ward', paying £12 for each pupil in advance to the hospital to offset the cost of board and lodging during the six-month course. The Nightingale midwifery scheme was intended to lead the way in the training of midwives. A Government-sponsored school for this purpose was 'a want long felt in England', in contrast to the situation on the continent. Florence hoped that the arrangement at King's would offer a prototype for the future, while providing a skilled midwifery service for the rural poor, training women from country parishes as midwives. After a century during which doctors had increasingly encroached on midwifery, claiming it as a legitimate part of their own province and thereby depriving women of a traditional means of earning a living, she also saw the plan as a way of providing 'medical women' with a branch of medicine entirely their own. It seemed obvious to her that no lying-in 'would be attended but by a woman if a woman were as skilful as a man . . .' There would be constant demand for proper nursing of women during their confinements, if only it was available. But, in the six years it lasted, the King's scheme met with only modest success (the total number of midwives completing the training in the first five years was no more than thirty). A large part of the problem stemmed from economic difficulties. A parish could not afford to subsidize the midwife during her absence (when she would have to forgo half a year's earnings). Nor could it guarantee her employment on her return.

What condemned the Nightingale lying-in ward to its relatively short-lived existence, though, were two major crises arising in swift succession, one which resulted in Mary Jones's resignation from St John's House, the other in the permanent closure of the ward. Mary Jones had long wished for greater self-regulation for her community, to protect it from the interference of the male council and bishop in its internal affairs. In 1867 a dispute occurred when the St John's sisters were denied the right to choose their own High Church chaplain, and matters quickly escalated into an unseemly power struggle in which Florence could not help but become involved. She tried to be evenhanded, while listening with growing impatience as William Bowman, her old friend from King's, and one of the doctors on the St John's House council, 'jawed away . . . till I am much more dead than alive' on the subject of regulations and possible nursing replacements. In the end she sided with Mary Jones against the council's assertion of its autocratic powers. Discipline and internal management of sisters and nurses could not be in any other hands than 'those of ONE female Head'. It was yet another example of men interfering where they were not wanted. '. . . I never would have created men,' Florence wrote in a fit of annoyance to Sutherland, 'never, never.' Her support didn't stop Mary Jones, and all but two of her sisters, leaving St John's House at the beginning of 1868. As far as Florence was concerned, that put an end to sisterhoods.

Almost simultaneous with these events was a sudden disease scare in the ward itself. In the summer of 1867 Florence had been alerted by a worried Mary Jones to an increase in the mortality of the women in the lying-in ward, caused by puerperal fever. Mary Jones, probably correctly as it turned out, believed that 'the unhappy post-mortem room', close to the ward, was 'the prime, if not the sole cause of the evil', while one of the medical staff took up the argument commonly advanced at this time that maternal mortality was likely to be high if a maternity ward was situated inside an ordinary hospital. The cause of puerperal fever was not known until 1902 (when it was identified as a form of the micro-organism streptococcus A). But published research from mid-century onwards, of which the individuals running the King's midwifery ward were unfortunately unaware, did point to a connection between medical students performing hospital autopsies before entering the lying-in ward and examining women in labour. Puerperal fever was cadaveric blood poisoning, and women and babies were dying as a result of particles from cadavers passed on from the hands of students and doctors. In fact, the percentage of deaths in the King's ward was not unacceptably high when compared with statistical returns from other institutions. It was below the 4 per cent average for lying-in hospitals, and well below the 20 per cent death rate at one point recorded by the Paris hospital La Maternité, whose midwifery training was highly praised, not least by Florence herself. Nevertheless, to Florence the King's statistics exhibited 'deplorable midwifery mortality', and in conjunction with the hospital authorities a decision was made to close the ward from January 1868. The Nightingale Fund's connection with King's was thus severed, and although the hospital had hopes of utilizing the Fund's income in opening another lying-in ward, nothing further came of the plan. Florence's scheme for training midwives similarly came to an abrupt halt. She continued to express interest in a training school, while recognizing that the growth in medical training for women was a threat to the independent existence of such a school.

However, Florence's concern about maternal mortality from puerperal fever, prompted by the cases at King's, encouraged her to investigate the subject further. A request from Vicky, the Crown Princess of Prussia, the Queen's eldest daughter, for Florence's assistance in plans for a nurse training school near Spandau, which was to include midwives, helped focus her ideas and ultimately became the impetus behind Florence's writing of her *Introductory Notes on Lying-in Institutions*. The Crown Princess was 'cultivating herself in knowledge of sanitary (& female) administration for her future great career', Florence reported to Sir John McNeill in December 1868. 'She comes alone like a girl, pulls off her hat & jacket like a five-year-old, drags about a great portfolio of plans, & kneels by my bedside correcting them'. She found Vicky 'quick as lightning', especially in her inquiries about the workings of lying-in huts for soldiers' wives, in which there had been as many as 800 confinements without a single case of puerperal fever.

Florence's *Introductory Notes* was finally published in 1871. Its appearance was delayed not only by all the other demands on Florence's time, but also by the difficulty posed in obtaining reliable statistics, and the severe attack of illness she suffered in the autumn of 1869, during which she left instructions to Dr Sutherland to edit a paper on the subject from all the materials she had 'so laboriously prepared'. Dedicated to Socrates, whose mother was said to have been a midwife, the finished work offers the usual prescriptions for improvements to sanitation and ventilation, while concluding that the effect of the lying-in institution on mortality rates was greater than such social factors as class, health or stamina. 'With all their defects, midwifery statistics point to one truth, namely that there is a large amount of preventable mortality in midwifery practice, and that, as a general rule, the mortality is far, far greater in lying-in hospitals than among women lying-in at home.'

If Mary Jones is all but forgotten, Jane Shaw Stewart, who, as Florence's candidate in 1861, had become the head of the Army's first female nursing service, has been to a great extent obliterated from the historical record. The story of Shaw Stewart's seven years as Superintendent-General at Netley, and at the Royal Herbert Hospital in Woolwich, has been described as veering 'between tragedy and farce'. It ended in disaster in 1868 when, in a humiliating sequence of events, Jane Shaw Stewart was obliged to resign following a War Office inquiry into the 'unsatisfactory' state of Army nursing, during which she was accused of imperious behaviour and violent temper.

The daughter of a Scottish baronet, and very much conscious of her membership of the patrician class, Jane was a year Florence's junior. She had come to venerate Florence as her heroine after meeting her just days before Florence set off for Scutari. Years later she recalled that 'memorable' occasion. 'I see you now,' she wrote nostalgically to Florence, 'in a black silk dress and a little white bonnet...' In the Crimea she had served with distinction, earning approbation from Florence which was just occasionally tempered by concern for Jane's unpredictable ways. After the war Jane had continued to obtain nursing experience in civilian hospitals, while carrying out research for Florence into hospital systems and layouts. 'I shall serve you until you wish my service ended,' she told her, 'or until I die.' A marked cooling in the women's relationship occurred after the publication, in 1858, of Florence's work on female nursing in military hospitals. This incorporated Jane's confidential memoranda on the subject, as well as excerpts from her letters without the author's permission. Jane was utterly horrified to find her words in print. Although the book was published anonymously, she considered Florence's action a 'Breach of trust'. Furthermore, she had begun to perceive her idol's feet of clay. She thoroughly disapproved of Florence working behind the scenes on Government commissions and legislation – and was not afraid of telling her so. She 'mourned over' Florence doing 'the work of men', and saw her post-war activities as in direct conflict with her own conception of what a 'lady's' role in nursing reform should be: '. . . silent, quiet, as well as laborious and trying work, in governing, training and organizing the women who nurse in hospitals' under the auspices of the Anglican Church. Florence was in danger of forsaking 'the glorious talent of action, of female action and direction, which you have received' for male principles of work. The Nightingale Fund, she had prophesied, would be 'a continual hindrance', and as for Florence's immersion in Indian affairs, how could this be an effective use of her time given that she had no 'knowledge or experience of India'? Florence grew accustomed to regular doses of this epistolary abuse, though Aunt Mai had stepped in at one point to insist that Jane give up writing to her, warning her that in future her letters would be opened and read by a third party.

Jane's acceptance of her appointment as Superintendent-General, shortly before Sidney Herbert's death, was made with a heavy heart. She did not see herself as in any sense a pioneer, but regarded herself instead as being called 'to serve God in the painful way of official duty' (to Florence's immense irritation, Jane had won the right to stipulate that all her nurses should be Anglicans). In October 1861, Jane arrived at Woolwich with a staff of six, moving to Netley in 1863, and then back to the newly opened Royal Herbert three years later. Things started to go wrong from the start. Like Florence before her, Jane insisted on the right as Superintendent-General to independent control of her nurses without interference from medical officers or the military governor. Her terms of reference, published in the official regulations, replicated Florence's privileged wartime relationship with the Secretary of State for War, with whom Jane communicated directly and to whom she was answerable. It represented an independent chain of female authority similar to that of the St John's House sisterhood; and, as in the case of St John's, it was a state of affairs that the male authorities within the institution immediately started to challenge. Jane Shaw Stewart's aristocratic hauteur made it all the easier for them to do so. The medical officers lost no opportunity to undermine her: refusing to allow her nurses to accompany them on their rounds, intriguing with disaffected members of her staff, and spreading stories of her supposed failings to the War Office.

Added to this was the broader question of how effective the female nursing at Netley and Woolwich actually was. Was it even really necessary? The War Office had consistently opposed the introduction of female nurses into Army hospitals, preferring a system of properly trained orderlies. Florence herself, with her anxious concern for propriety in military hospitals, had always been cautious about letting loose more than a small number of nurses in their wards. As a consequence, the nursing service at Netley and Woolwich, into the early 1880s, never consisted of more than about twelve women. Most of the personal tasks, especially those requiring close physical proximity to the patient, continued to be carried out by male orderlies. In the meantime, there was public criticism of the standard of the female intake from St Thomas's, and of their rapid turnover. In 1866 *The Times* reported that 'it appears to be generally considered that the introduction of lady nurses is an innovation from which no benefit can possibly be derived'.

Matters reached a head with the War Office inquiry held before a three-man tribunal over ten days in May and June 1868. It must have been a deeply embarrassing experience for the intensely private Jane Shaw Stewart as she was forced to listen to a string of allegations about her personal behaviour from witnesses who included members of her own nursing staff and the Commandant of Netley, Colonel Wilbraham. Nurse Henrietta claimed to have overheard the Superintendent-General say of the situation at Netley that 'rather than be subject to any restraint either in the wards or as regards the nurses she would rather see the place blown up'. Testimony was provided of her insulting and sometimes violent manner, and of how she clapped her hands and stamped her feet when angry. One of the doctors claimed that she had snapped her fingers at him and slammed the door in his face. Reading the closely printed pages of the tribunal's proceedings, Florence felt like 'a Chief Justice'.

To Mary Jones, she wrote 'of the most painful thing I ever had to do in my most painful life ... Mrs S. Stewart is accused of Anglicanism, "Foaming-at-the-Mouth", Manslaughter, "Snapping her Fingers", Insanity, <u>Drink</u>, Being Silent in an Omnibus, General Incivility, Not accepting an Invitation to tea, &c &c &c.' She had no doubt of Jane's efficiency as a nursing Superintendent, but said that she herself would have faced down these male opponents with a laugh rather than Jane's fury, seemingly forgetting her own feelings of oppression when dealing with adversaries in the Crimea, twelve years earlier. The result was, in any case, a foregone conclusion. Jane Shaw Stewart had to go. What, though, of the future for military nursing, and could the post of Superintendent-General 'be of any used to the service after such a scene as this?'

However, the office survived to have its dignity restored under Shaw Stewart's successor, Jane Deeble. Mrs Deeble was paraded before Florence at South Street before being dispatched for a short period of instruction under the St Thomas's matron, Mrs Wardroper. Florence was mildly unimpressed. Mrs Deeble was no doubt sincere and cour-ageous, but any medical man would be able to wrap her round his finger, and 'She will be engaged in planning a <u>nice tea</u> for the Nurses, while she lets the Nursing go to ruin . . .' This was unfair, but then Florence was habitually inclined towards harsher judgements of military nurses than of regular nursing recruits, perhaps because military nursing was a role that in some sense she continued to reserve for herself. There was in fact more to Mrs Deeble than this. Not the least of her advantages, in terms of her relations with the medical corps, was that she was the widow of an army medical officer, and therefore one of their kind, with none of the social superiority that had acted as a barrier in their dealings with Jane Shaw Stewart. Throughout the 1870s, Florence continued to pass an eagle eye over successive Fund candidates as they joined the staffs of Netley and Woolwich. But slowly the authority of the Superintendent of the Army female nursing service was whittled away. Mrs Deeble no longer reported directly to the Secretary of State for War; nor did she have exclusive power to appoint and dismiss her sisters, a right that eventually passed out of her hands into those of the Director-General of the Army Medical Department.

The South African and Egyptian campaigns of the early 1880s revived calls for the employment of women nurses in wartime, in a manner not dissimilar to the excitement of 1854. Writing in 1882 to Jane Shaw Stewart, who was serving on a hospital ship as part of the British Expeditionary Force in Egypt, Florence expressed a hope that 'the difficult & delicate work of re-construction of Military & War Hospital Nursing may be forwarded by this War'. But despite new regulations, and the extension of nurses to military hospitals throughout the country, the total number of army nurses remained limited: just seventy-two at the time of the outbreak of the Boer War. The 'whole system of female nursing in the army appears to have been clumsily grafted onto the old system . . . purely out of deference to public opinion and Miss Florence Nightingale', noted one doctor who had volunteered for war service at the end of the century. That graft would not take root until the First World War, when Florence's plans for military nursing, elaborated almost half a century earlier, finally came into being.

Agnes Jones died in February 1868 after not quite three years of dedicated nursing at the Liverpool Workhouse Infirmary. Her death from typhus was sudden and unexpected. Recovering from the shock of the news, Florence told William Rathbone that she regretted nothing. Agnes had thanked her 'over & over again' for having persuaded her to go to the Liverpool Workhouse. A month after Agnes's death, in a letter to Parthenope, Florence looked back on her protégée's achievement, and described it as a complete success. She had reduced 'the most disorderly hospital population in the world to a state of Christian discipline'; she had guided and overseen the work of 'eighty rather commonplace' nurses; and had converted the Vestry to her views – 'the first instance of the kind in England' – while disarming all opposition. How had she done this? Agnes was not, after all, Florence admitted, 'a girl of any great ability'. But she had managed to build up an 'unbounded influence' – recognized by everyone, the paupers, the Vestry, 'even the rascal governor' – based simply on 'the manifestation of the life which was in her, so different from the governing and ordering and driving about people principle'.

The Liverpool experiment was already bearing fruit. In the year of Agnes Jones's death, the St Pancras guardians in London followed Liverpool's example by appointing one of St Thomas's special probationers, a Scottish Presbyterian called Elizabeth Torrance, to the new 500-bed workhouse infirmary at Highgate. Miss Torrance sought to overcome the problem of pauper nurses by training her own. The shortage of trained nurses meant that pauper women would continue to be employed in their stead (the Royal Commission on the Poor Law, forty years later, was to show that paupers were still being used and that one-third of nurses in workhouses had inadequate training). But replacing pauper nurses with paid ones was now a far more realistic goal to work towards.

In the short term, the problem of finding a suitable replacement for Agnes Jones at Liverpool proved a severe headache, and one that was chiefly Florence's. Everybody expected her to manage the workhouse from her bedroom, she complained. Agnes's two aunts, who had come to the Brownlow Hill Infirmary to be present at her deathbed, stayed for three months to run the nursing. The vacancy was then filled by a Mrs Kidd, who sickened, and was subsequently dismissed. Her successor Louisa Freeman's tenure of the post was similarly short-lived. She wished to revert to the old system of subordinating the nurses to the Governor and, in so doing, had by 1870 apparently brought the infirmary to 'a deadlock'. The difficulty in finding a nursing superintendent was 'a miserable business', Florence told William Farr. 'I do think it is more difficult than it was to find a general in the Crimea. And this is what makes me so heartsick, that people talk & write & gabble & print, & think it will do for the "lower middle-class," and here am I in my old age trying in vain to supply a gap of this kind, but of any class! (a well-paid position too).'

The absence of larger numbers of women prepared to train as nurses was increasingly a bitter disappointment to her. Three years earlier, in an article written at Florence's behest, and published in the Cornhill Magazine, Harriet Martineau had bemoaned 'the dearth of Nurses'. The public interest in the subject aroused by the Crimean War had long since dissipated: 'We grew tired of hospital-romancing years ago,' as Martineau remarked. And this was a change reflected in the census returns for 1861, which revealed a falling off in the number of registered nurses when compared with the numbers recorded in the census of ten years earlier.

Agnes Jones's death gave Florence the opportunity to attempt to remedy this unhappy situation. The disastrous Shaw Stewart episode was in the process of being hushed up, but Agnes's example was there to be exploited for all it was worth. An article by Florence in Good Words – the highest circulation periodical of its time – appeared in the early summer of 1868. As a tribute to Agnes as 'the pioneer of workhouse nursing', it contained a rallying cry to the women of England to fill the want of nurses by taking up this 'independent and well paid calling', in addition to a bit of blatant advertising on behalf of the Nightingale Training School itself, giving the name of the secretary and the address of where to apply.

Entitled 'Una and the Lion', the article invokes the myth made famous by Ariosto and Spenser, while at the same time implying that paupers are far more difficult than lions to tame. Coated in a thick layer of sentiment, astutely directed at the magazine's popular but pious tone, the description of Agnes's brief life ends with a graveside scene in which young and old, even those who can scarcely move on their crutches, gather to scatter primroses, snowdrops and violets on the coffin. Yet Florence's clarion call can be heard, audible and clear, above this: 'All England is ringing with the cry for "Women's Work" and "Women's Mission". Why are there so few to *do* the work?' Some did respond to this impassioned entreaty, though it's uncertain how many actual new recruits the article attracted to the cause. The piece was also widely circulated in the United States, where it was printed in a pirated edition alongside *Memorials of Agnes Elizabeth Jones* by Josephine Higginbotham, Agnes's sister. This American edition included an introduction by the minister and abolitionist Henry Beecher Stowe, brother of Harriet. Harriet Beecher Stowe was herself moved to write to Florence to tell her how 'deeply touched and affected' she had been by reading 'your Una' (Stowe also let slip that Mrs Gaskell had once given her 'a drawing of your residence', presumably Lea Hurst, 'in which the very mirror of your room is marked', an odd disclosure that must have disconcerted Florence). In reply, Florence revealed how much she had disliked the family's memoir. She did not see Agnes in it: 'It is not her.' She had vigorously opposed the book both before its publication in 1871, when the manuscript was submitted to her, and afterwards when, to her fury, it was advertised using her name. 'It was worse than any miracle-mongering modern R. C. saint's life I ever saw . . . It gives no more idea of Agnes Jones than my cat does.' Florence had good grounds for fearing that the strength of Agnes's evangelical fervour would seep through in the memoir, and prove off-putting to prospective recruits. In one passage, Mrs Higginbotham described Agnes giving Bible classes for the infirmary inmates, seeking to lead sinners to repentance.

In truth, though, the religious tone and vocabulary of Florence's own pronouncements about nursing could just as easily have been counter-productive and discouraging to potential recruits. She was keen to emphasize that reformed nursing was a properly remunerated occupa-tion, but at the same time she warned that nurses should 'serve for a higher motive than pay'. In 'Una and the Lion', she went further, and admitted that 'there *have* been martyrs'. She described nursing as 'God's work more than ours', and placed a heavy accent on 'self-sacrifice'.

There had indeed been martyrdoms. Not just Agnes Jones, dead at thirty-five, but Jane Shaw Stewart, disgraced and humiliated, and Mary Jones, worn out, and unable therefore to contemplate the workhouse nursing that Florence was so anxious to press on her. These women were Florence's frontline troops, the 'daughters of God' who went 'forth to war', like the 'Son of God' in her favourite hymn, to fight against 'misery and wretchedness'.* But would any of them have been quite so willing to embark on such a physically exhausting, and sometimes dangerous, career without the impulse of a powerful religious motiv-ation? This was a question that was to hang uncomfortably in the air, in the final decades of the century, as a new generation of nurses came forward with more secular outlook and a stronger professional interest.

She felt old before her time. Her chronically poor health, of course, exaggerated this feeling. At the beginning of 1869, Florence was so unwell for seventeen nights in succession, with an attack on her chest, that she was able neither to lie down nor to sit up to speak. The opium injections muddled her thinking, and made her wonder for how much longer she would be able to keep a hold over her mind.

As Florence approached her half-century, in May 1870, there were signs that a new chapter was opening in her life. The relentless pace of hard work continued, though under the terms of their mutual compact, Jowett begged her not to kill herself with overwork, arguing that she should give up an hour of each day to 'some unprofessional occupation', and cease to speak evil of others – except 'when human nature can endure no longer'. Change was, in any case, being forced on her. Her

* 'The Son of God goes forth to war/A kingly crown to gain', quoted in 'Una and the Lion', was written by Reginald Heber (1783–1826), Bishop of Calcutta, with music by William Croft, and sung, in 1910, at both Florence's funeral and her memorial service in St Paul's Cathedral.

influence on the work of various Government departments was waning. In 1869, Douglas Galton, Florence's indispensable ally at the War Office, retired. Early in 1872, the Viceroy of India, Lawrence's successor, Lord Mayo, was assassinated. The next Viceroy, Lord Northbrook, left for India, much to Florence's disappointment, without first coming to see her. She often contrasted the days of Sidney Herbert and Palmerston, when she was closely concerned with Government business, with those of Gladstone and Disraeli, when she was beginning to be excluded from direct involvement. Gladstone, in particular, had generally resisted her appeals to interest himself in the causes closest to her heart. She had failed in persuading him to implement the War Office reforms in Herbert's place, and enjoyed only limited success in pressing her views about India on him.

Florence regarded herself as having been 'in office' since her departure for Scutari in October 1854. At the beginning of the 1870s, as she moved 'out of office', she would be able to turn the full weight of her attention for the first time to the Nightingale Training School at St Thomas's. She was not going to like what she found there.

Part Four
Queen of Nurses
1871–1910

The lady whose name will always remain associated with the care of the wounded and sick.

Queen Victoria, speaking of FN, at the ceremony to open the new
St Thomas's Hospital, 21 June 1871

. . . For 18 years I have done the Sanitary work for India: but, for the last 4, have been continually struck with this – What is the good of trying to keep them in health if you can't keep them in life?

FN to Richard Monckton Milnes (Lord Houghton), 25 November 1877

We are only on the threshold of nursing . . . Hospitals are only an intermediate stage of civilization, never intended at all events, to take in the whole sick population.

FN, 'Sick-Nursing and Health-Nursing' (1893)

17. Taking Charge

The new St Thomas's Hospital was formally opened by Queen Victoria on 21 June 1871, three years after she had laid the foundation stone. The battle to rebuild the hospital on a breezy, upland, suburban site was long since lost. Forty-four possible locations had been considered before Sir John Simon, the Chief Medical Officer at the Board of Health, and a surgeon at St Thomas's, had cannily swung the argument by negotiating the purchase of a prime London situation: eight-and-a-half acres facing the Houses of Parliament from across the Thames, with half the acreage reclaimed from the river. This mudbank, Florence said, was the worst possible site in London. But while the rebuilt St Thomas's would not enjoy the benefit of the purer air of the countryside, canvassed for by the sanitarians, it did conform to a strict application of the pavilion principle, the first English voluntary hospital to do so, and on a scale that was unrivalled. Seven pavilions, designed by the architect Henry Currey in fashionable Italianate style, were strung out along a central corridor. 'Are those the mansions of your aristocracy?' asked one American visitor who was taking tea on the Commons terrace opposite. Owing to a direct bomb hit during the Second World War, only three of the pavilions remain standing today, together with the chapel and Governors' Hall, all of them now dwarfed by a massive Seventies block.

In 1871, the feature of the new hospital that most stirred the imagination of contemporaries was, as the *Lancet* put it, 'its astounding bigness' (the feature that seems to have irritated many people was the elaborate urns ornamenting the parapets, which, someone suggested, seemed to be waiting for the ashes of the patients inside). The cost of the 588-bed building, the most expensive in Europe, was so great that the governors were forced to skimp on the furnishings. Wards were 120 feet long by twenty-eight feet wide by sixteen feet high. More than thirty feet between opposite windows, according to the rules laid down in *Notes on Hospitals*, might impair the cross-ventilation. The ward length was

determined by the number of beds – twenty-eight – providing a reasonable allowance of 1,900 cubic feet of air for each patient. The courts
between pavilions had to be 125 feet wide to ensure that each building
in turn didn't overshadow its neighbour, and cut off its supply of sunlight
and air. The length of the hospital, including outbuildings and medical
school, amounted to a quarter-of-a-mile, and the problem of staff maintaining contact with each other over such a distance would only be
partially solved when, in 1881, a system of what Florence termed 'Telephonic communication' was introduced.

The interior, in line with Florence's instructions, contained floors of
solid wainscot oak, while the walls of each ward were covered in Parian
cement, washable, and non-absorbent, unlike ordinary cement. The
colour was reportedly a little paler 'than that of red blotting paper';
after a few months it had grown patchy and had to be painted with
distemper. To ensure the 'boundless profusion' of fresh air, the windows
of every ward, specially built for St Thomas's in Sweden, were constructed in three sections, the lower two opening in the usual way, the
upper one, within a foot of the ceiling, acting as a conduit to clear the
collection of foul air. The three open fireplaces in each ward also drew
in air. The copious ventilation required by the pavilion principle was
produced by three exit systems, a combination of turrets, including
sturdy sanitary towers, and chimneys that gave the roofline a ragged,
instantly recognizable outline.

Florence excused herself from the opening ceremony because of ill-
health. She had overseen and approved Currey's plans from an early
stage, registering defects – the pavilions, she thought, were still too close
together – and sending Dr Sutherland to inspect the new buildings. In
the past she had sometimes imagined ending her days at St Thomas's,
nursed by Mrs Roberts. She revived the idea after the hospital had been
settled in its new home for a year, leaving Jowett to dismiss the plan as
an eccentric piece of whimsy, and to assert what was manifestly the
truth, that if admitted she would never be a patient, 'but a kind of
directress to the institution viewed with great alarm by the Doctors'.
Instead, relying on the designs, and on details picked from the minds
of informed correspondents, she had to conjure up a picture in her
imagination of this great hospital of air. In January 1882, Florence
finally paid an official visit to the Training School and one of St Thomas's
wards (she had been too ill to go, two years earlier, on the Nightingale

School's twentieth anniversary), and was welcomed by Mrs Wardroper as 'our dearly loved Chief'. Rumour made the most of embellishing the story of her visit. In 1888, it was reported in one church newspaper that 'long hours of standing' during her Crimean hospital work had affected Florence's spine, and that consequently 'she has been for some years past an in-patient at St Thomas's Hospital'.

———

The number of Nightingale School probationers almost quadrupled, from ten to thirty-eight, to meet the needs of the expanded hospital. There were now five distinct classes of intake: 'Ordinaries', who received £10 a year; 'Free Specials', many of them clergymen's daughters or educated women left in difficult circumstances, who received no salary; 'Free Specials' who received a small salary; 'Specials' who paid £30 a year for their room and board; 'Specials' who paid £52. All, except the last group, signed a four-year contract (later reduced to three years) requiring them to spend a year in training followed by three years in a public hospital selected by the Fund, to ensure that their training was not wasted on private nursing. In the face of St Thomas's insistence on the rise in probationer numbers, the fee-paying 'Specials' were vital to the Nightingale Fund's continuing ability to support its trainees while keeping within its income. Florence was adamant at the hospital's planning stage that St Thomas's provide accommodation that allowed, as far as possible, for all the probationers to live under one roof. The idea of the Nurses' Home was born. 'Ward training is but half the training,' she reminded Henry Bonham Carter, Secretary of the Fund Council (which was now headed by Sir Harry Verney). 'The other half consists in women being trained in habits of order, cleanliness, regularity and moral discipline.'

Henry Bonham Carter, Hilary's younger brother, was the linchpin of the Fund. His efficiency had first come to Florence's attention in 1856 when, as a barrister in his mid-thirties, he had sent out equipment to her for the reading rooms she was setting up at Scutari. 'Harry Carter,' she wrote approvingly, 'must, I believe, be a man of business.' Married, with twelve children, to Sibella Norman, the daughter of a director of the Bank of England, Henry gave up his practice at the Bar to become managing director of the Guardian Fire Insurance Company, but his legal training held him in good stead in his dealings with St Thomas's. Throughout the 1860s he was in regular contact with Mrs Wardroper and Richard Whitfield, the Resident Medical Officer, reporting back to Florence, who put her faith in his assessment of the School's development. However, despite his obvious importance to the Fund's affairs, Florence communicated with her cousin entirely by letter. After more than a decade of this treatment, Henry finally protested. In June 1873 he called at South Street, and saw Florence 'by her request', as he noted in his diary, 'for the first time for at least 14 years'. Subsequently, they held regular meetings; and in later years, a move by Henry and his family to Hyde Park Square put him within comfortable walking distance of Florence. To his children growing up, Henry was a remote, retiring character, and they grew accustomed to seeing little of him. 'Father often did not return until late, having so much to do with Miss Nightingale,' recalled his son Charles. When a crisis in the School broke, not long after St Thomas's reopened, Henry's management skills were essential both for setting the problems straight, and for maintaining the Nightingale Fund's reputation in public.

By 1871, the writing had been on the wall for some time. In 1860 St Thomas's had driven a hard bargain with the Fund. Florence's reluctance to expend more energy on the matter had led her to accept it, though at least a part of her reason for doing so – that the new hospital would be built on a site that met with her approval – had gone by the board, while other aspects of the bargain had begun to look increasingly like a poor exchange. In return for the Fund's payment of the cost of a specified number of probationers, St Thomas's had promised to provide these trainees with a far from clearly defined course of instruction. Warning noises of just how ill-defined this training was started to reach Florence's ears from the mid to late 1860s. During the hospital's time at its temporary home in Surrey Gardens, there was criticism in the press that rather than paying for the training of nurses, as the public had intended in donating money, the Nightingale Fund was being used to finance the running of St Thomas's. Critical voices concerning the School's training – or rather, the absence of it – were also heard from some of the lady probationers among the 'Specials'. Emmy Rappe from Sweden stayed just eight months at Surrey Gardens in 1866–7, before returning to Uppsala to take up a post as Matron. Florence's first impression of her was that she was 'a dreadful little Swede' with inadequate English, but Rappe went on to provoke her indignation by writing to one of her fellow countrywomen advising her that she would learn nothing about nursing by going to the Nightingale School. To Florence herself Rappe wrote that there had been not a single lecture in physiology or anatomy while she was at St Thomas's, and that the only reason for a nurse to go there was so that she could learn 'to be <u>obedient</u> and <u>humble</u> and not think so much of herself'. The following year, Maria Dinsdale and three other, unnamed, probationers made accusations of unkindness and arbitrary treatment against Mrs Wardroper. Like Rappe's complaints, their charges were blindly dismissed by Florence on the grounds that the students were antagonistic towards Wardroper, and as evidence that they lacked a true nursing vocation.

The testimony of Rebecca Strong, who attended the Nightingale School in the year following Emmy Rappe, confirms the picture of inadequate training. Writing in the 1930s, Strong remembered that 'Kindness, watchfulness, cleanliness, and guarding against bedsores were well ingrained', but that only a 'few stray lectures were given'. There was apparently a dummy on which to practise bandaging, and 'some ancient medical books', but little more. A more damning indictment of the School, and in particular of Mrs Wardroper's judgement in selecting suitable candidates, is recorded in the register of probationers entering St Thomas's in the first ten years. The drop-out rate is startling. Of the 180 names registered between 1860 and 1870, sixty-six did not complete their contract; four died in training; seven resigned with no reason given. Of the others, half were dismissed for misconduct, at least five of them for insobriety, while the rest were dismissed because of poor health, often with the comment 'not strong enough for work' (one nurse ended up in Bedlam after taking up her duties on the wards at St Thomas's). The high incidence of sickness among probationers may be explained by the insanitary conditions at Surrey Gardens, where the ward kitchen also served as the operating theatre. Among the dismissals were women suffering from syphilis and drug addiction: not at all the kind of candidates that the Nightingale School wished to attract.

Precisely at what point Florence and Henry Bonham Carter awoke to the seriousness of the situation isn't clear. Certainly the publicity surrounding the new St Thomas's attracted a large number of inquiries from other institutions, asking for nurses or advice about training, which may have alerted them to the fact that Mrs Wardroper was out of her depth and unable to cope. But more probably it was Florence's conversations with Elizabeth Torrance, who had trained as a 'Special' before her appointment, in 1869, as Superintendent of the new Highgate Infirmary, that instilled a real sense of crisis. In the course of taking up her post at Highgate, Miss Torrance paid several visits to South Street. Before long she had become something of a favourite. Florence appreciated Elizabeth Torrance's wit and spirit. Moreover, she valued and trusted the insights that Torrance was able to give her into the state of affairs at the Training School. 'I had rather have her opinion upon our women,' she told Henry Bonham Carter in the summer of 1871, 'than that of any woman now living.'

Torrance lifted the curtain on a situation at St Thomas's that displayed petty tyranny and neglect, with a heavy dose of human foibles and failings thrown in for good measure. Mr Whitfield no longer gave any lectures to the probationers, as he was paid to do, and practically no instruction was given on the wards. Furthermore, as Florence reported to Henry Bonham Carter, Whitfield was often the worse for drink. He made his rounds at night 'oftener tipsy than sober', and his relationship with Sister Butler was a standing joke among the staff. Mrs Wardroper was said not to know one probationer from another, and to be 'governing like a virago', while her entries on the character assessment sheet 'were made with as much caprice as if a cat had made them'. Wardroper and Whitfield's relationship veered wildly between mutual love and mutual loathing. Mrs Wardroper was frequently ill, perhaps as a result of a family tragedy. The detail here is unsubstantiated, but it was rumoured that she had lost her grip on matters after going to meet her daughter from a steamer returning to England. It was not her daughter that she met, however, but her daughter's coffin.

Florence was horrified. The Nightingale School probationers were being subjected to blatant exploitation by St Thomas's, 'doing half the hospital's work', instead of attending lectures and instruction. No wonder so many of them were falling ill. Nor was there any chance as things stood of developing a self-perpetuating system for training the superintendents of the future, who, in a sense, were more badly needed than the ordinary nurses. There was no training, as Florence succinctly put it, for those who were to train others.

How could this be resolved? The Fund took legal advice about removing the School from St Thomas's and beginning again. It was entitled to do this, but a nurses' training school would always have to be attached to a hospital, so there was the likelihood of a similar situation developing elsewhere. Staying put, though, also produced some seemingly intractable problems, not the least of which was that the Fund Council had no power to remove Mrs Wardroper. 'We were the making of St Thomas's,' Florence wrote ruefully as she agonized over a solution, 'St Thomas's now truly is the unmaking of us.'

The export of Nightingale nurses overseas hadn't been running smoothly either. The spread of Florence's fame abroad had led to a request, in 1866, from Sir Henry Parkes, the Colonial Secretary to New South Wales, for nurses to staff the Sydney Infirmary. Never mind that Parkes appeared to be ignorant of Florence's major nursing innovation, that a matron be in overall command of her nurses, nor that he proposed that a team of nurses be subordinated to the medical staff at Sydney (a point he was quickly put straight on). This was too good an opportunity to be missed as publicity for the Fund. One major problem stood in its way. No suitable Superintendent was available at this time. However, a 'Lady of education, experience and character', as Mrs Wardroper described her, soon presented herself. Lucy Osburn was a little past thirty, a blunt Yorkshirewoman with High Church leanings, and a distant cousin of Florence's on the Shore side. Osburn probably exaggerated the surgical nursing experience she had obtained in Jerusalem in the late 1850s; and her record at the Nightingale Training School in 1866–7, which included a visit to Liverpool to observe Agnes Jones's practice, was not outstanding. Florence, too, had her own personal reservations about Osburn, fearing that she was 'as hard as door nails', and would lack any maternal feelings for her nurses. Nevertheless, Lucy Osburn was the only possible candidate for the job, and in December 1867, she and a party of five nurses sailed for Australia. Florence received them before their departure. She could not help contrasting the five nurses – whom she liked 'so much better than I expected' – with 'the poor drinking rabble' she had taken to Scutari. One senses a pang of envy on her part that she was not going with them. While Florence stayed upstairs, Sir Harry Verney hosted a farewell tea party for Osburn and her team in the dining room at South Street, and hymns like 'Nearer, my God to Thee' were sung to encourage the nurses to go to Sydney in a 'prayer-ful spirit' rather than on 'a Matrimonial speculation'.

In Sydney, Osburn made a promising start. A week after her arrival, an assassination attempt was made on Queen Victoria's second son, Prince Alfred, Duke of Edinburgh, who was paying an official visit to the city. The bullet was successfully extracted, and Alfred was nursed back to health by Osburn and two of the Nightingale nurses, who were sent Queen Victoria's thanks for the care of her son, and acclaimed as 'fair sisters of charity'. It was a public relations triumph, especially as the Queen was about to lay the foundation stone of the new St Thomas's. Unfortunately, that triumph quickly faded after Lucy Osburn indiscreetly wrote a gossipy letter home about the incident which was circulated in the London clubs by a cousin. 'How could she?' Florence exploded to Mrs Wardroper. '. . . If that letter gets into the newspapers, she is "done for".' As it turned out, the letter was suppressed, and Osburn was able to withdraw the resignation she had immediately offered. However, there was no repairing the damage done to Osburn's standing in Florence's eyes. As Lucy Osburn clashed with the existing hospital administration, and was pilloried in the Sydney press for her suspected Catholic sympathies – she had asked to be called the 'Lady Superior' – Florence increasingly disowned her. Thousands of miles away, and dependent on a postal service between London and Sydney that took four months for letters to arrive, she fretted about Osburn's troubled relationships with the sisters accompanying her from England, unwisely claimed by Osburn to be inferior to the Australian ones employed at the Infirmary. 'They were not fit to look after themselves,' Osburn had written, 'let alone the patients.'

The crunch came in 1871 – just at the time when Florence was faced with unassailable evidence of Wardoper and Whitfield's failings, which meant that its impact was felt all the harder by her. At the end of their three-year contract all the English sisters, with the exception of Osburn herself and the most senior of her nurses, were dismissed. The inference that the nurses recruited in Australia were superior to those sent out from the Nightingale School was one that Florence deeply resented. The whole experiment was viewed by her as a complete debacle, and Lucy Osburn found herself 'cast off as a reprobate'. Osburn remained at the Sydney Hospital, returning to England in 1885. By that time she was regarded as an icon of Nightingale nursing, despite the fact that she had failed to fulfil Florence Nightingale's own hopes.

Canada was the destination of the only other team of nurses that the

Nightingale Fund sent overseas.* Led by Maria Machin, a Nightingale-trained nurse who was Canadian by birth, the five women left for Montreal in 1874. They had been requested by the administrators of the city's general hospital to establish a training programme for nurses there. However, continuing assurances that the 'hopelessly unhealthy' hospital would be rebuilt were never met. In Machin's first winter in Montreal, one of her team died of typhoid, and there was a subsequent history of ill-health among the nurses. There was also a long-running dispute about the high running costs of the hospital to which Machin's rapid turnover of staff was said to be making a signal contribution. After three years, Henry Bonham Carter ordered Maria Machin home. Despite the evidence that Machin's high-handed manner and lack of diplomacy had contributed to the difficulties she encountered in Montreal, not least with nurses who openly rebelled against her orders, Florence never attached any personal blame to her. Indeed, for many years she kept up a friendly correspondence with Machin, always regarding her as the most 'spiritual' of the Nightingales.

The problems Florence and the Fund experienced with Lucy Osburn were considered to reflect still further on Sarah Wardroper's poor judge-ment. In letters to Bonham Carter, Florence gave vent to a string of invective about St Thomas's hapless Matron. Mrs Wardroper wouldn't know 'a sheep's head from a carrot'; was incapable 'of any considered opinion or judgement whatever'; was 'the most utterly impractical, inconsiderate, untrustworthy, forgetful' person she had ever known; and was 'more of a slave-driver & less of a woman every day'. Henry Bonham Carter agreed, with lawyerly restraint. Mrs Wardroper, invited to South Street on several occasions in 1872–3 to attempt to sort out the mess, was more garrulous, with Florence worrying that 'her brain might go any day'. Wardroper spent one Sunday talking and crying 'over this miserable business', and saying that ' "the whole place was falling to pieces" ', which, Florence wrote, 'is just my own feeling you know.'

The first option, to take Miss Torrance from Highgate, make her the

---

* Although Nightingale nurses were never sent to the United States, three training schools for nurses based on the Nightingale model were opened in New York, Connecticut and Boston, in 1873. They all followed 'Miss Nightingale's uncompromising doctrine that all control over the nursing staff . . . should be placed in the hands of the Matron or Superinten-dent, who must herself be a trained nurse'.

mistress of the probationers and authorize her to teach students on the wards, was fiercely resisted by both Wardroper and Whitfield. Mrs Wardroper said that if Torrance came to St Thomas's she would be forbidden entry to the hospital. In the meantime, it was clear that Richard Whitfield would have to go. Henry Bonham Carter insisted on his resignation, and after writing an 'impertinent' letter – so impertinent that Florence immediately struck him out of her will – Whitfield departed. As a compromise, Elizabeth Torrance was introduced as a 'Home Sister'. In this position she would not have to tread on Mrs Wardroper's toes at St Thomas's, but would be confined to giving lectures in the Nurses' Home, and to supervising trainees when off duty. That it was in many ways an impossible job is confirmed by the rapid succession of four Home Sisters in the three years after Miss Torrance left suddenly at the end of 1872 to get married. Her departure left Florence shocked and crestfallen. Torrance's fiancé, Dr Dowse, the Medical Superintendent at Highgate, was, in Florence's opinion, an 'unmanly wretch'. Perhaps to soften the blow, Miss Torrance had told Florence that she was only marrying Dowse to prevent him from going 'entirely to the bad'. There were many conversations at South Street, as Torrance 'poured out the whole of her story with that wretched little Dowse'. If only he could have seen her with Miss Torrance, Florence wrote to Henry Bonham Carter after one such meeting, 'all emotion on her part, all tenderness on mine'. She wondered whether she should step in and break off the engagement on Torrance's behalf – 'as I believe she intended I should' – but then decided that that one couldn't take such action 'for any but a girl in her teens'. Miss Torrance subsequently married Dr Dowse, and her decision was inevitably received with ill feeling on Florence's part. Miss Torrance had thrown away a promising future (a married woman could not be a Nightingale nurse). Like others in the future who, to Florence's chagrin, chose marriage above nursing, she was regarded as a loss to the cause. In 1875, Mary Crossland arrived as Home Sister and remained for twenty-one years. Miss Crossland, a clergyman's daughter, was a woman of strong vocation. Her visits to South Street over the years were frequent, providing Florence with a regular flow of information about the running of the School and the teaching abilities of individual sisters on the wards.

John Croft, a senior surgeon at the new St Thomas's, was introduced to replace Richard Whitfield early in 1873. Croft's weekly lectures to the probationer nurses were designed to give a rigorous course of instruction, offering practical guidance and theoretical background for the year's training. Croft, an energetic forty-year-old, took these duties very seriously, promising Florence that he would be 'an active and faithful comrade'. She ordained that in the future 'all probationers must give their afternoons for the purposes of training' and that 'the Hospital must provide the means of carrying itself on without the services of the Probationers being absorbed entirely in Hospital drudgery'.

Croft continued to give an annual course of over fifty lectures up to his retirement in 1894. Ranging from basic nursing craft to more advanced instruction on applied anatomy and physiology, and specific diseases, they offer a bird's-eye view of an ongoing revolution in the hospital world. Anaesthetics and antisepsis – Joseph Lister's discovery of the use of a carbolic acid spray in theatre to keep airborne germs away from patients' wounds – were enlarging the possibilities of surgery, and making nurses schooled in hygienic practices all the more essential. At the core of Croft's instruction are the thirteen areas of practical nursing set down at the time of the foundation of the Nightingale School in 1860. These included the dressing of wounds, the application of fomentations, the making of bandages and beds – 'the counterpanes have to be kept 6 inches from the ground and both sides exactly even', noted Mary Cadbury, a member of the famous Quaker family, who was a probationer in 1873 – and the preparation of invalid diets. Additionally, a strict post-operative routine was being developed, in which the clinical role of the nurse was seen as increasingly vital (for instance, it was now the nurse, rather than the surgical dresser, who constantly checked dressings for bleeding). Probationers were also starting to attend autopsies for teaching purposes. Laura Wilson, a student in 1876, wrote home of her distress at the use of a human liver at one post-mortem demonstration.

What is especially interesting about Croft's curriculum is the way in which it borrows extensively from Florence's *Notes on Nursing*. Probationers were instructed to read designated chapters from the book 'at least four times', and the ideal of sanitary nursing prevailed. Wards had to be kept adequately ventilated with fresh air, while high standards of environmental cleanliness were expected to be followed. Although nurses were no longer expected to scrub floors, as in the pre-reform era, a number of other menial tasks awaited them, including the emptying and cleaning of bedpans, the washing of plates and dishes after meals, and the polishing of window ledges with oil and industrial meths. As for personal cleanliness, from 1878 probationers were expected to carry a bar of carbolic soap in their pockets.

The importance of close observation of the sick was equally Nightingale-inspired. In a passage strongly reminiscent of *Notes on Nursing*, Croft emphasized the necessity of taking into account physical signs like the regularity of breathing, the tone of the skin, and the odour and colour of expectorations. Scientific measurement of a patient's condition had been facilitated earlier in the nineteenth century, first by the invention of the stethoscope, and later by the introduction of the thermometer. Temperature-taking had begun as medical students' work, but by the late 1860s it had been taken over by the nursing staff. Croft also laid stress on two other aspects of nursing that were of great concern to Florence: the importance of patient-centred care, and the requirement for the nurse to develop a personal self-discipline which would enable her to meet emergencies calmly.

There can be little doubt that John Croft's teaching made a major contribution to the longer-term success of the Nightingale School, following the difficulties of its early years; and that his effective combination of the theoretical with the practical may well have compensated for the variable teaching performance by some of the sisters on the wards. Nevertheless, there were worries, expressed by Croft himself, that a number of the 'Ordinaries' were insufficiently literate to keep up with the lecturer while taking notes, testament to the wide range of ability among probationers, and to the problem of instructing them as one diverse group (Florence instituted two afternoons a week in reading, writing and spelling lessons for the less able). And Florence's own ambivalence about what exactly should constitute a nurse's body of knowledge hardly diminished as the years went by. Her early criticism of the lectures stemmed from a concern that Croft was intent on turning the brighter probationers into ancillary doctors – 'medical women', her old bugbear – rather than into nurses, which in its turn was a threat to her vision of the nurse as a sanitary missioner. Nursing and medicine, Florence had long been convinced, must never be mixed up. '. . . I would almost say,' she once wrote, 'that the less knowledge of medicine a hospital matron has, the better (1) because it does not improve her sanitary practice, (2) because it would make her miserable or intolerable to the doctors . . .' Yet, by the end of the 1870s, she was complaining that Croft's lectures, although 'excellent', were also too 'elementary' and unlikely therefore to attract women of the Special Probationer class to St Thomas's. There was perhaps a recognition here of the fact that training schools at other London hospitals were by then incorporating a greater degree of medical instruction into their courses for nurses, partly in response to doctors' demands.

On taking up his appointment, Croft had assured Florence that he wouldn't stagnate in the job. He kept abreast of the latest scientific developments, and was one of the first surgeons in London to adopt Listerian methods. Croft's influence may be discernible in Florence's own conversion to the use of antiseptic precautions in nursing. 'Always have chlorinated soda for nurses to wash their hands,' she wrote in the late 1870s, in an article for *Quain's Medical Dictionary*, 'especially after dressing or handling a suspicious case. It may destroy germs at the expense of the cuticle, but if it takes off the cuticle, it must be working.' By 1896, Florence would be anxious to promote the adoption of aseptic methods – the exclusion of germs rather than killing them by chemicals – after learning about them from information provided by the surgical nurse of a hospital in Finland. 'Asceptik [sic],' she noted, 'may be briefly put as <u>boiling</u> yourself . . . & everything within your reach, including the Surgeon.'

As a part of her closer involvement with the School, Florence began to conduct personal interviews with all the sisters, nurses and probationers attached to it. In May 1873, she told Mary Jones that she had spent 'the last 6 or 8 months' seeing one or two of the nursing staff every day. 'This not only compels me to give up a great deal of my Indian or War Office work, but takes out of me, I think, more than any thing did before.' She was particularly anxious to monitor Mrs Wardroper's assessments of individual probationers, which she often found to be starkly at odds with her own. Interviews usually took place at teatime. Florence received the nurse from her drawing-room couch, a shawl thrown over her feet. Dressed in black silk, she wore a fine net cap edged in lace tied under her chin. The size of the cake served to probationers with their tea was said to vary according to the poverty or otherwise of the nurse's dress.

Seeing the probationers for herself was one way of checking on their progress; reading the ward diaries they were obliged to keep was another, although Florence tended to be frustrated by the small insights that these provided into what the students were actually being taught. Once she had met a probationer, Florence would send for the Red Register. The Register contained a personal record sheet for every probationer, with fourteen headings, filled in on a monthly basis, reporting on the moral character of each nurse during training, and assessing her acquirement of a range of nursing skills. Beneath Mrs Wardroper's official verdict, Florence would append her own, sometimes pungent, remarks in red pencil. The degree of variation in the two women's judgements might beg the question of whether they were commenting on the same nurse. Of one young woman, who had been judged 'good' in most of the columns, Florence noted: 'Queer and rough ... If I were a patient I would not have her within a mile of me.' Of another, whom Mrs Wardroper had described as likely to make a good nurse, Florence presented this more considered report: 'deficient in truth, management and steadiness, a coarse low sort of woman but with capabilities which had she a stricter probation would have made her a more successful nurse and a better woman.' Frances Spencer, one of the Specials in 1872–3, was unable to keep order in the children's ward but otherwise received the seal of Florence's approval. She was 'cheerful, grateful, shy ... religious ... very feeling'. Moreover, she had just come from reading 'Una and the Lion'.

At the point when she was most exercised about the School's failings, Florence had briefly toyed with moving to a house in Birdcage Walk, off St James's Park, to place her within easier reach of St Thomas's. Although nothing came of this plan, she pursued other ideas to stamp her personal influence on the Nightingale Training School, and to provide probationers with a greater sense of *esprit de corps*. A collegiate atmosphere was encouraged in the residential home, where there were communal meals and evenings of musical recitals and poetry readings in off-duty hours from the hectic ward routine. From May 1872, Florence addressed her probationer-nurses collectively in an annual letter read aloud by Sir Harry Verney to the assembled School at St Thomas's. With the exception of a few years when she was ill or otherwise occupied, she was to continue this practice regularly until 1888, with three later letters produced for 1897, 1900 and 1905. Some of the addresses are very long, which must have made sitting through them quite an ordeal. A printed

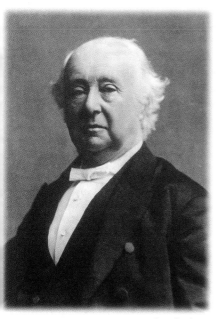

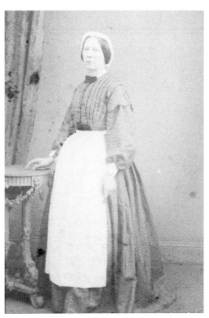

42. Benjamin Jowett, Master of Balliol College, Oxford from 1870 to 1893, who may have asked Florence to marry him.

43. Nurse Barker, the first recorded probationer, in 1860, at the Nightingale School of Nursing at St Thomas's Hospital.

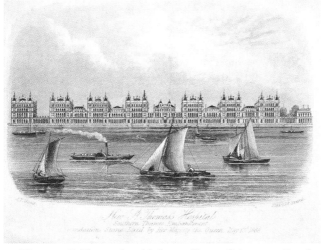

44. The new St Thomas's, with its pavilions of air, soon after the Hospital's opening by Queen Victoria in 1871.

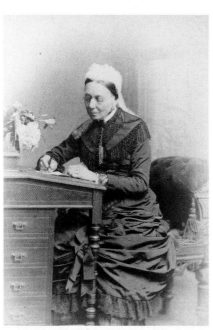

45. Sarah Wardroper, Matron of St Thomas's from 1854 to 1887, and Superintendent of the Nightingale School of Nursing.

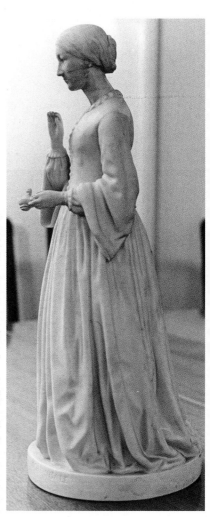

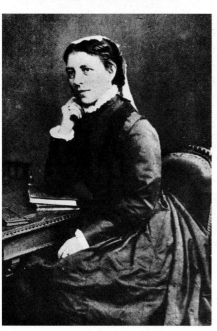

46. Lucy Osburn, who was sent to Australia in 1868 to spread Nightingale nursing doctrines at the Sydney Infirmary but fell out of favour with Florence.

47. One of the copies of Hilary Bonham Carter's statuette of Florence Nightingale, distributed among public institutions to accompany the dissemination of the Nightingale myth.

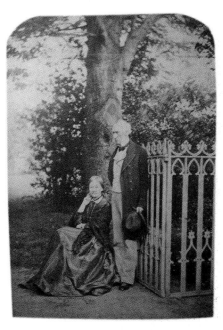

48. Parthenope with her husband, Sir Harry Verney, at Claydon, *c.* 1870.

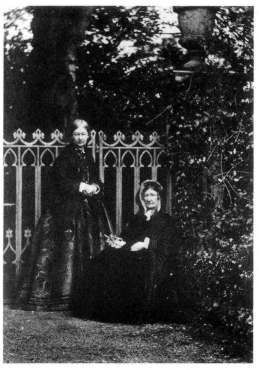

49. Fanny Nightingale in old age with Parthenope.

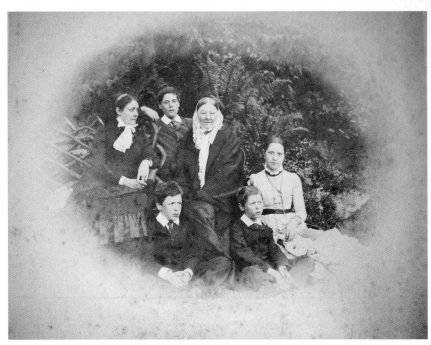

50. A previously unpublished photograph of Florence at Claydon, *c.* 1879, with members of George Lloyd Verney's family.

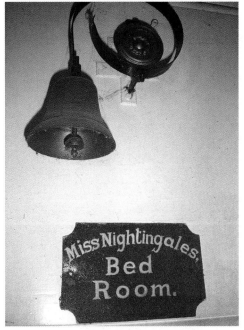

51. The servants' bell at Claydon for Florence's bedroom.

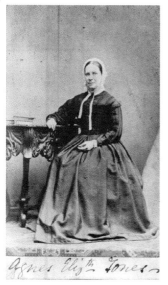

52. Agnes Jones of the Liverpool Workhouse Infirmary.

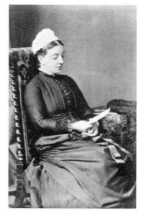

53. Angélique Pringle, one of Florence's favourites from St Thomas's.

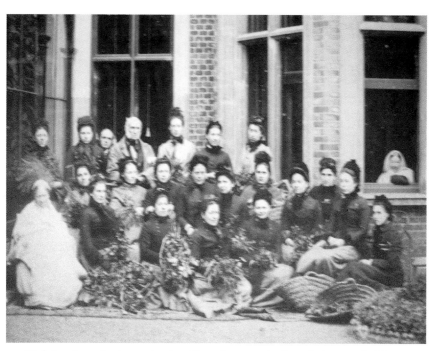

54. Nightingale probationers in the 1880s, photographed on their annual visit to Claydon. Florence can be seen looking through the window.

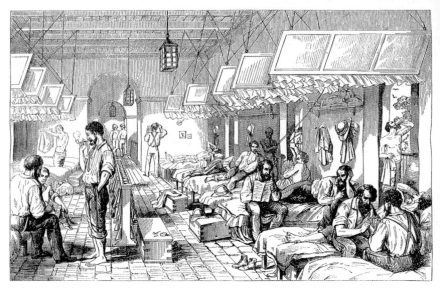

55. 'Daily Means of Occupation and Amusement'. A woodcut by Hilary Bonham Carter of a typical British army barracks in India, designed for Florence's *Observations* on the evidence presented to the Royal Commission on the Sanitary State of the Army in India, 1863.

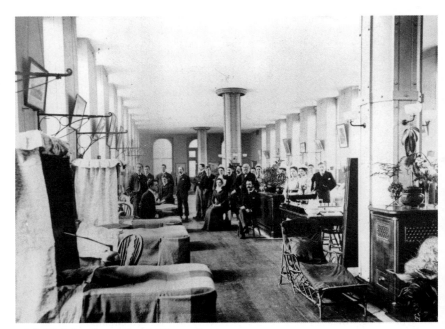

56. A Nightingale ward at St Thomas's.

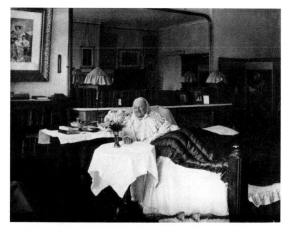

57. Florence in her bedroom at South Street. The Chalon portrait of Fanny Nightingale and her two young daughters can be seen hanging on the wall in the background. A photograph taken by Lizzie Caswell Smith, *c.* 1906.

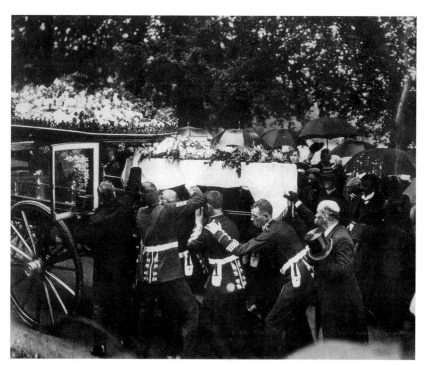

58. Florence's Nightingale's funeral on 20 August 1910. The churchyard of St Margaret's, East Wellow, was crowded with local people who had come to pay their respects to her.

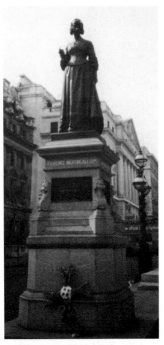

59. The statue of Florence Nightingale, by A. G. Walker, at Waterloo Place, London. It was unveiled with a marked lack of ceremony in 1915.

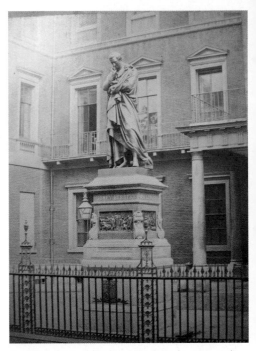

60. The statue of Sidney Herbert by J. H. Foley, shown at its original site, outside the old War Office in Pall Mall. Later it was moved to stand beside Walker's statue of Florence Nightingale.

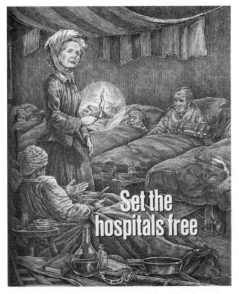

Set the hospitals free

61. The Iron Lady as the Lady with the Lamp. A cartoon from *The Economist*, 1988. In the late 1980s Nightingale iconology was occasionally employed when an internal market system was introduced to the financing of NHS hospitals.

copy, or lithographed facsimile of the manuscript, was given to each nurse present 'for private use only'. The language was kept deliberately simple to appeal to the widest audience possible; and stories, like that of the fall of General Gordon at Khartoum in the issue for 1886, were introduced as illustrations of moral precepts (in the case of Gordon, whom Florence regarded with an attitude little short of veneration as the embodiment of 'muscular Christianity', the story of his death was given as an example of humility, as well as of heroism). Edward Cook, after wading through all the repetition, extracted the gist of the addresses: 'that nursing requires a special call; that it needs, more than most occupations, a religious basis', for without it, hospital life becomes 'a very hardening routine and bustle'; 'that it is an art, in which constant progress is the law of life; and lastly, that the nurse . . . has of necessity a moral influence'. In order to counteract the militaristic image of the nurse promoted by Mrs Wardroper – who insisted on nurses standing to attention when she entered a ward – Florence's letters increasingly took on a gentler tone of maternal solicitude.

This expression of maternal concern for the welfare of her young can be seen most plainly in Florence's relationships with Angélique Pringle and Rachel Williams. Of all the student nurses who passed through St Thomas's, Pringle and Williams were the two for whom she reserved her deepest affection. Both had entered the Training School as Special Probationers before the era of the Croft reforms – Pringle in 1868, while St Thomas's was still at Surrey Gardens, Williams in 1871 – but both were women of outstanding intelligence with the ability to act on their own initiative. Physically and temperamentally they were polar opposites, though, having met on the wards at St Thomas's, they remained close friends for the rest of their lives. Angélique Pringle, known as 'the Pearl' or 'Little Sister', was tiny, modest and self-effacing. Rachel Williams, six years Pringle's senior, was a tall, stately woman, addressed by Florence as 'Goddess', and just occasionally as 'Goddess-baby', an acknowledgement of the petulant side to Williams's personality. Just as Jowett as Master of Balliol had his favourite undergraduates, Florence now had these two loyal devotees whom she adored, and who looked upon her as their 'Mother-in Chief'. She was able to take a relaxed pleasure in their friendship, savouring 'the vigour of your cruel splendid youth', as she wrote to Rachel Williams in October 1873, and contrasting it with 'the sadness of my much-tried age'. She was an 'old black

beetle', she told Williams on another occasion, and often had 'a shud-
dering sort of maternal feeling in wishing you "blessings"'.

Devotion was lavished on them. Once, when Pringle left South Street
without eating her dinner, it was sent after her in a cab. For Williams,
suffering the strain of overwork, there was a £10 cheque – 'my little
mother's gift' – as Florence's contribution towards a restorative holiday
'at Boulogne or . . . any other watering-place'. They repaid her with
visits, confidences, opinions of other nurses – and letters, which were
Florence's 'pure joy'. 'And life,' as she confessed to Williams, 'has not
many joys for me, my darling.' Inevitably, there was strong guidance,
too, about career choices. In 1872, the Nightingale Fund was
approached by the Edinburgh Royal Infirmary, which required a staff
of nurses. Mrs Wardroper managed to find nine who were suitable, and
sent them to Edinburgh under the leadership of Miss Barclay, another
Special of whom Florence had high hopes. With Florence's approval,
Angélique Pringle was selected as Assistant Superintendent. Pringle was
unhappy at this new position of responsibility but, as she informed
Florence, 'I am so glad to be your child, and to go where you want me.'
However, as Superintendent, Barclay soon found herself beset with
difficulties. The Edinburgh Infirmary was 'a lawless place', the doctors
were proving uncooperative, and the reputation of the hospital was so
bad that only 'scrubbers' applied to be nurses. Miss Barclay looked for
solace in alcohol and opium. By the autumn of 1873, there was no
alternative but to dismiss Barclay, replace her with Pringle, and bring
Rachel Williams up from St Thomas's to act as 'the Pearl's' assistant. In
an ironic twist as she was leaving, Miss Barclay warned Angélique
Pringle against the employment of drunken nurses.

Over a period of fourteen years as Superintendent, until she left to
succeed Sarah Wardroper on her retirement as Matron of St Thomas's,
Angélique Pringle established an outstanding training programme for
nurses and future Matrons at the Edinburgh Royal Infirmary, which
was in some ways an advance on what was offered at St Thomas's.
Florence's confidence in her had been well-founded. After three years at
Edinburgh, Rachel Williams won promotion and became Superintendent of St Mary's Hospital, Paddington. She then spent a rocky decade
attempting to win acceptance from the medical staff of her right to
engage and dismiss staff, before resigning in 1885.

Edinburgh was the most outstanding result of the Nightingale nursing in voluntary hospitals. But it was far from being the only success story. After a disappointing start, the system pioneered by the Nightingale Training School at St Thomas's, of sending out Special probationers as Superintendents after a year in hospital, was beginning to bear fruit. Already, in the summer of 1873, Florence was describing herself to Julius Mohl as 'immersed in a torrent of my trained matrons and nurses, going and coming . . .' By the beginning of the following decade, former Nightingale probationers had obtained the superintendence of a large number of London and provincial hospitals, including, among others, St Bartholomew's and the Westminster Hospital; Leeds Infirmary; Salisbury Infirmary; Lincoln Infirmary; Huntingdon County Hospital; the Royal Hospital for Incurables, Putney; the Southern Hospital, Liverpool – and there were more to come. 'The new order spread by geometric progression as each trained nurse trained others.' Most London teaching hospitals now had training schools for nurses, often with less rigid contracts than those imposed by St Thomas's, but the prestige of the Nightingale name ensured a continuing supply of well-educated candidates.

The ravages of old age were taking their toll on Florence's parents. In 1864, when Mr Nightingale was seventy and Fanny seventy-six, William Allingham, the intimate of Tennyson, had visited them at Embley in the company of Blanche Clough. He was struck by the sight of these two elderly people living alone in a great house, 'at the end of their days'. Florence, he wrote, 'they never see, and rarely, I think, hear from', though he noted the presence of Sir John Steell's bust of her in the hall. Allingham described William Nightingale as 'tall, thin, courtly, white-haired, with [a] blue swallow-tailed coat always buttoned; in manner very quiet and sad'. At Mr Nightingale's request, Allingham read one evening from *In Memoriam*, which seemed 'to impress him deeply'.

In fact, Florence and her father still met on his occasional visits to London; but meetings with her mother had all but ceased as the decline in Fanny's health made it difficult for her to leave home. 'I am grieved to say dear child that I am such a wreck in every way . . . ,' Fanny told Parthenope in the mid-1860s. 'I am thoroughly broken down – alas I can neither see [n]or understand & he [Mr Nightingale] cannot hear!' Describing their routine to his daughter, William wrote of 'Carriage at 3, till 4, then Newspaper till Dinner & Bed, as the clock strikes 10, but oh! the blank which annihilation of memory has caused'. Fanny was in the early stages of dementia. Attempting to maintain a grip on her fragmenting mind, she compiled long notes for herself, writing out her bitterness at Florence's decision to break away from her family, and of 'the daily & hourly sacrifice it entails'; and expressing her distress at the 'most painful and most untrue' reports that Parthenope had ever stood in the way of her sister's ambition, and determination to leave home.

In the autumn of 1866 Florence returned to Embley, for the first time in eight years. Exhausted by her exertions over Poor Law nursing, she finally gave in to pressure from Jowett to take some rest in the country while visiting her parents. 'You know Florence Nightingale has been a dozen weeks at Embley! – her mother being too infirm to go to her,' Harriet Martineau announced jubilantly to Richard Monckton Milnes – now Lord Houghton – at the beginning of 1867. Fanny's condition appeared to Florence to vary wildly: one day she was like a dying woman, the next walking like a girl of fifteen. However, she was shocked by the deterioration in her mother's formerly high standards as manager of her household. The 'dilapidation & extravagance' was visible 'even from my bed'.

A new pattern was set. For the remainder of the decade, and into the next, Florence paid prolonged visits to her parents at both their country homes. Sometimes Jowett arrived to spend a few days or a week with her. In the summer of 1867, Florence was at Lea Hurst, the home she had always loved best, for three months, and again, the following year, for a month. In 1869, she was at Embley from August to October. As Fanny's condition worsened, the calls on her time became greater, especially during her father's absences from home. In 1872, Florence was forced to spend much of the latter part of the year shuttling between London and Embley, to ensure that her mother was receiving proper care. Fears that her mother was suffering from neglect had increased after it was discovered that Fanny's maid Webb had locked her mistress in her room for most of the day to prevent Fanny from wandering about unsupervised. Parthenope was herself too ill, crippled with arthritis, to deal directly with the problem; and so, 'Upon me,' Florence wrote to Mary Jones in February 1873, 'the only one of the family who has any real work to do, the whole thing is thrown. Last year, I spent at Embley nearly eight months of it, & twenty-two hours out of every twenty-four in the room next to my mother's. The consequence was that my London work was ruined & I reduced to a sort of trembling corpse.'

However, despite all her complaints, Florence was torn between concern for her work, and a desire to help and care for her mother, to a greater degree than she could ever have anticipated. Fanny's failing memory caused her great distress. She had to remind her mother of the imminent approach of her golden wedding in 1868, and was upset that same year when Fanny forgot her birthday on 12 May. 'It is the first birth-day I have ever had without hearing from my dearest mum,' she wrote sorrowfully to Fanny the following day. But while her mother's short-term memory was fading, Florence also observed that Fanny had gained 'in real memory of the phases of the past, in appreciation of her great blessings, in happiness, real content & cheerfulness & in lovingness'. As for herself, she put aside past resentments about her family, trying hard not to let 'these things "corrode" into me now . . .'

On the morning of 5 January 1874, William Nightingale came down for breakfast at Embley. Finding that he had forgotten his watch, he started back upstairs to fetch it, but slipped and fell, hitting his head. He died instantly. The news reached Florence in London. 'I do not feel his death awful for <u>him</u>,' she wrote to Liz Herbert, a few days later.

. . . it is what he would have chosen – he was quite ready to part with his life – he always wished to go out of the world quietly – it was part of his single-minded character . . . But is very dreary not to have seen him once more, that none of us were by him at the last: not a last word or farewell . . . No one knows what a break up it is to us, for me especially; I had only just received the idea that I might survive my mother; I never once thought that <u>I</u> should survive <u>him</u> . . .

Her grief is sweet & gentle: she begged to go in & 'kiss him' but yielded when she was told that it was only his 'old garment' there . . . We had been anxious for her, not him, & I actually had the invalid carriage ordered every day for a fortnight to go down to her. He wrote himself to prevent me – on account of my weakness. I had not seen so much of them as usual this last year: work was so heavy in London & I had been only two months with them at Lea Hurst.

Florence was too unwell to attend her father's funeral, held at St Margaret's in East Wellow, with tenants from the Embley estate forming the cortège. When Selina Bracebridge died, a few weeks later, it seemed that another line was being firmly drawn under the past. Charles Bracebridge had died in the summer of 1872. 'Dearest ever dearest friend,' Florence had written to Mrs Bracebridge; 'It does seem so long between the times I hear from you and of you.' Learning that Selina Bracebridge was seriously ill at the beginning of 1874, Florence asked Sir Harry Verney to visit her on her behalf. 'She was more than mother to me,' she told Sir Harry and Parthenope as word came of her death at the end of January, '& oh that I could not be a daughter to her in her last sad months. What should I have been without her?' Sorting through a cupboard at Lea Hurst at the end of the year, she came across the letters she had written from Rome and Egypt a quarter of a century earlier, 'very dear to me now on Mrs Bracebridge's account'.

Under the terms of 'Mad' Peter Nightingale's will, the entailed Nightingale estate, consisting of Embley and Lea Hurst, passed on Mr Nightingale's death to his sister Aunt Mai and her husband Uncle Sam. For Florence and Parthenope, there was the protracted business of clearing both houses and deciding how much of their contents should be left to the new owners. There was friction with Aunt Mai, who had decided that, ill herself and with an ailing husband, she was unable to take in Fanny at Embley and look after her. Most of all, it was heartrending to see Fanny, weeping in a confused state, because she could not understand why she was being banished from her home of fifty years. The question of where Fanny was going to live preoccupied everyone, but there seemed to be no easy solution in sight. 'I am utterly exhausted,' Florence declared. 'Not a day passes without the most acute anxiety & care. Oh the cruel waste of time, of all real work.' In August 1874, she took her mother to stay at the Verneys' at Claydon House for several weeks. Florence had often been asked there, but had resisted all invitations. Parthenope and Sir Harry remained in London, so Florence wrote to Mrs Turnham, the housekeeper, in advance of her arrival, warning her that '. . . I shall give you a great deal of trouble: I am a troublesome inmate in another person's house: too great an Invalid to be away from home.' Nevertheless, the change was recuperative for both of them. Fanny went out almost every day, and was able to watch a local cricket match from a garden chair. Florence opened the window of her room and listened to the sound of hymns and chants floating across the lawn from Claydon church. 'I shall be very sorry to leave your beautiful place,' she wrote to Sir Harry on her last day, 'its silence and peace, its trees, & these lovely & comforting rooms . . .'

Florence was unwilling to leave the care of her mother to strangers, but the difficulties this created bore down heavily on her, as she assumed responsibility for her mother for months at a time. Miss Parish, the companion she and Parthenope had engaged, was quickly deemed untrustworthy: 'Either she drinks or she has a screw loose.' Adeline Paulina Irby, who had trained at Kaiserswerth out of admiration for Florence, and subsequently spent much of her life bringing aid to the Slavonic Christian refugees in Bosnia-Herzegovina, stayed with Florence and her mother on several occasions in 1874 and 1875, and shouldered some of the burden. However, it was William Shore Smith – 'my boy Shore' – now married with four young children , who came to Florence's rescue by generously inviting Fanny to live with him and his family in London at York Place for six months, and allowing her to return to Lea Hurst for prolonged periods. In familiar surroundings, Florence reported that her mother was 'like a new being'.

But inevitably there were still times when Florence's watchful care was called for, and an overwhelming sense of the old frustration came flooding back to her. In June 1875, when Fanny became ill while staying with Shore in London, Florence decided to rent a house at Abbotsleigh, Church Road, in Upper Norwood as an unlikely venue for her mother's recovery. 'I am "out of humanity's reach" in a red villa like a monster lobster,' she wrote to Mary Mohl.

Stranger vicissitudes than mine in life few men have had: vicissitudes from slavery to power, & from power to slavery again. It does not <u>seem</u> like a 'vicissitude', a villa in Norwood, yet it is the strangest I yet have had. It is the only time for twenty-two years that my work has not been the first reason for deciding where I should live & how I should live. Here it is the <u>last</u>. It is the caricature of a life.

18. A Taste of Heaven in Daily Life

The end of 1874, like its beginning, had been overshadowed by the death of another friend from Crimean days. The Reverend Mary Clare Moore, Superior of the Convent of Mercy at Bermondsey, whose 'silent sympathy & trust' had supported Florence at Scutari, and without whose nursing experience Florence believed that the whole enterprise would have failed, died shortly before Christmas. They had met rarely, probably no more than three or four times at South Street in the intervening years, but had kept up a regular correspondence, with Florence continuing to depend on Clare for her sympathy and support. In Clare's last days, Florence ordered food for the other sisters at Bermondsey, concerned that they were worn out 'with watching & sorrow' as they gathered around their Mother Superior's bed, repeating the name of Jesus. She herself was left feeling 'motherless' after Mary Clare Moore was gone.

Florence admired Clare's mind as the most religious she had ever known. They may have been separated by disagreement on many doctrinal points – though Florence claimed that Mary Clare Moore was the only Roman Catholic she had encountered who had never tried to convert her – but they spoke freely about religion to one another. They also shared a profound belief that the essence of a religious life should consist of active work undertaken in accordance with God's will. Temperamentally, the two women could hardly have been less alike. Florence longed to imitate Clare's imperturbable spirit. She was 'not like my dear Revd Mother who is never ruffled', she once admitted regretfully. As a child, Clare had possessed a violent temper, which she eventually overcame to the extent that as an adult she was often reluctant to express an opinion for fear of causing offence. She understood only too well Florence's struggles to subdue her own outbursts of anger and self-pity, and her tendency to see conflict in all around her, while recognizing that the part Florence played in the affairs of the outside world was far more likely to aggravate such personality traits, than her own kind of life within a religious community. 'I am so careful & troubled & have such a want of calmness about His work & His poor – as if they were my work & my poor instead of His,' Florence wrote to Clare as she grappled with the problems of the Liverpool Workhouse Infirmary in the months following Agnes Jones's death. To Clare, as to no one else, not even to Benjamin Jowett, Florence revealed her loneliness in the decade before her interest in the nursing school introduced a new stream of younger people into her life. It was nothing less than 'solitary imprisonment'. Writing from her 'little cell' in December 1866, she told Clare that Christmas was worst. She was always 'quite alone' at that time of year: 'even more so than at other times in London'.

For spiritual nourishment, Clare sent religious books – received 'with a great parcel of thanks'; some by saints from the Catholic mystical tradition, many of them writing against the backdrop of the religious and social upheaval of the Reformation. Florence still regarded Roman Catholicism as beset with error, but in the record of the personal faith of St John of the Cross, for example, the sixteenth-century Carmelite friar and disciple of St Teresa of Avila, she saw a reflection of her own 'dark night' of the soul. In 1865 she apologized to Clare for having kept her copy of a French edition of the life and writings of John of the Cross for so long, but she was finding him 'to have had the most wonderful practical knowledge of the ways of God in the heart of man'. John, who had faced opposition, even imprisonment in the 1570s, because of his membership of the reformed Discalced Carmelite community, helped Florence to come to terms with feelings of discouragement and isolation as she battled against officialdom during the hectic period of reform dominating her life in the 1860s. The self-sacrifice John endured in order to follow what he perceived as the will of God emboldened her, and gave her the courage to believe that her suffering was divinely sanctioned.

Florence similarly derived guidance and consolation from the texts by three female saints that Mary Clare Moore sent her. She quoted prayers by the fourteenth-century Catherine of Siena, who had offered her bodily sufferings to God in return for the reform of the medieval Church, and observed to Clare that 'St Catherine did not see the reformation she desired. And I shall not see the reformation of the Army. But I can truly say that, whatever I have known our Lord to desire of me, I have never refused Him (knowingly) anything.' The life of Catherine of Genoa in the fifteenth century was also 'very singular & suggestive'. Catherine had been the 'Directress' of the Pammetone Hospital in Genoa, where she was noted for her skills as a manager and treasurer, and for the emergency measures she took when plague struck the city in 1493. In Teresa of Avila, Florence discovered a reformer of passionate temperament who suffered from frail health for much of her life and struggled against a strong desire to be admired by others.

The books loaned by Clare encompassed works by familiar writers, in addition to those by the more obscure. The Spanish mystical tradition was well represented, along with books by seventeenth-century French Jesuit writers like Seurin and Lallemont, and by Francis Xavier and Francis de Sales, two patron saints of the Sisters of Mercy. More recent literature included *Spiritual Conferences*, an extraordinary compendium of mystical theology and hagiography across nineteen centuries by Frederick William Faber, a founder of the London Oratory (who insisted on addressing the Virgin Mary as 'Mamma'). Many of these writers were mystics. Like Florence, they had asked the question, 'Where shall I find God?' and found the answer, 'In myself.' They had embarked on a life's journey to place themselves 'in a state for Him to come and dwell in me', which, as Florence said, was the 'whole aim of the Mystical Life . . . all Mystical Rules in all times and countries have been laid down for putting the soul in such a state'.

But it was towards those mystics who had worked actively in the world that Florence found herself drawn by instinct and experience, and for whom she expressed the greatest admiration. It should come as no surprise to learn that she retained a deep suspicion of mysticism as it was commonly understood: a withdrawal from the outside world into a life of prayer and contemplation, punctuated by moments of ecstasy and self-mortification. This 'rule of passive conformity' was adhered to 'in the most complete perfection'. Yet these mystics 'did nothing' beyond 'a few little manual works' to keep themselves in physical good order.

Florence's 'true doctrine of mystics', by contrast, would place the accent not on devotion, but on 'work and suffering for the love of God'. We are called upon not merely to think about ideals, 'but to do and suffer for them'. A mystical state, so defined, is a permanent condition, and not a sudden 'call' or spark of insight. How much happier she personally would have been, Florence commented – and a better woman, too – if she had spent her life 'thinking only of the Ideal . . . instead of struggling daily, hourly, with the selfishness, indifference, wilful resistance, which are all that surround me now . . .' It was the difference, she thought, between swimming against a strong current, with the waves closing over your head, and standing on the bank, looking at the blue sky.

Out of all this reading, at the start of the 1870s, came the idea for a new book. This was to consist of Florence's selection of passages from the classics of the mystic tradition, prefaced with an extensive introduction of her own. Jowett was keen to encourage her. He regarded any project of writing that was unconnected with Florence's administrative work as a means of diverting her from the profound depression she sometimes lapsed into, now that her days of influencing matters at the War Office were over. She had done much good 'to the health & moral condition of the Army', he assured her in September 1872, but her position had always been an unsatisfactory one, dependent as it was upon 'the goodwill of the Minister'. 'A straightforward work' in which she was dependent on herself would be of greater service than 'the administration of any public office . . .' Jowett was not himself familiar with mystical writing, and was initially repulsed when he sampled some of Teresa of Avila's work. But the analogies between certain mystical texts and his beloved Plato were undeniable. Concurrent with her work on the mystics, Florence was helping Jowett to revise his edition of Plato's *Phaedrus*. She admired its closing prayer as an expression of her own sense of the mystical state: 'Give me beauty in the inward soul, and may the outward and inward man be at one.'

She entitled her selection 'Notes from the Devotional Authors of the Middle Ages, Collected, Chosen, and Freely Translated by Florence Nightingale' – though in fact not all the passages are from the Middle Ages, and many of them date from the early modern period. Florence's translations were generally made from French versions of Italian or Spanish writers, while in certain cases she withheld the names of the authors, presumably so as not to reinforce readers' anti-Catholic prejudices. Her introductions and commentary provide further evidence of her wide reading: the writers quoted from include Erasmus, Wesley, Newman, while the eponymous hero of Daniel Defoe's *Robinson Crusoe* is introduced as an example of a man who finds God's presence in solitude, which more than compensates him for his solitary state. By the spring of 1873, Jowett was reading some of the translations, and perhaps irritating Florence by suggesting that the quotations from Teresa of Avila should be shortened, in case modern readers found them 'too rhetorical & egotistical'.

There is little doubt that at one stage Florence intended to publish the book. The surviving manuscript contains various instructions to the printer, directing him to omissions and indicating the size of the preferred typeface. Even more perhaps than for *Suggestions for Thought*, she had hoped that it would find a sympathetic audience. However, unlike its predecessor, 'Notes from the Devotional Authors' didn't even get as far as a proof stage. It may be that the death of Florence's father, at the beginning of 1874, cut across its completion, and removed much of her enthusiasm for the project. Not only did the practical demands arising from his death deprive her of time in which to write, she had also lost the individual whose opinions on religious subjects, even when she didn't agree with him, had been a regular source of stimulus to her throughout her life (moreover, she appears to have found Jowett wanting in certain respects as a replacement). Or, just as probably, she may have become dissatisfied with the form the book was taking. In 1937, more than a quarter of a century after Florence's death, Rosalind Vaughan Nash, as one of the Nightingale executors, approached the Society for Promoting Christian Knowledge, to inquire whether they might be interested in publishing the unfinished manuscript. Their response was discouraging, not least because, by that date, direct translations from the Spanish were freely available.*

This rejection led to the destruction by Vaughan Nash of some of the translations, but enough of the commentary has been preserved to give us an outline of what has recently been called Florence's 'spirituality of the active life'. Evelyn Underhill, the scholar of mysticism and spiritual life, writing in 1914, in her book *Practical Mysticism*, saw Florence both as 'one of the greatest and most balanced contemplatives of the nineteenth century', and as a figure acting 'under mystic compulsion' like Joan of Arc. In 'Notes from ... Devotional Authors', Florence attempts to resolve the central problem that was especially pertinent to her own life: how to find the proper relationship of action and union

---

* Aldous Huxley's anthology of the great religious and metaphysical systems of the world, *The Perennial Philosophy*, published in 1946, contains generous selections from the works of the great Catholic mystics, and possesses a flavour of Florence's incomplete work.

with God. She begins with a strange injunction: 'This book is not for anyone who has time to read it.' Mystical books, she continues, are for 'hardworked people' like herself, to inspire their daily work; they are not for ' "mystical people", contemplative people . . . unoccupied people'.

A spiritual ideal must be embodied in everyday life. 'If we . . . keep the spiritual Ideal for Sundays or for prayers, it is like people who go to hear Bach's Passion music at Westminster Abbey and think their enjoyment devotional feeling.' There will be no heaven, Florence insists, unless we make it for ourselves. Like Teresa of Avila and John of the Cross, we must ask God to give His will to us. Prayer is not for asking God what we want – because since God is immutable we are unable to change His mind – but for asking Him what He wants us to do. We must surrender our will completely to God's, 'Uniting oneself with His work by observing what His universal laws are, as the only means of carrying out His work'. We shouldn't waste time wondering whether or not our intentions are pure, and in accordance with God's will, but in each action 'stake one's existence in carrying out that action'. There will be challenges and obstacles, but these are only to be expected, and we ought to be ready 'to go down "into hell" for God's service'. To work out perfection through God's laws necessarily implies the existence of evil and suffering. Christ on the cross is the highest expression of God – not 'in the vulgar meaning' of the atonement – but in the way that God, as fellow-sufferer, hangs on the cross every day 'in every one of us'.

Florence believed that the passive and the active life could be united, though she admitted that such a union had never been achieved, partly because the active life was so much a product of modern science. However, supposing, she asks, we look upon the Bengal sanitary commissioners as God's true missionaries in India (truer than St Francis Xavier, a Jesuit missionary, who had preached and converted in India in the sixteenth century)? It might seem a shocking idea, and one that would undoubtedly repel some religious people – as well as later providing Lytton Strachey with the basis for his snide remark that Florence Nightingale thought that God was a sanitary engineer – but in cleaning out a foul drain are they not carrying out God's work; and are we not just as bound by one of God's laws to clean out a drain, and save the population from typhus, as we are by the commandment 'not to steal'?

According to Florence, religion should infuse the intellectual work of

the day, even its scientific discoveries, and 'the practical intellectual
work of all of us'. In advancing these ideas, she was simply advocating
to the outside world what had long been manifestly true for herself: that
religious faith should exist, not on the periphery of an individual's
existence, as an excuse for shirking responsibilities; but at its very centre,
guiding and informing our actions in daily life.

———

Just how Florence's own relationship with God was integrated into her
everyday existence may be glimpsed in the brief diary she kept for 1877,
the only such record that survives for the latter part of her life. This
little book, whose entries for most days are restricted to a bare few
lines, describes her daily routine, of books read, and articles and letters
written; and domestic responsibilities, including expenditure on household matters, like fire insurance. Throughout its pages Florence refers
to the comings and goings of visitors on essential business, like Henry
Bonham Carter and Sarah Wardroper. There is a visit from her old
friend Clarkey, a widow since the death of Julius Mohl a year earlier,
and always a vociferous complainant whenever she thought Florence
was neglecting her in favour of her work. Benjamin Jowett arrives eight
times in the course of the year to take communion with her. She notes
her bouts of ill-health. A 'Terrible night' leaves her feeling very ill the
next day; on another occasion she has a 'Strong impression of death on
lying down'. She sets aside time from her work for overseeing the care
of her mother, and deals with a host of tribulations connected with
her servants, occasionally expressing remorse when she feels she has
mistreated them. In July, Florence goes to Lea Hurst for two months
with Fanny Nightingale. While there, she supervises the disinfecting of
the room of the footman, who has recently died from smallpox, and
sends an account of his last hours to the dead man's mother. Mr White,
one of the cats she has brought with her, scratches her maid Fanny, and
then, a few days later, bites another servant, Lizzie, so that the doctor
has to be called out to apply a caustic fomentation and poultice to the
wounded area.

Anniversaries are kept assiduously: in February, Florence marks the
fortieth since her call to service; at the beginning of November, the twenty-
third anniversary of her landing at Scutari. These are not so much tokens
of memory, more affirmations that she has acted in accordance with
God's will. On six occasions 'The Voice' is recorded as speaking to her

(four of these visitations come at night), and at various other points in the diary the reader suddenly becomes aware that a dialogue with God is taking place. Much of this dialogue is concerned with Florence's work for India, then occupying a large proportion of her time. Other parts of it are filled with a surprising degree of self-reproach and self-doubt ('O God in Thee have I never trusted, therefore I am rightly confounded') – though, on one occasion, she turns to questioning God Himself ('O God, are you sure you are doing all you can for the Bosnians?').

However, the predominant note in Florence's relationship with God is the same here as it had been thirty years earlier, at the time of her travels in Egypt. Is she willing to give up her own name and reputation for God? 'Take O take from me ever the wish to impress, cause of my unrest,' she begs Him. When she receives bad news about the provision of nurses at the Royal Herbert Hospital, she realizes that she has felt disappointment in her own name, and not in God's. At the age of fifty-seven, she still feels divided between a love of self and a love of God. Even her work can become 'an idol, a Moloch', preventing her from confronting her pride.

———

There are several references in the diary to the 'Great Famine' which was ravaging Madras and other parts of south-west India. On 16 August 1877, Florence asks God: '. . . can nothing be done for these poor people in the Indian famine?' Such a vast human tragedy reinforced a sense of her own impotence. Gone were the days when she might have had the influence – or the energy – to agitate for a Royal Commission to investigate the plight of the Indian population. Now she had to rely on her brother-in-law, Sir Harry Verney, to make his interventions in Parliament on her behalf. 'My mind is full of the dying Indian children,' Florence wrote to Edwin Chadwick in September, 'starved by hundreds of thousands from conditions which have been made for them, in this hideous Indian famine . . . How I wish that some one would now get up an agitation in the country . . .' She had been sent photographs of five or six victims – one of them 'a living skeleton in its mother's skeleton arms' – but had hidden them away. 'I could not bear to look at them.'

Major famines swept across India every decade or so in the second half of the nineteenth century. A prolonged period of drought and the failure of the monsoon rains could result in catastrophe, while excessive monsoon rains and flooding could prove just as devastating, leading to the widespread destruction of crops. A starving population, too poverty-stricken to have laid up reserve stocks in advance, was left defenceless against disease. The terrible Orissa famine of 1865–6, which killed roughly a million people, was the first major famine to occur after Florence had started her work on the sanitary reform of the Indian Army, and the first to alert her to the seriousness of the problem. The Government in London failed to take steps in time to introduce precautions in the form of stocks of grain supplies, and so did the local government. Sir Cecil Beadon, the Governor of Bengal, situated just to the north of Orissa, had informed the Viceroy, Sir John Lawrence, that the situation was not as serious as preliminary reports suggested, and had promptly retreated to the hills of Darjeeling as crisis struck. The findings of a lengthy Government inquiry were debated in the House of Commons in 1867, and Beadon, and officials like him, were criticized for 'walking in a dream', and for putting the risk of losing lives below the risk of losing money.

As many as 29 million Indians were to die under British rule as a consequence of the almost perpetual famine conditions. It would take the end of Empire, and the declaration of Indian Independence in 1947, for the onset of regular famine to cease. The British Raj was at a loss to explain the frequency of famine, often unable to coordinate local power to act effectively, and, crucially, unprepared to adopt interventionist policies that ran counter to their espousal of a free market economy. Meanwhile, revenues from India's national wealth, which might have been diverted to help the native population recover from famine, funded the expensive colonial establishment, and paid for Britain's spate of frontier wars in Afghanistan and Abyssinia, even though India herself had no interest in becoming involved in these conflicts.

From the early 1870s, Florence's work on India had started to shift away from her earlier concentration on sanitary reform towards the far more intricate problems – the 'hundred-headed Hydra', as she called it – associated with the poverty of the Indian peasant, the *ryot*. She continued to monitor the progress of the Army Sanitary Commission, the institution central to the control of all sanitary measures in India, but now realized that only a limited amount could be achieved for civil sanitation through these official channels, given the lack of will among British officials to bring about change. Moreover, her growing awareness of the threat posed by famine to vast sections of the population, and of the complex land revenue system which was keeping the Indian peasant in conditions of abject poverty, and pushing him to the edge of extinction, made her appreciate the preposterousness of expecting improvements in sanitation to tackle the problem at its root. After all, one could hardly ask a person to keep clean when he or she was dying of starvation and disease. In a paper delivered on Florence's behalf at a meeting, in Norwich, of the National Social Science Association, in 1873, she declared that '... one must live in order to be a subject for sanitary consideration at all, and one must eat to live. If one is killed off by famine one certainly need not fear fever or cholera.' This paper, 'Life or Death in India', was a sequel to the one that Florence had written, ten years earlier, to publicize the findings of the Royal Commission on the Health of the British Army in India, and demonstrates the shift in her focus. It starts by giving credit to the advances that have been made in lowering the death rate of British soldiers, but then turns to devoting two-thirds of its length to the plight of the people of India themselves.

Florence's programme to save the Indian peasant rested on two main issues: the need for irrigation and water transit as a famine-preventive measure; and the reform of the land tenure system, which permitted the *zemindars*, the landlords, to exploit the peasant cultivators of their land, and to drain them financially. After considerable research, dating back to the late 1860s, Florence had reached the conclusion that irrigation works and canals would provide considerable aid for both the production and transportation of food. They would allow Government to anticipate periods of crisis by reducing the shortage of supplies, thereby alleviating the suffering of the *ryot*. There had been a long-running debate about whether or not to invest in irrigation work throughout the history of nineteenth-century India, predating the transfer of power from the East India Company to the Crown. Under successive viceroys, the principle of irrigation was largely accepted, but there were disputes about how the construction of the irrigation canals was to be financed: should it be through private investment, or state-guaranteed works, with funds raised by increased taxation of the *ryot*, or a special water rate? There were arguments, too, about the design of the canals themselves: were they to be navigable canals, in which case they required higher levels of water, or were they to be primarily used for irrigation? And against all this, there was the continual pressure on the Government to spend the money on railways instead.

To Florence, the answer appeared straightforward. The way to rescue the Indian peasant from poverty, and from some of the harsher results of famine, was to irrigate his land. Her leading ally in this cause was Sir Arthur Cotton, whom she acknowledged as 'the master, almost the father in modern times of the art of irrigation'. One of Cotton's greatest achievements, at the beginning of the 1850s, was his design for a system of distributive canals to cross the Godavari River in the Madras Presidency, which had helped to mitigate the effects of famine in the area. In 1864, Cotton had returned to England and become a determined campaigner for the improvement of water communications in India, emphasizing the great importance of irrigation works and the development of a system of inland waterways. He encountered much antagonism to his views, and was accused by his opponents of having water on the brain. Even Florence believed Cotton to be lacking in moderation. He gave the public 'strong alcohol', she once said, in comparison to her 'watered milk'. However, his expertise was vital to Florence's grasp of the subject, while her support for his ideas was used by Cotton to publicize his work, when he found that the general press was refusing to publish his letters about the Indian famine of 1877.

Florence's efforts to win the support of Lord Salisbury, Secretary of State for India in Disraeli's Government, from 1874–8, for public works of irrigation ultimately proved unsuccessful. Salisbury had briefly held the same office in the previous decade, at the time of the Orissa famine. He had felt some moral responsibility for the British Government's failure to take measures in time to help the starving, and had demanded that irrigation schemes be put in place without delay (his successor rejected the plans on the grounds that they weren't remunerative enough). Subsequently, though, Salisbury had begun to have doubts about the effectiveness of irrigation as a measure of famine prevention. He argued that in irrigating a district, the land could become marshy, encouraging malaria and fever, and pointed to the *ryot*'s unwillingness to take water from the irrigation canals. It was still the Government's intention to pursue a policy of irrigation, Salisbury said, in a speech made in 1875, but it would be undertaken with 'more frugality than was our intention several years ago'. Florence criticized Salisbury for allowing 'the most industrious peasantry' in the world to continue their work without adequate investment 'from 'Western capital, Western engineering, English public works'; but, during his period in office, she kept up the pressure on him, convinced that 'Lord Salisbury's worst' was better than any other Secretary of State for India's best. She sent him statistics for the cost of irrigation works, agreeing with him that reliable figures were hard to come by; and pressed him to appoint a commission or committee of inquiry. However, despite her confidence in Salisbury, he left office without having established a definite way forward. It would take the 1899 famine in western India, unprecedented in its extent and virulence, to alter the climate of opinion. In 1900, the new Viceroy, Lord Curzon, finally appointed an Irrigation Commission in a speech which went a long way towards conceding that the pro-irrigation lobby had been right. This Commission reported in 1904, twenty-eight years after Florence had originally suggested it.

But just as she had recognized that better sanitation was of little use if the *ryot* was no longer alive to enjoy the benefits of clean water and better drainage, Florence also understood the futility of increasing the productivity of land by irrigation if the profits went to the *zemindars* and moneylenders, rather than to the peasants themselves. In involving herself in issues relating to the land tenure system and the occupancy rights of *ryots*, Florence was entering a complex and controversial area, which bore a close resemblance to the condition of the Irish peasantry in the second half of the nineteenth century (both Irish and Indian peasants had, of course, been severely depleted by the scourge of famine). Like his Irish counterpart, the Indian *ryot* had experienced high taxation, eviction from the land, and exploitation at the hands of landowners who were often absentee landlords. The 1793 Permanent Settlement, which applied to Bengal and other parts of northern and eastern India, was an agreement reached between the British Government and the *zemindar* class. Under this arrangement, the *zemindars* held their land by paying a fixed rate of revenue to the Government. However, the amount of rent to be paid by the peasant cultivators of the land to the *zemindars* was left unassessed. In practice this gave unscrupulous landowners the power to exact as much rent as they wanted from the hapless *ryot*. In cases where the *ryot* was unable to pay, he was evicted from his holding. Although the Bengal Rent Act of 1859 had at last afforded the *ryots* some protection, including the rights of occupancy if they had cultivated the same piece of land continuously for twelve years, this law was difficult to enforce, and what the *zemindars* were unable to take legally they set about trying to obtain illegally. Widespread oppression of the *ryots* followed. By the end of the 1870s, at the time when Florence had begun to consider the problem, there had been peasant revolts and protests in parts of Bengal; and this agrarian tension was only heightened when, in 1878, the Government brought in a new bill to facilitate the collection of rent arrears for the *zemindars*.

Much of Florence's information about the land tenancy dispute came from a young Bengali lawyer from Calcutta called Prasanna Kumar Sen. In February 1878, Sen had written to her about the arrears bill, enclosing a book on the subject, and seeking her support for the *ryots*' cause. Florence had responded by asking him to collect facts for her, 'individual and personal histories of ryots'. This request was repeated in further correspondence with Sen between 1878 and 1882, soliciting details of *zemindar–ryot* relations, and of the illegal taxes being imposed on the peasant population. 'English people will not read Reports in general,' she told Sen in December 1878,

nor generalities, abstractions, statistics, or <u>opinions</u>, such as most Reports are full of. They want <u>facts</u> . . . Give us detailed facts. We want to rouse the interest of the <u>public</u>: for behind the Cabinet in England always stands the House of Commons & behind the House of Commons always stands the British public. And these are they we want to interest: and these can only be interested by narratives of real lives.

In her work for India, Florence depended on 'the plain unvarnished evidence of plain witnesses'. Her introduction to the Bengal Social Science Association, whose honorary membership she accepted in 1870, brought her into contact with the English-educated elite of Bengali society. These middle-class Indians were Florence's first-hand witnesses to conditions that blighted the lives of those at the bottom of Indian society. She also corresponded regularly with four or five officials in India, who provided her with facts and figures from different parts of the country. In England, a host of members of the Council of India, some current, some retired, gave her the benefit of their expertise, like General Rundall, the ex-Inspector-general of Indian Irrigation, or A. W. Croft, who had headed the board for public education in India. Sir Louis Mallet, Permanent Under-Secretary of State at the India Office, was always a sympathetic source of information, even when he disagreed with her; while Sir Bartle Frere, a former Governor of Bombay, who returned to London in 1867 to join the India Council and Sanitary Committee, became not only a trusted consultant and adviser, but a good friend as well.

It was sometimes said that Florence had more facts at her fingertips than the War Office and the India Office put together, and there were times when officials at the India Office had to admit that her information was more reliable than theirs. In 1878, Florence's estimate of 5 to 6 million deaths in the recent famine quickly came to be regarded as closer to the actual number than the official figure of 1,250,000. Not surprisingly, there was resentment of this in Government circles – 'the official mind is much disturbed', one India Office insider wrote to her – and Florence found herself accused of meddling. Attempting, in 1878, to gain access to the untabulated data in the India Office relating to irrigation returns, she received a sharp rebuff from a member of the Revenue Department. The department minute acknowledged that Florence's 'advice and intelligent philanthropy is universally recognised', but advised 'that to open the records of a public office to the free inspection of a private individual, however distinguished for character and ability, would constitute a very inconvenient precedent'.

Meanwhile, Florence was putting those facts to good use. Throughout the 1870s, she published a stream of papers and pamphlets on famine and irrigation, and land tenancy reform. She used the letter pages of newspapers, and periodicals like the *Illustrated London News*, to publicize her views, with signed letters alerting the public to the conditions in which the Indian peasant lived, and urging the authorities to bring in reforms to make a difference. She was giving a voice to the ordinary people, living in the villages of India, who constituted 80 per cent of the country's population, acting as 'the Government's conscience', and using her reputation in an attempt to embarrass them into taking action. Not everyone close to Florence believed in the wisdom of her approach. In 1874 she showed a draft of her work on the land tenure system, which accused the Government of being indifferent to the human cost of famine, to Benjamin Jowett. With donnish precision, he criticized it for its 'jerky & impulsive' style, and for the way in which it appeared to place exaggeration above pure reasoning. He further argued that publication of the book would do harm to her position with officials at the India Office, including Lord Salisbury, and that 'if your book was deemed rash or inaccurate you would be discredited ... & you would lose influence'. Although its material formed the basis for several subsequent articles, Florence put the book to one side, and it was never published.*

Four years later, though, Florence decided to throw caution to the winds. She was surer now of her facts, and of the inferences to be drawn from them. She was also in deep despair about the apathy of the British Government's attitude to the 'Great Famine'. Florence's article, 'The People of India', which appeared in August 1878 in the journal *Nineteenth Century*, was derided by some officials as a 'shriek'. But it caused a stir, and uncomfortably jolted the India Office out of some of its complacency. 'We do not care for the people of India,' was Florence's opening remark. 'This is a heavy indictment: but how else account for the facts about to be given? Do we even care enough to know about their daily lives of lingering death from causes which we could so well remove?'

In the words which she used to sign off her letters to Prasanna Kumar Sen, Florence had become 'the Ryot's faithful servant'.

The months that Florence spent with her mother at Lea Hurst, in the latter half of the 1870s, following William Nightingale's death, were a homecoming in more ways than one. For the first time in over twenty years, she was an active member of a large family. Usually Florence was at Lea Hurst in July or August, in time to greet her mother, who arrived with Shore, his wife, Louisa, and their children, from their house in London. She stayed until the final months of the year, sometimes remaining there alone with Fanny after the Shore Smiths had departed. Shore's devotion to her mother more than repaid the care that Florence had taken of him as he was growing up. The happiness of Fanny's last years, she told him later, was largely 'due to you & yours'. Shore's own health was poor. In his mid-forties, he had retired from his clerkship at the House of Commons, but struggled on an income of £5,000 per annum to maintain both Nightingale country properties, in addition to his London home. His parents, Aunt Mai and Uncle Sam, were themselves in failing health, and rarely well enough to make the journey from

---

* In 1914, however, Sir William Wedderburn, a founding member of the Indian National Congress, was allowed by Florence's executors to examine the proof, and published a summary of its findings in the *Contemporary Review*.

Combe Hurst to stay with him. As a result, Embley, and sometimes the Hurst, were let for large parts of the year.

Shore's and Louisa's children, two boys and two girls, were welcoming and affectionate towards their cousin Florence, who became an honorary aunt. Sam, the eldest, would train as a doctor at St Bartholomew's. Rosalind, or Rosie as she was known, just a year his junior, was an especial favourite of her great-aunt Fanny, to whom she always showed a 'protecting care'. Determined and independent-minded, Rosalind was adored and admired in equal measure by Florence herself. In 1881, at the age of twenty, Rosalind won a place at Girton College, Cambridge. '. . . Remember that when your brain is tired, it is not saving time to force it on, but rest it for ¾ hour,' was Florence's advice to the new student. 'Take a brisk walk is best, or read an entertaining book or play a bit of Mozart. Tennis greatly to be approved of, but not for ½ hour's relaxation . . .'

Back at Lea Hurst, Florence turned her attention to the running of the local school that her parents had founded, and to the foundation of a new coffee house which, in an area strong in Methodism, forced the closure for a time of the local pub. As a young woman she had found a sense of purpose in visiting the sick poor in the villages surrounding the Hurst. Over the years, she had kept in touch with local families, many of whom she had known since childhood, through a network of inform-ants, including former employees of the Nightingales. During her pro-longed periods at Lea Hurst in the 1870s, Florence re-established personal contact with the villagers, especially with the tenants in the Lea cottages; and, in conjunction with the local doctor, Christopher Dunn, formed a remarkable arrangement of health care for members of the community, funded from Florence's personal benevolence. As well as providing some of these neighbours with extra food – meat, milk, and cocoatina, a nourishing drink – Florence paid for hospital stays, medi-cines and cleaning help, and hired private nurses where necessary. From London, she continued to keep a careful eye on the progress of those she described in letters to Dunn as 'our patients'. In essence, this was a partnership, and one that lasted until Dunn's death in 1892 (when Florence engaged Dr George MacDonald to succeed him). Having made home visits, a service for which she paid him quarterly, Dunn wrote Florence lengthy reports on individual cases, and together they discussed the possibilities for treatment, either in person, while she was staying in

Derbyshire, or by mail. In the winter of 1876, for example, Florence asked Dunn to call on Mrs Swindell, a typhoid patient, and Widow Henstock, 'who is said to have vomited blood a few days ago'. She also requested that he might visit Lizzie Holmes, a maid at the Hurst, 'now & then, & should you wish her to return to Buxton [for a water cure] when the spring returns I shall be too glad to send her'. The following summer, Adelaide Peach, a sufferer from pericarditis, was a cause for concern on account of her bedsores. 'Would you wish her to be put on a water bed or water pillow, & if so where could either be had?' Florence asked Dunn. As for that 'silly girl', Rose Wren, she 'will never keep on the cold-water bandage (or think that it does her any good) ... Would you like it to be put on as a compress with oiled silk & bandage over it?'

In 1878, Florence was alarmed to learn of the 'abominable' nursing care of bedridden patients at the Devonshire Hospital at Buxton. This was the nearest hospital to Lea and Holloway, where villagers and cottagers for whom Dr Dunn and Florence were caring were regularly admitted. Her information came from Mrs Limb, the widow of the local stonemason. Florence had paid for Mrs Limb's admission to the Devonshire to receive treatment for her severe rheumatism, but was disturbed to discover afterwards that she had been placed in a ward with five other women, who were left all night without care. Other reports established that patients were discouraged from waking the nurse at night, and, furthermore, that they were 'in bodily fear of the management'. Investigating the situation cautiously at first, Florence enlisted the help of Dr Dunn and Sir Harry Verney. Within a year, the Devonshire had been subjected to a Nightingale-style course of improvement. Finding that the dismissal of the matron and steward had done nothing to remedy the care of bedridden patients at night, Florence appealed for the assistance of the Duke of Devonshire, the hospital's patron, and a council member of the Nightingale Fund. The Devonshire family was proud of Derbyshire's Nightingale connection – on her return to England in 1856, Florence had been presented with a model in silver of Athena the owl by the Duke's predecessor – but Florence was initially worried about the Duke's ability to carry out a full-scale inquiry, and concerned that he should be seen to be acting on his own initiative, without using her name. In fact, although Florence supplied the Duke with a questionnaire to use in his inquiry, about the number of nurses, the matron's pay and training, and the number and type of wards, she managed to remain in the background. A properly qualified matron was introduced, and Florence concluded to Dr Dunn that 'the Nursing for <u>helpless</u> patients is now what it ought to be'.

In the final ten days of January 1880, Fanny Nightingale's condition suddenly worsened. At the beginning of the month, Florence was with her mother in London as they marked the anniversary of her father's death, six years earlier. Four times Fanny looked at a photograph of William Nightingale's monument in St Margaret's churchyard, and repeated its inscription. On 20 January she went out in her carriage, and the next day came downstairs at Shore's house in York Place, where she was living, for the last time. Outside, a thick winter fog enveloped everything, and at night Fanny coughed incessantly, and struggled painfully to breathe. Shore 'strove for her life as if his own depended on it'. Although he was far from well himself, he got up in the night to feed her, knowing that she might take food from him. 'He was so happy when he could get two or three teaspoonfuls or a morsel of sponge cake into her mouth,' Florence wrote to the surgeon Sir William Webb, in a close analysis of her mother's condition. 'But, after doing this to please him, she would take an opportunity to put it all out again . . .' The end came soon after midnight on 2 February, a month before her ninety-second birthday, with Shore and his wife at Fanny's side. In her final hours Fanny listened to her favourite hymns and prayers. Her pulse had been strong, and the doctor had confidently predicted that she had days to live, so that Florence was not with her mother when she died, and did not see her again until after she was dead. 'She looked then and afterwards fifty years younger, like a picture there is of her at Embley with us two as children' (later Florence regretted seeing photographs of Fanny on her deathbed, as they left her with a more distressing memory). Neither daughter was well enough to brave the freezing February air as Fanny was lowered into the ground next to her husband. A small group of family and loyal servants were at the graveside, and the churchyard crowded with villagers and tenants. The coffin was surmounted with a huge wreath from the nurses at St Thomas's.

'She knew me without knowing me,' Florence wrote of her last visits to her mother. On the penultimate occasion, just days before she died, Fanny addressed her as 'Filomena', the name of the heroine in the poem by Longfellow, which Florence had inspired. Sorting through Fanny's possessions after her death, Florence was moved to discover that she had kept her old Crimean hospital sash. It must have felt like a mother's blessing on her work at last.

19. Battle of the Nurses

She was exhausted. 'For six years & six weeks I have had not one day's rest of body or mind,' Florence wrote of the period since her father's death when she had borne the main responsibility for her mother. In the days following the funeral, people were coming and going at South Street, and staying for hours, 'when all one longs for is silence'. The Queen sent her condolences. Never one to miss an opportunity, Florence replied with a 'lingering' account of Fanny's last days, and asked leave to address the Queen about India (permission was granted, though Victoria ignored the substance of Florence's letter, merely responding with the gift of Theodore Martin's recently completed *Life* of the Prince Consort). As one of the executors of her mother's will, Florence was involved in the winding up of Fanny's estate, and in the distribution of legacies, including £1,000 to each of her daughters, together with some stocks and shares. She and Parthenope disagreed about the wording for Fanny's memorial in the churchyard at East Wellow. Florence withdrew her mother's age from her draft at Parthenope's request – 'though it greatly loses in pathos thereby' – and bowed to her sister's insistence on greater simplicity for the inscription. The last of the older generation of Smiths, 'those ten vigorous brothers & sisters', were slowly dying out. Aunt Patty had died a decade earlier; Uncle Sam went 'painlessly & calmly' in the autumn of 1880, leaving Aunt Mai alone at Combe Hurst; Julia, three years later, while Joanna, Hilary and Henry Bonham Carter's mother, outlived all her siblings, dying at the age of ninety-three, in 1884.

Advised by her doctors to rest out of London, Florence spent three weeks in the middle of February 1880 at the Granville Hotel, on the seafront at Ramsgate. She could not leave her work behind, and inevitably a crisis, this one concerning the nursing at Netley, was not long in following her. But, as she reported to Parthenope, she did not feel worse. She enjoyed watching the white-capped waves crashing in upon the shore, a sight she had not seen for almost a quarter of a century, though the hotel was 'too London-y & I don't like acting the "lady" '. Florence was back at South Street for a month, working 'at high steam pressure, but with every sail set', though finding that 'the crazy old vessel won't stand it'. In early April she accepted an invitation from her old friend Louisa Ashburton to stay at her home at Seaton, in Devon. She was there for a month, designing a scheme for a nurses' provident society, while looking out over the Jurassic coastline along the bay, and mourning the death of a friendly thrush which had been eaten by a hawk.

In spite of the immense strain imposed on her during her mother's last years, Florence's overall health had started to improve. She continued to be plagued by serious joint pain, which led to a consultation later in the decade with a new doctor, Thomas Brunton of St Bartholomew's, famous for his experiments in pharmacology, who prescribed a course of potassium bromide and massage therapy; but the muscle spasms linked to spondylitis had all but ceased, relieved by injections of subcutaneous opium. And while she still suffered regularly from insomnia and bad headaches, the great weight of depressive feelings, of worthlessness and failure, had gradually lifted. By the early 1880s, she was less subject to the attacks of irritability, frustration and emotional instability which we now recognize as symptomatic of brucellosis in its most chronic form. There was a new benevolence about her, a generosity of spirit and openness reminiscent of the younger Florence of pre-Crimean days. No one perhaps was more surprised by this change in temperament than Florence herself. In a letter to Madame Mohl in the summer of 1881, not long after her sixty-first birthday, Florence remembered how, in the wake of the deaths of Sidney Herbert and Clough, twenty years earlier, she had grown accustomed to watching for her own death, 'as no sick man ever watched for the morning'. Now, however, she found that she craved it less. 'I want to do a little work a little better before I die.'

Work, of course, continued to take precedence over everything else, and her health remained useful as a protective shield against any unwarranted or unwelcome demands that might be made on her. 'People don't know how weak I am,' she wrote in June 1881, as she began interviewing the St Thomas's trainees employed as nurses at the new, 760-bed, Marylebone workhouse infirmary. Nevertheless, in limited respects, Florence's horizons were widening. She enjoyed carriage drives in Hyde

Park, or sometimes further afield: a round trip to Westminster Abbey, for instance, along the Embankment, back past the Abbey and home again to South Street. She also made a number of public appearances. Admiration for the former Viceroy Sir John Lawrence made her attend his funeral in the Abbey, in July 1879, where she heard Dean Stanley proclaim Lawrence as 'An Indian Statesman'. In January 1882, Florence visited the Nightingale Training School for the first time; and on 13 November that year she accompanied Sir Harry Verney to Victoria station, to watch the arrival of the Foot Guards from the first Egyptian campaign, as a nephew of Sir Harry's, Colonel Philip Smith, commanding a regiment of the Grenadiers, was among those returning. Florence took a particular interest in the event, having been consulted about the selection of nurses for the short-lived campaign. '. . . Anyone might have been proud of these men's appearance,' she wrote, her emotion rising, as it always did with anything connected to the ordinary soldier, ' – like shabby skeletons, or at least half their size – in worn but well-cleaned campaigning uniforms; not spruce, or showy, but alert, silent, steady . . . A more deeply felt and less showy scene could not have been imagined.' Five days later, she was the guest of Prime Minister Gladstone at a Royal Review of returning troops, which took place at Horse Guards Parade. Florence sat between Gladstone and his wife on a stand erected in the garden of Ten Downing Street. 'Not far from the dais,' Queen Victoria recorded in her diary, 'I recognized Florence Nightingale, whom I had not seen for years . . .' She sent Florence a message to say how well she had looked, and asked her to the opening, the following month, of the Royal Courts of Justice, which Florence also attended.

Walking, after years of being bed- or sofa-bound, was becoming easier for Florence, though she preferred to take exercise unaccompanied: '. . . I have only strength to walk if I am quite alone & unnoticed,' she explained to Sir Harry. Relatives, unexpectedly coming across the ambulant figure of someone they had grown accustomed to thinking of as a reclusive invalid, regarded the sight with something of a shock. Young Charles Bonham Carter, one of Henry's massive brood, remembered the surprise of seeing Cousin Florence for the first time, walking with the aid of a stick in the garden of the family home at Ravensbourne. Several years later, Rosalind Shore Smith and one of her brothers had a similar experience when they came upon Florence in the grounds at Embley:

We did not know she was out, or we should have kept out of the way, for, in her many years of retired work, she never saw anyone unprepared, and never saw more than one person at a time, on account of the state of her heart and nerves. I saw the reason, for she flushed at seeing us, and for once looked slightly disturbed . . . We passed on almost at once. She had been sailing along down the little glade through which the Long Walk runs, and I saw then how beautifully she walked. Anyone who has seen Queen Alexandra walk knows what a charming sight human progression can be. Florence Nightingale's walk was that of a taller woman, but it was as graceful.

Florence's adoption of Claydon, at the Verneys' request, as her primary home in the country was symbolic of this new sense of liberation. In the summer of 1881 she stayed there for the first time since her mother's death, and thanked Sir Harry afterwards for 'the enjoyment of this beautiful house and gardens'. Over the course of the next thirteen years, Florence was to return on many occasions, most often in August and September. A bedroom and dressing room were set aside for her use, known by the household as 'the F wing', and she had her own bells in the servants' hall which she could ring whenever she needed assistance. Her cats accompanied her, though it could prove hazardous transporting them on the train journey. Returning to London from Claydon, in the autumn of 1885, Florence was alarmed when Quiz, a Persian kitten, jumped out of the window on to the track at Watford, and scampered out of sight. 'I summoned all the stationmasters in England to my assistance,' Florence announced with a dramatic flourish. 'He of Watford' was sent back along the line to find Quiz, and telegraphed Florence later that evening: 'Cat found not hurt.' Quiz spent the night in the Euston parcels office and was returned to her grateful mistress the next morning, shocked but 'alive & singing'.

Florence admired the enormous care that her sister had taken in overseeing the restoration of Claydon House from its former dilapidated state. She loved sitting in the Blue Room best, gazing on its 'Great Western Sky'. To please the Verneys – and to compensate for G. F. Watts's failure two decades earlier – Florence agreed to sit for her portrait to the artist W. B. Richmond, who had painted other members of the Verney family (the finished half-length oil shows a well-rounded face beneath a lace scarf tied at the chin, and currently hangs in Florence's former room at Claydon). Parthenope and Sir Harry respected her privacy in the house, often barely encountering Florence for days at a time. It had taken 'self-denial', Florence told her sister in May 1886, not to come down to the library to have a conversation with her, but she had been obeying her doctors' instructions 'that I would not put my feet to the ground or sit or stand for some days'. Several months later, she refused Parthenope's invitation to a concert in the saloon. 'Sir Harry must not come, offering me his dear arm, and saying: "you <u>must</u> come down, because I ask you, into the saloon." I shall probably never be able to come downstairs at all, except to doddle out quite alone & unseen into the garden occasionally.' One social event, however, was inscribed on the summer calendar. This was the day out at Claydon for the Home Sister and Nightingale probationers of the year from St Thomas's. 'We have come back to our work,' runs a vote of thanks to the Verneys from one group following their visit, 'refreshed by the sweet country air and the kindnesses shown to us, and encouraged to future & stronger efforts in our hospital by the indirect contact we have experienced with our Chief and model whose great example we have always before us.' Only a favoured few were interviewed by Florence, but W. A. C. Egan, a probationer in 1881–2, recalled Florence standing at an open window, waving as nurses left for a carriage drive with Parthenope in the afternoon.

As at Lea Hurst, so at Claydon, Florence cared for other people's health as well as her own. With the local doctor, Philip Benson, she formed an alliance similar to the one she had established with Dr Dunn in the villages near the Hurst, paying for Sir Harry's employees to have medical consultations, and following up in her guise as 'an old Nurse' on the patients' progress. Mrs Robertson, a member of the Claydon household, saw Benson, at Florence's urging, about a pain in her groin, and was put up at South Street while she was in London, having a truss fitted. Florence heard one of the maids, Emily Baker, 'breathing hard like a steam engine' as she lit the fire in her dressing room, arranged for her to be seen by Benson, and asked him, 'do you think she <u>laces</u> too tightly?'

The younger Verneys – Sir Harry's three surviving sons, their wives, and children – gave Florence the opportunity of experiencing the pleasures of extended family life to the full, rather than simply its frustrations.* She

* Emily Verney, Sir Harry's daughter, who had corresponded with Florence and established a warm relationship with her, had died in 1872, at the age of twenty-nine.

entered into their lives, involved some of them in her work, and lent a sympathetic ear to their problems. Edmund, Sir Harry's eldest son, now in his early forties, and partially disabled after a shooting accident on the family estates, had retired from the Navy following active service in the Crimea and Indian Mutiny, and further commands on the Pacific seaboard of Canada and in West Africa. He was subsequently elected as Liberal MP for North Buckinghamshire, his father's old seat, and represented Brixton on the first London County Council in 1889. George Hope Verney, who pursued an Army career, was the middle brother, and the one Florence knew least well; but the youngest, Frederick – or 'Mr Fred' as she called him – was Florence's favourite, and, later, her collaborator in various schemes for rural health. She had watched Fred grow up, corresponding with him while he was a schoolboy at Harrow, and applauding his early efforts to become a clergyman, though he never proceeded to holy orders after being ordained as a deacon, and opted to train as a lawyer instead. Fred sought Florence's advice about his plans for working-men's clubs in northern industrial cities, and she undoubtedly saw in him the fusion of faith and social action that was so fundamental to her own beliefs. Like Edmund Verney, Fred later became a councillor and was elected to Parliament.

Edmund and Fred married sisters, Margaret and Maude, the daughters of Sir John Hay Williams, a Welsh baronet. Florence had received Edmund and Margaret Verney at South Street in 1869, soon after their marriage, and quickly came to appreciate the new Mrs Verney's resilience and sterling qualities as an administrator, not least on the local school boards in the villages around Claydon. An intimacy, formed at first through correspondence, developed between the two women, and by the early 1880s Florence was addressing her in letters as 'Blessed Margaret', or even 'Dearest Blessed Margaret'. Margaret's sister Maude married Fred in 1870 (confined to bed, Florence regretted that her wedding present to the couple would have to be a 'fipun' note). Maude, too, became a confidante. She visited South Street – where she was even permitted to perform on her Stradivarius – and made her home at Sunningdale, in Berkshire, available for Florence when she was recovering from illness. The children from both marriages were a constant source of great pleasure and amusement for 'Aunt Florence', as well as being recipients of a generous stream of gifts from her. Ruth, Edmund and Margaret's eldest child, was among Florence's godchildren, as were Gwendolen and Kathleen, Fred and Maude's two daughters. While staying at Claydon in 1886, Florence sent daily reports to Maude in London about the health of young Gwendolen and her brother Ralph, who, along with their governess, had gone down with an attack of measles. 'You understand that they are both now in the inner nursery . . .,' Florence informed her, 'Gwendolen in bed, of course, with her doll & two picture books, but without a trace of apparent illness. Dolly "has <u>not</u> got measles"!!! Aunt Florence's orders were to come back & read to them . . . Of course she obeyed her general & general's sister – "Them's my orders."'

Florence participated vicariously in the excitement of a General Election through the parliamentary campaigns fought by Edmund and Fred Verney. 'Our maids are all in the [Liberal] colours, red, & the four cats are marching in with their four tails up & in four red necklaces,' she wrote to Parthenope and Sir Harry as news came of Gladstone's victory in 1880 (though Edmund had lost at Portsmouth). '. . . May God continue the election for the Liberal interest as He has begun it!' Family ructions over Home Rule for Ireland, however, required all Florence's powers as a conciliator. Sir Harry opposed Home Rule, while Edmund and Fred adopted the Gladstonian position in its favour. Disagreement between father and sons became at one stage so great that Edmund and Margaret Verney had to rent separate lodgings near Claydon during the 1885 election, in which Edmund was seeking to replace Sir Harry, who had retired from his North Buckinghamshire seat. Florence did her best to resolve matters – she and Parthenope were similarly divided, she for Home Rule, her sister for the Unionists – while understanding the difficulties. 'I feel with you more than you can imagine,' she told Edmund later, ' – it is indeed the greatest difficulty in political life since 1832 [and the Great Reform Act].'

Six years later, Florence would be instrumental in reconciling Sir Harry with his eldest son as a sex scandal rocked the Verney family. In May 1891, Edmund was convicted on a charge of conspiring to procure a minor – a nineteen-year-old woman, then legally a minor – for immoral purposes, and sentenced to a year's imprisonment. The trial revealed that Edmund had been leading a double life as a 'Mr Wilson', and that he had persuaded the young woman, Nellie Baskett, to meet him in Paris. She had refused to have sexual relations with him, but it was clear that Edmund had succeeded in seducing other women. He was forced immediately to resign as MP and councillor, in the midst of a public outcry against him. Margaret Verney forgave him, and Florence interceded for Edmund with Sir Harry, asking him to ensure that people shouldn't think that 'his <u>father</u> doubts his repentance'.

The lengths to which Margaret was prepared to go in caring for Parthenope, who was afflicted by the devastating combination of severe rheumatism and arthritis, and cancer in its early stages, more than earned her the nickname of 'Blessed'. At the end of 1882, Parthenope had suffered her first major collapse. For Sir Harry, in his eighties and in far from good health himself, it was a terrible blow. He sobbed at the sight of Parthenope's distress, and lay awake at night listening to his wife's cries of pain. Diagnosis of Parthenope's condition was complicated by the fact that she changed her doctor so often. 'She has had 10 Doctors in little more than 5 months!' Florence reported with amazement to Sir Harry, in November 1882. In December, Margaret Verney came to Claydon to supervise Parthenope's care, and to take charge of carrying out the orders of Dr William Ogle, a physician from the Derbyshire Royal Infirmary whose work was well known to Florence, and whom she respected. The improvement under this regime was marked, although the Verneys could not be persuaded to give up their homoeopathic doctor – or 'quack' as Florence referred to him. By the spring of 1884, Florence thought Parthenope was 'quite herself' again. 'I am sure she has the use of her right hand <u>much</u> more . . .,' she wrote to Margaret, to whom she awarded much of the credit for having rescued her sister. 'She sees many people, too many. She has the use of her mind & she is often without pain, thank God, for hours together.' To Parthenope, Florence sent her own prescription for conserving health: avoid getting tired; see no one except by appointment, apart from Sir Harry; and for 'the safest atmosphere', have an open fire '& a window open <u>at the top</u>'.

A period of remission was vital to Parthenope's completion of what had become the major passion of her life, a history of the Verneys during the English Civil War, based on the bundles of family letters, diaries and accounts from the seventeenth century, preserved at Claydon. With the help of Margaret Verney, and two other young friends, Catherine and Frederica Spring Rice, Parthenope tackled the enormous task of sorting and classifying the documents, a task made all the more difficult, as well as physically painful, by the crippling effects of rheumatoid arthritis on her hands. There was a cruel irony in the fact that Parthenope, who had once devoted so much energy to copying letters in her sister's cause, was now often unable to transcribe material for work of her own. At first, she overcame difficulties to some extent by using a stylographic pen; but latterly the condition of her hands was such that she could barely turn over the pages of the letters themselves, let alone hold a pen. In 1885 Parthenope published a short article on the history of Claydon for the Buckinghamshire Archaeological Society. Four years later, having relied heavily on Margaret's skills as researcher and amanuensis, she presented the manuscript of the first volume of the *Memoirs of the Verney Family during the Civil War*, as a gift for Sir Harry's eighty-eighth birthday.

Parthenope's often agonizing pain, which increased its hold as the decade wore on, made her extremely irritable, and sometimes impossible to deal with. While still able to write by hand, she was in the habit of sending 'outrageously discourteous' letters to members of her family, which Florence did her best to excuse on her sister's behalf, as the products of a mind that did not always know what it was doing. When both sisters were in South Street, Florence set aside every Sunday afternoon to see Parthenope; and when well enough, in all but the severest weather, Parthenope would be carried the short distance from the Verneys' home to the drawing room at number 10 to sit with Florence. A new spirit of tenderness had entered Florence's relationship with Parthenope, as she contemplated her sister's sadly crippled state, and recollected her own experience of excruciating pain. 'Grieved you are so bad,' she wrote to Parthenope, in December 1888, signing off with her assurance that 'Dear Pop – I am always thinking of you . . .'

Florence had done as much as she could to maintain personal relationships with successive Viceroys of India, following the departure of Sir John Lawrence at the end of the 1860s. She had initially been appalled by the appointment of Lawrence's successor, Lord Mayo, who lacked any experience of India. 'He's a good & sensible man,' she had written of him, 'but he knows absolutely nothing.' Mayo, however, had won her over by demonstrating his interest in irrigation and canal-building schemes; and, after his assassination in 1872, Florence had mourned him as someone who was 'not only willing but wanting . . . to do all he could'. The next Viceroy, Lord Northbrook, who had served under Sidney Herbert at the War Office, treated Florence with respect, but otherwise kept her at a distance, failing to call on her before his departure for India. The policies of Lord Lytton, Disraeli's appointee in 1876, were simply anathema to her. Lytton's new ethos of imperialism, symbolized by the lavish ceremonial durbar that marked his arrival in India, his passing of the Vernacular Act – a tacit form of racial discrimination, which subjected newspapers published in Indian languages to censorship – and his 'forward' policy towards Afghanistan, which provoked the Second Afghan War, were viewed by Florence, with others of progressive opinion in Britain, as retrograde steps which could only prove disastrous. Lytton's period of office, the most turbulent in viceregal history, was to act as a strong stimulus to the rise of Indian nationalism, and the eventual foundation, in 1885, of the Indian National Congress.

Florence's hopes rose dramatically with Gladstone's appointment of Lord Ripon as Viceroy, following the Liberal victory of 1880. For she had worked with Ripon, or Lord de Grey as he was then known, at the War Office two decades earlier, having successfully agitated for him to succeed Sir George Lewis as Secretary for War in 1863. She did not doubt his proficiency in sanitary matters, while his knowledge of Indian affairs was not in question either, as Ripon had served as Secretary of State for India for a short time during Lawrence's viceroyalty. 'Dear Lord Ripon,' Florence wrote to him soon after he went to India as Viceroy, 'May I venture to recall to your kind remembrance one Florence Nightingale, & to ask you a favour for "auld lang syne" at the War Office?'

Much of Ripon's time in India would be devoted to undoing the harm done by his predecessor to native perceptions of British rule in India. His first and most urgent concern was to extract the army from Afghanistan, terminating the 'forward' policy of Disraeli's Government. Ripon's subsequent attempts at introducing liberal measures were often met with resistance by conservative elements at home, and by Anglo-Indians in India, who regarded him as an Empire wrecker. But many ordinary Indians would come to look upon him as their saviour. His radical credentials were solid. As a young man he had been associated with the Christian Socialists; as an older one, he was involved in the Co-operative movement. He always argued that considerations of right and justice outweighed those associated with political aims or force. Like Florence, Ripon believed that the future for India ultimately lay in self-government, and he attempted to institute a number of political, social and educational reforms to prepare Indians for the task of administering for themselves. Ripon's greatest achievement would be a Bill, passed in May 1884, just before he left India, introducing a measure of decentralization at the municipal level, and encouraging the growth of a political consciousness among native Indians.

Florence has been described as Ripon's 'morale-booster'. Certainly she spurred him on, lobbying him on issues that were important to her, as well as providing information and detail on subjects on which they shared a common mind. They didn't agree on everything: she could never persuade him, for instance, to accept her view of the primacy of irrigation canals over railways. But in many other areas, she was able to give him her support. Ripon arrived in India at a time when land tenancy reform in Bengal was still a burning issue. His efforts to give the *ryot* fixity of tenure, fair rents and free sale met with studied opposition from the Government in London, and from officials in India, who denounced it as 'socialistic'. It was another two years before an amended bill was presented for consideration, and a further two before a watered-down version of the original, making a number of major concessions to the *zemindars*, was passed as the Tenancy Act – by which time Ripon had left India. Meanwhile, Florence had written an article backing up Ripon's position, read out for her by Fred Verney at a meeting of the East India Association, chaired by Sir Bartle Frere, in June 1883. In 'The Dumb Shall Speak and The Deaf Shall Hear, or the Ryot, the Zemindar, and the Government', Florence outlined the reforms she considered necessary to a system by which the peasant cultivator was kept at the mercy of the landlord. She also lambasted those who chose to ignore the problem and maintain the status quo: 'the interests involved are so enormous that we prefer to turn away our head, saying that we cannot understand them. We will not "look them in the face;" we shut our eyes; they are too big for our vision.'

While the Bengal Tenancy Bill was being argued over, Ripon's administration was making more definite progress with improvements to agricultural practice in India. For her part, Florence wanted to see the introduction of proper agricultural training for Indian Civil Service candidates. This would enable them to arrive in India equipped with a range of relevant practical knowledge – about soil conservation, for example, or animal physiology relating to breeds and diseases of cattle – to assist the peasant in the cultivation of his land. Jowett collaborated

with her on a programme of lectures to be established at Oxford for
these candidates. To Arnold Toynbee, then a lecturer in economics at
Balliol, Florence expressed her hope 'that something of instruction on
Agricultural and technical science, including Forestry, may direct your
students' attention ... to what are the peculiar wants of India – a
knowledge often absent in her rulers ... The future of India depends,
more than anything else, on the rulers we bring up ...' In India itself,
Florence had made contact with W. R. Robertson, the Principal of the
Madras Agricultural College, in an attempt to discover the kind of
training that Indian students received in agriculture, and to inquire about
the most effective ways of disseminating information about modern
farming methods throughout the villages. She researched the idea for an
agricultural bank to offer cheap loans to the *ryots* on a cooperative
basis, and won Ripon's support for a trial scheme.

The catalyst for Ripon's resignation as Viceroy, in 1884, before the
end of his term of office, was the Ilbert Bill. This piece of legislation –
named after Sir Courtney Ilbert, who originally presented it before the
Council of India – formed part of Ripon's broad vision to remove the
restrictions that existed on racial grounds from Indian society (he had
already repealed the controversial Vernacular Act). It proposed giving
the power to Indian magistrates and district judges to exercise jurisdiction over European subjects. The uproar it created, among a wide section
of the Anglo-Indian population, the British press and opposition MPs
at home, was unprecedented. Lord Salisbury, the current leader of the
Conservative Party, summed up the case for opponents of the Bill when
he asked a Birmingham audience how they would feel if they were 'in
some distant and thinly populated land, far from all English succour,
and your life or honour were exposed to the decision of some tribunal
consisting of a coloured man'.

It seemed that, all at once, anyone with a grudge against Ripon's
administration – particularly Anglo-Indians suspicious of his plans to
share power with the natives – was noisily demonstrating against him.
Florence wrote to Ripon that, in her 'long & busy life', she had never
seen 'such an instance of mania as seems to have seized London against
the so-called "Ilbert Bill" '. But she begged him to hold firm against the
anti-Bill lobby, and those intent on destabilizing his own position. Ripon
responded by telling her how 'pleasant it is in the midst of much obstruction and misconception to learn that one, whose opinion I value so

highly, understands so thoroughly the spirit in which I am labouring and the aims which I have set before me'. He would, however, need all the support in England that he could muster, for 'my adversaries will leave no stone unturned to secure the overthrow of my plans'.

Florence left no stone unturned to speak up in Ripon's favour. Her article, 'Our Indian Stewardship', which appeared in the December 1883 issue of *Nineteenth Century*, set out the argument for Ripon's viceroyalty. What he was doing in India, she reminded readers, was fulfilling the pledge made by Victoria, the Queen-Empress, in her proclamation to the people of India: '. . . that there are to be no race distinctions, that where there is fitness the employment of natives and Europeans is to be alike; that race is not to be a qualification or disqualification'. Florence also wrote to the Queen herself, politely reminding her of those words from her 'gracious Proclamation'.

The Ilbert Bill was finally passed in January 1884, though with a significant compromise that allowed European subjects in India trial by jury. Ripon had by then decided to resign. As he passed through the streets of Calcutta to board ship for his return journey to England, he was greeted with a tumultuous reception from crowds of Indians, bidding him farewell. In London, Florence's efforts to raise a hero's welcome for him were met with a distinct lack of enthusiasm.

The Ilbert Bill had raised some uncomfortable questions about the nature of British rule in India. Ripon's departure left Florence with forebodings that a new Viceroy might overturn liberal reforms, like the Tenancy Act, which were still waiting to be implemented. In the event, these fears were unfounded. Ripon's successor, Lord Dufferin, proved an enlightened Governor-General, restoring the confidence of the Indian Civil Service, badly shaken under his predecessor's rule, while promising educated Indians a greater share in provincial government. Dufferin's experiences as a landowner in Ireland during the 1840s famine had given him a practical sympathy with tenants' rights, and his administration introduced a number of measures to protect the Indian peasant from exploitation. He was also sympathetic to Florence's concerns for wider sanitary reform in India. Much had been done for the big cities, but the villages were still a 'blot' on the sanitary record of the country. Dufferin admitted to being largely ignorant about sanitation, but told Florence that if she gave him instructions, 'the powder', he would 'fire the shot'. Similarly, in

1888, when Lord Lansdowne succeeded Dufferin, he sought Florence's advice before leaving to be installed as Viceroy. Lansdowne, Lord Salisbury's protégé, was one of Jowett's pupils. He would never be 'a great Liberal', Jowett admitted, but he might make an eminent statesman. 'Could you write me down, in simple words only,' Jowett asked Florence, 'the principal questions which a Governor-General should consider & perhaps the titles of some books which he should read e.g. irrigation, Instruction in Agriculture.'

However, the focus of Florence's work for India, following Ripon's departure, would start to shift once more. She kept open her official channels to the Viceroys and Secretaries of State, especially in maintaining the pressure on them to introduce sanitary improvements. She continued to publish articles and letters, highlighting issues she considered important for India. But, in the final phase of her involvement in Indian affairs, she would also make renewed attempts to establish contact with ordinary Indians, to involve them in rural sanitation, and to educate Indian women, particularly, about the importance for their families' health of a clean water supply, good drainage, and the avoidance of overcrowding.

This shift was partly a consequence of Florence's frustration, and loss of patience, at the pace of reform that could be achieved by her conventional methods of lobbying and influence, partly a recognition of the fact that the massive scale of the task of keeping the population of India in good health was beyond the capacity of any government, even one possessing the will to take action. Ripon's term of office had taught her how difficult it was for a progressive Viceroy to work against the reactionary forces of the status quo. The appointment, in 1885, of Lord Randolph Churchill – contemptuously referred to by Florence as 'the "Boy with the drum"' – as Secretary of State for India, in Salisbury's caretaker Government, was a reminder of the extent to which governmental change could be responsible for inflicting damaging setbacks. Once in office, Lord Randolph had sanctioned drastic economic cutbacks, which immediately threatened the future work of the Sanitary Commissioners out in India. It was now Ripon's turn to offer Florence consolation. 'There are waves,' he told her, 'the thing is come in upon waves. You would have done nothing for the Army Medical and Sanitary Service if it had not been for the crash in the Crimea.' Although, he continued, the wave was currently 'against interest in India', if there was another Russian scare, all eyes would be on India again. 'Then will be the time.'

Before his departure from India in 1888, Lord Dufferin did institute a system of Sanitary Boards, intended to supervise and control sanitary works in rural and urban areas. The scheme was sent to Florence for her approval, but she criticized it on the grounds that it depended for its success on the willingness of the local government to act. What she envisaged was the re-establishment of the village *panchayats* – local government bodies – and the granting of authority to the village heads-man to punish those who disobeyed the government's orders. She pointed to the town of Ahmedabad, part of the Bombay presidency, where local people, by using their own intiative, had successfully raised money to introduce a new water supply. The pressing requirement, in Florence's view, was to educate Indians in this kind of self-help.

The foundation of the Indian National Congress, in 1885, naturally won Florence's support. Conceived as a forum for political and civic dialogue between educated Indians and the British ruling class, the Congress initially acted like a safety-valve in the wake of all the disturb-ance and ill-feeling caused by the Ilbert Bill. As a national representative body, it marked a new era of unified political consciousness for rising Indian nationalists, supported by British Liberals with a background of working in India, like A. O. Hume and Sir William Wedderburn, two of its founders. Florence met and corresponded with both these men. 'We are watching the birth of a new nationality in the oldest civilization in the world,' she wrote to Wedderburn, as she waited on the Congress's critical first steps, concerned that the first session might lapse into per-sonal attacks between members (Muslims were outnumbered six to one by Hindus). At South Street, during the General Elections of 1885 and 1886, Florence received delegates from India who were in Britain addressing public meetings and lobbying candidates sympathetic to the cause of India. In the 1886 election, she sent a letter to be read out to the electors of Holborn in support of Dadabhai Naoroji, a founder of the Indian National Congress, fighting the seat under the Liberal banner. Naoroji was unsuccessful this time in Holborn – though Florence's letter was met with loud cheers – but, two years later, became MP for the constituency of Central Finsbury.

Florence had begun her work of exporting hygiene to India as a means of strengthening the British Army in its role as defender of the

British Empire. Now, three decades on, she lent her voice, without hesitation, to the beginnings of a movement to make India independent of British rule. 'India is not standing still,' she had written to Gladstone in 1884, in a letter intended to bolster the continuance of Ripon's reforms.

We have talked much about giving her 'Western civilization'. Western Civilization has given her, whether we will or no, western powers ... with western power must we not give them gradually western responsibilities? If we did not would they not take them?

For a brief time during his viceroyalty – no more in fact than a few days – the post of Ripon's private secretary had been filled by General Charles Gordon. Gordon's popular renown, based on the widespread cult of him as a Christian military hero, had originated in the 1860s with his victory over the Taiping rebellion in China. His later appointments included one as Governor-General of Equatoria, in the south of Egyptian-occupied Sudan, where he had succeeded in suppressing the slave trade. Intensely religious, with piercing grey-blue eyes, Gordon was famous for his ability to inspire confidence in his soldiers, and for spending his own money on their care and comfort. He was irreverent of authority, believing that his first duty was to the subjects of the Empire rather than to the imperial power itself, and deeply fatalistic, more than happy to place his destiny in the hands of God. He devoted his spare time to the charitable work of tending the sick in the workhouse infirmaries, and feeding, clothing and educating young street urchins, whom he took into his house at Gravesend. All these characteristics commended him to Florence. If she saw anything of the egotism and self-righteousness which so exercised other contemporaries, she never mentioned it. What continued to impress her most about Gordon was his 'disinterestedness'. In the spring of 1880, Gordon had written to Florence about the neglect of patients in military hospitals by orderlies. This situation had been brought to his attention by his cousin Amy Hawthorn, wife of a colonel in the Royal Engineers, who wanted Gordon's help in bringing the matter to the War Office's attention. 'I have had a letter ... about the bad nursing of the orderlies in military (station) hospitals . . .,' Florence told Sir Harry Verney. 'I can hardly read the signature, C. E. Gordon? . . . Is this the Colonel Gordon of the Sudan & Upper Nile – a truly great man?'

Florence duly approached the Secretary of State for War, Hugh Childers, who failed to be convinced by the evidence of the case. But out of this failure, a friendship between Florence and Gordon began to flourish. 'I gained the hearts of my soldiers (who would do anything for me),' he told her, in a description that was bound to go straight to Florence's own heart, 'not by my justice, etc., but by <u>looking after them when sick or wounded, and by continually visiting the hospitals</u>.' He called on her, sent her 'a little book of comfort' before leaving for India in May 1880, and saw her on his return to England, shortly before he set off again, this time to Syria, where, armed with a Bible, he would follow in the footsteps of Jesus, and convince himself that he had identified the 'Place of the Skull', where Christ had been crucified.

To Florence, Gordon was another footsoldier in the service of God, like those in a verse of her favourite hymn, 'The Son of God Goes Forth to War'. They both gained spiritual guidance from Thomas à Kempis's *Imitation of Christ*. And for Florence, perhaps, there was the vicarious thrill of Gordon's martyr-like certainty that he was destined to make the ultimate sacrifice for God. She expressed her impatience, though, at what she regarded as Gordon's waste of his manifest talents. 'My life truly to me is a straw . . .,' he wrote to her at one point while prevaricating over his future. She had hoped to persuade him to go back to India, but he explained that he could never 'accept the shibboleth of the Indian or colonial official classes. To me, they are utterly wrong in the government of the subject races. They know nothing of the hearts of those peoples and oil and water would as soon mix as the two races.' Instead, at the beginning of 1884, Gordon accepted a mission from the King of Belgium to eradicate the slave trade in his Congo territory. He had no sooner arrived in Brussels when he received the call to return to the Sudan to save the beleaguered garrison at Khartoum from the forces of the Mahdi. In early February 1885, as rumours reached London by telegraph that Gordon had been speared to death by Dervishes, Florence wrote to Mrs Hawthorn of her conviction that Gordon's 'was literally a Christlike life'. For many years, Florence marked the day of Gordon's death. She actively commemorated his life and example by advising the committee of a boys' home at Woking, in Surrey, founded in Gordon's name. In a public letter to raise funds for this home, she wrote that Gordon's battlefield in time of peace 'was the hospital, the workhouse, the slums . . . the ragged schools'; in time of war, he was a

Paladin, in the best chivalric tradition, and his fighting 'was sympathy and benevolence in action'.

The Gordon relief campaign under Lord Wolseley, which, to the fury of the British public, arrived at Khartoum too late to save their hero, was the impetus behind another official request for female nurses to be sent out to Egypt. Some nurses, having proved themselves effective during earlier fighting in 1882, remained out there, and to their number was now added a new team of recruits. In conjunction with the Princess of Wales's branch of the National Aid Society, whose committee comprised, among others, Lady Rosebery, Lady Salisbury and Mrs Gladstone, Florence worked to select nurses and superintendents to lead them. Rachel Williams, who had recently resigned as Matron of St Mary's, Paddington, was chosen to take seven nurses to Suez. Florence had had initial reservations about 'Goddess's' suitability for the post, largely on account of Williams's stormy temperament and the possible effects of the climate on her health, but used her influence, nevertheless, with the Director-General of the Army Medical Services, Sir Thomas Crawford, to secure her a good posting. Several St Thomas's nurses went with Rachel Williams, among them Maria Machin and Elizabeth Dowse, the former Miss Torrance, recently widowed and received back into the fold.

Florence's excitement at their departure was palpable. She had the Williams party to breakfast on the morning of their voyage, and inspected their uniforms. She presented them with copies of a popular life of Gordon and, with a twinkle in her eye, gave an india-rubber travelling bath to one former probationer, Sister Hicks, who had once reminded her that cleanliness was next to godliness. In their cabins on board the *Navarino*, the nurses found a bouquet of flowers for each of them, with a message wishing them 'God-speed from Florence Nightingale'. Florence followed the campaign closely in *The Times*, and wrote to Rachel Williams by every mail. 'We are still, of course, without direct tiding of you which we yearn for,' she wrote to Williams at the end of March 1885. 'The terrible hand to hand fighting which is now going on every day at Souakim but which, one trusts, will be over before this reaches you, makes us suppose that there will soon be wounded under your careful & devoted hands.' In July Florence was still writing regularly, assuring Rachel Williams that her example, and that of the other nurses, would be enough to prevent the orderlies – 'not hopeless but untrained' – from neglecting patients. Later that month, Florence told Williams that she had seen a painting of General Gordon called 'The Last Watch', depicting him watching from the ramparts at Khartoum. In it she discerned a 'far-off look in his eyes of solemn happiness' at his imminent reunion with God.

Rachel Williams was home by the end of the year, and engaged to a doctor, Daniel Norris, whom she married in December 1885. Her great friend Angélique Pringle, a guest at the wedding, reported the radiance of the bride, though nothing could allay Florence's disappointment at the loss to marriage of another trained superintendent. Meanwhile, it was the end of an era at the Nightingale School at St Thomas's. In 1886, Mrs Wardroper, who was over seventy, announced her decision to retire as Superintendent and Matron of the Hospital. She was presented with a silver salver – though some former probationers refused to allow the inscription to describe them as pupils, on the grounds that Wardroper had never taught them anything – and a pension from the Fund of £100 a year. A booklet by Henry Bonham Carter was published, lauding the School's achievements. Early failures were tactfully omitted, and St Thomas's was portrayed as the mother house of Nightingale nurses scattered across the globe, and of whole training schools grown up under its inspiration. Angélique Pringle, Florence's favourite, who had made such a brilliant success of her time at the Edinburgh Infirmary, was Mrs Wardroper's obvious successor. She took some persuading, but was finally welcomed to St Thomas's in the autumn of 1887. It did not take long, however, for a crisis to emerge. In the latter half of 1888, Pringle revealed, to Florence's horror, that she was inching towards conversion to Rome. Florence was alarmed by Pringle's obvious mental exhaustion, but moved quickly to counsel against such a momentous step. 'Do you think a growing inclination for the Church of Rome a sign of madness?' Angélique Pringle asked, in response to a letter in which Florence had described her as being 'in a far more dangerous state than if you were ill'. She felt an 'unspeakable fear' about paining Florence, but after months of self-questioning finally reached the decision to con-vert. She resigned as Matron, and was received into the Roman Catholic Church in August 1889. Florence did her best to conceal her personal hurt, but it comes across all too evidently in a letter to Sir Harry, beneath the force of her protestations. Pringle, she wrote, 'thinks that the "personal bereavement" to me of herself is what influences me, as if I <u>could</u> have the unutterable baseness (in what I feel – I hope I exaggerate – shakes our work almost to the foundations) of thinking of <u>my</u> loss!!' Louise Gordon, a Nightingale nurse from Leeds, took Pringle's place. Despite Florence's bitter disappointment, she did not cast off Angélique Pringle, and they remained close for the rest of Florence's life.

Her object, Florence had told Jowett as Pringle's final decision hung in the balance, had been to infuse 'mystic religion' into nursing, making women 'handmaidens of the Lord'. Clearly, though, as the Pringle case showed, 'some visible organisation' was still necessary. 'The best & ablest woman I know is going to join the Church of Rome for no other reason.'

But nurses and their aspirations were changing. Throughout the 1880s, the numbers involved in nursing had grown massively, as the idea of women seeking work had itself become steadily more acceptable. Training schools had even started to turn away applicants, though the high drop-out rate remained. Nursing was at last regarded as a respectable occupation for women. Florence did not necessarily view all the implications of these changes favourably. She disliked the sentimental glamour – 'all that ministering angel nonsense' as she had once called it – so often attached by press and public to those who cared for the sick, particularly as it created misleading expectations among uninitiated probationers. And she feared the consequences for the future of nursing as it became ever more fashionable and its roots in the idea of 'the life of a calling' decreased. 'We have fallen . . . I will not say upon evil times,' Florence told Frances Spencer, Angélique Pringle's successor as Matron at Edinburgh, 'but upon <u>modern</u> times.'

For their part, the generation of nurses emerging in the second half of the 1880s and early 1890s were uncomfortable with the older definition of nursing, espoused by Florence and other earlier reformers, as a religious vocation. In line with the position taken by school teachers – the most important occupation for single women at the end of the nineteenth century – many former lady pupils inclined towards a new professional status for nurses. In 1887, Ethel Bedford Fenwick, a former Matron of St Bartholomew's Hospital, and the leader of a campaign to lobby for the state registration of nurses, was one of the founders of the British Nurses' Association at a meeting of matrons at her house in

Wimpole Street. The central plank of the BNA's programme was the introduction of a register to establish a distinction between trained and untrained nurses. Florence vehemently opposed the proposals as likely to do great damage to the cause of nursing. The battle lines were drawn for the next seven years.

In practical terms, there appeared to be good reason for the introduction of a register of nurses. There were by now a large number of hospitals throughout Britain offering training for nurses, but the quality of that training varied widely. A central body, with properly accredited powers, would be able to decide which hospitals were giving adequate training, and which were not. However, Mrs Bedford Fenwick and her cohorts had another major goal in mind. They wanted to exclude working-class nurses, and make nursing a profession for ladies only. Under their plan, nurses in training would be paid no salary, and would be charged the sum of five guineas to be examined in writing, certificated and, finally, registered. In this way they hoped to deter those they viewed as undesirable from entering the profession while, at the same time, encouraging middle-class entrants, with a liberal education 'and a refined home training'. Enhanced social status was a clear aim of those lobbying for registration. They hoped to achieve parity with the medical profession; and misguidedly – because they didn't fully understand the implications of the legislation – planned to use the Medical Act of 1858 as their model (Bedford Fenwick had recently married a doctor who participated actively in his wife's campaigns).

Florence objected to the use of a written examination to test a nurse's suitability for admission to the register. An exam tested memory, but not the moral and personal character of the nurse on which Florence had always laid such emphasis, nor indeed the application of that knowledge to patients on the wards. 'The idea of the new-fangled people,' she said, 'seems to be to put nurses on the level of dictionaries – a dictionary can answer questions.' Moreover, she recognized the use of written exams as a ploy to catch out working-class applicants who were insufficiently literate to score highly in them. Yet without the recruitment of probationer nurses from ordinary backgrounds, nursing as a profession would grind to a halt. There were simply not enough ladies to take their place. At a later stage in the debate, Sydney Holland of the London Hospital would forcefully back up this argument by pointing out that 'We have exhausted the numbers of Florence Nightingales in the world . . .'

The BNA's cosy relationship with the medical profession, the way in which it placed nurses' training under doctors, and did little to differentiate nursing from medicine, threatened Florence's half a lifetime of work to establish nursing as an occupation independent of men, run by women from top to bottom. Bedford Fenwick might publicly announce that doctors would not be permitted to exploit nurses or exert unwarranted control over them, but in practice the power of the medical profession within the BNA would enable doctors to exercise undue influence over the curriculum of the registered nurse, especially when it came to ensuring that the knowledge a nurse gained in training could not possibly threaten medical supremacy.

Florence did not rule out some system of registration for nurses in the future, based on certifying them individually on an apprenticeship model rather than by examination. But she argued that, for the time being, nurses were not well enough educated to take part in any registration scheme (the benefits of compulsory, free, elementary education in Britain would only begin to be felt in the early years of the twentieth century). Nursing needed to continue its 'quiet progress' without interference from outside regulators.

She regarded Bedford Fenwick, a flamboyant character with a penchant for expensive clothes, with deep suspicion, believing her to be unscrupulous in her methods, especially when it came to claiming greater levels of support than the BNA in fact possessed. As the standard bearer of reformed nursing, Florence's views still commanded great authority, particularly among hospital matrons who had originally trained at St Thomas's. They flocked to the anti-registrationist side, bringing their nurses with them. However, Mrs Bedford Fenwick, who had never been a Nightingale trainee, owed Florence no such allegiance. A number of other factors influenced nurses as they took sides in the argument about registration. Some matrons at provincial hospitals saw registration as a way of achieving parity with the smart London hospitals; some opposed it because they feared that their training would be found wanting, and they would be denied approval as a training school; still others were set against because it challenged the matron's authority to control the training of her own probationers.

It was to be the last great battle of Florence's life, but experience had taught her to tread cautiously. Above all she was concerned not to split nursing irreversibly into two camps divided against one another. Royal patronage of the BNA also restrained her from publicizing her opposition too forcefully after Princess Christian, Queen Victoria's third daughter, accepted the Presidency of the Association ('they are trying to make a Nurses' Republic with a Princess at its head,' Florence noted). In 1888, Florence published a pamphlet she had written, *Is a General Register for Nurses Desirable?*, under Henry Bonham Carter's name. Its true authorship, or at least the real spur behind its argument, must have been obvious to informed commentators like the editor of *Nursing Record*, the journal of the BNA, who criticized the author of the pamphlet for not caring whether a nurse dropped her h's, and whether she was bred in the scullery or the drawing room. As the debate grew more heated, even Florence would not be free from personal attack in the medical press. 'She has long looked upon the active world from the distance which the sick room imposes between the sufferer and those who toil,' was the remark in one *Lancet* editorial.

The row over state registration worried and absorbed her. Jowett thought that it was 'a comparative trifle, among all the work which you have done', and begged her not to be over-anxious. But Florence saw it as a crisis, of the kind that afflicted all social movements at a defining point in their development. She mustered all the support and influence she could, first opposing the BNA's application to be registered a public company, and then assisting William Rathbone with the preparation of his evidence against registration for his appearance before a House of Lords committee investigating the condition of hospitals. The committee's report did not recommend the formation of a register. Matters reached a climax in 1892, when, having obtained permission from the Queen to use the title 'Royal', the BNA further petitioned the Queen for a Royal Charter, and pledged a register for nurses with three years' hospital training. Florence and the anti-registrationists moved into action. Thousands of matrons, nurses and doctors signed a letter of protest, headed by Florence's signature. A hearing before a committee of the Privy Council took place in November 1892, and the verdict was announced the following May. A Royal Charter was granted to the association, but the right to maintain a register was withheld. There was nothing in the charter which gave any nurse the right to call herself 'chartered' or 'registered', merely the permission for trained nurses to have their names included on a list, if they so chose. Both sides claimed to have won, but in reality it was a tactical victory for Florence and the antis.

The nursing profession would not finally achieve state registration until 1919, almost a decade after Florence's death. But, as she had foreseen, registration would bring nursing neither the freedom to control its own destiny, nor protection from the risk of interference by the medical profession.

In February 1887, Florence had marked the fiftieth anniversary of her call to service. Later that same year, Queen Victoria celebrated the Golden Jubilee of her accession to the throne in 1837, and in deciding on how to spend the £70,000 donated by the women of England as a Jubilee gift, Victoria gave a significant fillip to a cause close to Florence's heart: district nursing. The money was allotted to a national scheme, the Queen Victoria Jubilee Institute for the nursing of the sick poor in their own homes by trained nurses. The Queen took pride in referring to 'my nurses', and in the design of a distinctive uniform with a badge, of which Florence did not approve.

Florence had resolved, more than two decades earlier, 'to give herself to District Nursing' after working closely with William Rathbone on the establishment of an experimental programme in Liverpool. By 1867, Liverpool had been divided into eighteen districts, each with its own nurses. In 1875, the movement had taken a significant step forward with the foundation of a District Nursing Association in London. The Metropolitan Nursing Association, established after a detailed survey carried out under Florence's supervision reported on the existing provision and requirements for district care in the city, was headed by Florence Lees, a Nightingale nurse who had seen distinguished service in the Franco-Prussian War. After completing the standard year's training as Lady Probationers at St Thomas's – for a district nurse had always to be 'of a yet higher class' than the hospital nurse – the MNA trainees worked an eight-hour day: six hours in their district with the two other hours filled with lectures or reading. District nursing was considered more demanding than its hospital counterpart, with added responsibilities. A district nurse, in the absence of a doctor, had often to work on her own initiative. She had to take all the case notes for him, and be 'his staff of clinical clerks, dressers, and nurses' all rolled into one.

In district nursing, and the associated idea of health missionaries that she was to develop at the beginning of the 1890s, lay many of Florence's hopes for the future of health care. In 1867 she had described the nursing of the sick poor at home as the ultimate destination of all nursing. Hospitals, she recognized, had taken great strides forward in the course of her lifetime. But although they were no longer seen as simply a 'box to hold patients in', hospitals were still not the best place for the sick poor, except for severe surgical cases, and a constant watch had to be kept to ensure that patients suffered no harm from the sanitary arrangements of the building. There could be no excuse for complacency. Even St Thomas's, with its pavilions of air, had been revealed, in a report of 1878, to be far from hygienic. 'It is now a well-known rule,' Florence had written in a note to herself: 'keep no patient in hospital a day longer than is absolutely necessary ... And even this may be days too long. The patient may have to recover not only from illness or injury but from hospital.'

In the last phase of her working life, Florence would redouble her efforts to bring her philosophy of preventative care into ordinary people's homes. Hospitals belonged to a stage of imperfect, 'or rather of non-civilization'; they would undoubtedly disappear, she said, as society became more Christian. Florence looked forward to the eventual abolition of all hospital and workhouse infirmaries. But, she added, 'it is no use to talk about the year 2,000'.

20. Lustre on the Name

Parthenope died at Claydon on 12 May 1890, Florence's seventieth birthday. The sisters had met for the last time a week earlier in London, when Parthenope had been carried into the drawing room at 10 South Street in a state of great suffering. 'You contributed more than anyone to what enjoyment of life was hers,' Sir Harry wrote to Florence on 15 May. '. . . You and I were the objects of her tender love and her love for you was intense. It was delightful to me to hear her speak of you and to see her face, perhaps distorted with pain, look happy when she thought of you.' In August, Florence went to stay at Claydon, remaining there until early in the New Year. Sir Harry was nearly ninety, failing in health and memory. She encouraged him to overcome his despondency, took over the running of the household, and helped with the management of the estate. 'Claydon is sad & strange,' she wrote, ' – all the same yet all changed.' Parthenope's great pride, her history of the Verney family during the English Civil War, was being seen through the press by Margaret Verney, who would follow Parthenope's two volumes with two of her own, taking the story down to the end of the seventeenth century. With a preface by the Civil War historian Samuel Gardiner, who had encouraged Parthenope's work, the *Memoirs of the Verney Family* was published in 1892. Parthenope's wish that the book should appear in Sir Harry's lifetime had been fulfilled. A short biographical sketch by Margaret Verney, which opened the first volume, stated that Parthenope would 'be chiefly remembered hereafter as the sister of Florence Nightingale'.

Florence's immediate family was now all gone. The previous decade had also delivered a dying blow to some of her most important friendships, forged long ago in the past. From Paris, in May 1883, came news of the death of Clarkey, still spirited and witty at ninety, though sadly bereft without her beloved husband Julius Mohl. Just over two years later, Richard Monckton Milnes, Lord Houghton, died, also in France where he was on holiday. For Florence his passing brought with it many bittersweet memories of his courtship of her, together with thoughts of how very different her life would have been had she married him. The death of Aunt Mai, in January 1889, disturbed her perhaps more. Aunt Mai, a 'humble mind of high & holy thought' as Florence called her in a personal note of farewell, had sacrificed much to nurture her niece's talents and enable them to flourish. Yet, for both women, their intense relationship had fostered an unhealthy dependence during Florence's early years of illness, resulting in a brief but bitter period of estrangement. In Mai's old age, Florence tried to make amends by assuring her aunt of her appreciation of that sacrifice. 'Let me say, my dearest Aunt Mai . . . how much I am always with you . . . in spirit,' she had written in the autumn of 1888. 'On 12 August I was with you all the day remembering how thirty-five years ago you brought me up to Harley St. On 7 August how you brought me back to Lea Hurst thirty-two years ago.'

The disappearance of Florence's friends and colleagues during the following decade appeared to confirm her in the status of survivor. For so long she and those closest to her had lived in expectation of her impending demise, but, although she still sometimes spoke of herself as at death's door, she was starting to outlive them all. Dr Sutherland, who had collaborated more closely with her than anyone else, died in July 1891. He had retired three years earlier, leaving Florence to put pressure on the War Office to ensure that he was replaced on the Army Sanitary Committee by someone with similar expertise. To the end, Sutherland had lost none of his capacity to irritate her. A request that he provide her with background material for Lord Ripon on Indian sanitary matters had been met with Sutherland's response that the Viceroy would have to wait, as he was too busy peering at a cholera bacillus through the lens of a new microscope he had bought himself from Vienna. It was some-how typical of Sutherland's ability to cause her consternation that, in 1888, she was told that he had died when in fact he hadn't. Florence was horrified to think that she could have been unaware of his passing. When Sutherland did actually die, she was eager to pay public tribute to him in the master–pupil terms she had once applied to her relationship with Sidney Herbert, though in Sutherland's case there could be no doubt of the enormous influence he had had in shaping Florence's work. '. . . I was his pupil both in sanitary administration and practice,' she told the editor of The Times, G. E. Buckle, '& am anxious for my master's fame.' Sutherland's own final words to his wife reportedly included a wish that she give Florence his love and blessing. It was the conclusion of a remarkable thirty-year partnership.

In October 1893 Florence received a further serious blow with the death of Benjamin Jowett. His first serious attack of illness, a form of pulmonary disease, had occurred in 1887, and in the autumn of that year he had been taken ill while visiting Florence at South Street. In October 1891, Jowett suffered a heart attack, and for several days hovered on the brink of death. Regaining full consciousness, he dictated to his secretary a letter to Florence, rejecting her offer to visit him at Oxford, which might be 'too much for both of us & not really wise'. As he recovered strength, he received a letter from her, gently berating him for having been careless with his health. '. . . You live on your head for years. You entirely ignore the effect on the nerves & the effect of the strained nervous system on the action of the heart and on sleep . . . Nature sends in her bill. And that bill always has to be paid . . .' In November, Florence paid her projected visit to Balliol. She took the short train ride to Oxford from Claydon, where she was staying, and was met at the station by the carriage belonging to Sir Henry Acland, the Regius Professor of Medicine. Unused to sitting down to a meal with more than one person, she refused lunch, and spent little more than an hour with Jowett in the Master's lodgings.

'You are never out of my mind for long,' Jowett wrote to her the following May. '. . . I want to hold fast to you, dear friend, as I go down the hill. You and I are agreed that the last years of life are in a sense the best and that the most may be made of them even at the time when health & strength seem to be failing.' Jowett's final message to Florence was sent less than a fortnight before his death, on 1 October 1893. He had called on her in London only to find that she had gone to Claydon. He had just time for a few words, he said. 'How greatly am I indebted to you for all your affection. How large a part has your life been of my life.' She, too, remembered the 'genius' of his friendship.

From the mid-1870s, Florence and Jowett had discussed the foundation at Oxford University of a Chair in Statistics. A few years before his death, Jowett returned to the idea, proposing that they each contribute £2,000 for the endowment of a professorship. This, according to Florence, would educate future politicians and civil servants in the uses of statistics. A number of University figures had been approached for their views, including Alfred Marshall, the Balliol economist, and Francis Galton, whose analysis of data had made an important contribution to the science of human genetics. Galton had gone so far as to draw up a list of matters to which a future Professor of Statistics might address himself, including public health, the effect of punishment upon crime, and the interpretation of statistics relating to India. But in the end the Oxford authorities were reluctant to establish a Chair in a subject for which there was no Final Honour School, and Florence revoked the £2,000 bequest she had made to the University in her will because she feared that the money would be used to sponsor a statistical essay prize rather than to teach statistics. Florence and Jowett's joint proposal for a Chair in Statistics has been appropriately – and teasingly – described by the editors of Jowett's letters as 'a substitute for the lack of offspring of a marriage that never took place'.

Sir Harry Verney died four months after Jowett, in February 1894. Aged ninety-two, he had been out riding just a week before his death ('Remember, you have promised not to ride out in the cold,' Florence had cautioned him the last time this habit of his had been brought to her attention. '. . . Don't remember to forget.') She felt the loss of 'his courage, his courtesy, his kindness'. In August, Florence mourned the death, 'good & simple like himself', of her beloved Shore. In twelve months she had lost 'the three nearest to me'.

She was slowly taking her farewell of the places that mattered to her most. Lea Hurst had been let for a decade in 1883, and Florence did not visit it again after her mother's death; but she returned to Embley in 1891, for the first time since her father's death and, for a final occasion, in the autumn of 1893. Three years later the house was sold. It was sad, she said, to have been turned out of Hampshire. She was at Claydon one more time after Sir Harry's death, for a four-month stay in the winter of 1894–5, as the guest of Edmund and Margaret Verney. Subsequently the trip was considered too tiring for her, and her visits ceased altogether. None the less, Florence remained at the heart of the Verney family, receiving Sir Harry's sons and their wives, and his grandchildren, at South Street and keeping in contact regularly by letter with Margaret and Maude. This closeness to the Verneys was viewed jealously by members of her own family, like Shore's younger son Louis, who claimed unfairly that the Verneys only cultivated Florence for her money.

The younger members of her extended family elicited Florence's sympathy, and she in turn devoted time to listening to their problems. Young Arthur Clough, the poet's son, confided a string of broken romances to her before he settled down and married a Miss Freshfield, daughter of the mountain explorer. She was concerned about the future of Shore's daughter Rosalind. On coming down from Girton, Rosalind had become a journalist, writing on suffrage and labour questions, as well as involving herself in the Women's Co-operative Guild. Her vegetarianism struck Florence as odd, but she did her best to comply with Rosalind's dietary requirements, on one occasion sending her a parcel of 'six "vegetables" ', and doing her 'humble best' to collect 'grasses' for her to eat when she came to dinner at South Street. In 1892 Rosalind married Robinson Vaughan Nash, another journalist interested in labour issues, later the *Manchester Guardian*'s correspondent in India. Mr Nash, according to Florence, had everything to recommend him 'except money'. It was a 'unique, singular marriage', she told Margaret Verney, 'with absolutely no <u>certain</u> provision'. The couple were going to live 'at the East Pole of London, separated from us by 5 millions of people, but not from the Easterns among whom they are going to labour'.

Florence had mellowed. If people were aggravating, she wrote in a note to herself, 'that is a call to us for patience & self-control & not to be aggravating in return'. From the vantage point of old age, she was even able to look back on the discontent of her life as a daughter at home before the Crimean War, and see it as tiresome rather than painful. In 1895, on her seventy-fifth birthday, she wrote that 'There is so much to live for. I have lost much in failures and disappointments, as well as in grief but . . . life is more precious to me now in my old age.'

While staying at Claydon in 1891, Florence had embarked on a new experiment relating to the problems of rural health. There had been scattered references in her letters since the 1870s of an idea for 'health missioners' or 'sanitary nurses', who might educate women in rural communities about measures to promote good health and the prevention of disease in the home. In some respects, this was a return to the themes that Florence had set out, thirty years earlier, in her edition of *Notes on Nursing* directed specifically at the labouring classes. County Councils, established in 1888, had been given the power to spend money on 'technical education'. Frederick Verney was the chairman of the Techni-

cal Education Committee of North Buckinghamshire, and with his help
and influence, the training of Lady Health Missioners was classified as
part of technical education, and money earmarked for a course of
lectures. Dr De'Ath, the medical officer of health for the county, undertook this training, which was practical as well as theoretical. Taking his
pupils to the villages in the vicinity of Claydon, he introduced them to
the local women, and pointed out improvements that might be made to
the sanitary conditions and home cleanliness of their cottages. On passing an independent examination, the ladies were given certificates as
Health Missioners and authorized to visit and lecture in the villages.
This scheme, starting in 1892, involved Florence in much work, in which
she was assisted by Fred, Margaret and Maude Verney. In 1894, Maude
delivered Florence's paper on 'Rural Hygiene' to the Conference of
Women Workers at Leeds. In a letter to Dr De'Ath, Florence explained
the basis of the idea. Just as the district nurse visited the cottage 'to
nurse & to teach the Patient by the family with her own head & hands
– so would the Health Nurse (Missioner) teach what to do in the cottage
for health with her own head & hands'.

The Health Missioners project in the villages near Claydon paralleled
on a smaller scale the work that Florence had been doing for India since
the late 1880s. In letters to members of the Indian National Congress,
she continually put forward programmes for 'collective cleanliness
carried out collectively'. Villagers needed to be taught that disease was
preventable, and that it was 'not so much the want of money as the want
of knowledge that produces bad sanitary conditions'. Lectures in village
schools, using magic lantern shows, were one suggestion, the introduction of sanitary primers another. In collaboration with the Vicereine,
Lady Dufferin, Florence had involved herself in various schemes for the
promotion of female health care and education in India. The Dufferin
Fund, established in 1885, had revolutionized access to modern health
care for Indian women, introducing cottage hospitals, female wards in
larger hospitals, all under the administrative control of women doctors.
Most importantly, the Fund paid for the training of not only doctors,
but also nurses and midwives, two decades after Florence's recommendations for nurse training in India had first been sought by Sir John
Lawrence and then rejected.

Florence's vision of a public health system for the future, emphasizing
the supreme importance of collective action to safeguard the health of

others, is contained in one of her last major statements to the outside world. In early 1893, Angela Burdett-Coutts, among the wealthiest women in Britain and a distinguished philanthropist, persuaded Florence to write an article on 'Sick-Nursing and Health-Nursing', as part of the British contribution to the women's section at the Columbian Exposition World's Fair, taking place later that year in Chicago. The Columbian Exposition was organized to highlight the 400 years of human progress since Columbus's voyage of discovery in 1492, and for the first time in an international world fair, women's contribution to the benefit of humankind was being represented through exhibits, events and meetings. An official exhibition building, christened the 'Women's Hall', had been designed by an award-winning woman architect, Sophia Haydon, and a board of lady managers appointed to help plan the international participation of women at the exposition.

Florence was advised by Henry Bonham Carter that she should avoid allowing the issue of registration of nurses to play too prominent a part in her paper. However, not only Ethel Bedford Fenwick, but also her American ally, Isabel Hampton, nursing superintendent of the Johns Hopkins Hospital in Baltimore, was taking part in an International Nursing Congress that had been convened at the Columbian Exposition. Florence must therefore have realized the importance of stating her opposition to registration once more, this time to a world forum. This she duly did, arguing that the qualities of a good nurse could not be judged by examination, 'while the best nurse may come off worse'. What stands out as prescient among the ideas presented in the paper is Florence's assertion that the 'art of health-nursing' – the cultivation of good health – is as important as the 'art of sick-nursing'. Her stress on prevention rather than cure – on nursing as a proactive as well as a reactive occupation – together with her recognition of the healing properties of nature itself, has a remarkably modern ring to it.

. . . A new art and a new science has been created and within the last forty years. And with it a new profession – so they say, we say, calling . . . the art of nursing the sick. Please mark – nursing the sick; NOT nursing sickness . . . What is health nursing? . . . the cultivation of health . . . What is Sickness . . . Nature's way of getting rid of the effects of conditions which have interfered with health. It is nature's attempt to cure. We have to help her . . . What is health? Health is not only to be well, but to use well every power we have ... What is nursing? Both kinds of nursing are to put us in the best possible conditions for Nature to restore or preserve health ...

The legend kept Florence's fame alive. In her seventies, fan letters continued to arrive for her from around the world. At Sir Harry's persuasion, in 1891, she had allowed Mr Payne of Aylesbury to take her photograph at Claydon, but had immediately regretted the decision as the result had been 'a plague' of unwelcome requests, 'to have my photograph & an interview with me, & a history of my life from myself, including the dolls I played with!!' There was a buoyant industry in popular biographies of her. These books concentrated on Florence's early years, emphasizing the sacrifice of her privileged life – while conveniently overlooking the fact that such an existence had possessed no attraction for her – and relating the by now familiar tales of the young Florence nursing her sick dolls, and tending to the injured sheepdog, Cap. Such stories sometimes developed a life of their own, most bizarrely in the case of Mentona Moser, daughter of Freud's first patient, Fanny Moser, and later a member of the Swiss Communist Party. In 1903, Mentona reacted against the stifling luxury of her own background by publishing a pamphlet entitled *The Upbringing of Women of the Upper Classes: Considerations and Recommendations*, in which she used Florence as a model, urging young girls to seize control of their lives, and to educate themselves about the social world and the nature of poverty.

Florence had no patience with her legend, or with anyone seeking to promote it. But she could always be relied on to spare a kind word for old soldiers, especially Crimean veterans, who sought her out. In 1887, she was evidently moved by a letter from a soldier called Samuel Atkins, who had been wounded at the Battle of Inkerman, as she took special pains to preserve it. Atkins had been sent to the Barrack Hospital at Scutari with wounds in the right arm and ribs.

After being under the doctor's treatment for a time [Atkins told Florence] he said that the next day he must cut my arm off, and I told you ... and you told me I had not better have it off as there was no danger and that they could not take it off without my permission and that my arm would look better in my sleeve than the sleeve would look in my waistcoat pocket.

Atkins had insisted on keeping his arm, and wanted to thank her 'from the bottom of my heart for all your kindness to me and all other suffering ones . . . in the Hospital'.

In the summer of 1890, Florence agreed to deliver a message in support of the veterans of the Charge of the Light Brigade through the medium of Thomas Edison's phonograph machine. A public scandal had erupted in May when it was revealed that many veterans of the Charge were destitute. The Secretary for War had told Parliament that he could not offer assistance, and in response the *St James's Gazette* had set up the Light Brigade Relief Fund. Florence's was one of three recordings made to support the fund (the others were a reading by Tennyson of his famous poem *The Charge of the Light Brigade*, and a recording of the trumpeter and veteran Martin Lanfried sounding the charge as heard at Balaclava). On 30 July, Edison's assistant Colonel George Gouraud arrived at South Street to make a forty-one-second recording of Florence as she delivered the words, 'When I am no longer even a memory, just a name, I hope my voice brings to history the great work of my life. God bless my dear old comrades of Balaclava and bring them safe to shore. Florence Nightingale.'

The recording gives an impression of a grand old actress before her final curtain, speaking in a voice that Florence had herself once described as 'little' and 'silvery'. The original wax cylinder, recently restored by digital technology, features two recordings by Florence of the same speech. On her first attempt she stumbles on her words, and there is a long pause between the sentences. The second reading, first produced commercially in 1935 on a 78 rpm record, was heard by the writer and politician Harold Nicolson at the beginning of the Second World War. 'She says the last words,' he wrote, 'as if she was signing her signature on a cheque. "Florence" (pause) "Nightingale" (defiantly).'

Among the events organized to celebrate Queen Victoria's Diamond Jubilee in 1897 was an exhibition of the Victorian Era, held at Earls Court, the idea of an entrepreneurial showman called Imre Kiralfy. The section on trained nursing centred on Florence Nightingale, and Lady Wantage, an acquaintance of Florence's and a pioneer of the British Red Cross, was delegated to obtain Florence's portrait and some relics of the Crimean War from Florence herself. The initial approach was refused with a splutter of invective. 'Oh the absurdity of the people and the vulgarity!' Florence wrote.

The 'relics', the 'representations' of the Crimean War! What are they? They are, first, The tremendous lessons we have had to learn from its tremendous blunders and ignorances. And next they are Trained Nurses and the progress of Hygiene. These are the 'representations' of the Crimean War. And I will not give my foolish Portrait (which I have not got) or anything else as 'relics' of the Crimea. It is too ridiculous. You don't judge even of the victuals inside a public-house by the sign outside. I won't be made a <u>sign</u> at an Exhibition.

In a letter to Edmund Verney, she developed her idea further. The real 'relics' of the Crimean War were the Royal Commission on the Health of the Army, which had provided for 'great improvements in the soldier's daily life'; the training of nurses 'both in character & technical skill & knowledge'; and hygiene and sanitation, 'the want of which in the military & medical authorities caused Lord Raglan's death & that of thousands of our men from disease'.

But in the end, Florence relented. She had 'such a respect' for Lady Wantage that it was impossible to refuse her. Moreover, she took her point that the Royal Commission's Report was perhaps a little dry for the purposes of an exhibition. Florence lent the marble bust by Steell, while her Crimean carriage was located, 'all to pieces', in an Embley farmhouse, where it had lain since the sale of the Nightingales' home. '. . . That wretched Russian car . . . ,' Florence remarked to Henry Bonham Carter, '<u>hangs</u> round my <u>neck</u>.' She did, however, score one significant victory over the organizers of the exhibition. Her 'relics' were displayed, not in the historical section, but in a contemporary setting, among the latest nursing equipment, as if to emphasize that the significance of her life's work lay not with the past, but as a part of the ongoing progress of health care for the present and in the future.

Slowly her faculties began to fail, and after 1896 Florence seldom left her bedroom at South Street. She had first reported problems with her eyesight in 1887, and by the opening years of the new century could read and write only with the greatest difficulty. She had to accustom herself to being read to, an activity she had once despised so much. Her firm, clear handwriting deteriorated, and for longer pieces of writing in the 1890s she was forced to rely on the services of a band of lady 'typewriters'. In September 1895, she started to complain, like her mother before her, of 'a want of memory'. At first, she was forgetful of dates and names, but gradually a mist of uncertainty surrounded her.

While she was still able, Florence worked on. 'I have my hands full, & am not idle,' she assured Henry Bonham Carter in 1895, 'though naturally people think that I have gone to sleep or am dead.' Indeed, her death was reported in the press on more than one occasion. She continued to correspond with nurses and matrons – though her opinion of the later batches of probationers at St Thomas's was that they were 'Louder & nastier' – and in 1896 was involved in an experiment by Lord and Lady Monteagle to introduce trained nurses into Irish workhouses. A stream of visitors, family members and nurses, still called at South Street. After 1898 these visits were curtailed to a few close relatives, and old favourites like Angélique Pringle. A companion, Alice Cochrane, was engaged in 1902; and when she left to get married two years later, Elizabeth Bosanquet took her place. A nurse was also eventually hired. Florence did not make an easy patient. '. . . When the nurse had tucked her up for the night, she would often reverse the parts, get out of bed and go into the adjoining room to tuck up the nurse.'

Florence's eightieth birthday in May 1900 was marked by congratulatory messages from the United States and Japan, as well as from Europe. The South African War, with its echoes of the Crimean conflict almost fifty years earlier – the overcrowded hospitals and neglected British soldiers, the public outcry demanding female nurses – revived Florence's place in the national memory. One celebratory article spoke of the 'sunlit summit' of Florence's old age, 'reverenced, admired and beloved by the whole world'. There was 'a lustre on the name . . . which no lapse of time can dim'. The Nightingale name itself would not long outlive Florence. Shore's sons, Samuel and Louis, had chosen to become Shore Nightingales, but both were unmarried and childless. With Louis's death in 1944, the name of Nightingale would die out.

Queen Victoria's death, in January 1901, was observed with full mourning by the household at 10 South Street. Florence told Henry Bonham Carter's wife, Sibella, that she had wanted to do something 'to show that one cares . . .' Later that year, Queen Alexandra, the new King's consort, sent Florence birthday greetings. In 1904, Edward VII conferred the title of a Lady of Grace of the Order of St John of Jerusalem on Florence. But the King initially resisted the proposal, recommended by the Prime Minister, Sir Henry Campbell-Bannerman, that Florence be awarded the Order of Merit, the monarch's personal reward created by Edward soon after his accession. 'He has always been opposed to women being given the order,' the King's private secretary, Lord Knollys, wrote to Campbell-Bannerman in June 1907. Five months later, however, following further representations on Florence's behalf, Edward changed his mind.* Colonel Sir Douglas Dawson was selected to deliver the insignia of the Order of Merit to South Street. Since Florence was not well enough to see Dawson, the reward was received for her by Louis Shore Nightingale. After the brief ceremony on 5 December, Dawson wrote to Miss Bosanquet. He considered it an honour to have been chosen by the King for the duty, 'the more so as my father was killed in the Crimea, at the battle of Inkerman'. Two months later, Florence was the recipient of another award. At a ceremony at the Guildhall in London, she was given the Freedom of the City of London, received again on Florence's behalf by her cousin Louis. 'I do not think that Miss Nightingale took in the nature of the Ceremony,' Henry Bonham Carter wrote later. 'She remarked that she was not worthy of the honour or something to that effect.'

By the autumn of 1909, Florence was no longer able 'to give her attention to anything without great effort . . .' There was 'no real suffering', reported Miss Bosanquet, 'but a gradual failure of all the powers', and she was no longer equal to receiving visitors 'beyond the 2 or 3 relatives who come habitually'. When Florence received a photograph, kindly sent by Edmund Verney, of the cypresses at Claydon, grown from cones which she had brought back with her from Scutari, there appeared for an instant to be a flicker of recognition. She died in her sleep, at about two o'clock in the afternoon, on 13 August 1910. Death, she had confidently predicted in her final years, would not bring rest to the weary. Instead, it would undoubtedly be an opportunity for yet more 'immense activity'.

* It is more than likely that Vaughan Nash, Rosalind's husband, was one of the supporters, perhaps even the proponent, of the idea. Following a career in journalism, Nash was brought into Ten Downing Street by Campbell-Bannerman, in 1905, as an assistant private secretary. In 1908 Nash was promoted to principal private secretary by Campbell-Bannerman's successor, H. H. Asquith.

Part Five
Icon

21. A Hard Nut to Crack

Anyone passing London's Waterloo Place, off Pall Mall, early on the morning of 24 February 1915 would have been witness to a ghostly spectacle. At precisely seven thirty, three workmen from the Office of Works arrived on the site with a hand-cart and several ladders, and, in a scene completely devoid of ceremony, unveiled a statue of Florence Nightingale, shaking the snow from the canvas covering as they did so. The three men then departed as quietly and unobtrusively as they had come.

The decision to forgo a formal unveiling of this public statue – the first in London of a woman other than royalty – could almost be construed as an acknowledgement of Florence Nightingale's own desire for anonymity. But in fact, in the wake of the battles of Mons, Marne and Ypres, Asquith's Government had deemed 'any grand ceremony' in wartime as inappropriate. The idea that Waterloo Place should be renamed Crimea Place was also rejected: it might wound the 'susceptibilities' of the British Government's Russian allies (though, as one civil servant pointed out, it might equally be viewed as a compliment to their other allies, the French, by 'submerging' the name of Waterloo). At the eleventh hour, the very survival of the new statue had been threatened when it was discovered that a gas main beneath the site was threatening to blow.

Plans to commemorate Florence Nightingale with a statue were first mooted by the organizers of a Memorial Fund set up in her name in the months immediately following her death, and given public sanction at an open meeting at the Mansion House in March 1911. Various locations were proposed, including one in front of the National Gallery, but final selection of a site was complicated by the need to give precedence to the ongoing plans for another national memorial in the vicinity, to the late King, Edward VII, whose death, in May 1910, had preceded Florence Nightingale's by three months. In the end, the area adjacent to

John Bell's Guards Memorial (known commonly as the Crimea Memorial) in Waterloo Place was chosen, and at the inspired suggestion of Sydney Holland (later Lord Knutsford), treasurer of the Nightingale Memorial Fund, it was decided to move Foley's statue of Sidney Herbert, which had once stood in the quadrangle by the old War Office in Pall Mall, to stand next to the one of Florence Nightingale. 'I believe Sidney Herbert wanted to marry her,' Holland wrote with cavalier disregard for biographical truth. 'Anyhow it is a pretty thought to put them side by side. He who had the bravery to send her out & stick by her when there & she who went.' To accommodate this coupling, it was necessary to move the Guards Memorial forty feet back from the entrance to Waterloo Place towards Regent Street. A triangle effect was the result, producing one of the capital's finest sculptural groupings, with the Nightingale statue to the west, the Herbert one to the east, and the larger memorial looming behind them.

The commission for the new statue was awarded, in May 1912, to A. G. Walker (later responsible for the statue of Emmeline Pankhurst in Victoria Tower Gardens). The finished work stands on a pedestal, ten feet ten inches high. The statue itself is nine feet high, and depicts Florence Nightingale as the Lady with the Lamp, walking at night through the wards of Scutari (a miniature version sits today in the White Drawing Room at Ten Downing Street). 'The face,' reported *The Times*, 'reflects Florence Nightingale's characteristic qualities of strength of will irradiated by an expression of great sweetness and sympathy.' Bronze panels at the foot of the statue show Nightingale at the hospital door as wounded soldiers arrive, meeting with senior officers, and advising a doctor standing before a row of beds occupied by the wounded, and in old age surrounded by her nurses. There was 'no excuse for too florid a treatment', the Office of Works had agreed. Nevertheless, the figure in the statue holds a Grecian oil lamp, not the folding Turkish lantern that Florence Nightingale would have used at Scutari. Not long after the unveiling, a Mr MacAlpine of Finchley wrote to the Office of Works to suggest that a light be placed in the lamp. His suggestion was politely declined.

Despite its unceremonious unveiling, the statue soon became a familiar landmark. The following year, on Florence Nightingale's birthday – 12 May – Arthur Benson, Master of Magdalene College, Cambridge, was walking to the Athenaeum when he noticed to his disgust that the

Nightingale statue, opposite his club, had been 'enclosed in a structure
of laurel, and a flat cake of yellow flowers put behind her head – meant
for a halo, but looking like an odd umbrageous hat'. The attempts of
the English to honour people, Benson continued, 'are very infantile . . .'
As London went mad with rejoicing during the Victory March in 1919,
one drunken soldier was observed up on the statue's pedestal, with his
arm round Florence Nightingale's waist. He was making a speech to the
crowd, which most people were ignoring, that 'the bloody war wouldn't
have been won without the help of women like good old Florence'.

———

Official biographers had proved something of a curse for Florence
towards the end of her life, so much so that she compared the experience
of dealing with them to one of Dante's Purgatories. In 1894, Evelyn
Abbott who, with Lewis Campbell, had been appointed to write Benjamin Jowett's biography, approached Florence to ask if he could read
some of Jowett's letters to her. In her response, Florence prevaricated.
She did not give Abbott her outright refusal, but made it clear that she
considered that it would be 'treacherous to show them even to you'.
Nevertheless, she decided to cooperate with Abbott, sending him packets
of selected letters with the proviso that nothing should be printed without her consent, and that her own name was not to appear in the finished
book, published in 1897. Much worse was the alarm she felt at Lord
Stanmore's projected biography of Sidney Herbert, commissioned by
Liz Herbert, with Gladstone's encouragement, at the beginning of the
1890s, but not published until 1906. Stanmore had the right background. His father had been Lord Aberdeen, Prime Minister at the
outbreak of the Crimean War, and Stanmore had himself known Herbert
well, though not on terms of personal friendship. What, however, distressed Florence about Stanmore's book was Liz Herbert's decision to
hand over all the letters Florence had written to Sidney Herbert, 'without
my KNOWLEDGE or consent'. She was further angered by Stanmore's
subsequent request to see Sidney Herbert's side of the correspondence,
and consulted Frederick Verney about her position with regard to
copyright. Florence once again attempted to stall the biographer,
then allowed Stanmore to see some letters, while continuing to hold
back many more. Stanmore's retaliation was spiteful and scathing, and
marked a new development in the history of Florence's public reputation. 'It is impossible to speak in too high terms of Miss Nightingale's

great qualities and equally great work,' he wrote in the chapter of his *Memoir* devoted to Herbert's part in the Crimean War, 'but as every medal has its reverse and every picture its shadows, it cannot be denied that these great capacities were accompanied . . . by a jealous impatience of any rival authority, and an undue intolerance of all opposition or difference of opinion.' Florence Nightingale's 'great qualities', Stanmore concluded, 'were combined with some womanly weaknesses'.

The contrast between Stanmore's estimate of Florence's character, and the sentimental school of Nightingale biography, extolling her as a secular saint with a litany of the usual stories of self-sacrifice, could not have been greater. Two years before the appearance of Stanmore's life of Herbert, Sarah Tooley had taken advantage of the renewed interest surrounding Florence's life and career by publishing the fullest biography to date. The predominant tone of Tooley's book may be surmised from its introduction, where Tooley mentions a recent contest conducted by the editor of *Girl's Realm* to find the most popular heroine in history: Florence Nightingale had been the overwhelming winner, receiving more than 120,000 of the 300,000 votes polled. Stanmore and Tooley were, of course, addressing widely different readerships. But the dichotomy between the well-worn, though seemingly indestructible myth, and the flesh-and-blood reality of a complex, even flawed personality, had been publicly exposed for the first time.

Sir Edward Cook, the man chosen by the Nightingale executors to write Florence's own official biography, was to prove cleverly adept at navigating a course between these two extremes of interpretation. 'The real Florence Nightingale was very different from the legendary, but also greater,' Cook announced on the second page of his two-volume biography, published in 1913. 'Her life was built on larger lines, her work had more importance, than belong to the legend.'

Cook's *Life of Florence Nightingale* is remarkable, not least because it is the first authorized biography in the Victorian Lives and Letters tradition which accords a woman the same level of distinction and attention normally reserved for statesmen or generals. Born in 1857, Cook had been a journalist on the *Pall Mall Gazette*, succeeding W. T. Stead as editor before moving to the *Daily News*, where his editorship was brought to an abrupt end by a disagreement with the paper's proprietors over his determinedly imperialist stance during the South African War. The consuming interest of Cook's existence, though, lay in the life and works of John Ruskin. In the years before the First World War he devoted as much time as he could to the preparation of a monumental edition of Ruskin's writings, in collaboration with Alexander Wedderburn, before embarking on a Ruskin biography.

Cook's diary records that, in January 1912, he received a visit from Arthur Clough, one of the Nightingale executors, wanting to know if he would write Florence's official biography. In July of that year, Cook was in dispute with Louis Shore Nightingale about 'a preposterous contract of service agreement'; but by September he had started to research the book intensively. He made trips to Embley and Claydon, and to St Thomas's. He visited Henry Bonham Carter for some rather 'rambled reminiscences', and dined with one of Florence's doctors from her last years, Sir Thomas Barlow, who told him that Florence had suffered from 'hysteria', and that she had been misled by some of her physicians into taking to her bed, and had stuck to it 'from habit'. The Verneys had refused Louis Shore Nightingale's invitation to contribute material; but Cook was able to take full advantage of the unsorted boxes of Florence's papers, eventually to find a permanent home at the British Museum, which were being stored by Rosalind Vaughan Nash at her house in Hampstead. Mrs Nash, once described as resembling one of the genteel Amazons from Mrs Gaskell's *Cranford*, was the most important influence on the finished work, directing Cook's attention to material, and filling in gaps with her own memories and stories that had been handed down to her.

Cook was an astonishingly quick worker. By the end of 1912, he had already reached 1858 in Florence's story. He laboured enormously hard. On a single day in February 1913, he recorded working on the book for eleven and a half hours. In May he reached the final chapter, and on the nineteenth noted in his diary, 'Finished FN.' Cook had completed the research and writing of two volumes, amounting to 1,000 pages, in just nine months. *The Life of Florence Nightingale* was published by Macmillan that November.

'Perhaps I over-emphasised the harder and stronger feelings of Miss Nightingale's character,' Cook wrote to Margaret Verney, whose wish to publish a more intimate study of Florence, using her own correspondence with her, and the Smith and Nightingale letters at Claydon, was shortly to be rejected by Florence's executors on the grounds that such a book would conflict with 'F.N.'s strong dislike' of publicity. 'I gather that you rather think I did. I can only plead in extenuation that these were the features which seemed to me to have been too much over-laid by the sentimental "legend".' Indeed, Cook had been at pains to distance himself from the image of the 'Plaster Saint', emphasizing Florence's 'resolute and masterful' qualities, and – in an echo of Stanmore – writing of his subject as 'not lightly turned from her course, impatient of delay, not very tolerant of opposition'. He had been extraordinarily candid by the standards of the time about Florence's fraught relations with her mother and sister ('the intolerable sister', as one of his early readers, Violet Markham, described her). He had given due weight to aspects of Florence's post-Crimea work, like her efforts to improve the health of India, of which most of the reading public of the time would have been wholly ignorant. Only in regard to the Training School at St Thomas's had he tactfully trod an official line, portraying Florence as the only begetter of modern nursing, and establishing the misleading impression that the Nightingale School was immediately successful, rather than a difficult compromise worked out over time between the hospital officials, who wanted to use probationers as extra pairs of hands to scrub wards, the doctors, who wanted to keep nurses accountable to them, and the Fund Council, who wished to found a proper system of nurse training.

'Such a long journey', mused Flora Masson, a former Nightingale trainee, after reading Cook's *Life*, 'with its sheltered places, its highest mountain-tops early on the way, & the long, long populously level plains to the end.'

Nearly a century after it was written, Sir Edward Cook's biography remains the unsurpassed account of Florence Nightingale's public life. Almost all of the fifty or so biographies of Nightingale that followed Cook's, in the course of the twentieth century, may be said to emanate directly or indirectly from it. And while it's doubtful that many people nowadays read Cook's *Life* from cover to cover, his attempt to overturn the sentimental legend attaching to Florence Nightingale had a profound influence on a book that is still widely read, and which, moreover, is often proclaimed as a defining text of modern biography, and of twentieth-century iconoclasm: Lytton Strachey's *Eminent Victorians*, first published in May 1918, and containing an essay on Nightingale as the second of his four Victorians, sandwiched between Cardinal Manning and Dr Arnold (the fourth was General Gordon). In his preface,

Strachey warmly acknowledged his debt to Cook, and exempted his *Life* of Nightingale from the criticisms of style, tone and content he had made of other 'Standard Biographies' of the time. Cook was Strachey's single most important source, and one that he mimicked on the opening page of the essay, where Cook's phrase about the real Florence Nightingale was reworked with irony, to become: 'And so it happens that in the real Miss Nightingale there was more that was interesting than in the legendary one; there was also less that was agreeable.'

Strachey had a more personal interest in Cook's biography, for he had initially been approached to write the book himself. On reflection, this is perhaps not as surprising as it at first sounds. In the decade since coming down from Cambridge in 1905, Strachey had established himself as a writer of promise, mainly through a series of review-essays in the *Spectator* and the *Edinburgh Review*. Furthermore, the Strachey family possessed their own Nightingale connections, through their extensive service as administrators in India. Florence had corresponded with Lytton's father, Richard Strachey, during his time as head of the country's Public Works Department, while his uncle, Sir John Strachey, had kept her supplied with detailed information on numerous aspects of Indian life. Sir John had occupied several key posts in the British Raj, including the Presidency of the Bengal Sanitary Commission and the Lieutenant-Governorship of the North West Provinces, and had won Florence's praise for his 'immense energy, practical ability and determination'.

Lytton Strachey had yet to find the subject for the masterpiece that his Bloomsbury friends expected of him, but recognized that the genre of the official biography was not for him. Instead, from 1912 onwards, he had started to plan a collection of short biographies, originally entitled 'Victorian Silhouettes', 'written from a slightly cynical standpoint'. Florence was to be the only woman to make the final list. 'I have just been reading the book I might have written,' he told his brother James in January 1914, after finishing Cook's *Life* of Nightingale. 'I'm glad I didn't, as I couldn't have satisfied anybody. She was a terrible woman – though powerful. And certainly a wonderful book might have been made out of her, from the cynical point of view.' To his mother he admitted finding Cook's biography 'extremely interesting', but that Nightingale herself, though 'capable', was 'rather disagreeable in various ways – a complete egoist, and also full of a very tiresome religiosity, and

I don't think really intelligent'. By the time he had finished the Manning essay at Christmas 1914, Strachey had decided to include Nightingale in his new book, melting down Cook's epic to fit the dimensions of a taut five-act drama. The research and writing of the Nightingale essay took six months, from January to June 1915, its progress hampered by Strachey's bouts of ill-health, his anxiety about the war, and by the fact that Florence Nightingale was proving 'rather a hard nut to crack'. However, on 23 June he was able to report chirpily that 'F. Nightingale has at last been polished off . . .' In the spring of 1916, Strachey stayed with Virginia and Leonard Woolf at Asheham. 'Last night,' Virginia Woolf wrote to her sister on 22 April, 'he read us his Florence Nightingale, which is very amusing.'

Amusing it certainly is, but for the generations raised on the storybook myth, the portrayal of Florence Nightingale in *Eminent Victorians* was also provocative and truly shocking, while at the same time never less than enlightening. Strachey's Nightingale, seen first as a great bird of prey, and later as a tigress in the forest waiting to pounce, does not treat human beings as sentient creatures, but rather as objects to be manipulated to her own ends. In the scheme of *Eminent Victorians*, she embodies the Victorian spirit of humanitarianism, though paradoxically her own humanity is sacrificed in the process of pursuing humanitarian goals. According to Strachey, Nightingale had suppressed her genuinely erotic nature, transforming herself into a megalomaniac, who 'would think of nothing but how to satisfy that singular craving of hers to be *doing* something'. Through this deep and brooding neurosis, Nightingale becomes for Strachey a symbol of a type of woman who sublimates her sexual feelings in pursuit of power over men.

Lytton Strachey cannot help but be enthralled, though, by Florence Nightingale's dominating will, which he clearly finds irresistible, even as he is exposing what he sees as the fundamental inhumanity of her power. Max Beerbohm wrote that while Strachey 'recognised the greatness of Florence Nightingale, the necessary grit that was at the core of it rather jarred on him'; while Strachey's own biographer, Michael Holroyd, considers that Strachey's ambivalence towards Nightingale, and his lack of a consistent line, only adds to the essay's complexity. His admiration for all that Nightingale accomplished at Scutari is manifest. However, when he attempts to reconcile this admiration with his underlying theme of the legendary humanitarian, cut off from humankind,

Strachey's use of hyperbole betrays him and he succeeds only in creating 'a schizophrenic monster': 'at one moment a saintly crusader in the cause of hygiene, at the next a satanic personality, resorting to sardonic grins, pantomime gestures and sudden fits of wild fury'. More recently, Frances Partridge described as 'absurd' the notion that the Nightingale essay 'is complete debunking', pointing out that 'He says enormously admiring things about her – her tact, efficiency, the way she moved mountains and got everything going.'

There's something else that gives the Nightingale essay its staying power. In contrast to Strachey's Manning, Arnold and Gordon, 'Florence Nightingale' takes no enormous liberties with the truth, though naturally Strachey did embroider details in order to poke fun at individuals – like poor Clough – as well as to heighten the dramatic effect. One only has to compare it with Strachey's treatment of Manning – derived from the biography of Manning by E. S. Purcell, which was tantamount to a character assassination – to see how much Strachey depends on Cook for his veracity. Cook provided him with a solid, accurate source into which he could lower his celebrated little bucket. However, in 1928, a decade after the original publication of *Eminent Victorians*, Rosalind Vaughan Nash took advantage of the appearance of a cheap edition to publish an article calling the author to account for his smaller departures from the truth, and taking him to task on twelve specific points of error and misjudgement. One of these was Strachey's description of Nightingale's 'fury', her 'terrible rage', and 'demoniac frenzy'. On the contrary, insisted Nash, Nightingale's pronounced characteristic was her 'gift of calm'. 'I remember well her manner in speaking of things she disapproved. The words came out a little more quickly than usual. The voice was the same sweet voice, but on a rather lower note. There was nothing in the least acrimonious or uncontrolled . . .'

But to one, unidentified, member of the Clough family the effect of Strachey's portrait on Florence Nightingale's posthumous reputation seemed mostly positive, through its introduction of Cook's research to a wider audience. 'A large part of the essay is a very vivid résumé of Cook – & he makes the picture stand out strikingly & truly. He has got a wrong impression in certain very essential matters – but a great part of his picture is true . . . [Strachey has] made people generally aware of her & realize that she was a great figure & an amazing one whereas they had forgotten about her . . .' In other ways, though, the explosion of the myth surrounding Nightingale was obviously less beneficial. There was a sudden decline in works of popular biography about her, particularly those addressed to young girls. Her name appeared less frequently on lists of famous women, while the obligatory question which had appeared on schoolgirls' examination papers before the war, asking for an account of her life, now disappeared. According to James Pope-Hennessy, Strachey's sexual innuendo had taught 'adolescents to snigger' at her name. As the twentieth century wore on, a trace of this innuendo would be increasingly present in popular discussion of Florence Nightingale's life and personality, in the widespread, though unfounded, assumption that she must have been a lesbian, or in the bizarre story handed down among generations of American nursing students that she died from syphilis. For the modern age, Florence Nightingale's celibacy continues to be almost as puzzling as her rejection of celebrity.

Perhaps the natural heir to Lytton Strachey's Nightingale is the character bearing her name in Edward Bond's surreal sixties play, *Early Morning*. Bond's Florence Nightingale has a lesbian affair with Queen Victoria, who rapes her, disguises her sex by wearing a kilt and speaking in a bad Scottish accent, and nurses soldiers by providing them with sexual favours. It was Bond's use of sexual metaphors, especially in relation to the Nightingale character, that caused the strongest objections to the play at the time of its first performance in 1968, exactly fifty years after Strachey had first raised the spectre of Nightingale's sexual repression. In Britain, *Early Morning* was the last play to be banned in its entirety by the Lord Chamberlain, while Methuen balked at publishing it out of fear of libel suits stemming from Bond's prefatory remark that 'the events of this play are true'.

In general historical terms, nursing as a profession has had little truck with a feminist call to arms. If anything, nurses have tended to see themselves as dominated by other women, rather than put upon by men. Florence Nightingale herself had displayed ambivalent feelings on the subject of women's rights. Yet it did not take long, at the beginning of the twentieth century, for the movements for women's suffrage in Britain to claim Florence as one of their own. Marion Holmes, a member of the Women's Freedom League, the militant, though non-violent, organization that had split from the Pankhurst-led Women's Social and Political Union, issued *A Cameo Life-Sketch* of Nightingale in 1913, which announced that it should go 'without saying' that Florence was 'a convinced Suffragist'. Suffragettes as well as suffragists used Florence's name and image in their propaganda. Among the striking banners designed by the artist Mary Lowndes for the 1908 public demonstration by the National Union of Women's Suffrage Societies is one emblazoned with 'Florence Nightingale' and 'Crimea' in large capitals, with the nurses' tower at Scutari depicted underneath. In performances staged around Britain before the First World War of Cicely Hamilton's *Pageant of Great Women*, written to demonstrate women's capacity for leadership, Florence Nightingale was predictably among the dramatis personae. She was portrayed as one of 'The Warriors', as opposed to the heroic type of woman exemplified by Grace Darling, or the saintly one by Elizabeth Fry. At the *Pageant*'s première at London's Scala Theatre, in November 1909, Nightingale was played by Ellen Terry's sister Marion. Subsequently, the role was taken by both suffrage militants and nonmilitants: Lady Constance Lytton at Bristol, for example, Charlotte Despard, the leader of the Women's Freedom League, in a production at Swansea.

It was the appearance, though, at the end of the 1920s, of 'Cassandra', Florence's impassioned commentary on the desperate lives of midnineteenth-century women of her class, which signalled Florence Nightingale's acceptance into the fold by the generation of younger feminists who had recently achieved voting parity with men with the passing of the 1928 Equal Franchise Act. Hitherto 'Cassandra' had been accessible only in the limited number of private copies of *Suggestions for Thought*, which Florence had had printed almost seventy years earlier. In the decade following Florence's death, her executors had arranged for the essay to be set up in type again, this time as a separate booklet. However, only with the publication, in 1928, of Ray Strachey's short history of the Women's Movement in Britain, *The Cause*, which included 'Cassandra' as an appendix, did the essay became generally available for the first time. Ray Strachey – coincidentally Lytton Strachey's sister-in-law – was a veteran suffragist, a campaigner for women's employment and equal pay, who had been one of the first women to stand for Parliament after the vote was won. Her book was instantly acclaimed a classic, while 'Cassandra' gradually acquired the status of a focal feminist text, an important documentary link between women's earlier struggles for their personal, legal and political liberties, and the full-blown fight for emancipation that emerged in the first decades of the twentieth century. To a younger feminist like Vera Brittain, the publication of 'Cassandra' appeared to deal a final blow to the 'monstrous legend' of the Lady with the Lamp. In an article for the *Manchester Guardian*, published in January 1929, Brittain applauded Nightingale for having produced 'a protest against the wastage of her powers', adding that 'Cassandra' 'was as consistent an exponent of this attitude as any feminist could wish'. This insight into a Florence Nightingale who suffered while chafing against the restrictions on her personal liberty offered feminists a more sympathetic figure to identify with than either of the earlier Nightingale incarnations of sentimental angel, or dictatorial reformer 'of the most ruthless and aggressive type'. Indeed, Brittain, who had served for four years during the First World War as a VAD nurse at a variety of civilian and military hospitals, admitted to having previously detested the woman she referred to as 'the founder of modern nursing', largely because of the 'ferocious hatred' that Brittain had felt towards the civilian hospital authorities she had encountered during the war. 'Cassandra' allowed her to recognize the contrast between Florence Nightingale's 'rebellious spirit, her administrator's grasp of essentials, and the bigoted narrowness of some of her successors'.

The newly published 'Cassandra' also offered inspiration to Virginia Woolf, whose aunt Caroline Stephen had once corresponded with Florence about the pros and cons of religious sisterhoods in nursing. Woolf was writing *A Room of One's Own*, and considering the ways in which, historically, women writers had found their creativity stifled by a lack of education and economic independence, family tyranny and demands on their time. Florence's example was especially pertinent to her discussion of the last of these, the vital necessity of time and privacy for women's creative work. 'Women,' Florence had written, 'never have an half hour . . . that they can call their own . . .' In Woolf's early drafts, Florence Nightingale assumes an even more significant role than in the final published text. She provides a key to the 'great revolution'; some guide to the question of what had finally led women to 'forsake their station in the drawing room beside the tea pot', and 'actually go on foot . . . [to] regions of busy life which Charlotte Brontë dreamt of with such passion but was never to see'.

The guns roared in the Crimea ... the limbs of living men were torn asunder ...
Meanwhile, a single shell crossed the seas ... penetrated into peaceful villages
... sought out a peaceful manor house ... and crashed through the drawing
room. The mahogany panels were shivered for ever. Out stepped a single figure
– a solitary woman. In one hand she bore a roll of lint; in the other a lamp. Her
name was Florence Nightingale. The reign of women's servitude was over.

This new, feminist-friendly Nightingale required a further authorized
biography. Ida O'Malley, a friend of Ray Strachey's, who had assisted
with research for The Cause, was chosen. O'Malley (pronounced
O'Mailey) was in her fifties, the Oxford-educated daughter of a soldier
in the Royal Horse Artillery, and a mother who spent much of her life
as a permanent invalid. A devout High Church woman, she was a close
friend of Maude Royden, the first campaigner for the ordination of
women (a cause which would have undoubtedly won Florence's support), and had been involved in the suffragist movement before the First
World War. O'Malley's biography, which appeared in 1931, covered
Florence's life down to the end of the Crimean War, using some of the
Verney papers at Claydon that had been denied to Cook, and presenting
'a more personal and familiar account' than had been available to date, in
a readable, accessible style. If O'Malley ever intended to complete the
story with a second volume, it remained unpublished at her death in 1939.

Stage and screen were meanwhile making their own contribution to the
public's perception of Florence Nightingale. The first film biography,
Florence Nightingale, was produced in Britain in 1915. A four-reel silent
feature, it was directed by Maurice Elvey, and starred Elizabeth Risdon
in the title role. The film is now lost, but in promotional material was
described as 'biographical rather than dramatic'. The screenplay was
suggested by episodes from Cook's Life, and apparently opened with
a scene from Florence's childhood, in which she is shown bandaging a
doll. It ended with the elderly Florence receiving the Order of Merit.
One caption referred erroneously to Florence as the 'Founder of the
Red Cross', signifying that one of the film's primary objectives was
possibly to encourage young women to volunteer their wartime services
to the British Red Cross. A still photograph shows Risdon as Nightingale
the moral crusader, raising her hand and warning soldiers against the
dangers of drink.

In the theatre, the first major stage treatment of Florence's life appeared in the United States, in 1922. This three-act play, *Florence Nightingale*, by Edith Gittings Reid, an American writer known mainly for magazine articles and short biographies of medical subjects, never reached the New York stage and was probably rarely performed, though its script was published and reviewed. It contrasts 'the highbrow rhetoric of the Nightingale legend' with the language of 'a down-to-earth heroine'. The supporting cast of characters provides a romantic commentary on Nightingale's work at Scutari, which the heroine herself frequently punctures with heavy doses of reality. 'Florence has a vision of a woman's love flowing over the red fields of the wounded,' Mrs Nightingale says at one point; to which Florence responds, 'Mama, mama! My vision is of soap and splints and food and sheets – clean sheets.'

The Nightingale play that was to have a far greater impact on audiences on both sides of the Atlantic opened at the Arts Theatre in London for three weeks in January 1929, before moving for a long run to the Garrick Theatre; at the end of 1931, it transferred to the Broadway stage. This was *The Lady with a Lamp* by Reginald Berkeley, a considerable triumph in London and New York for Edith Evans in the leading role. Berkeley was a playwright, novelist and screenwriter, whose radio play *Machines*, about the threat of machinery to modern life, was banned by the BBC in 1930 for being 'of a propaganda nature'. He had already written a biographical novel – later made into a film – about the heroism of Edith Cavell, the wartime nurse executed by the Germans in 1915 for assisting in the escape of Allied soldiers. *The Lady with a Lamp*, by far Berkeley's most successful play, demonstrates his concern with the social function of art in its very first scene, set on the terrace at Embley in the late 1840s. There, William Nightingale, Lord Palmerston and Sidney Herbert discuss – with interjections from a perplexed Fanny Nightingale – the value of Carlyle's tract *Past and Present* ('He's making a big reputation as a thinker'). The questioning by Carlyle of the ease and indolence of the upper-middle-class way of life, into which Florence Nightingale had been born, foreshadows the play's underlying theme of Nightingale as a pioneer of work for women (highlighted by some of Berkeley's earlier titles, 'Woman Power', 'Sex and Power' and 'Sigh No More Ladies'). Bernard Shaw's influence on Berkeley's marriage of drama with the playwright's social and political convictions was hinted at by the critic Ivor Brown, who referred to the Florence of *The Lady with a Lamp* as a 'St Joan of Sanitation whose girlhood voices give one clear call to drains'.

Berkeley drew on Lytton Strachey for his characterization of Florence Nightingale, especially in his emphasis on the darker side of her personality. Strachey, who saw the play in the summer of 1929, considered it to be 'entirely based on E.[minent] V.[ictorians] except for some foolish frills added by the good gentleman'. These 'foolish frills' chiefly consisted of the introduction of scenes involving a character called Henry Tremayne, Florence's suitor, based on Richard Monckton Milnes, to whom Cook had alluded, though not by name (Milnes was finally unmasked as having proposed marriage to Florence by Ida O'Malley). Tremayne, played at the Garrick by John Gielgud, is rejected in a scene of awkward romanticism ('No, Henry, no, I won't surrender . . . I have had a call'), but then turns up at Scutari as a wounded soldier and dies in Florence's arms. Much of the dramatic tension, in another departure from historical truth, derives from Florence's conflict with Liz Herbert. Liz, who is jealous of Florence's predominant part in her husband's life, is in turn scorned by Florence for her inability to disguise that jealousy. 'Liz, dear, I'm really very, very sorry for you,' Florence says at one point, as Liz harangues her about the effects of Florence's 'terrible slave-driving will' on her husband's health. 'It must be awful to be unable to disassociate men from the seraglio.'

In spite of its title, *The Lady with a Lamp* contains no scenes of Florence as a nurse, apart from the brief one in which Tremayne dies. The accent in scene four, set at Scutari in the first winter of the war, is on her performance in purveying the hospitals, and in dealing with the obstacles she faces from officialdom, personified by the recalcitrant purveyor Mr Bamford. Here she shows an iron will and uncompromising determination in cutting through the red tape, which is standing in the way of efficiency and 'putting a premium on stupidity and death'. The stage directions introducing Florence in the next scene, set seven years later, in the Burlington Hotel, demonstrate the extent of Berkeley's debt to Strachey. At forty-one, Florence is described as 'in the prime of her mental powers'. But 'Seven years' rigid repression of sex . . . have clamped her features into an ascetic mask, fixed the lines of her mouth in a hard line, and soured her sense of humour into an acid irony.' In an alternative ending, which was never performed, Berkeley revealed his intention of examining the complex character behind the legend. Two nurses tend Florence in her final hours. The older nurse says simply, 'She's a saint.' The younger of the two replies, 'Saint! Oh, I know these saints. They're usually sinners who've gone soft on it . . . I don't believe in making idols of people. They've got their faults like you and me. Why not be frank about it?' To which the older nurse replies, 'I have never heard anyone say before that Florence Nightingale had a fault.'

Berkeley's play did not present a 'bloodless myth', wrote the critic in the *Daily Telegraph*. Rather, it was about a 'living woman . . . a great woman, with the defects of her qualities . . .' Louis Shore Nightingale raised objections on behalf of the Nightingale executors, writing to inform *The Times* that neither the executors, nor any member of Florence Nightingale's family, had been in any way responsible for the production, nor had they been consulted about it. Berkeley riposted with a letter to the paper, stating that he was 'unaware of any obligation on a writer to consult the executors of the wills of historical personages before a noble life is reverently shown to the public'.

The success of *The Lady with a Lamp* led Hollywood to produce its own version of the Florence Nightingale story. Warner Brothers' *The White Angel*, directed by William Dieterle in 1936, was a follow-up to Warners' *The Story of Louis Pasteur*, released the previous year. Once again, Strachey's essay was a major source for the selection of scenes from Nightingale's life that lent themselves to dramatization. This time, though, the main character was presented more sympathetically. In place of Strachey's demonic Nightingale, the familiar, legendary figure of the Lady with the Lamp was reinstated, perhaps to make her more palatable to nurses who were regarded as a significant part of the film's prospective audience. For the same reason, 'the Nightingale Pledge', written by American nurses, a doctor and a clergyman, in 1893, for use in a nursing training school in Detroit, was introduced in a glaring anachronism at the end of the film, when Florence Nightingale meets Queen Victoria, and is overheard reciting the pledge.

Kay Francis, the actress playing Nightingale, was an unlikely choice for the role. She was well known to American filmgoers for her portrayal of rich, sophisticated, big city women, attired in expensive clothes and jewellery, who often succumbed to the temptation of adultery. Francis's performance in *The White Angel* is handicapped by her lisp and American accent. In a scene showing her tending to a wounded soldier, she holds him more as a lover than a nurse, and appears to be on the verge of kissing him. The *White Angel* was an expensive flop, and Hollywood has yet to return to Florence Nightingale as subject matter for a big-budget production.

Reviewing Margaret Goldsmith's waspish biography of Nightingale, another book, published in 1937, that owed much to a Stracheyan perspective, the *Times Literary Supplement* acknowledged that the process of cutting the legend down to size might be getting out of hand. 'Now there seems to be a good deal of danger that the Crimean heroine's capacity for sharpness and sarcasm and her dictatorial efficiency will be as much exaggerated as her tenderness was in Victorian oleographs.' Four years later, Cecil Woodham-Smith, a woman in her early forties, who had written pot-boilers while her children were young, embarked on the research for a biography of Florence Nightingale, which was intended to reassert some measure of balance. The book was to be the largest-scale life of Nightingale of any since Cook's. 'She is a woman of remarkable intelligence,' Michael Sadleir, Woodham-Smith's editor at Constable, wrote to Ellin Salmon, Edmund Verney's eldest daughter, 'and will I think produce an outstanding book, which will not in any way be a pious monument or an essay in white-washing, but will really tell the truth about Miss Nightingale's great qualities and great failings.' Woodham-Smith possessed the social cachet which enabled her to gain privileged access to the British Library's Nightingale Papers while they were in Wales for safe keeping during the Second World War. At Claydon, she charmed Sir Harry Verney, the eldest son of Edmund Verney, who had succeeded his father as fourth baronet in 1910, and was given permission to use the extensive Nightingale collection there. Sir Harry, just nine years old at Parthenope's death in 1890, had always been vocal in his dislike of his step-grandmother, in marked contrast to his veneration of Florence (he had only known Parthenope at her most cantankerous, during her worst bouts of arthritis). He was undoubtedly the source of several unflattering stories about Parthenope which he fed to a gullible Woodham-Smith, who later reproduced them in her book, including the most commonly repeated one, that the original Sir Harry had only asked Parthenope to be his wife after Florence had refused him.

After nine years' research and writing, Cecil Woodham-Smith's *Florence Nightingale* was published in the autumn of 1950, an event marked by the display, in the window of Harrods, the department store in Knightsbridge, of the carriage in which Nightingale had been driven around the Crimea (known to generations of nurses at St Thomas's, where the carriage was preserved, surviving bomb-inflicted damage during the Blitz, as 'Florrie's Lorry'). The book was instantly acclaimed. Ralph Partridge called it a 'great' biography, while Raymond Mortimer commended the author for having 'selected the facts impartially ... inviting us to form our own opinions'. It sold widely in Britain in many reprints of the Constable hardback and, later, as a Penguin paperback; and its success heralded a new kind of blockbuster historical biography that was to come to fruition in the course of the next two decades.

There can be no doubt of Cecil Woodham-Smith's admiration for Florence Nightingale. She generally shows a reluctance to make judgements, while drawing on a vast range of primary material to place Nightingale in the best light. The underlying reasons for Woodham-Smith's hero-worship – and she generally refers to her subject as 'Miss Nightingale', an odd kind of distancing device in itself – may have been twofold. First, Woodham-Smith's father, Colonel James FitzGerald, was an Indian Army officer who had served during the Mutiny, and Woodham-Smith had grown up with an awareness of the part played by Florence Nightingale in reducing the number of deaths among British soldiers in India. Secondly, Cecil Woodham-Smith had been something of a rebel as a young woman. She was expelled from school, and, in 1917, rusticated for a term from St Hilda's College, Oxford, for joining Irish Republican demonstrators in the street (Colonel FitzGerald was Irish, and his daughter felt a great sense of identity with her Irish heritage, as she was to show in a subsequent work on *The Great Hunger* of the 1840s). This attitude of rebellion may have led her to identify in turn with Florence Nightingale's own struggles to escape the claims of family in her attempts to gain nursing experience in her twenties. It may also account for Woodham-Smith's tendency to exaggerate and over-dramatize the early frustrations of Nightingale's home life. This was an aspect of the book criticized by the historian W. H. Greenleaf, in a somewhat patronizing article, published in 1959, entitled 'Biography and the "Amateur Historian"'. Greenleaf took Woodham-Smith to task for her many errors of transcription, which suggested to him 'an intolerable degree of carelessness'; he drew attention to her reliance on

Cook, in both substance and presentation; and he noted that Cook's more balanced narrative of Nightingale's conflict with her family 'is infinitely to be preferred ... [Cook] recognizes that there was at least something to be said for the long-suffering Nightingale family and their point of view'. Additionally, Woodham-Smith had committed the cardinal sin, which Cook had warned against, of interpreting Florence's written notes and letters, so often filled with explosions of anger, as if they were indicative of her spoken word, and of ignoring many examples of her expressions of love and concern for her mother and sister.

None the less, after more than half a century, Cecil Woodham-Smith's *Florence Nightingale* has retained its place as, if not the most authoritative biography (a distinction that belongs still to Cook), then certainly the most dramatically vivid and enjoyable narrative of Nightingale's life. The film rights were snapped up by an American producer who planned a feature with the stage actress Katherine Cornell taking the lead. The film was never made. Instead, a British film biopic, directed by Herbert Wilcox and starring his wife Anna Neagle – who added Nightingale to the roll call of real-life heroines she had portrayed, including Queen Victoria, Edith Cavell and Amy Johnson – was released at the end of 1951. *The Lady with the Lamp* credited Reginald Berkeley's play as its source, but in fact very little of Berkeley remains in the screenplay, and strikingly absent as well are any hints of the acidic, repressed character that he had drawn. Anna Neagle's Nightingale is a plucky heroine, insufferably noble as she wafts through the corridors at Scutari carrying her lamp, pausing only to wipe the brows of the suffering wounded. As one critic noted, the film was no more than 'the old fiction of the Victorian Lady Bountiful calling with the soup'. Neagle's Sidney Herbert was Michael Wilding, a pairing that unavoidably brought to mind their earlier screen partnership in a string of wartime musical comedies. Much of the film was shot at Lea Hurst, Embley, and Broadlands, Palmerston's old estate. In the course of her research, Anna Neagle came across Athena the owl, stuffed, and proudly displayed in a glass case on the mantelpiece of the Mayfair home of Mr Mitchelhill, the new owner of Lea Hurst.

The pendulum has continued to swing backwards and forwards between the reductive extremes of saint and sinner ever since. There has been a constant stream of biographies, for adults and children, novels (among

them an entertaining contribution by Richard Gordon, famous for his
Doctor books, in which Florence is portrayed as a brilliant administra-
tor, but also outed as a lesbian), plays for television and radio, musicals
and operas (a chamber opera was performed at the Elora Festival in
Ontario, in 1992, and another is forthcoming, commissioned by the
Royal Opera House in London for its Linbury Studio). Actresses who
have essayed the role for television and radio include Helen Hayes, Irene
Dunne, Sarah Churchill, Julie Harris – who, as Nightingale in the 1965
NBC TV drama *The Holy Terror*, by James Lee, suddenly tears off a
wig, at the Ambassador's ball in Constantinople, to reveal her complete
baldness – Janet Suzman and Jaclyn Smith (a case of one of TV's
Charlie's Angels portraying an angel of the ministering variety).

Thirty years after Cecil Woodham-Smith's biography had acquired a
reputation as the so-called 'definitive' study of its subject, there came an
assault on Florence Nightingale's good name and character which made
Strachey's essay seem 'almost bland and benevolent by comparison'.
Florence Nightingale: Reputation and Power, by F. B. Smith, an Australian historian, published in 1982, is character assassination masquerad-
ing as a serious history, a polemic infected with unpleasant traces of
misogyny which often degenerates into snide debunking. So intent is
Smith on proving that Nightingale was a fantasist, a bully and a liar that
he resorts to making statements that are demonstrably untrue, while a
close inspection of the citations in his endnotes often reveals them to be
saying something quite different from the inferences he has drawn from
them – or in some cases, the complete opposite of what he claims they
say (Smith ignored the two largest collections of family material, at the
Wellcome and Claydon, which makes some of his assertions about
Florence and her family less than authoritative, to put it mildly). Yet
despite this frenzied act of literary iconoclasm, Smith cannot finally bring
himself to deny that Florence Nightingale managed to save many lives.

The strength of the legend is such that for some, it seems, the only
way to counter it is with something equally uncomplicated and one-
dimensional. The final decades of the twentieth century saw the launching of two projects to further understanding of Nightingale's life and
achievements. The Florence Nightingale Museum was opened in 1989,
in the shadow of St Thomas's, 'to promote an understanding and
appreciation of Florence Nightingale's legacy and its continuing influence on nursing and people's health'. The museum's permanent exhib-

ition centres on the Nightingale memorabilia guarded faithfully for many years by Rosalind Vaughan Nash. At their height, attendance figures have come close to 300 visitors a day, many of them from Japan and the United States.

The *Collected Works of Florence Nightingale*, a mammoth sixteen-volume printed edition of selections from Nightingale's correspondence, together with many previously unpublished, or long unavailable, books, pamphlets and articles by her, was conceived in the mid-1990s, and the first volume was published in 2001 (comprehensive electronic publication will eventually follow). The project's editor is Lynn McDonald, Emeritus Professor of Sociology at the University of Guelph, in Ontario, who first encountered Nightingale during her research into theorists of nineteenth-century social science. When publication of the *Collected Works* is complete, it will enable us to see Florence Nightingale for the first time in all her many different guises, as both a more complex and a more rounded historical figure.

The effort of transcribing all Florence Nightingale's known unpublished correspondence is a Herculean task. A librarian at the British Library, observing Lynn McDonald's industry and commitment, was once overheard viperously to remark, 'She thinks she *is* Florence Nightingale.'

Remarkably, the winds of biographical interpretation that buffeted Nightingale's reputation throughout the twentieth century left little mark for decades on the nursing profession's own conception of its dominating iconic figure. A decision was reached at a meeting of the International Council of Nurses in Cologne, in 1912, to commemorate Florence Nightingale with 'an appropriate memorial'. Florence's old adversary in the registration battle, Ethel Bedford Fenwick, was one of the leading proponents of the idea. 'Miss Nightingale,' she told delegates at a banquet to mark the conclusion of the congress, 'was above all nationality, and belonged to every age and country.' The endowment of a living memorial to Florence Nightingale was proposed; an educational foundation, to be established in Britain, which would benefit not only the nurses of the world, but also the sick whom they served. However, war intervened before the scheme could be organized, and it was not until 1931 that the Florence Nightingale International Foundation was set up, to support the advancement of nursing education and research.

At St Thomas's – known to former Nightingales as the 'Mother House' – the appointment, in 1913, of Alicia Lloyd Still as Matron of the Hospital and Superintendent of the Nursing School ensured a strong degree of continuity with traditions established in Florence Nightingale's lifetime. Lloyd Still saw herself as in a direct line of succession, having been the last Nightingale nurse to be sent to South Street to receive her charge as Ward Sister 'from the hands of the Foundress herself'. Emphasis continued to be placed on character formation and personal dedication. Morning prayers took place in each ward. Nursing probationers at St Thomas's were encouraged to think of themselves as the elite ('You are an extraordinarily lucky gel, I must say, to be taking your training in the Nightingale School,' Lloyd Still told selected candidates, while other training schools repeated the adage, 'Tommy's for snobs'). And where the tradition didn't exist, Lloyd Still saw fit to invent one. In 1925, the Nightingale Badge was introduced, to be worn, and treasured, by nurses who had received their certificates, an invention which ignored the fact that Florence Nightingale had always objected to medals and badges, not least on the grounds that they were unhygienic. During Lloyd Still's tenure of office, which lasted for nearly a quarter of a century, lip-service continued to be paid to the preventative aspect of modern medicine – Nightingale's 'health-nursing' – though there was little St Thomas's could do to resist the overall trend in nurse training towards nurses becoming doctors' assistants, a development that Florence Nightingale, with her idea of 'sanitary missioners', had always been set against.

The upheaval and uncertainty in the world of nursing in Britain, caused by the recommendations of no fewer than eight successive government reports, in the space of six decades, on the profession's future, gradually eroded many of Florence Nightingale's own tenets. The 1966 Salmon Report swept away the Matron and the Nightingale Ward system in an attempt to improve the status of nurses, transforming them, according to the new management babble, into 'ward managers'. Project 2000, conceived in 1988, went further, bringing about the greatest revolution in nurse training since state registration seventy years earlier. The historical tension between theory and practice was resolved in favour of the academy, as the training of nurses was absorbed into higher education as part of the university model. Traditional hospital-based nursing schools were closed. The Nightingale School ceased to exist in 1991, with the last batch of nurses receiving their badges five years later. Training for nurses was removed from the bedside to be taught instead in universities and colleges of higher education. The old apprenticeship system was gone forever. The new preoccupation with studying has meant that, for many trainee nurses, there is no longer enough time to be concerned with basic hospital routines of cleanliness and hygiene.

It was against this background of wholesale change that Britain's nurses finally turned on Florence Nightingale as the source of all the ills of their profession. In 1999, delegates at the annual conference of Unison, Britain's largest trade union representing nurses, declared that she had held back the nursing profession for too long. 'All over Eastern Europe, statues of Lenin are being taken off their pedestals . . .,' said one aggrieved health visitor supporting a motion to move the celebration of International Nurses' Day from 12 May, Nightingale's birthday. 'It is in the same vein that the nursing profession must . . . start to exorcise the myth of Florence Nightingale.' Among the welter of accusations directed against Nightingale, most of them of dubious veracity, was one that she had 'not so much kept nurses under the thumb as under the boot'. There may be no credible way to draw a link between Florence Nightingale and the problems of contemporary nursing, as Patricia D'Antonio has said. However, there can be no doubt that, at the end of the century, the figure of Nightingale had become 'a lightning rod for all the profession's discontents'.

But the legend goes on drawing us in, more than 150 years after it first captured the imagination of the world. On a May afternoon in 2005, I sat in a Westminster Abbey burnished gold with sunlight for a service to commemorate the life of Florence Nightingale. The congregation at this annual event consists mostly of nurses and nursing students, together with representatives of the Red Cross and the military. At the climactic point in the service, a procession of nurses makes its way to the high altar, carrying a lighted Grecian lamp. At the sacrarium, the lamp is handed from a sister to a staff nurse, signifying the passing on of knowledge, as well as the emergence of the light of humanity from darkness. It is then offered to the Dean of Westminster, who places it on the high altar.

Some have argued that such a service in a great national church is the last thing that Nightingale would have wanted. She would have scorned the perpetuation of the myth associated with her name. She might also have questioned, as she often did, the place of ceremonial and ritual in organized religion. To a twenty-first-century onlooker, the commemoration in Westminster Abbey appears to do a disservice to all the many other dimensions of Florence Nightingale's life and work, by confining her to her best-known and most traditional role, as a nurse.

One does not have to look far today to see that many of Florence Nightingale's greatest concerns remain ours too. In the closing months of 2007, news stories continually surfaced, revealing deep-seated problems in health care she would certainly have recognized, and which would have alarmed and exercised her. The shameful neglect of British troops, injured in Iraq and Afghanistan, by the Government at home, is one; reports of a sharp rise in worldwide rates of maternal mortality, another. Most worrying to much of the population of the United Kingdom is our reported failure to keep hospitals clean and free from infection. If we were to derive one simple lesson from Florence Nightingale's life and work, it would stem from this single unifying thread: that society has a collective responsibility for the health of all its members. Florence Nightingale may have had no time for symbols, but for us the lamp still burns.

Select Bibliography

A complete bibliography would require at least a volume to itself. The following books and articles are ones that I have found especially helpful, or which are cited in short form in the notes. Place of publication, unless otherwise stated, is London.

Abbott, Evelyn, and Lewis Campbell (eds), *The Life and Letters of Benjamin Jowett. MA, Master of Balliol College, Oxford*, 2 vols, John Murray, 1897.

Abbott, Jacob, *The Corner-stone, or, A Familiar Illustration of the Principles of Christian Truth*, T. Ward, 1834.

Abbott, Jacob, *The Way to Do Good: Or The Christian Character Mature*, T. Tegg, 1836.

Abel-Smith, Brian, *A History of the Nursing Profession*, Heinemann, 1960.

Abel-Smith, Brian, *The Hospitals 1800–1948: A Study in Social Administration in England and Wales*, Heinemann, 1964.

Adams, Elmer C., and Warren Dunham Foster, *Heroines of Modern Progress*, New York: Macmillan, 1921.

Allchin, A. M., *The Silent Rebellion: Anglican Religious Communities 1845–1900*, SCM Press, 1958.

Allingham, William, *A Diary, 1824–1889*, Penguin, 1985.

Armstrong, Emma, 'Art and War Reportage in the Crimean War I: the *Illustrated London News*', in *A Most Desperate Undertaking. The British Army in the Crimea, 1854–56*, ed. Alastair Massie. National Army Museum, 2003.

Arnold, David, *Colonizing the Body. State Medicine and Epidemic Disease in Nineteeth-Century India*, Berkeley: University of California Press, 1993.

Asquith, Margot, *The Autobiography of Margot Asquith*, ed. Mark Bonham Carter, Eyre & Spottiswoode, 1962.

Attewell, Alex, 'Throwing light on Florence Nightingale. Of lamps and lanterns', *International History of Nursing Journal*, 7 (2003), 94–7.

Aytoun, W. E., 'The Conduct of the War', *Blackwood's Magazine*, 77 (1855).

Bakewell, Michael, *Lewis Carroll. A Biography*, Heinemann, 1996.

Baly, Monica, *Florence Nightingale and the Nursing Legacy*, 2nd edn, Whurr Publishers, 1999.

Barrell, John, 'Death on the Nile: Fantasy and the Literature of Tourism 1840–1860', *Essays in Criticism*, XLI (April 1991), 97–127.

Barrett Browning, Elizabeth, *Letters of Elizabeth Barrett Browning*, ed. Frederic G. Kenyon, 2 vols, Smith Elder, 1897.

Barrett Browning, Elizabeth, *Aurora Leigh*, ed Margaret Reynolds, Ohio: Ohio University Press, 1992.

Baylen, J. O., 'The Florence Nightingale/Mary Stanley Controversy: Some Unpublished Letters', *Medical History*, 18 (1974), 186–93.

Beerbohm, Max, *Lytton Strachey* (the Rede Lecture), Cambridge: Cambridge University Press, 1943.

'Benevolent Institutions: Establishment for Gentlewomen During Illness', *The Pen*, 7 (23 July 1853), 98–103.

Benson, A. C., *Diary*, ed. P. Lubbock, Hutchinson, 1926.

Berkeley, Reginald, *The Lady with a Lamp* in *Plays of a Half-Decade*, Victor Gollancz, 1933.

Biswas, Robindra Kumar, *Arthur Hugh Clough*, Oxford: Clarendon Press, 1972.

Blackwell, Elizabeth, *Pioneer Work in Opening the Medical Profession to Women: Autobiographical Sketches*, Longmans, 1895.

Blake, Mrs Warenne, *An Irish Beauty of the Regency*, John Lane, 1911.

Boase, Frederic, *Modern English Biography*, Truro: Netherton & Worth, 1892.

Bonham Carter, Victor, *In a Liberal Tradition. A Social Biography*, Constable, 1960.

Bostridge, Mark, ' "Like a True Woman". Self-Sacrifice and Parthenope Nightingale', *Times Literary Supplement*, 5173 (24 May 2002), 14–15.

Boyd, Julia, *The Excellent Dr Blackwell. The Life of the First Female Physician*, Stroud: Sutton, 2005.

Boyd, Nancy, *Josephine Butler, Octavia Hill, Florence Nightingale. Three Victorian Women Who Changed Their World*, Macmillan, 1982.

Bracebridge, Selina, *Panoramic Sketch of Athens*, Coventry: Henry Merridew, 1836.

The British Film Catalogue. Volume 2: Non-fiction films, ed. Denis Gifford, Fitzroy Dearborn, 2000.

Brittain, Vera, ' "The Lady of the Lamp". Florence Nightingale as Feminist', *Manchester Guardian*, 16 January 1929.

Brittain, Vera, *Testament of Youth. An Autobiographical Study of the Years 1900–1925*, Victor Gollancz, 1933.

Brown, Thomas J., *Dorothea Dix. New England Reformer*, Cambridge, Mass.: Harvard University Press, 1998.

Bullough, Vern L., Bonnie Bullough and Marietta P. Stanton (eds), *Florence Nightingale and Her Era. A Collection of New Scholarship*, New York: Garland, 1990.

Bunsen, Frances von, *A Memoir of Baron Bunsen Drawn Chiefly from Family Papers by His Widow*, 2 vols., Longmans, 1868.

Calabria, Michael D., and Janet A. Macrae (eds), *Suggestions for Thought by Florence Nightingale. Selections and Commentaries*, Philadelphia: University of Pennsylvania Press, 1994.

Calabria, Michael D., *Florence Nightingale in Egypt and Greece. Her Diary and 'Visions'*, Albany: State University of New York Press, 1997.

Cannadine, David, *History in Our Time*, Penguin, 2000.

Carlyle, Jane, *The Collected Letters of Thomas and Jane Welsh Carlyle*, Kenneth J. Fielding et al. (eds), vol. 30, July–December 1855, Duke University Press, 2002.

Chorley, Katharine, *Arthur Hugh Clough: The Uncommitted Mind. A Study of His Life and Poetry*, Oxford: Clarendon Press, 1962.

Churchill, Winston, *A History of the English-speaking Peoples*, vol. 4, Cassell, 1962.

Clifford, Deborah, *Mine Eyes Have Seen the Glory. A Biography of Julia Ward Howe*, Boston: Little, Brown, 1979.

Clough, Arthur Hugh, *The Correspondence of Arthur Hugh Clough*, ed. F. L. Mulhauser, 2 vols, Oxford: The Clarendon Press, 1957.

Clough, Arthur Hugh, *The Poems of Arthur Hugh Clough*, ed. F. L. Mulhauser, Oxford: Clarendon Press, 1974.

Cockin, Katharine, 'Cicely Hamilton's Warriors: dramatic reinventions of militancy in the British women's suffrage movement', *Women's History Review*, 14 (2005), 527–41.

Cohen, Bernard I., 'Florence Nightingale', in *Scientific American*, 246 (March 1984), 128–33, 136–7.

Cooper Willis, Irene, *Florence Nightingale. A Biography*, George Allen & Unwin, 1931.

Cope, Zachary, *Florence Nightingale and the Doctors*, Museum, 1958.

Cope, Zachary, *Six Disciples of Florence Nightingale*, Pitman Medical Publishing, 1961.

Croston, James, *A Pilgrimage to the Home of Florence Nightingale*, Whittaker & Co., 1862.

Davies, John, *Florence Nightingale, or the Heroine of the East*, Arthur Hall, 1856.

Davis, Elizabeth, *Autobiography of Elizabeth Davis*, 2 vols, ed. Jane Williams, Hurst & Blackett, 1857.

Davis, Richard W., *Dissent in Politics 1780–1830. The Political Life of William Smith M. P.*, Epworth, 1971.

Dereli, Cynthia, 'Gender Issues and the Crimean War: Creating Roles for Women?', in *Gender Roles and Sexuality in Victorian Literature*, ed. Christopher Parker, Scolar Press, 1995.

Diamond, Marion, and Mervyn Stone, 'Nightingale on Quetelet', *Journal of the Royal Historical Society* (Series A), 144 (1981), 66–79, 176–213, 332–51.

Disselhoff, Julius, *Kaiserswerth. The Deaconess Institution of Rhenish Westphalia, Its Origin and Fields of Labour*, Hatchards, 1883.

Dock, L., and M. Stewart, *A Short History of Nursing from Earliest Times to the Present Day*, New York: Putnam, 1920.

Dossey, Barbara, *Florence Nightingale. Mystic, Visionary and Healer*, Pennsylvania: Springhouse, 2000.

Dossey, Barbara, et al., *Florence Nightingale Today: Healing, Leadership, Global Action*, Maryland: American Nurses Association, 2005.

Duberly, Fanny, *Mrs Duberly's War. Journal & Letters from the Crimea*, ed. Christine Kelly, Oxford: Oxford University Press, 2007.

Edge, Frederick Milnes, *A Woman's Example and a Nation's Work: A Tribute to Florence Nightingale*, Ridgway, 1867.

Eliot, George, *The George Eliot Letters*, vol. 2, ed. G. Haight, Oxford: Oxford University Press, 1954.

Ellis, Sarah, *The Daughters of England, their Position in Society, Character and Responsibilities*, Fisher, Son, & Co., 1842.

Erb, Peter C., and Elizabeth J. Erb, 'Florence Nightingale For and Against Rome. Her Early Correspondence with Henry Edward Manning', *Recusant History*, 24 (1999), 472–506.

Essays and Reviews, Parker, 1860.

Establishment for Gentlewomen During Illness, Nissen & Parker, 1853.

Eyler, John M., *Victorian Social Medicine. The Ideas and Methods of William Farr*, Baltimore: Johns Hopkins University Press, 1979.

Faber, Geoffrey, *Jowett: A Portrait with Background*, Faber, 1957.

Forbes, Bryan, *Ned's Girl. The Authorised Biography of Dame Edith Evans*, Elm Tree Books, 1977.

Forster, E. M., *Marianne Thornton*, Edward Arnold, 1956.

Forster, Margaret, *Significant Sisters: The Grassroots of Active Feminism 1839–1939*, Secker & Warburg, 1984.

Fox, Caroline, *The Journals of Caroline Fox 1835–1871*, a selection ed. Wendy Monk, Elek, 1972.

Gaskell, Elizabeth, *The Letters of Mrs Gaskell*, ed. J. A. V. Chapple and Arthur Pollard. Manchester: Manchester University Press, 1966.

Gaskell, Elizabeth, *Further Letters of Mrs Gaskell*, ed. J. A. V. Chapple and Alan Shelston, Manchester: Manchester University Press, 2003.

Gibbs, Philip, *The Pageant of the Years. An Autobiography*, Heinemann, 1946.

Giffard, J. T., *Constance and 'Cap' The Shepherd's Dog. A Reminiscence*, Harrison, 1861.

Gladwyn, Turbutt, *A History of Derbyshire*, Cardiff: Merton Priory Press, 1999.

Godden, Judith, *Lucy Osburn, a lady displaced. Florence Nightingale's envoy to Australia*, Sydney: Sydney University Press, 2006.

Goldie, Sue, *A Calendar of the Letters of Florence Nightingale*, Oxford: Wellcome Institute for the History of Medicine, 1983.

Goldin, Grace, 'Building a Hospital of Air: The Victorian Pavilions of St Thomas' Hospital, London', *Bulletin of the History of Medicine*, 49 (1975), 512–35.

Goodman, Margaret, *Experiences of an English Sister of Mercy*, Smith, Elder, 1862.

Gordon, Richard, *The Private Life of Florence Nightingale*, Heinemann, 1978.

Gourlay, Jharna, *Florence Nightingale and the Health of the Raj*, Aldershot: Ashgate, 2003.

Greenleaf, W. H., 'Biography and the "Amateur" Historian: Mrs Woodham-Smith's *Florence Nightingale*', *Victorian Studies*, 2 (1959), 190–202.

Greville, Charles, *The Greville Memoirs, 1814–1860*, vol. 7, ed. Lytton Strachey and Roger Fulford, Macmillan, 1938.

Griffin, Eric R., 'Victims of Fiction: Research Notes on "The Love Story of Florence Nightingale and John Smithurst"', *Wellington County History* 5 (1992), 45–52.

Guppy, Shusha, 'Frances Partridge', in *Looking Back*, New York: Paris Review Editions, British-American Publishing, 1991.

Hall, Mrs S. C., 'Something of What Florence Nightingale Has Done and Is Doing', *St James's Magazine*, I (April–July 1861), 29–40.

Handley, Jenny, and Hazel Lake, *Progress By Persuasion. The Life of William Smith 1756–1835*, privately printed, 2007.

Harben, Niloufer, *Twentieth-Century English History Plays: from Shaw to Bond*, Basingstoke: Macmillan, 1988.

Haskins, C., *History of Salisbury Infirmary*, Salisbury, 1922.

Hawthorne, Nathaniel, *The English Notebooks, 1856–1860. The Centenary Edition of the Works of Nathaniel Hawthorne*, vol. 22, ed. Thomas Woodson & Bill Ellis, Ohio: Ohio State University, 1997.

Hebert, Raymond G., *Florence Nightingale: Saint, Reformer or Rebel?*, Malabar: Robert E. Krieger, 1981.

Helmstadter, Carol, 'Robert Bentley Todd, Saint John's House, and the Origins of the Modern Trained Nurse', *Bulletin of the History of Medicine*, 67 (1993), 282–319.

Helmstadter, Carol, 'Passing of the Night Watch: Night Nursing Reform in the London Teaching Hospitals, 1856–1890', *Canadian Bulletin of Medical History*, 11 (1994), 23–69.

Helmstadter, Carol, 'Early Nursing Reform in Nineteenth Century London: A Doctor-Driven Phenomenon', *Medical History*, 46 (2002), 325–50.

Helmstadter, Carol, 'Florence Nightingale's Opposition to State Registration of Nurses', *Nursing History Review*, 15 (2007), 155–66.

Herbert, Elizabeth, *How I Came Home*, Catholic Truth Society, 1893.

Hirsch, Pam, *Barbara Leigh Smith Bodichon. Feminist, Artist and Rebel*, Chatto & Windus, 1998.

The History of Embley, Romsey: Embley Park School, 1995.

Hobson, W. F., *Catharine Leslie Hobson, Lady-Nurse, Crimean War, and Her Life*, Parker & Co., 1888.

Holmes, Marion, *Florence Nightingale. A Cameo Life-Sketch*, Women's Freedom League, 1913.

Holroyd, Michael, *Lytton Strachey. A Critical Biography*, 2 vols, Heinemann, 1967–8.

Hornby, Emilia, *Constantinople during the Crimean War*, Richard Bentley, 1863.

Housman, Laurence, 'Florence Nightingale', in *The Great Victorians*, ed. H. J. Massingham and H. Massingham, Ivor Nicholson, 1932.

Howse, Carrie, ' "The Ultimate Destination of All Nursing": The Development of District Nursing in England, 1880–1925', *Nursing History Review*, 15 (2007), 65–94.

Hoy, Suellen, *Chasing Dirt. The American Pursuit of Cleanliness*, Oxford: Oxford University Press, 1995.

Hubble, Douglas, 'William Ogle of Derby and Florence Nightingale', *Medical History*, 3 (July 1959), 201–11.

Huntsman, R. G., Mary Bruin and Deborah Holttum, 'Twixt Candle and Lamp: The Contribution of Elizabeth Fry and the Institution of Nursing Sisters to Nursing Reform', *Medical History*, 46 (2002), 351–80.

Jenking, Christine, *The Bracebridge Family and Atherstone Hall*, Atherstone: Bracebridge Court, 2000.

Jensen, Debra, 'Florence Nightingale's Mystical Vision and Social Action', *Scottish Journal of Religious Studies*, 19 (1998), 69–81.

Jewitt, Llewellynn, *A Stroll to Lea Hurst, Derbyshire, the Home of Florence Nightingale*, Derby, 1855.

Jones, J., *Memorials of Agnes Elizabeth Jones, by Her Sister*, Strahan, 1871.

Kalisch, Beatrice J., and Philip A. Kalisch, 'Heroine out of Focus: Media Images of Florence Nightingale', 2 parts, *Nursing & Health Care*, 4 (April–May 1983), 181–7, 270–78.

Keele, Mary (ed.), *Florence Nightingale in Rome: Letters Written by Florence Nightingale in Rome in the Winter of 1847–1848*, Philadelphia: American Philosophical Society, 1981.

Keen, Norman, *Florence Nightingale*, Ripley, Derbyshire: Footprint Press, 1982.

Kenny, Anthony, *Arthur Hugh Clough. A Poet's Life*, Continuum, 2005.

King, A., 'Hospital Planning: Revised Thoughts on the Origin of the Pavilion Principle in England', *Medical History*, 10 (1966), 360–73.

Kinglake, A. W., *The Invasion of the Crimea. Its origin, and an account of its progress to the death of Lord Raglan*, 8 vols, Edinburgh: Blackwood, 1863–7.

Kopf, Edwin W., 'Florence Nightingale as Statistician', *Publications of the American Statistical Association*, 15 (1916–17), 388–404.

Lawrence, George Alfred, *Sword and Gown*, John W. Parker & Son, 1859.

Leslie, Shane, 'Forgotten Passages in the Life of Florence Nightingale', *Dublin Review*, 161 (October 1917), 179–98.

Lesser, Margaret, *Clarkey: A Portrait in Letters of Mary Clarke Mohl (1793–1883)*, Oxford: Oxford University Press, 1984.

Litchfield, Henrietta (ed.), *Emma Darwin: A Century of Letters 1792–1896*, 2 vols, John Murray, 1915.

Luddy, Maria (ed.), *The Crimean Journals of the Sisters of Mercy 1854–56*, Dublin: Four Courts Press, 2004.

MacCarthy, Fiona, *Byron. Life and Legend*, John Murray, 2002.

MacDonnell, Freda, *Miss Nightingale's Young Ladies*, Angus & Robertson, 1970.

Mackerness, E. D., 'Frances Parthenope, Lady Verney (1819–1890)', *Journal of Modern History*, 30 (June 1958), 131–6.

MacQueen, Joyce Schroeder, 'Florence Nightingale's Nursing Practice', *Nursing History Review*, 15 (2007), 29–49.

Maggs, Christopher (ed.), *Nursing History: The State of the Art*, Croom Helm, 1987.

Mantripp, J. C., 'Florence Nightingale and Religion', *London Quarterly Review*, 157 (1932), 318–25.

Martineau, Harriet, *Eastern Life: Past and Present*, 3 vols, Edward Moxon, 1848.

Martineau, Harriet, *England and Her Soldiers*, Smith, Elder, 1859.

Martineau, Harriet, 'Nurses Wanted', *The Cornhill Magazine* (March 1865), 409–25.

Martineau, Harriet, *Harriet Martineau's Letters to Fanny Wedgwood*, ed. Elisabeth Sanders Arbuckle, Stanford: Stanford University Press, 1983.

Martineau, Harriet, *The Collected Letters of Harriet Martineau*, ed. Deborah Anna Logan, vols 3–5, Pickering and Chatto, 2007.

Masson, Flora, *Victorians All*, W. & R. Chambers, 1931.

Maurice, C. Edmund, *Life of Octavia Hill*, Macmillan, 1913.

Mayne, Ethel Colburn, *The Life and Letters of Lady Byron*, Constable, 1929.

McDonald, Lynn, 'Florence Nightingale Revealed in Her Own Writings', *Times Literary Supplement*, 5907 (8 December 2000), 14–15.

McKellar, Elizabeth, *The German Hospital Hackney. A Social and Architectural History 1845–1987*, Hackney Society: 1991.

Memoirs of a Highland Lady. The Autobiography of Elizabeth Grant of Rothiemurchus, afterwards Mrs Smith of Baltiboys, 1797–1830, ed. Lady Strachey, John Murray, 1911.

Merle, Gabriel, *Lytton Strachey (1880–1932). Biographie et critique d'un critique et biographe*, 2 vols, Lille: Lille University, 1980.

Mills, J. Saxon, *Sir Edward Cook KBE. A Biography*, Constable, 1921.

Mitford, Nancy (ed.), *The Stanleys of Alderley. Their Letters between the Years 1851–1865*, Hamish Hamilton, 1968.

Mitra, S. M., *The Life and Letters of Sir John Hall*, 2 vols, Longmans, 1911.

Monteiro, Lois A., 'On Separate Roads: Florence Nightingale and Elizabeth Blackwell', *Signs*, 9 (1984), 520–33.

Montgomery, William, *The Prophecy of Ada late Countess of Lovelace on her friend Florence Nightingale*, G.Emery & Co., 1856.

Moser, Mentona, *Die weibliche Jugend der oberen Stände Betrachtungen und Vorselläge*, Zurich: Druck und Verlag von Schulthess & Co, 1903.

Nash, Rosalind Vaughan, 'Florence Nightingale according to Mr Strachey', *Nineteenth Century*, 103 (February 1928), 258–65.

Nash, Rosalind Vaughan, 'I Knew Florence Nightingale', *The Listener*, 14 July 1937, 61–3.

Neagle, Anna, *An Autobiography*, W. H. Allen, 1974.

Neeley, Kathryn A., *Mary Somerville. Science, Illumination and the Female Mind*, Cambridge: Cambridge University Press, 2001.

Nicolson, Harold, *Diaries and Letters 1939–45*, Fontana, 1971.

Nightingale, Florence, *Notes on Matters Affecting the Health, Efficiency, and Hospital Administration of the British Army, founded chiefly on Experience of the Last War*, Harrison & Sons, 1858.

Nightingale, Florence, *Notes on Hospitals*, 3rd edn, Longman, Green, Longman, Roberts and Green, 1863.

Nightingale, Florence, *Notes on Nursing*, ed. Victor Skretkowicz, Scutari Press, 1992.

Nightingale, Florence, *Florence Nightingale to Her Nurses: a selection from Miss Nightingale's addresses to probationers and nurses of the Nightingale School at St Thomas's Hospital*, Macmillan, 1914.

Nightingale, Florence, 'Cassandra', in Ray Strachey, *The Cause. A Short History of the Women's Movement in Great Britain*, Bell, 1928.

Nightingale, Florence, *Selected Writings of Florence Nightingale*, ed. Lucy Seymer, Macmillan, 1954.

Nightingale, Florence, *Florence Nightingale at Harley Street: Her Reports to the Governors of her Nursing Home, 1853–4*, with an introduction by Sir Harry Verney, Dent, 1970.

Oliver, Hermia, 'The Shore Smith Family Library: Arthur Hugh Clough and Florence Nightingale', *The Book Collector*, 28 (1979), 521–9.

O'Neil, Robert, *Cardinal Herbert Vaughan: Archbishop of Westminster, Bishop of Salford, Founder of the Mill Hill Missionaries*, Tunbridge Wells: Burns & Oates, 1995.

Osborne, Sidney Godolphin, *Scutari and Its Hospitals*, Dickinson Brothers, 1855.

Palmer, Irene S., *Florence Nightingale and the First Organized Delivery of Nursing Services*, New York: American Association of Colleges of Nursing, 1983.

Pickering, George, *Creative Malady: Illness in the Lives and Minds of Charles Darwin, Florence Nightingale, Mary Baker Eddy, Sigmund Freud, Marcel Proust, Elizabeth Barrett Browning*, Allen & Unwin, 1974.

Poovey, Mary, *Uneven Developments. The Ideological Work of Gender in Mid-Victorian England*, Chicago: University of Chicago Press, 1988.

Poovey, Mary (ed.), *Florence Nightingale: Cassandra and Other Selections from Suggestions for Thought*, New York: New York University Press, 1993.

Pope Hennessy, James, *Monckton Milnes. The Years of Promise 1809–1851*, Constable, 1949.

Pope Hennessy, James, *Monckton Milnes. The Flight of Youth 1851–1885*, Constable, 1951.

Pugh, Evelyn, 'Florence Nightingale and J. S. Mill Debate Women's Rights', *Journal of British Studies*, 21 (1982), 118–38.

Pugh, P. D. Gordon, *Staffordshire Portrait Figures and Allied Subjects of the Victorian Era*, Woodbridge: Antique Collectors' Club, 1987.

Quain, Richard, *A Dictionary of Medicine*, Longmans, 1882.

Quetelet, L. A. J., *Physique Sociale, ou essai sur le développement des facultés de l'homme*, 2 vols, 2nd edn, Brussels: Muquardt, 1869.

Rappaport, Helen, *No Place for Ladies: The Untold Story of Women in the Crimean War*, Aurum, 2007.

Rappe, Emmy, *God Bless You, My Dear Miss Nightingale. Letters from Emmy Carolina Rappe to Florence Nightingale*, ed. Bertil Johansson, Stockholm: Bertil Johansson, 1977.

Rees, Joan, *Writings on the Nile: Harriet Martineau, Florence Nightingale, Amelia Edwards*, Rubicon, 1995.

Richards, Laura E., *Florence Nightingale: The Angel of the Crimea*, New York: Appleton, 1909.

Richards, Laura E., and Maud Howe Elliott, assisted by Florence Howe Hall, *Julia Ward Howe 1819–1910*, Boston: Houghton Mifflin, 1916.

Richards, Laura E. (ed.), 'Letters of Florence Nightingale', *Yale Review*, 24 (December 1934), 326–47.

Richards, Laura E., *Samuel Gridley Howe*, New York: D. Appleton-Century, 1935.

Rickards, E. C., *Felicia Skene of Oxford. A Memoir*, John Murray, 1902.

Roberts, Andrew, *Salisbury. Victorian Titan*, Weidenfeld & Nicolson, 1999.

Robinson, Jane, *Mary Seacole. The Charismatic Black Nurse Who Became a Heroine of the Crimea*, Constable, 2005.

Rosenberg, Charles E., 'Florence Nightingale on contagion: The hospital as moral universe', in *Explaining Epidemics and other Studies in the History of Medicine*, Cambridge: Cambridge University Press, 1992.

Ross, J. C., and J. Ross, *A Gifted Touch. A Biography of Agnes Jones*, West Sussex: Churchman Publishing, 1988.

Rossetti, Dante Gabriel, *The Correspondence of Dante Gabriel Rossetti*, ed. William E. Fredeman, Cambridge: D. S. Brewer, 2002.

Roxburgh, Ronald, 'Miss Nightingale and Miss Clough. Letters from the Crimea', *Victorian Studies*, 13 (1969), 71–89.

Royle, Trevor, *Crimea. The Great Crimean War 1854–1856*, Little, Brown, 1999.

Russell, W. H., *The British Expedition to the Crimea*, Routledge, 1858.

Samuel, Raphael, *Theatres of Memory. Volume 1: Past and Present in Contemporary Culture*, Verso, 1994.

Sattin, Anthony (ed.), *Letters from Egypt: A Journey on the Nile 1849–50*, Barrie & Jenkins, 1987.

Seacole, Mary, *Wonderful Adventures of Mrs Seacole in Many Lands*, introduction by William L. Andrews, Oxford: Oxford University Press, 1988.

Sen, P. R. (ed.), *Florence Nightingale's Indian Letters*, Calcutta: M. K. Sen, 1937.

Shepherd, John, *The Crimean Doctors. A History of the British Medical Services in the Crimean War*, 2 vols, Liverpool: Liverpool University Press, 1991.

Shirreff, Emily, *Intellectual Education and Its Influence on the Character and Happiness of Women*, John Parker, 1858.

Showalter, Elaine, 'Florence Nightingale's Feminist Complaint: Women, Religion, and Suggestions for Thought', *Signs*, 6 (1981), 395–412.

Showalter, Elaine, 'Miranda and Cassandra: The Discourse of the Feminist Intellectual', in *Tradition and the Talents of Women*, ed. F. Howe, Urbana: University of Illinois Press, 1991.

Shrimpton, Charles, *La Guerre d'Orient. L'Armée Anglaise et Miss Nightingale*, Paris: Galignani, 1864.

Skelley, Alan Ramsay, *The Victorian Army at Home. The Recruitment and Terms and Conditions of the British Regular, 1859–1899*, Croom Helm, 1977.

Small, Hugh, *Florence Nightingale: Avenging Angel*, Constable, 1998.

Smedley, Pat, 'Nightingale Nursing 1872–1890. The Practice Perspective', unpublished research paper.

Smith, F. B., *Florence Nightingale: Reputation and Power*, Croom Helm, 1982.

Smith, Julianne, '"A Noble Type of Good Heroic Womanhood"', *Nineteenth-Century Prose*, 26 (Spring 1999), 59–80.

Smith, Sydney, *Selected Letters of Sydney Smith*, ed. Nowell C. Smith, Oxford: Oxford University Press, 1981.

Snyder, Katherine V., 'Nofriani Unbound: The First Version of Florence Nightingale's "Cassandra"', *Victorian Literature and Culture*, 24 (1996), 251–88.

Sorabji, Cornelia, *India Calling. The Memories of Cornelia Sorabji, India's First Woman Barrister*, ed. Chandarn Lokugé, Oxford: Oxford University Press, 2001.

Soyer, Alexis, *A Culinary Campaign*, ed. M. Barthorp and E.Ray, Lewes: Southover Press, 1995.

Speirs, Edward M., *The Army and Society 1815–1914*, Longmans, 1980.

Spencer, Jenny, *Dramatic Strategies in the Plays of Edward Bond*, Cambridge: Cambridge University Press, 1992.

Spink, W. W., *The Nature of Brucellosis*, Minneapolis: University of Minnesota Press, 1956.

Stanley, A. P., *Memoirs of Edward and Catherine Stanley*, John Murray, 1880.

[Stanley, Mary], *Hospitals and Sisterhoods*, John Murray, 1854.

Stanmore, Lord, *Sidney Herbert. A Memoir*, 2 vols, John Murray, 1906.

Steegmuller, Francis (ed.), *Flaubert in Egypt. A Sensibility on Tour*, Michael Haag, 1983.

Stephen, Barbara, 'The Shores of Sheffield and the Offleys of Norton Hall', *Transactions of the Hunter Archaeological Society*, 5 (January 1938), 1–17.

[Stephen, Sarah], *Passages from the Life of a Daughter at Home*, Seeley, Burnside, 1845.

Stephen, Sir James, *Essays in Ecclesiastical Biography*, 4th edn, Longman, Green, Longman & Roberts, 1860.

Sticker, Anna (ed.), *Florence Nightingale: Curriculum Vitae*, Kaiserswerth: Diakoniewerth, 1954.

Stigler, Stephen M., *The History of Statistics. The Measurement of Uncertainty before 1900*, Cambridge, Mass.: Harvard University Press, 1986.

Stone, Richard, 'Florence Nightingale and Hospital Reform', in *Some British Empiricists in the Social Sciences 1650–1900*, Cambridge: Cambridge University Press, 1997.

Strachey, Lytton, *Eminent Victorians. The Definitive Edition*, foreword by Frances Partridge, introduction by Paul Levy, afterword on Florence Nightingale by Mark Bostridge, Continuum, 2002.

Strong, Rebecca, *Reminiscences*, Edinburgh: privately printed, 1935.

Sullivan, Mary C. (ed.), *The Friendship of Florence Nightingale and Mary Clare Moore*, Philadelphia: University of Pennsylvania Press, 1999.

Summers, Anne, *Angels and Citizens. British Women as Military Nurses 1854–1914*, Routledge & Kegan Paul, 1988.

Summers, Anne, *Female Lives, Moral States. Women, Religion and Public Life in Britain 1830–1900*, Newbury: Threshold Press.

Taylor, Fanny, *Eastern Hospitals and English Nurses. By a Lady Volunteer*, Hurst & Blackett, 1856.

Taylor, Jeremy, *Hospital and Asylum Architecture Design in England 1840–1914. Building for Health Care*, Mansell, 1991.

Terrot, Sarah Anne, *Nurse Sarah Anne: With Florence Nightingale at Scutari*, ed. Robert G. Richardson, John Murray, 1977.

The only and unabridged edition of the life of Miss Nightingale (The Heroine of European philanthropy; wherein is not only given a faithful biography of her charitable and humane life in England, but is also continued to the end of the war), Coulson, 1855.

Thompson, Paul, *William Butterfield*, Routledge & Kegan Paul, 1971.

Tooley, Sarah, *The Life of Florence Nightingale*. S. H. Bousefield, 1904.

Tuke, Margaret J., *A History of Bedford College for Women 1849–1937*, Oxford: Oxford University Press, 1939.

Twain, Mark, *Mark Twain's Letters*, ed. Edgar Marquess Branch et al., vol. 3, Berkeley: University of California Press, 2000.

Underhill, Evelyn, *Practical Mysticism. A Little Book for Normal People*, Dent, 1914.
Van der Peet, Rob, *The Nightingale Model of Nursing*, Edinburgh: Campion Press, 1995.
Verney, F. P., *Stone Edge*, Smith, Elder, 1868.
Verney, F. P., *Lettice Lisle*, Smith, Elder, 1870.
Verney, F. P., *The Grey Pool and Other Stories*, Simpkin & Marshall, 1891.
Verney, F. P., *Memoirs of the Verney Family during the Civil War*, ed. Margaret M. Verney, vols 1–2, Longmans, 1892.
Verney, Sir Harry C. W., 'The Perfect Aunt: F. N. 1820–1910', *Journal of the Royal Army Medical Corps*, 107 (January 1961), 8–10.
Vicinus, Martha, *Independent Women. Work and Community for Single Women 1850–1920*, Virago, 1985.
Vicinus, Martha, and Bea Nergaard (eds), *Ever Yours, Florence Nightingale. Selected Letters*, Virago, 1989.
Vicinus, Martha, 'Tactful Organizing and Executive Power: Biographies of Florence Nightingale for Girls', in *Telling Lives in Science. Essays on Scientific Biography*, ed. Michael Shortland and Richard Yeo, Cambridge: Cambridge University Press, 1996.
Wake, Roy, *The Nightingale Training School 1860–1996*, Haggerston Press, 1998.
Webb, Beatrice, *The Diaries of Beatrice Webb*, ed. Norman and Jeanne MacKenzie, one-vol. abridgement, Virago, 2000.
Webb, R. K., *Harriet Martineau. A Radical Victorian*, Heinemann, 1960.
Wells, S. R., *New System of Physiognomy*, New York: Fowler & Wells, 1866.
Widerquist, JoAnn G., 'The Spirituality of Florence Nightingale', *Nursing Research Record*, 41 (1992), 49–55.
Widerquist, JoAnn G., ' "Dearest Friend", The Correspondence of Colleagues Florence Nightingale and Mary Jones', *Nursing History Review*, 2 (1993), 25–42.
Widerquist, JoAnn G., 'Sanitary Reform and Nursing. Edwin Chadwick and Florence Nightingale', *Nursing History Review*, 5 (1997), 149–60.
Wieslander, Henning, 'Florence Nightingale och Hennes Svenska Ungdomsväninna', *Samfundet Orebro stadts och länsbiblioteks vänner*, Meddlenade, 12, 12–75.
Wilkinson, John, *Modern Egypt and Thebes*, 2 vols, John Murray, 1843.
Williams, Gary, *Hungry Heart. The Literary Emergence of Julia Ward Howe*, Amherst: University of Massachusetts Press, 1999.
Williams, Perry, 'Religion, respectability and the origins of the modern nurse', in Roger French and Andrew Wear, *British Medicine in an Age of Reform*, Routledge, 1991.
Wood, Miriam, 'Thomas Nightingale of Lea. Lead Merchant 1665/6–1735', *Derbyshire Miscellany*, 11 (1987), 81–7.
Woolf, Virginia, *The Letters of Virginia Woolf*, ed. Nigel Nicolson, vol. 2, Hogarth Press, 1976.
Woolf, Virginia, *Women and Fiction*, ed. S. P. Rosenbaum, Shakespeare Head, 1992.
Worboys, Michael, *Spreading Germs. Disease Theories and Medical Practice in Britain, 1865–1900*, Cambridge: Cambridge University Press, 2000.
Young, D. A. B., 'Florence Nightingale's fever', *British Medical Journal*, 311 (23 December 1995), 1697–1700.

Notes

ABBREVIATIONS

BJ   Benjamin Jowett
Cook   Sir Edward Cook, *The Life of Florence Nightingale*, 2 vols: I. 1820–1861;
              II. 1862–1910, Macmillan, 1913.
CW   *The Collected Works of Florence Nightingale*, ed. Lynn McDonald, Ontario:
              Wilfred Laurier University Press, 2001–; 10 vols to date: 1. *An Introduction
              to Her Life and Family*; 2. *Spiritual Journey*; 3. *Theology*; 4. *Mysticism and
              Eastern Religions* (ed. Gérard Vallée); 5. *Society and Politics*; 6. *Public
              Health*; 7. *European Travels*; 8. *Women*; 9. *Health in India* (ed. Gérard
              Vallée); 10. *Social Change in India* (ed. Gérard Vallée).
FN   Florence Nightingale.
FN Museum   Florence Nightingale Museum, London.
FaN   Fanny Nightingale.
Goldie   *'I Have Done My Duty': Florence Nightingale in the Crimean War, 1854–56*,
              ed. Sue M. Goldie, Manchester: Manchester University Press, 1987.
Jowett   *Dear Miss Nightingale. A Selection of Benjamin Jowett's Letters 1860–1893*,
Letters   ed. E. V. Quinn and J. M. Prest, Oxford: Clarendon Press, 1987.
'Memoir'   Unpublished draft memoir of Florence Nightingale, to the outbreak of the
              Crimean War, by Parthenope Nightingale, *c.* 1857. Claydon 389.
O'Malley   I. B. O'Malley, *Florence Nightingale 1820–1856: A Study of Her Life Down
              to the End of the Crimean War*, Thornton Butterworth, 1931.
PN   Parthenope Nightingale (later Verney).
PRO   Public Record Office (now part of the National Archives).
WEN   William Nightingale.
W-S   Cecil Woodham-Smith, *Florence Nightingale*, Constable, 1950.

The indispensable guide to the 200 or so books, pamphlets and articles that make up Florence
Nightingale's own published writings is *A Bio-Bibliography of Florence Nightingale*, compiled by W. J. Bishop, and completed by Sue Goldie (Dawsons, 1962). Where possible, I
have used the texts printed in the *Collected Works*. Where these are not yet available, I have
used other editions listed in the select bibliography.

MAJOR ARCHIVAL SOURCES

BL   British Library Additional Manuscripts. Nightingale Papers. Donated to the
              library in three main tranches of material: 1) Add MSS 43393–43403; 2)
              45750–45849; 3) 47714–47767. There have been smaller supplementary

	gifts and purchases since. See *British Museum Quarterly*, XV (1941–50), 28.
Claydon	Nightingale Papers at Claydon House, Buckinghamshire. Numbers refer to the bundles in which Margaret, Lady Verney, and her son, Sir Harry C. W. Verney, originally arranged the papers, and in which they are still kept. The collection falls into three parts: 1) Family papers inherited by Parthenope, Lady Verney, including the extensive correspondence of her parents William and Fanny Nightingale with members of the Smith and Shore families. 2) Letters from Florence Nightingale to her family. 3) Letters about Florence Nightingale from members of her family. A checklist is available at the Wellcome Library in London.
CUL	Papers of William Smith MP and the Smith family. Cambridge University Library Add. MS 7621.
LMA	London Metropolitan Archives. Collections of letters written by or to Florence Nightingale deposited by the Florence Nightingale Museum Trust and the Nightingale Fund Council.
Verney	Verney Family Papers at Claydon House, Buckinghamshire.
Wellcome	Florence Nightingale material in the Wellcome Library for the History and Understanding of Medicine, Euston Road, London. Includes photocopies of Florence Nightingale's letters at Claydon (8991–9015), other Claydon material by Florence Nightingale (9016–9029), and a selection of material at Claydon by persons other than Florence Nightingale (9030–9082). Also copies of Nightingale material held at repositories throughout the world (9083–9109), and other miscellaneous Nightingale letters and papers.

Other primary sources are detailed in the notes. I have used printed texts of Florence Nightingale's letters where available, but have also relied on my own transcriptions, most notably for material in the British Library and the Wellcome Library.

Epigraph Mary Mohl to PN, 16 February [1853]. Claydon 240.

PROLOGUE

p. xix As the cortège: Descriptions of FN's funeral in *The Nursing Times*, 27 August 1910; *The Times*, 22 August 1910; *Daily Graphic*, 22 August 1910.

'**Though there was no suffering':** Elizabeth Bosanquet to Margaret Verney, 24 September 1910. Claydon 363.

Irene Cooper Willis: Cooper Willis, *Florence Nightingale*, 246.

p. xx wish for a private funeral: Expressed in FN's will. CW1, 858.

presence of photographers and cameramen: A short 35mm film was made of FN's funeral procession by the Warwick Trading Company, though its current whereabouts are unknown. See *The British Film Catalogue*, 2, 164. There are photographs in Hampshire Record Office.

'**with the universal desire . . . one would have wished':** Louis Shore Nightingale to Margaret Verney, 23 August 1910. Claydon 363.

Private John Kneller: Reported in the *Nursing Times*, 27 August 1910, 706.

p. xxi the historian Raphael Samuel: Samuel, *Theatres of Memory*, 27.

'**Has there':** Housman, *The Great Victorians*, 357.

Nightingale cradle: A design for one of these is in the FN Museum.

'**acting Florence Nightingale':** Mark Twain, to Olivia Langdon, 17/18 May 1869, *Mark Twain's Letters*, 240.

tops polls: For instance, see *The Times*, 8 January 2004.

p. xxii 'Good public!': FN, Note [1857]. BL 43402/178. CW5, 232.

David Young: Young, 'Florence Nightingale's fever'.

p. xxiii 'without irreverence': FN to Margaret Verney, 2 December 1885. Wellcome 9010/123. *CWI*, 654.

'Long before Thatcher': Cannadine, *History in Our Time*, 206.

'Might we not': FN to Margaret Verney, 2 January 1895. Wellcome 9015/13.

CHAPTER I: THE RIDICULOUS NAME
OF NIGHTINGALE

p. 3 Villa La Colombaia: Parts of the villa, including the northern tower, date back to the fifteenth century, with additions in the course of the next 200 years. Since 1957 the villa has belonged to a religious order of sisters, the Adorers of the Blood of Christ. A plaque on the wall overlooking the Via di Marignolle commemorates the villa as FN's birthplace. A monument (by I. W. Sargent) and mural tablet to FN in the first cloister of the Franciscan church of Santa Croce also records her association with the city.

'so rumbustical': WEN to Ben Smith, 12 April 1820. CUL 7621/361.

p. 4 I found a house': Elizabeth Barrett Browning, *Aurora Leigh* (1857), ed. Reynolds, Book Seven, lines 515–6, 476.

'inside piano stools': Smith, *Florence Nightingale*, 200.

'to cover Australia': FN to Margaret Verney, 27 May 1895. Wellcome 9014/45.

p. 5 smaller holdings: For a preliminary list of these, see *CWI*, 870–73.

significant gaps: Among the more regrettable of these is the absence of the extensive correspondence between the Mohls and FN, destroyed in 1946 by FN's cousin Rosalind Vaughan Nash. Only six letters were preserved in the BL collection, though another extensive set of letters is today in the Woodward Biomedical Library. According to Vaughan Nash (BL 46385/22), 'There was much repetition & the interest of the letters had much diminished.' But one suspects that the letters may have been destroyed because they were critical of members of FN's family. Vaughan Nash had already admitted to feeling guilty about the destruction of some of FN's papers following the publication of Cook's biography. In a letter to Joan Bonham Carter of 10 August 1931 (BL 46385/95), Vaughan Nash confessed that 'More should be kept than we decided on keeping when we first began to destroy papers, in the belief that Cook's biography was final.'

during the Second World War: Goldie, Introduction to *A Calendar of the Letters of Florence Nightingale*, 10.

'& after my death': FN to PN, n.d., [August 1853]. Wellcome 8994/41.

'I have alas!': FN to Henry Manning, 25 February 1860. BL 45797/102.

Nightingale's will: Reprinted in *CWI*, 852–61.

p. 6 'I earnestly wish': FN to WEN, 2 February 1862. BL 45790/247.

'Well might Sir Cornwall Lewis': FN to Margaret Verney, 23 April 1896. Wellcome 9015/71.

Flora Masson remembered: Masson, *Victorians All*, 121.

Footnote: Margaret Verney reported that PN had been 'most anxious' that these family letters should never be mixed up with FN's papers, 'or be given her', because FN might destroy them. After PN's death in 1890, Sir Harry Verney, PN's widower, had locked them up (Margaret Verney to Louis Shore Nightingale, 13 February 1914. BL 72832A/94). Yet it is clear that while sorting PN's papers at Claydon after her death, Margaret Verney told FN of her discoveries of 'packets of letters' belonging to the Nightingale parents. See M. M. Verney, 'Talks with Miss Nightingale in the Blue Room at Claydon, October 1890'. Claydon 390.

'Experience appears': Vicinus and Nergaard, eds, *Ever Yours, Florence Nightingale*, 6.

p. 7 'La Vie de Florence Rossignol': This has disappeared since O'Malley used it extensively in her first chapter. Three pages from another of FN's early journals, describing a visit to Chatsworth and Haddon Hall, in 1828, with her cousin Henry Nicholson, are at Claydon

461. For a description of the occasion, see FN to Sarah Christie [1828]. Wellcome 8991/
10.

'I think one's feelings' Quoted in O'Malley, 88.

'That power': FN, Diary, 7–8 May, 1850. Calabria (ed.), *Florence Nightingale in Egypt and Greece*, 59.

'confoundedly cheap': FN to Mary Mohl, 7 February [1851] BL 43397/303. *CW8*, 556.

'firm and beautiful': Harriet Martineau to Fanny Wedgwood, 13 March 1860, *Harriet Martineau's Letters to Fanny Wedgwood*, 190.

'dash off': William J. Bishop, 'Florence Nightingale's Message for Today', in Hebert, *Florence Nightingale: Saint, Reformer or Rebel?*, 197.

p. 8 Jowett once chastised her: BJ to FN, 11 August [1874], *Jowett Letters*, 261.

'the ruin of the family': Julia Smith to WEN, 2 June 1819. Claydon 4.

p. 9 William Smith: For an account of Smith's political career, see Davis, *Dissent in Politics*. See also Handley and Lake, *Progress By Persuasion*, for an authoritative account of Smith's family life.

'no system': *The Parliamentary History of Great Britain*, XXXIII, 583.

'as if to prove': Stephen, *Essays in Ecclesiastical Biography*, 543–4.

financial aid: In commemoration of Samuel Smith's kindness to Flora Macdonald, a needlecase made by her and comprising pieces of her own gown was presented to the Smith family by Macdonald's daughter, Mrs Macleod, in 1809. It is on show today at Claydon House.

p. 10 'future destination': Samuel Smith to William Smith, 17 October 1769. Quoted in Davis, *Dissent in Politics*, 6.

p. 11 'the open sore of the world': 'Addresses to Probationers', 26 May 1875, in *Florence Nightingale to Her Nurses*, 93. FN was quoting the words of David Livingstone.

childhood scrapbooks: From 1827. Claydon 27.

'prosperous and pious': The phrase is E. M. Forster's, from his *Marianne Thornton*, 23.

ties with the Thornton family: The connection continued among Smith's children and grandchildren. Marianne Thornton, Henry's daughter, first met FN as a baby in Paris on her way back to England with her parents, in late 1820. Verney 10/317 preserves Marianne Thornton's later correspondence with PN.

p. 12 'to procure': William Smith to WEN, n.d. [mid-1820s]. CUL 7621/141.

'heart-stirring laughter': Stephen, *Essays in Ecclesiastical Biography*, 528.

Essex Street Chapel: The chapel was built for Belsham's predecessor, Theophilus Lindsey, who resigned from the Church of England and conducted his first service using a Unitarian revision of the Book of Common Prayer in April 1774. Today Essex Hall, the headquarters of the General Assembly of Unitarian and Christian Churches, stands on the site of the Essex Street Chapel in London WC2.

Unitarianism: For a clear introduction to Unitarianism at this date, see Webb, *Harriet Martineau*, 65–90.

Joseph Priestley: Priestley fled to America. William Smith attended his farewell sermon at Hackney in 1794.

'the head of the Unitarian Church': Quoted in Davis, *Dissent in Politics*, 211.

'the dissenting king': Sydney Smith to Francis Jeffrey, April 1820, *Selected Letters of Sydney Smith*, 94–5. A contemporary squib, quoted in the *Dictionary of National Biography*, lampooned William Smith as a supporter of worthy causes: 'At length, when the candles burn low in their sockets,/Up gets William Smith with his hands in his pockets,/On a course of morality fearlessly enters,/With all the opinions of all the dissenters.'

p. 13 'when no chapel': Anonymous obituary of William Smith. Claydon 2.

Frances was deeply religious: Unlike her husband, Frances Smith appears never to have become a Unitarian, remaining true to her parents' Presbyterian faith. Her taste for religious disputation led Thomas Belsham to dedicate to her his *Review of Mr Wilberforce's Treatise, entitled A Practical View of the Prevailing Religious System of Professed Christians. In letters to a Lady*, London: J. Johnson, 1798.

twelve children: 'Smith Pedigree'. CUL 7621/73. Fanny was born at Clapham on 28 February 1788. A neighbour of the Smiths, paying an evening visit to Parndon in the summer of 1808 noted: 'He [William Smith] is a very sensible, pleasant man, and she is not unentertaining and seems a really good sort of woman. She is a little of a *blue-stocking*, but really not unpleasant. They have ten children, five of each sort, and we were introduced to Patty's, Joanna's, Julia's, Octavia's [sic] etc., etc., till I thought there was no end of them.' (Mrs Warenne Blake, *An Irish Beauty of the Regency*, 106).

Parndon Hall: Also known as The Mount, the house was demolished in 1832. All that remains today is part of the original wall beside the old road from Harlow to Royden.

6 Park Street: Now 16 Queen Anne's Gate, the offices of the Council for Religious Liberty.

art collection: 'List of pictures at 6 Park Street', Verney 10/51. Smith was able to take advantage of the sale of several large French aristocratic collections as a result of the French Revolution. His copy of *Mrs Siddons* is today in the Huntingdon Art Collection in the United States.

p. 14 '. . . Horses, Pictures': Patty Smith to FaN, 14 December 1842. Wellcome 9038/8.

'where the cotton': Frances Smith, 'Various Tours', I, 121. CUL 7621/6.

'Music, French': Quoted by Barbara Stephen, unpublished 'Family History of the Smiths', chapter X, 9. CUL 7621/71. The Smiths were advised on their history reading by the poet and essayist Anna Barbauld.

'Julia dwells much': Frances Smith to FaN, n.d. [1812]. Claydon 6.

'You are in general': Frances Smith to Octavius Smith, 14 August 1804. Claydon 2.

p. 15 'very much affected': FaN, Diary, 11 May 1812. CUL 7621/15.

Patty could remember: Both Patty and Julia left memoirs uncompleted at their deaths (CUL 7621/13). For Patty's memories, see also Stephen, 'Family History', chapter V.

'crush at Carleton House': Patty Smith to FaN, 27 June 1811. Claydon 5.

'little dark man': Julia Smith, quoted in Stephen, 'Family History', chapter X.

'a most extraordinary man': From the diary of Joanna Smith, August 1806, quoted in Stephen, 'Family History', chapter X.

'She is daily': Frances Smith to William Smith, n.d. [1809?]. CUL 7621/241.

'she was very much': Anne Smith to Patty Smith, 24 April 1804. Quoted in Stephen, 'Family History', 16.

'a good deal of shopping': FaN, Diary, 1 February 1812. Claydon 401.

p. 16 'the poor children': FaN, Diary, 10 December 1812. Claydon 401.

'I considered him': Ben Smith to FaN, [n.d.]. Claydon 15.

'very thoughtless': James, Earl of Caithness, to William Smith, 2 March 1816. Claydon 10.

'highly improper': Frances Smith to FaN, 16 March 1816. Claydon 10.

'look as well': William Smith to FaN, 20 March 1816. Claydon 10. Sinclair had married Elizabeth Tritton by 1818. He reached the rank of Lieutenant-Colonel in the army and died in 1856.

p. 17 The Shores: See Stephen, 'The Shores of Sheffield and the Offleys of Norton Hall'.

'a lad of about ten': Quoted in Stephen, 'Family History', chapter VII, 6.

p. 18 profits of lead and cotton: The Nightingales operated the largest lead-smelting works in the county. The Cow Hay smelting mills at Lea were owned by Thomas Nightingale (1666–1735) in partnership with John Spateman. Nightingale's interests were taken over by his second son, Peter (1704–63), who built a new cupola at the Cow Hay mill in the 1740s. His son, known as 'Mad Peter' (1736–1803), combined these lead-smelting interests with those of cotton. In 1783, he built a cotton-spinning mill in association with Thomas Smedley (probably at the intersection of the Lea Brook and Littlemoor Brook). Smedley later established the hosiery manufacturing business which passed to his son John and exists to this day at Lea Mills. Gladwyn, *A History of Derbyshire*, vol.4, 1432, 1492, 1506. Records of the Nightingale Estates, from the seventeenth century onwards, are at the Derbyshire Record Office (D 1575). See also Wood, 'Thomas Nightingale of Lea'.

thin and lanky: 'rather thin and long, of the Shore make', as FN described her cousin Bertha Smith. FN to PN, [postmarked 19 February 1837]. Wellcome 8991/88.

born in Sheffield: WEN was baptized at the Upper Chapel (Presbyterian), Norfolk Street, Sheffield, on 6 March 1794. PRO RG4/3207 f47RH.

Trinity College, Cambridge: For details of WEN's career at Trinity, see *Trinity College, Admissions*. Vol. IV, 1801–1850, edited by W. W. Rouse Ball and J. A. Venn, London: Macmillan, 77, and *Alumni Cantabrigienses*, Cambridge, 1953, 501. The evidence of the Head Lecturer's Book, 1801–1900, suggests that either WEN was below standard or, more probably, he was something of a dilettante. In 1811, he was recorded in the fifth class; in 1812 in the sixth (out of a possible eight or nine classes). Trinity College, Cambridge Archives.

'a term or two': *Memoirs of a Highland Lady. The Autobiography of Elizabeth Grant of Rothiemurchus*, 298. See the draft of an account of WEN's life by PN, *c.* 1874. Claydon 314.

Edinburgh University: Arts and Medical matriculation listings.

p. 19 **'assume and take upon'**: PRO PROB 11/1399 f66RH. At the same time WEN requested 'Armorial Ensigns duly assigned to be borne by him and Descendants by the said Name of Nightingale . . .'. Claydon 213.

'the ridiculous name': *Memoirs of a Highland Lady*, 298.

Stray references: For instance, 'Shore is still with us . . .'. Frances Smith to Patty Smith, 2 August 1811. CUL 7621/276.

'affectionate correspondence': Ben Smith to FaN, [April 1817]. Claydon 16.

'I am always saying': William Shore to FaN, [May 1818]. Claydon 11.

'May God': Frances Smith to FaN, 2 June 1818. Claydon 12.

'thinks Nightingale': Julia Smith to Patty Smith, 16 June 1818. Claydon 4.

They were married: Westminster City Archives 61 m/f.

'roaring': Julia Smith to FaN, [June 1818]. Claydon 12.

p. 20 **'Don't you think'**: William Shore to WEN, 2 June 1818. Claydon 12.

Kynsham Court: Sometimes spelt Kinsham, the house still stands today. For a description, see MacCarthy, *Byron. Life and Legend*, 190–91.

had cried so much: M. M. Verney, 'Talks with Miss Nightingale in the Blue Room at Claydon, October 1890'. Claydon 390.

'. . . It was a little disappointment': Frances Gale to Joanna Carter, 23 April 1819. Claydon 214.

p. 21 **'As for the sex'**: William Smith to WEN & FaN, 11 May 1819. Claydon 2.

'what a hard name': 'Journal of my little life – Frances Parthenope Nightingale' (by FaN). 28 May 1819. Claydon 214.

'quite a <u>Buty</u>': William Smith to WEN, 18 May 1819. Claydon 2.

'The cruelty': WEN to Joanna Carter, 13 May 1819. CUL 7621/405.

'a cargo of bad news': Julia Smith to FaN, 11 May 1819. Claydon 4.

'torment': Julia Smith to FaN, 30 July 1819. Claydon 4.

'my poor mother': Julia Smith to WEN, 2 June 1819. Claydon 4.

'so injured': FaN to Anne Nicholson, [November 1819]. Claydon 100.

'Villa called Colombaja': Lease dated 23 March 1820. Claydon 214.

wetnurse: Contract for Umiliana Pistelli as wet nurse. Claydon 20.

p. 22 **Dr Williams's Library**: Established in 1742 to give the records of non-conformist births and baptisms the same standing as Anglican registers.

recorded Florence's birth: PRO RG5/83 f57.

the size of a family: FN, BL 45839/119.

CHAPTER 2: POP AND FLO

p. 23 'a pretty piquante': Julia Smith, 'Recollections', CUL 7261/13.

p. 25 'one seems on the Devil's pinnacle': Mrs Gaskell to Catherine Winkworth, [11–14 October 1854], *The Letters of Mrs Gaskell*, 307–8.

'A perfect 3 months': WEN to FaN, 17 January 1832. Claydon 26.

'my solace': WEN to FaN, [?1847]. Claydon 73.

'the young squire': According to PN's account in her 'Memoir'.

p. 26 'scratting': For instance, CW3, 344.

'true but modest . . . world': Croston, *A Pilgrimage to the Home of Florence Nightingale*, 4, 22.

'a large number': Jewitt, *A Stroll to Lea Hurst*, 14. Jewitt's scrapbook of material relating to FN's life is in the Derby Local Studies Library.

Footnote: FaN, Diary, 27 July 1846. Claydon 67.

p. 27 'the new phase of Methodism': WEN to FaN, [postmarked 30 July 1851]. Claydon 69.

'Poor Fanny': Julia Smith to [?] Joanna Bonham Carter, [n.d.], CUL 7261/455.

'a capital and convenient': Quoted in *History of Embley*, 11. A tithe map (PRO IR 30/31/268) shows that WEN was the sole landowner in East Wellow.

'This looks': Patty Smith to Eliza [?], 7 July 1825, CUL 7621/324.

p. 28 'Mr N.': Lady Palmerston to FaN, [n.d.]. Verney 10/167.

p. 29 'multitudinous aunts': PN to FaN, [1840s]. Claydon 83.

'great clan of cousins': 'Memoir'.

'What energy': Miss Aiken to Lady Coltman, 31 October 1854. Claydon 290.

'hard, cold': Jane Carlyle, *The Collected Letters of Thomas and Jane Welsh Carlyle*, 219.

'angry with his son . . . himself': M. M. Verney, 'Talks with Miss Nightingale in the Blue Room at Claydon, October 1890'. Claydon 390.

p. 30 'in thralldom': Frances Smith to FaN, 6 November 1832. Claydon 26.

'was such a large': M. M. Verney, 'Talks with Miss Nightingale . . .' Claydon 390.

'the tabooed family': This phrase was coined by George Eliot. *The George Eliot Letters*, 2, 45.

probably corresponded: No letters between FN and Barbara Bodichon have come to light, though CW8, 858 gives the impression that correspondence between them was not unknown. See also FN to Louisa Shore Smith, 12 June 1891 (CUL 7621/70), written on Bodichon's death.

'very good friends': Mai Smith to FaN, [1830s]. Claydon 26.

'miserable education': Mai Smith to FaN, [1830s]. Claydon 26.

'She's got an oddness': FaN, Note. Claydon 401.

'with all her might': 'Memoir'.

'as precious': Mai Smith to FaN, [n.d.]. Claydon 95.

p. 31 'the numbers of my kind': FN to WEN, 26 October 1850. BL45790/107. CW1, 232–3.

'A Chronology': BL 72836A. It covers the years 1781–1864.

'a troublesome companion': Ben Smith to FaN, 27 March 1818. Claydon 198.

'a place': Patty Smith to FaN, [n.d.] Claydon 303.

'Stormy Ju': FN to FaN, [1845]. Wellcome 8992/111.

p. 32 'the most generous': Henry Crabb Robinson, 7 October 1848. Quoted in Tuke, *A History of Bedford College for Women*, 43–4.

'We children': M. M. Verney, 'Talks with Miss Nightingale . . .' Claydon 390.

earliest surviving letter: FN to Mary Shore, 14 October 1827. Wellcome 8991/1. CW1, 410.

p. 33 'two leopards': FN to Mary Shore, 2 July [1828]. Wellcome 8991/9. CW1, 411.

'Take any word': FN to PN, 4 April [1828]. Wellcome 8991/8. CW1, 280.

'large as half a tea tray': FN to PN, [postmarked 8 November 1833]. Wellcome 8991/67. *CW*1, 282.

'She does not look': FN to Mary Shore, 30 March [?] 1830. Wellcome 8991/6. *CW*1, 412.

coins: FN's collection of thirty-eight coins is at the FN Museum (0721). It contains examples of English Kings and Queens, as well as of Emperors of Rome, and of Ptolemy III of Egypt.

Woodarch's: FN's copy of this book, given to her by Marianne Nicholson, is in the FN Museum (0031). The FN Museum also has a collection of FN's shells (0018), as does Nottingham University.

'Answer me': FN to Mary Shore, 30 March [1828]. Wellcome 8991/6. *CW*1, 412.

'Please give me an answer': FN to Mai Smith, [n.d.]. Wellcome 8991/12.

'Why don't you': FN to PN, 29 March [1830]. Wellcome 8991/49. *CW*1, 281.

p. 34 'overflowing with fun': 'Memoir'.

'When the two': 'Memoir'.

'a little more yielding': FN to FaN, 13 March [1830]. Wellcome 8991/47.

'more good-natured': FN to FaN, 24 February [1830]. Wellcome 8991/44.

'smelling-bottle': FN to FaN, 14 December 1828. Wellcome 8991/18.

writing slate: Now in the FN Museum (0079).

'I promise': FN to FaN, [January 1830]. Wellcome 8991/42. *CW*1, 109.

Arnaud Berquin's: Oliver, 'The Shore Smith Library', 527.

p. 35 childhood library: A collection of FN's childhood books is preserved in the Osborne Collection at Toronto Public Library.

'the religious instruction': FaN to Sara Christie, [?1827]. Claydon 7.

'has not shown': FaN to Sara Christie, [?1827]. Claydon 7.

p. 36 conundrum that Florence wrestled with: For instance, in 1872, following the appearance of an article on 'Blood Relationships' by the geneticist Francis Galton, in the journal *Nature*, FN commented to Mai Smith, on 30 August 1872, that 'You and I have often discussed the extraordinary variety there is between sisters or between brothers born under almost exactly the same circumstances, specifying for want of a better, the difference between my sister & me' (BL 45793/219).

'I find so much': Emily Taylor to FaN, 24 November 1830. Claydon 240. Taylor was a hymn writer, and the founder of a school which emphasized the teaching of singing.

'I do figures': FN to FaN, [1828]. Wellcome 8991/10.

'till . . . I had the spirit': Quoted in O'Malley, 25–6.

'self-love': Sara Christie to FaN, 10 February 1831. Claydon 240.

'a voluble': 'Memoir'.

'She does not care': Joanna Bonham Carter to FaN, [1830]. Claydon 26.

'I do not like': Emily Taylor to FaN, 14 September [1830]. Claydon 240.

p. 37 'operate upon them': Emily Taylor to FaN, 24 November [1831]. Claydon 240.

'no taste': FaN to Emily Taylor, [1831]. Claydon 240.

'She was just': FN, 'Lebenslauf', 24 July 1851. *CW*1, 90.

tragic news: Sara Collmann, née Christie, was buried, on 4 February 1832, in the graveyard of Hampstead Parish Church, in north London.

'cultivation of my intellect': FN, 'Lebenslauf', *CW*1, 90.

Florence imagined running away: FN, Draft Novel, BL 45839/34. *CW*8, 114.

p. 38 she came to the conclusion: FN to BJ, [June 1869], *Jowett Letters*, 168.

'without covering': M. M. Verney, 'Talks with Miss Nightingale . . .' Claydon 390.

commonplace book: BL 45848.

'My father': FN to Rosalind Vaughan Nash, [?] July 1898. BL 45795/228.

p. 39 'Warrington Smyth': *Journals of Caroline Fox*, 12 June 1857, 224–5.

'worked patiently': 'Memoir'.

'not the means': WEN to PN [?1835]. Claydon 354.

'I sometimes': WEN to PN, 25 April 1835. Claydon 354.

p. 40 'Mama went': FN to Henry Nicholson, [after 14 January 1829]. Wellcome 8991/22. CW1, 462.

'very fine countenance': Hawthorne, *English Notebooks*, June 1856–May 1857, 80–81.

Fanny's pocket diaries: Claydon 401.

p. 41 'in trade': Patty Smith to FaN, 14 June 1859. Claydon 89.

'trimmings and tassles': John Dunn to WEN, 14 February 1829. Claydon 19.

'a most excellent manager': FN to [?] Julia Smith, 3 October 1871. BL 728832A/77.

'a kind of conscience quieter': FN, Note, BL 45801/5. CW5, 259.

A coffee house: J. Whitty to FaN, 27 February 1844. Claydon 28.

p. 42 '1100 of the most wretched': FaN, Diary, 10 April 1840. Claydon 104.

'habit of general derangement': WEN to FaN, 7 June 1830. Claydon 26.

'perfectly at your Highness's service': WEN to FaN, 3 June 1830. Claydon 26.

'a better husband': FN to [?] WEN, [1870]. Wellcome 9004/50. CW1, 196.

'be at the home': FN to [?] Julia Smith, 3 October 1871. BL 728832A/77.

'perambulations': WEN to FaN, [?1847]. Claydon 73.

p. 43 'buying shells': PN to FaN, [1834]. Claydon 29.

'our quiet little world': FN to FaN, [1834]. Wellcome 8991/73. CW5, 331.

'WEN MP': PN to WEN, [1834]. Claydon 29.

'We must win': WEN to FaN, [1834]. Claydon 30.

'And this Nightingale': Election Bill, 'The Nightingale'. Claydon 29.

p. 44 'Flo's lively feelings': WEN to FaN, [1834]. Claydon 30.

'information for the Wilberforces': Patty Smith to FaN, 24 November 1853. Claydon 284.

Fanny's journal: 24 April 1840. Claydon 104.

'a great man . . . no governess': FN to FaN, [1834]. Wellcome 8991/73. CW5, 332.

'Books, Books, Books': WEN to FaN, 20 January 1842. Claydon 23.

'for promoting the purity': Claydon 27.

p. 45 'the habit of his life . . . to look after': FN, Note, 7 January 1851, BL 43402/64–5. CW1, 97.

a degree of contempt: FN later criticized her father's 'sluggishness of character & impatience of mind . . .' (BL 728832A/77). A member of the Clough family recalled that, in middle age, 'She was not kind to Uncle N., twitted him with not having helped her [to escape from the confines of family life]. She didn't care for his scrappy sort of metaphysical conversation.' (BL 728832A/97).

'13 dolls': Mrs Gaskell to Emily Shaen, [27 October 1854], *Further Letters of Mrs Gaskell*, 113–14.

'when she had': 'Memoir'.

'to magnify': Cook I, 13.

p. 46 'No story': *The Nation*, 21 March 1908, 903.

'his pleasure grounds': FN to FaN, 19 January 1845. Wellcome 8992/73. CW1, 120.

'The Constance': Giffard, *Constance and 'Cap'*, 31. Giffard came to the Burlington Hotel, where FN was living in 1860–61, to read his 'most touching' tale to WEN and Mai Smith. Mai Smith to FaN, [c. 1860]. Wellcome 9049/33.

p. 47 'a sort of mysterious': FN to Dr Murdoch, December [1889]. BL 45809/235 [typed copy]. CW5, 822. In a letter to 'Uncle Toby' of the Dicky Bird Society, published in *Newcastle Chronicle's Weekly Supplement*, 16 February 1895, FN gave sound practical advice on the feeding of birds during the winter months, and protested against the destruction of certain species.

nineteenth-century tradition: See Vicinus, 'Tactful Organizing and Executive Power'. In his retelling, Lytton Strachey obscured the fact that Cap was a working dog by transforming him into one of FN's pets.

in some versions becoming entangled: For example, Adams and Foster, *Heroines of Modern Progress*, 120.

copies of which: *The Nation*, 21 March 1908, 903.

'the creeper-covered': *Morning Post*, 22 August 1910. According to this report, the shepherd's descendants were called Snellgrove.

'her special tendency': *Nursing-Times*, 20 August 1910, 683.

'the first idea': FN, 'Lebenslauf', CW1, 90.

p. 48 '16 grains': Cook I, 14.

'Such a dear kind boy!': FN to Miss Brydges, [June 1829]. Wellcome 8991/30. CW1, 428.

'made a good night': FN to Mai Smith, 16 May [1829]. Wellcome 8991/27.

'His complaint': FN to Miss Brydges, [June 1829]. Wellcome 8991/30. CW1, 428.

p. 49 'a baby of her own': Quoted in O'Malley, 35.

'Dear Flo': FaN to WEN, [February 1836]. Claydon 38.

'thought & reflection': Mai Smith to FaN, [postmarked 21 April 1836]. Claydon 38.

'every woman': FN, Preface to *Notes on Nursing: What It Is and What It Is Not*. CW6, 30 (1861 edition).

Fanny's letters: And also the letters to FaN from her aunt Maria Coape, written in the 1830s, while she was staying at Lea Hurst, which demonstrate the Nightingale family's involvement in the care of the local sick. Claydon 15.

entry for May 1830: Quoted in O'Malley, 33.

p. 50 'she was often missing': Mrs Gaskell to Catherine Winkworth, [11–14 October 1854], *The Letters of Mrs Gaskell*, 306.

'Flo has been very busy': PN to Mary Shore, [postmarked July 1836].

'when as a girl': *Lancet* (1860), i, 634.

Florence's insistence: Hilary Bonham Carter to FaN, [1860]. Claydon 37.

'the general chorus': FaN to PN, [postmarked 28 January 1837]. Claydon 31.

'the agitation': FN to PN, [postmarked 30 January 1837]. Claydon 354.

'Your merry tidings': FN to PN, [1837]. Claydon 31.

p. 51 'nurse, governess': FN to PN, 12 February 1837. Wellcome 8991/86.

'I have papers': FN, *Suggestions for Thought*, II, 26. On prayer, see also Calabria and Macrae (eds.), *Suggestions for Thought . . . Selections and Commentaries*, 126–9.

p. 52 '2 men to row us': FN to FaN, 12 July 1830. Wellcome 8991/55.

'a very good sermon': FN to FaN, 19 May 1832. Wellcome 8991/64.

'not of the church of England': FaN to Sara Christie, [?1827]. Claydon 7.

p. 53 Another letter: Patty Smith to FaN, [1827]. Claydon 7.

patron of the local parish church: On choosing a successor to J. T. Giffard at East Wellow, see Sam Smith to WEN, 25 October [1838]. Claydon 33. While at Embley, FN also attended services at Romsey Parish Church.

'rites and ceremonies': Cook II, 233.

reportedly read the works: See Calabria and Macrae (eds), *Suggestions for Thought . . . Selections and Commentaries*, xxi.

Priestley's Necessarian philosophy: For an account of Necessarianism, see Webb, *Harriet Martineau*, 80–86.

p. 54 'dull': Calabria and Macrae (eds), *Suggestions for Thought . . . Selections and Commentaries*, xxii.

Sixty years later: FN to Maude Verney, 10 December 1895. BL 68888/138. CW8, 927.

'Let it be your distinct': Abbott, *The Corner-Stone*, 403. Abbott's books were popular among English Unitarians. See *Further Letters of Mrs Gaskell*, 168, n. 15.

'God spoke to me': Quoted in Cook I, 15.

p. 55 innate suspicion: 'St Teresa in the sixteenth century, says that "Christ said" to her (metaphorically of course) . . .'. FN, unsigned note. Wellcome 9023/47. CW4, 81.

'impressions': See, for instance, CW2, 431.

'the passing fancy': FN to FaN, 31 August [1851]. BL 45790/141. CW1, 129.

'it was the most': 'Memoir'.

CHAPTER 3: PINK SATIN GHOSTS

p. 56 'Consult the Edinbro': Lucy Johnson to PN and FN, 26 August [1837]. Claydon 31.
'a formidable step': Maria Coape to FaN, 1 June [1836]. Claydon 31.
p. 57 'little Flo': Patty Smith to FaN, [1855]. Claydon 305. Patty describes FN in Chalon's
    painting as 'leaning against your [FaN's] knee'. Cook II, 467, misidentifies FN as the
    child on her mother's knee.
White's painting: Now in the National Portrait Gallery's collection (3246).
Fanny's diaries: Claydon 401.
'your sister's figure': Lady Palmerston to PN, [n.d.]. Verney 10/167.
'peculiarly graceful': 'Memoir'.
gnashing them: FN to Sir Edwin Saunders, 10 April 1867. Private collection.
p. 58 'a strong feeling': Cook I, 15.
'the journal': FN to Marianne Nicholson, [postmarked 30 October 1837]. Claydon 66.
    CW7, 10. This journal, now missing, was used by O'Malley, 44–64.
'a caravan about the continent': Harriet Martineau to Fanny Wedgwood, 7 January [1843].
    Harriet Martineau's Letters to Fanny Wedgwood, 42.
p. 59 'We have some of us': PN to Joan Bonham Carter, [September 1837]. Claydon 66.
'the dull plains': FN to Marianne Nicholson, [postmarked 30 October 1837]. Claydon
    66. CW7, 10.
'Nothing but quadrilles': FN to Marianne Nicholson, 20 December [1837]. Wellcome
    8991/93. CW7, 12.
p. 60 'an Arabian Nights . . . so enchanting': Quoted in O'Malley, 48.
annotated libretti: Forty-four surviving libretti, annotated by FN, are in the archives of
    Wayne State University in Detroit.
'rather too terrible': CW7, 16.
'balls to infinity': FaN to Joanna Bonham Carter, 10 February 1838. Claydon 66.
p. 61 'the Iliad of history': FN to PN, 16 May 1852. Wellcome 8993/88.
'It is not possible': Fanny Allen to Emma Allen, 24 February 1816. Litchfield (ed.), *Emma
    Darwin*, I, 94.
'seems to be founded': Quoted in Cook I, 17.
p. 62 'still walks . . . whited sepulchres': Quoted in O'Malley, 57.
p. 63 'Miss C': Patty Smith to FaN, 24 September 1838. Claydon 33.
'best friend': FN to Patty Smith, 18 January [1839]. Wellcome 8991/100. CW7, 57.
'a most extraordinary': FN to Mary Shore, 2 February [1839]. CW7, 59.
'curious séance': FN to Patty Smith, 13 December [1838]. Wellcome 8991/98. CW7,
    51–2.
p. 64 'quite right': Patty Smith to FaN, 14 December 1842. Wellcome 9038/8.
'She never had a breath': FN, draft letter, 3 March 1886. Woodward Biomedical Library,
    A.60. CW8, 600.
'improve her conventional manners': Lesser, *Clarkey*, 17.
'How delicious': ibid., 71–2.
p. 65 '*There's* the beginning': ibid., 73.
'mind with these young things': Mary Clarke to FaN, 10 October [1845]. Claydon 28.
'We have quite enough': FN to Mary Shore, 2 February [1839]. Wellcome 8991/101.
    CW7, 38.
'very unstatesmanlike': FN to Patty Smith, 18 January [1839]. CW7, 56.
'dull insipid': FaN to Julia Smith, 21 September 1838. [Copy]. Chiddingstone Castle.
    CW7, 34.
p. 66 'You should never have': FaN to Anne Nicholson, [1839]. Claydon 30.
'from morning till night': FaN to Mary Shore, [1839]. Claydon 34.
'was not nearly so much': FN to Mary Shore, 10 May [1839]. Wellcome 8991/102. CW1,
    413–4.

'and its re-establishment ... lost my voice': FN to Selma Benedicks, 13 May [1839]. Wieslander, 'Florence Nightingale', 35. *CW7*, 628.

p. 67 'one unlucky piano': PN to Sophie [?], [June 1839]. Claydon 34.

'rapid change': FN to Mary Shore, 3 March [1838]. Wellcome 8991/96. *CW7*, 22.

'Everything that catches': Fanny Allen to Elizabeth Wedgwood, 11 [November] 1847. Litchfield (ed.) *Emma Darwin*, II, 107.

'hard labour': Mary Clarke to FaN, [n.d.]. Claydon 223.

'Only think dearest': Quoted in O'Malley, 38.

p. 68 'prying propensities': Annabella Noel-King to PN, 23 August 1858. Claydon 277.

'She made my old bones': FN to WEN, [1844]. Wellcome 8992/69. *CW1*, 221.

had lost an eye: Laura Nicholson, Journals. Hampshire Record Office, F6981–8.

'a scrummage ... rooms: FN to PN, [October 1839]. Wellcome 8991/105. *CW1*, 289.

'I might distend ... vicious': FN to PN, [October 1839]. Wellcome 8991/106. *CW1*, 291.

p. 69 as many as fifteen servants: The 1861 Census records the employment of fifteen servants at Embley.

'We are working hard': FN to PN, [Autumn 1839]. Claydon 34.

'early play fellow ... rest': FN to Selma Benedicks, 1 January 1840. Wieslander, 'Florence Nightingale', 40. *CW7*, 633.

They found': Sam Smith to FaN, [1840]. Claydon 45.

Footnote: Patty Smith to FaN, [1840]. Claydon 36.

p. 70 'looks woefully': FN to FaN, WEN and PN, [February 1840]. Wellcome 8992/4.

'to ask if you': Mai Smith to FaN, [1840]. Claydon 220.

'would ever be a fine': Mai Smith to FaN, [1840]. Claydon 220.

'I feel that if': Mai Smith to FaN, [1840]. Claydon 220.

p. 71 'the risk of an outbreak': Mai Smith to FaN, [March 1840]. Claydon 220.

'a creature so nearly': FN to FaN and WEN, [Spring 1840]. Wellcome 8992/22.

'a most awful ... to dinner': FN to PN and FaN, [Spring 1840]. Wellcome 8992/10.

'raving mad about the longitude': Quoted in Neeley, *Mary Somerville*, 46.

'poring over': PN to FaN, [n.d.]. Claydon 299.

'cordial friend': Patty Smith to FaN, [?1835]. Claydon 22.

p. 72 'by night working': FN to PN, 9 September [1851]. Claydon 124. *CW1*, 308.

'has taken to mathematics': PN to Mary Clarke, 3 July [1840]. Typed copy BL 46385/1 [misdated to 1846].

'doing a little Algebra': FN to [?, n.d.]. Wellcome 8992/35.

Footnote: The idea that Sylvester gave FN private instruction in mathematics seems to stem from an obituary of Sylvester that appeared in the magazine of his old college, St John's, Cambridge. See J.W., 'James Joseph Sylvester Sc.D.', *The Eagle*, 19 (1897), 597.

p. 73 'very fair': FN to Marianne Nicholson, 20 December [1837]. Wellcome 8991/93. *CW7*, 12.

'the very great love': Marmaduke Wyvill to WEN, 25 August [1840]. Claydon 104.

'If I am not mistaken': Marmaduke Wyvill to FN, 25 August [1840]. Claydon 104.

'some things': FN to PN, [October 1840]. Wellcome 8992/21.

'vulgar expression': FN, 'Cassandra', 412.

'Biography of Ellen M': [c. 1840]. Wellcome 9027. *CW5*, 800–805.

'Ladies' work': Quoted in W-S, 40.

p. 74 'slack': Maria Coape to FaN, 18 November 1839. Claydon 15.

'dreadful deal': FN to FaN, [1841]. Wellcome 8992/35.

'My mind': Quoted in W-S, 44.

Parthenope later recalled: 'Memoir'.

'The horrors': FN to Blanche Smith, 21 March [1844]. Balliol College, Oxford, 301.

p. 75 'the glassy surface': FN to Hilary Bonham Carter, [c. 25 April 1846]. BL 45794/98. *CW1*, 433.

'an uncommonly gay time': FN to Mary Shore, [January 1842]. Wellcome 8992/31.

'of doing the office': FN to FaN, 6 February 1843. Wellcome 8992/43.

'as I have': FN to FaN, [January–February 1843]. Wellcome 8992/40.

p. 76 'Parthe's letters': FN to FaN, 15 February 1843. Wellcome 8992/38.

'Helen is sitting': FN to PN, [February 1843], Wellcome 8992/40.

'very ill': FN to Selma Björkenstam, 11 September 1842. CW7, 636.

'experience': FN to WEN, [1844]. Wellcome 8992/44.

'one of the most': FN to FaN, [1844]. Wellcome 8992/46.

p. 77 'an evergreen branch': FN to FaN, [1844]. Wellcome 8992/75.

fleshed-out account: W-S, 46.

doctoring unrelated material: W-S, 86, transcribes part of a sentence in FN's note of Christmas Eve 1850 (BL 43402/53–55) as referring to 'Henry's death'. In the original document the note reads 'Mary's death'.

'acquaintance': FN, 'Cassandra', 412.

theoretical objection: FN later obtained statistics to prove the high incidence of inter-marriage among Quakers, and their consequent insanity. See FN to Hilary Bonham Carter, [1847–8]. BL 45794/149.

closeness to Henry: Years later FN included Henry Nicholson in a note as one of her 'failures in . . . the relations of life'. BL 45844/36.

'fâites-lui': FN to PN, [postmarked 30 January 1837]. Claydon 354.

p. 78 admitted that his departure: FN to PN, [Autumn 1840]. Wellcome 8992/20.

'Henry is 31ˢᵗ': FN to PN, [1841]. Wellcome 8992/32.

'kind-hearted pity': Patty Smith to FaN, [c. 1855]. Claydon 303.

'with pain': George Nicholson to FaN, 5 April 1854. Claydon 339.

p. 79 'as the only note': FN to PN, [1844–5]. Claydon 116.

'read and burn': FN to PN, 7 October [1848]. Wellcome 8993/2. CW1, 301.

'that foolish Marianne': FN to FaN, 16 July 1851. BL 45790/136. CW1, 127.

'no unkindness': Quoted in O'Malley, 104.

'Some of our youthful friendships': 'Addresses to Probationers', 23 May 1873, in Florence Nightingale to Her Nurses, 35.

'Pray write to me': FN to Hannah Nicholson, [1844]. BL 45794/1. CW3, 339.

'mysterious power': FN to Hannah Nicholson, [April–May 1846]. BL 45794/31. CW3, 345.

p. 80 'only the pure in heart': FN to Hannah Nicholson, [September 1844]. BL 45794/13. CW3, 341.

'to whom all unseen': Quoted in Cook I, 46.

'The "kingdom of heaven is within" ': FN, Suggestions for Thought, II, 38.

'happiness of working': FN to Hannah Nicholson, 22 May [1846]. BL 45794/33. CW3, 346.

'Are not our': FN to Selma Benedicks, 13 June [1846]. Wieslander, 'Florence Nightingale', 13. CW7, 653.

'a queer feeling': FN to PN, [January 1845]. Wellcome 8992/71.

p. 81 'the plain prosaic now': FN to Hannah Nicholson, 10 July [1844]. BL 45794/7. CW3, 340.

'a strange ideal': 'Memoir'.

'pink satin ghosts': FN to Hilary Bonham Carter, [c. 25 April 1846]. BL 45794/100. CW1, 434.

'London is really': FN to Hannah Nicholson, [February 1846]. BL 45794/20. CW3, 343.

'the Duke and Duchess': FN to PN, [October 1839]. Wellcome 8991/106. CW1, 291.

'innumerable Howards': Quoted in O'Malley, 84.

p. 82 'a procession of one': FN to Frederick and Maude Verney, 7 February 1888. BL 68885/168.

'Should war's dread': Quoted in Cook I, 142. Ada Lovelace's poem was later set to music by William Montgomery as The Prophecy of Ada.

Her concern: FN to Louisa Ashburton, 14 April 1861. National Library of Scotland, CW8, 720.

uncomfortable: From the late 1860s, Louisa Ashburton was the patron and lover of the sculptor Harriet Hosmer. She was also later embroiled in a relationship with Robert Browning.

p. 83 Nicholsons to ask: Anne Nicholson to FaN, [postmarked 21 November 1835]. Claydon 30.

    '**I should get**': FN to PN, [1845]. Wellcome 8992/89A.

    '**which he did**': FN to PN, [1846]. Wellcome 8992/127.

    '**dine with us**': Lord Palmerston to WEN, [Summer 1842]. Verney 10/167.

    '**A most bland . . . a character**': Quoted in Pope Hennessy, *Monckton Milnes. The Years of Promise*, 43.

    '**We all liked him**': Quoted in O'Malley, 106.

p. 84 'calm dignity of deportment': Bunsen, *A Memoir of Baron Bunsen*, 2, 22.

    '**a red face**': Quoted in Pope Hennessy, *Monckton Milnes. The Years of Promise*, 47.

    '**but a village apothecary**': FN to WEN, 24 August 1863. Wellcome 9000/123. CW3, 366.

p. 85 The German Hospital: The '<u>Dalston</u> plan' was later described by FN as the 'beau ideal of hospitals'. FN to Selina Bracebridge, 14 February [1853]. Typed copy. FN Museum. CW8, 529.

    '**What can an individual**': Quoted in O'Malley, 87.

    '**Dr Howe**': Quoted in ibid., 93.

p. 86 a pivotal moment: It is portrayed as such, for instance, by Howe's daughter, Laura Richards, in a biography of FN, written for children, which she published in 1909. Richards, *Florence Nightingale: The Angel of the Crimea*, 34–5.

    '**festering**': Williams, *Hungry Heart*, 232.

    '**if he had been engaged**': Clifford, *Mine Eyes Have seen the Glory*, 82–3.

    Words for the Hour: Quoted in Williams, *Hungry Heart*, 187–9.

p. 87 she imagined herself: FN to Hannah Nicholson, 24 September [1846]. BL 45794/43.

CHAPTER 4: THIS LOATHSOME LIFE

p. 88 'a regular life': FN to WEN, [1844]. Wellcome 8992/69. CW1,221.

    '**decidedly instructive**': FN to FaN, [November 1844]. Wellcome 8992/62.

    '**very cordial & ladylike**': FN to FaN, [1844]. Wellcome 8992/65. CW1, 118.

    '**many an algebraical hour**': FN to FaN, [1844]. Wellcome 8992/67.

    '**& all sports**': FN to WEN, [1844]. Wellcome 8992/69. CW1, 221.

    '**that the most real**': FN to PN, 8 February 1845. Wellcome 8992/76. CW1, 297.

p. 89 '. . . When I look': FN to PN, 8 February 1845. Wellcome 8992/76. CW1, 499.

    '**carte blanche**': Mai Smith to FaN, [1845]. Wellcome 9038/35.

    '**deliberate**': FN to PN, [1845]. Wellcome 8992/68.

    '**pure & devoted enough**': FN to PN, [February 1845]. Wellcome 8992/72.

    '**all anxious ideas**': Hilary Bonham Carter to FaN, 17 July 1845. Claydon 223.

p. 90 'a giant among pygmies': FN to FaN, 7 February 1852. Claydon 122. CW1, 415.

    '**idolatrized**': WEN to FaN, [n.d.]. Claydon 354.

    '**early good training**': Mai Smith to WEN, [n.d.]. Wellcome 9049/50.

    '**She died a hero**': FN to Julia Ward Howe and Samuel Howe, 26 December 1845. Richards, 'Letters of Florence Nightingale', 332. CW8, 795.

    '**Mrs Gamp scene . . . I make of it**': Quoted in O'Malley, 109.

p. 91 'a sensible & agreeable': FN to WEN, [1845]. Wellcome 8992/116. CW1, 227.

    '**as much as if**': FN to Hilary Bonham Carter, 11 December 1845. Cook I, 44.

    Mary Clarke was to describe: In March 1863. Lesser, *Clarkey*, 169.

p. 92 **'vanity and selfishness'**: FN, Note, November 1845. BL 43402/34. CW2, 366.

'of my living': Quoted in Cook I, 44.

'Forgive me': FN, Note, November 1845. BL 43402/34. CW2, 366.

'poor mind': FN, Note 1 December 1845. BL 43402/34–5. CW2, 366–7.

'for ameliorating': FN to Julia Ward Howe and Samuel Howe, 26 December 1845. Richards, 'Letters of Florence Nightingale', 334. CW8, 797.

p. 93 **'to perform menial duties'**: Haskins, *History of Salisbury Infirmary*, 19–20.

'some sort': FN to Julia Ward Howe and Samuel Howe, 26 December 1845. Richards, 'Letters of Florence Nightingale', 335. CW8, 797.

p. 94 **Second footnote**: Dickens's preface to the 1849 edition of *Martin Chuzzlewit* (1844).

p. 95 **night nurse**: From the start of her professional career at Upper Harley Street, in 1853–4, FN would largely dispense with the old night nurse system. Later, at Scutari, she would forbid the practice of night nursing among her nurses, and would make her rounds of the wards alone at night (sometimes with a maid). The attempt to bring an end to the employment of the night nurse was reflected in the practice of other reformed nursing systems, for instance that of the Anglican sisterhood, St John's House, which was among the first to introduce a more integrated system in which nurses undertook both the day and the night watch.

p. 96 **'she had never known'**: FN to WEN, 22 February 1854. BL 45790/157. CW1, 238.

liked later to recount: FN to Grand Duchess of Baden, 31 March 1879. BL 45750/169. CW8, 837.

training at Westminster: see Helmstadter, 'Passing of the Night Watch', 33.

'She may often': Quoted ibid.

p. 97 **'may not the age'**: Quoted in O'Malley, 112.

The Fry Sisters: See Huntsman, Bruin and Holttum, 'Twixt Candle and Lamp' for the most detailed modern survey of Fry's Institution of Nursing Sisters.

p. 98 **'The first grasping'**: Tooley, *Life of Florence Nightingale*, 49.

well known to . . . William Smith: For example, John Gurney (1749–1809), Fry's father, was Deputy Chairman of the Dissenting Deputies with Smith. Fry's brother, to whom she was especially close, Joseph John Gurney (1788–1847), corresponded with FaN in the 1820s. E.g. J. J. Gurney to FaN, 26 June 1823. Claydon 21.

'trudge to & from': Patty Smith to FaN, [postmarked August 1822]. Claydon 22. Patty kept abreast of Fry's movements. In March 1839 she reported to FaN that 'Mrs Fry is in Paris'. Claydon 25.

one of her spiritual mothers: FN, Note, [c. 1870–72]. BL 45843/306.

intended to employ: FN to Selina Bracebridge, 14 February [1853]. Typed copy. FN Museum. CW8, 527.

p. 99 **'Practically'**: FN to H. W. Acland, 20 January 1867. Convent of Mercy, Birmingham. CW8, 96.

far from unique: Consider the example of Agnes Gladstone, daughter of W. E. Gladstone and his wife, Catherine. Although Mrs Gladstone was involved in the selection of nurses during the Crimean War, and praised those who allowed their daughters to nurse at Scutari or the Crimea, she steadfastly refused to allow Agnes to take up nursing. Agnes remained at home and did not marry until late in life.

p. 100 **Lucy Osburn's father**: MacDonnell, *Miss Nightingale's Young Ladies*, 23. More recently, Godden, *Lucy Osburn*, 53, has argued that William Osburn's objections to his daughter becoming a Nightingale probationer were based on his fears that she had become 'a Catholic stooge'.

'utterly ignorant': Henry Hunt Piper to WEN, [?1855]. Claydon 285.

a cautionary tale: For instance, Emily Southward Hill reported in 1858 that a 'Miss B.' had been offered the Secretaryship of the Children's Hospital. '. . . But her father and mother say that no daughter ought to leave home except to be married, or to earn her own living, witness Florence Nightingale, who has returned a mere wreck . . .' Maurice, *Life of Octavia Hill*, 126.

'with composure': FN to WEN, 18 January [1846]. Goldie, *A Calendar of the Letters of Florence Nightingale*, 2 260 1/46. The original MS of this letter appears to be missing.

p. 101 **Hospital of St Stephen's:** The Hospital of St Vincent's, St Stephen's on the Green, Dublin, was served by the Irish Sisters of Charity.

'moves with her': Quoted in Cook I, 59.

p. p. 000 **she kept a watch:** 'Memoir'.

'up to my chin': FN to Mary Clarke, 10 July [1846]. BL 43397/295.

p. 102 **'quota of amusement':** 'Memoir'.

'She is silent': WEN to FaN, [n.d.]. Claydon 354.

'neither science': WEN to FaN, [1840s]. Claydon 27.

'Flo astonishes': WEN to FaN, [November 1844]. Wellcome 9038/29.

'Oh if one has': FN, Note, 1 December 1845. BL 43402/34–5. CW2, 366.

'Dreaming always': FN, 'Cassandra', 406.

p. 103 **'the multiplicity':** Ellis, *Daughters of England*, 12. Mrs Ellis also wrote books addressed to the women, wives and mothers of England.

'. . . we know her': FN to Julia Ward Howe, 28 July [1848]. Richards, 'Letters of Florence Nightingale', 342–3. CW5, 774.

'dreams of attainment': Beatrice Webb, *Diaries*, 13 August 1882, 22.

sense of unreality: Beatrice Webb, *Diaries*, 24 April 1883, 31.

'aside the reins': FN to Hilary Bonham Carter, [1846]. BL 45794/135. CW1, 441.

confounded Florence's worries: Edinburgh Academy records.

p. 104 **'And so':** FN to Hilary Bonham Carter, [*c.* 25 April 1846]. BL 45794/103. CW1, 435–6.

'My happiness': FN to Selma Björkenstam, 30 September 1846. Wieslander, 'Florence Nightingale', 66. CW7, 661.

'And mayst thou': FN to PN, 18 April [1847]. Wellcome 8992/132. CW1, 300.

a wild swan: This famous remark was attributed by Lytton Strachey, and subsequently by many other writers, to Fanny Nightingale, though, in fact, it originated with Parthenope. In a letter written to Catherine Winkworth, during her stay at Lea Hurst in October 1854, Mrs Gaskell quoted Parthenope as making the comparison (*The Letters of Mrs Gaskell*, 307–8); and in a letter to Ellen Tollet, 7 October 1856, Parthenope herself alludes to Andersen's story of the 'Ugly Duckling', and says 'We are a duck's nest & have hatched a wild swan . . .' (BL 45791/279).

'none of that': FN, Note, [1840s]. Wellcome 8992/141. CW1, 96.

p. 105 **'not of other':** WEN to FaN, [1840s]. Claydon 27.

'fed on sugar-plums': FN, BL 45839/23.

expressed the opinion: Litchfield (ed.), *Emma Darwin*, I, 111.

'd'un de ses enthousiasmes': Ferdinand Françoise to FaN, 12 December 1846. FaN replied to Françoise on 4 March 1847. Verney 10/146.

'Mr Milnes': FN to William Shore Smith, 2 October [1846]. BL 46176/37.

'intellect, position': FN, 'Lebenslauf', CW1, 91.

'to her': FN to Selma Björkenstam, 30 September 1846. Wieslander, 'Florence Nightingale', 66. CW7, 662.

p. 106 **'Mr Milnes is lively':** Fanny Allen to Elizabeth Wedgwood, 27 December 1847. Litchfield (ed.), *Emma Darwin*, II, 114.

'The poetic parcel': FN to William Shore Smith, [postmarked 17 September 1846]. BL 46176/32. CW5, 665.

'For all ordinary': Richard Monckton Milnes to FN, [?1846]. Claydon 396.

Footnote: FN Museum (0773).

p. 107 **'a very bad hat':** FN to William Shore Smith, [postmarked 17 September 1846]. BL 46176/33. CW5, 666.

'a college man . . . afterwards': FN to Mary Clarke, [9 June 1847]. BL 43397/283–8. CW5, 668–9.

'inexpressible grief': Mary Clarke to FaN, 20 August [1847]. Claydon 39.

p. 108 'love given': FN to Mary Mohl, 13 October [1847]. BL 43397/298–300. CW8, 551–3.

'slow circulation': Mai Smith to PN, [1847]. Claydon 274.

p. 109 'I cannot but think': Selina Bracebridge to FaN, [1847]. Claydon 240.

'liberal country gentleman': This was Thomas Carlyle's description of WEN, but applies equally to Charles Bracebridge. Thomas Carlyle to Margaret Carlyle, 12 April 1851. *The Collected Letters of Thomas and Jane Welsh*, 26, 219.

A writer of sorts: Bracebridge was the author of pamphlets on the Irish Poor Law Bill (1838), on building a new jail in Warwick (1845) and, later, on the affairs of Greece (1850). In 1862, he published *Shakespeare No Deerstealer*.

'Is not one line': FN to Jane Smith, 21 September [1847]. Edinburgh University Library. CW5, 744.

a promising artist: There is an album of Selina Bracebridge's sketches of Turkey in the Searight Collection in the Victoria and Albert Museum. See also her *Panoramic Sketch of Athens*.

p. 110 'As long as one': Quoted in O'Malley, 125.

'more than mother': FN to Selina Bracebridge, 8 February 1873. Royal College of Nursing, Edinburgh. CW8, 538.

'the creators of my life': FN, Note, [1872]. BL 45784/90.

a visit to the museum: FN to William Shore Smith, 19 July [1846]. BL 46175/15.

'a winter in Rome': FN to Hilary Bonham Carter, 20 October 1847. BL. 45794/130.

'It seems': Quoted in Cook I, 70.

'I shall be': Richard Monckton Milnes to WEN, [1847]. Wellcome 9038/59.

p. 111 'a true angel': FN to Hilary Bonham Carter, [22 October 1847]. BL 45794/132.

'prosed & gossiped': FN to FaN, WEN and PN, 2 November [1847]. Wellcome 9016/5. CW7, 70.

'softly plashing': FN to FaN, WEN and PN, 11 November 1847. Wellcome 9016/7. CW7, 87.

CHAPTER 5: TO BE HAPPY IN MY OWN WAY

p. 112 'To Be Happy in My Own Way': FN to PN, 19 August [1851]. Wellcome 8993/45. CW1, 305.

'the dust ... grief': FN to FaN, WEN and PN, 11 November 1847. Wellcome 9016/7. CW7, 86–7.

p. 113 'So now ...': FN to PN, 11 November 1847, Wellcome 9016/8. CW7, 91.

'the father of liberty': FN to PN, 11 November 1847, Wellcome 9016/8. CW7, 90.

'a Communion of Saints': FN to PN, 14 November 1847, Wellcome 9016/11. CW7, 98.

'the least unsuccessful': FN to FaN, WEN and PN, 1 February 1848, Wellcome 9016/50. CW7, 243.

'their priests': FN to FaN, WEN and PN, 28 February 1848, Wellcome 9016/59. CW7, 278.

she would ridicule: FN, Note, [1871] BL 45843/104. CW3, 94.

'accidental developments': FN to PN, 28 December [1847]. CW7, 182.

p. 114 'Are you afraid': FN to FaN, WEN and PN, 31 December 1847, Wellcome 9016/32. CW7, 188.

'want of art': FN to PN, 17 December 1847. Wellcome 9016/24. CW7, 156.

Footnote: CW7, 342.

'horrible green gates': FN to FaN, WEN and PN, 20 December 1847, Wellcome 9016/26. CW7, 165.

p. 115 'the joy': Henry Colyar to William Empson, 17 January 1848. Keele (ed.), *Florence Nightingale in Rome*, 151.

'dear Flo's': Selina Bracebridge to FaN, [1847]. Claydon 38.

'Rowland Hill': FN to FaN, WEN and PN, 28 December [1847], Wellcome 9016/30. CW7, 181.

'particularly agreeable': FN to PN, 23 January 1848, Wellcome 9016/43. CW7, 213. On FN and Margaret Fuller, see Showalter, 'Miranda and Cassandra: The Discourse of the Feminist Intellectual'.

'how pleasant it is': FaN to PN, [1847]. Wellcome 9038/50.

'dragged out': FN to PN, 2 December 1847. Wellcome 9016/19. CW7, 130.

'doing society': FN to PN, 13 December 1847. Wellcome 9016/23. CW7, 148

'intimacy': FN to Julius Mohl, 21 November 1869. Woodward Biomedical Library. CW7, 328.

p. 116 'the sunshine': FN to FaN, 29 November 1847. Keele (ed.), *Florence Nightingale in Rome*, 73.

'... He achieved': FN, Note, 31 August 1896. CW5, 517-18.

p. 117 'inborn republican': FN to FaN, WEN and PN, 8 March 1848. Wellcome 9016/61. CW7, 285.

'quite appreciates': Selina Bracebridge to FaN, [1847-8]. Claydon 240.

'Lady Lightning': O'Neil, *Cardinal Herbert Vaughan*, 53.

'ever increasing': Sidney Herbert to Elizabeth Herbert, [1846-7]. Herbert Papers, Wiltshire Record Office, F4/51.

later account: Elizabeth Herbert, 'Account of Sidney Herbert'. Herbert Papers, Wiltshire Record Office, F6/98/16.

p. 118 'but because': FN to Julia Howe, 26 December [1845]. Richards, *Letters of Florence Nightingale*, 331. Wilton Church (1841-5), built by T. H. Wyatt and D. Brandon at a cost of £20,000.

'formal, empty': Herbert, *How I Came Home*, 50.

'He is about': FN to WEN, 26 January [1848]. Wellcome 9016/46. CW7, 228.

'an easy transit': FN to WEN, [28 January 1848]. Wellcome 9016/47. CW7, 237.

p. 119 'I cannot': FN to FaN, 11 January 1848. Wellcome 9016/36. CW7, 195.

'a course of convents': FN to FaN, 18 January 1848. Wellcome 9016/39. CW7, 206.

'dirty': FN to PN, 23 January 1848. Wellcome 9016/43. CW7, 218.

'a hopeless case': FN to FaN, 25 January 1848. Wellcome 9016/45. CW7, 224.

The convent: The convent of the Societé du Sacré-Coeur-de-Jésus, of which the Madre was maîtresse, still stands at the top of the Spanish Steps in Rome.

p. 120 'rough humility': FN, [16 February 1848]. Wellcome 9016/54. CW7, 262.

Dickens's article: Reprinted in CW5, 769-70.

'It is no good': Quoted in O'Malley, 144.

'the whole history': FN to PN, 17 February 1848. Wellcome 9016/56. CW7, 269.

her Bible: CW2, 6-7.

p. 121 dialogue: Quoted in O'Malley, 144-5.

'the strong woman': Laure de Ste Colombe to FN, 24 February 1856. Claydon 302. CW7, 341. Ste Colombe died in 1886.

'If 1848 ... a trigger against the Austrian first': FN to FaN, WEN and PN, [25 March] 1848, Wellcome 9016/65. CW7, 292-4.

p. 122 'the kingdom of heaven': FN to Julia Ward Howe, 28 July 1848. Richards, 'Letters of Florence Nightingale', 337-8. CW7, 316.

'artistic': FN to FaN, WEN and PN, 10 April [1848]. Wellcome 9016/67. CW7, 299.

'Everything here': FN to WEN, 2 February [1849]. Claydon 230. CW1, 230.

'petition': Liz Herbert to FaN, 28 June 1848. Wellcome 9038/54.

p. 123 'owing to her': FN to [?, 1848]. Wellcome 8993/9. CW8, 653.

'Mr Herbert': Selina Bracebridge to FaN, [early 1850s]. Claydon 240.

'everything that is painful ... London': Quoted in O'Malley, 149-50.

p. 124 'My God': Quoted in W-S, 74.

'Mama was so': FN to PN, [6 October 1848]. Wellcome 8993/1. CW7, 675.

'a new & horrible . . . one's time': FN to PN, 22 October [1848]. *CW7*, 676.

p. 125 **'a highly popular'**: Quoted in Cope, *Florence Nightingale and the Doctors*, 58.

'Your friend': FN to Richard Monckton Milnes, 29 November [1848]. Beinecke Rare Book and Manuscript Library. *CW7*, 677.

p. 126 **'I hope Mrs Nightingale'**: Fanny Allen to Emma Darwin, 3 February 1849. Litchfield (ed.), *Emma Darwin*, II, 121.

'the life next most valuable': Mai Smith to FaN, [1852–3]. Claydon 282.

'Richard was himself': FN, Diary, 17 July 1850. Calabria (ed.), *Florence Nightingale in Egypt and Greece*, 72.

'I have an intellectual . . . marry him': FN, Note, 24 December 1850. BL 43402/53–5. *CW2*, 383.

p. 127 **'He would hardly speak'**: Quoted in O'Malley, 174.

she wrote to Milnes: FN to Richard Monckton Milnes, 20 March 1851. Houghton Papers, Trinity College, Cambridge, 18/126. CW1, 552–3.

p. 128 **'gloom'**: Mai Smith to FaN, [1852–3]. Claydon 282.

'very glad': FN to Georgina Tollet, 31 January 1852. Claydon 369. *CW8*, 745.

'more than once': Richard Monckton Milnes to FN, 30 March 1869. Houghton Papers, Trinity College, Cambridge, 18/121.

through his verse: Richard Monckton Milnes, 'A Monument for Scutari', *The Times*, 10 September 1855. The poem praises the 'hero-sufferers' who 'unmurmuringly passed away'. The last stanza contains Milnes's tribute to FN. PN to Richard Monckton Milnes [1855]: 'Your sonnet is so beautiful that we cannot hold our tongues. It expresses what we are all feeling – deeply & sadly.' Houghton Papers, Trinity College, Cambridge, 18/152.

'the idol': From a missing notebook [early 1850s]. *CW8*, 528.

'in tongue or pen': FN to Lady Galway, 25 September 1889. Houghton Papers, Trinity College, Cambridge, 18/146. *CW5*, 489.

a private request: Richard Monckton Milnes to PN, 30 October [1854]. Claydon 255.

p. 129 **other possible suitors**: No evidence survives to support the story that FN declined a proposal from John Smithurst (1802–67), a clerk at St John the Baptist Church at Dethick, near Lea Hurst, nor that she encouraged him to become a missionary in Canada, where he ministered to the Red River Settlement from 1839 to 1851. The legend of Smithurst's relationship with FN, however, is perpetuated in the stained glass windows of him and FN at St John's Anglican Church, Elora, Ontario, where Smithurst was rector. See Griffin, 'Victims of Fiction: Research Notes on "The Love Story of Florence Nightingale and John Smithurst" '. In a letter to her uncle, Sam Smith, FN later claimed that she 'could have had as many husbands as Mahomet's mother'. (BL 45792/252).

'futur': FN to PN, [6 October 1848]. Wellcome 8993/1. *CW7*, 675.

'this man who wants . . . Abraham': FN to FaN, 1 December 1853. Wellcome 8994/65. *CW1*,138.

p. 130 **'an attack'**: FN to PN, 22 October [1849]. Wellcome 8993/4, *CW1*, 302.

'Miss Nightingale': Johnny Stanley to Lady Stanley, 20 October 1854. Mitford, *The Stanleys of Alderley*, 92.

never attempted to influence: FN, 'Lebenslauf', 24 July 1851. *CW1*, 91.

gossip: Patty Smith to FaN, [1849]. Claydon 397.

'We have talked': FaN to Selina Bracebridge, [September 1849]. Wellcome 9038/61.

p. 131 **'linen gingham gowns'**: FN to FaN, [September 1849]. Welcome 8993/27.

'the *dernier mot*': Quoted in Cook I, 84.

'excavating the temple': Wilkinson, *Modern Egypt*, I, 66.

'a Nile voyage': Martineau, *Eastern Life*, I, 86.

'Bless you': FN to FaN, 2 November 1849. Wellcome 8993/26.

Giovanni Belzoni: FN's copy of Belzoni's *Travels* (1824), a gift from FaN on FN's fifth birthday, is in the FN Museum (0264).

at Heliopolis: FN to FaN, WEN and PN, [24-25 March] 1850. Wellcome 9017/28. CW4, 435.

p. 132 privately published: FN, *Letters from Egypt* (for private circulation only). A. & G. A. Spottiswoode, 1854.

'a mistake': FN to FaN, WEN and PN, 11 February 1850. Wellcome 9017/22. CW4, 350.

'the model establishment': FN to FaN, WEN and PN, 7 November 1849. Wellcome 9019/4. CW4, 129.

p. 133 'valuable lessons': FN to FaN, WEN and PN, 19 November 1849. Wellcome 9019/9. CW4, 147.

'hopeless': FN to FaN, WEN and PN, 24 November [1849]. Wellcome 9018/8. CW4, 156.

'English family': Steegmuller (ed.), *Flaubert in Egypt*, 35.

'a single sensation': FN to FaN, WEN and PN, 27 November [1849]. Wellcome 9017/3. CW4, 160.

p. 134 'capital invention': FN to FaN, WEN and PN, 4 December 1849. Wellcome 9017/4. CW4, 174.

'who never moves . . . divan incumbent': FN to FaN, WEN and PN, 9 December 1849. Wellcome 9017/4. CW4, 175-81.

'a sort of torpor': FN to FaN, WEN and PN, 9 December 1849. Wellcome 9017/4. CW4, 182-3.

p. 135 'colourlessness': FN to FaN, WEN and PN, 2 January 1850. Wellcome 9017/12. CW4, 240.

'one almost fancies': FN to FaN, WEN and PN, 11 December [1849]. Wellcome 9017/4. CW4, 184.

'who thought and felt like us': FN to FaN, WEN and PN, 14 December 1849. Wellcome 9017/6. CW4, 192.

'wretched': FN, Diary, 2 February 1850. BL 45846. CW4, 323.

'voluntary abasement': FN to FaN, WEN and PN, 2 January 1850. Wellcome 9017/12. CW4, 239.

Mungo Park and James Bruce: Park (1771-1806) was one of Britain's great African explorers. Bruce was an African traveller, and the author of *Travels to Discover the Source of the Nile* (1768-73).

'the sort of city': FN to FaN, WEN and PN, [22 December] 1849. Wellcome 9017/8. CW4, 202.

p. 136 'To see human beings': FN to FaN, WEN and PN, 2 January 1850. Wellcome 9017/12. CW4, 239.

'South Sea savages': FN to FaN, WEN and PN, [6 January 1850]. Wellcome 9017/13. CW4, 246.

'frogs, camels': Barrell, 'Death on the Nile', 105. Lucie Duff Gordon (1821-69), who settled in Egypt in the early 1860s, and wrote a series of *Letters from Egypt* (1865) to her family, was perhaps the first English traveller to demonstrate an enthusiasm and understanding of the contemporary Egyptian way of life.

'that horrible Egyptian present': FN to FaN, WEN and PN, 17 January 1850. Wellcome 9017/16. CW4, 262.

'the impossibility': FN to Dr Fowler, 26 December 1849. Wellcome 9017/10. CW4, 214.

'one God': FN to FaN, WEN and PN, 29 December 1849. Wellcome 9017/10. CW4, 222.

p. 137 'Egypt is beginning': FN to FaN, WEN and PN, 17 January 1850. Wellcome 9017/16. CW4, 270.

'The evil is not': FN to FaN, WEN and PN, 17 January 1850. Wellcome 9017/16. CW4, 258.

'Or will a nation': FN to FaN, WEN and PN, 29 December 1849. Wellcome 9017/10. CW4, 229.

'like its own': Quoted in Rees, *Writings on the Nile*, 112.

'spoiled it all': FN, Diary, 26 January 1850. BL 45846. CW4, 302.

'in the very face of God': FN, Diary, 17 January 1850. BL 45846. CW4, 274.

'from this slavery': FN, Diary, 20 January 1850. BL 45846. CW4, 283.

p. 138 'Karnak': FN, Diary, 16 February 1850. BL 45846. CW4, 369.

'God called me': FN, Diary, 28 February 1850. BL 45846. CW4, 408.

March 3: FN, Diary, 3–12 March 1850. BL 45846. CW4, 436.

p. 139 'panoramic': FN to FaN and PN, [13 April 1850]. Wellcome 8993/33. CW4, 466.

'a cork model': FN to PN, 29 April 1850. BL 45790/15. CW7,377.

Athena: 'Got our owlet'. FN, Diary, 8 June 1850. Claydon 460. CW7, 425. Athena was FN's second owl. In February 1845 she had recorded the death of her first: FN to WEN, [February 1845]. Wellcome 8992/74.

'tangled cotton': Patty Smith to FaN, [1852]. Wellcome 9038/68.

'A few hints': FN, Fragment, [June 1850]. Claydon 122. CW7, 446.

'It was always God': FN, Diary, 30 April 1850. BL 45846.

'think only': FN, Diary, 12 May 1850. BL 45846.

'misspent': FN to FaN, 12 May 1850. Claydon 121. CW7, 397.

p. 140 a number of extracts: FN, BL 43402/38.

'Reading Cowper's life': FN, Diary, 27 May 1850. BL 45846.

'physically and morally ill': FN, Diary, 17 June 1850. BL 45846.

'if you don't': FN to FaN, WEN and PN, 12 July 1850. Claydon 122. CW7, 466.

'spirit . . . wanted': FN, Diary , 9 July 1850. BL 45846.

earliest surviving photograph: The original is at Claydon.

p. 141 'could see': FN to FaN, WEN and PN, [10–17] July 1850. Claydon 122. CW7, 464.

CHAPTER 6: YOUR VAGABOND SON

p. 142 Kaiserswerth: On Kaiserswerth's history, see FN, *The Institution of Kaiserswerth on the Rhine, for the Practical Training of Deaconesses*, 1851, CW7, 493–511, and Disselhoff, *Kaiserswerth*.

'More are eagerly': FN, *The Institution of Kaiserswerth*, CW7, 511.

p. 143 'hope was answered': FN, Diary, 1 August 1850. BL 45846.

'I hope you have': Selina Bracebridge to FN, 3 August [1850]. Claydon 92. CW7, 490.

p. 144 'free from vows': FN, *The Institution of Kaiserswerth*, CW7, 493.

'one of the means': ibid., CW7, 499.

'poor & ugly . . . Fliedner's character': FN to WEN, 15 August [1850]. Claydon 124. CW1, 232.

'feeling so brave': FN, Diary, 13 August 1850. BL 45846.

p. 145 'As I have undertaken': FN to Theodore Fliedner, 19 August 1850. Kaiserswerth Diakoniewerk. CW7, 512 (translation from French).

'I often wonder': Charlotte Brontë, *Shirley*, chapter 12.

'to cultivate her powers': FN, *The Institution of Kaiserswerth*, CW7, 492.

'If . . . there . . . to obey it': ibid., CW7, 495–6.

p. 146 a thorough search: FN to Messrs Dulau, 24 September 1897. Bishop and Goldie, *A Bio-Bibliography of Florence Nightingale*, 125.

'I think Kaiserswerth': FN to WEN, Note on back of envelope. Claydon 124. CW1, 232.

'dear people': FN, Diary, 21 August 1850. BL 45846.

p. 147 'make no mention': Selina Bracebridge to FN, 3 August [1850]. Claydon 92. CW7, 491.

'The opinion of the world': Selina Bracebridge to Mai Smith, [n.d.]. Claydon 274.

p. 148 'your Flo': Hilary Bonham Carter to PN [1849–50]. Claydon 37.

'Dear Flo's vocation': Mary Mohl to PN, [n.d.]. Claydon 77.

'intellectual': WEN to FaN, [1850]. Claydon 73.

'the intense satisfaction': [?] to PN, 26 August 1850. Claydon 240.

p. 149 'I can hardly': FN, Note, [?1851]. BL 43402/64.

'to rub her': FN to FaN and WEN, [1850]. Wellcome 8993/34.

'it excites her': FN to Mary Mohl, 7 February [1851]. BL 43397/304. CW8, 558.

'my selfishness': WEN to FaN, [early 1850s]. Claydon 77.

'for even': Mai Smith to FN, [early 1850s]. BL 45793/87.

'in this undisturbed way': Mai Smith to Blanche Smith, [October 1850]. BL 72826/9.

p. 150 'if trimmed': FN to FaN, 11 November 1850. Wellcome 8993/36.

'avalanche of water': FN to FaN, [2 December 1850]. BL 45790/121.

Another account: Joanna Bonham Carter to FaN [1850]. Claydon 23.

'the House of Mourning': FN to WEN, 26 October 1850. BL 45790/107.

'the axis': FN to [?] 17 November [1850]. Claydon 26.

'the poor mother ... in those regrets': FN to Georgina Tollet, 17 November [1850]. Claydon 369. CW8, 748.

p. 151 'like gin drinking': FN, Note, 24 December 1850. BL 43402/54. CW2, 383.

'I have no desire': FN, Note, 30 December 1850. BL 43402/55. CW2, 384.

'I feel myself perishing': Reported by Aunt Mai in a letter to FaN, [1850]. Claydon 274.

'Young ladies all': Punch, VI (1849), 226.

p. 152 'She can distinguish': Quoted in Boyd, The Excellent Doctor Blackwell, 136.

p. 153 'in the delicious air ... husband': Blackwell, Pioneer Work, 184–5.

'dined & drank': FN to FaN, 8 May [1851]. Wellcome 8993/42.

'who is about': Quoted in Blackwell, Pioneer Work, 186.

their names appear: The page is reproduced in McKellar, The German Hospital, 20.

'Write to me': FN to Elizabeth Blackwell, [postmarked 1 March 1852]. CW8, 22.

p. 154 'I have no faith': FN to Mary Mohl, 7 February [1851]. BL 43397/303. CW8, 556.

'to diminish ... struggle': FN, Note, 8 June [1851]. BL 43402/68–73.

p. 155 'danger': WEN to FaN, 18 August [1851]. Claydon 69.

a much later account: FN, Note, [1857]. BL 43402/182. CW5, 233.

'a very desirable thing': FN to FaN, 16 July 1851. BL 45790/135. CW1, 126.

p. 156 'a state secret': Quoted in W-S, 91.

'a profound silence': Selina Bracebridge to PN, 20 July [1851]. Claydon 274.

'on the Apothecary station': Selina Bracebridge to PN, 17 August [1851]. Claydon 274.

'Oh what pluck': Mai Smith to FN, [July–August 1851]. BL 45793/77.

'I know that': FN to FaN, 8 August, [1851]. BL 45790/138. CW1, 128.

'perpetual': FN to Henry Bonham Carter, 24 July 1867. BL 47714/223. CW7, 598.

p. 157 'Cupped': FN, Diary, 21 July [1851]. Wellcome 9025/76. CW7/521.

'very quietly': FN, Diary, 4 September [1851]. Wellcome 9025/78. CW7, 537.

'dead beat': FN, Diary, 21 July [1851]. Wellcome 9025/76. CW7/522.

'9–11 a.m.': FN, Diary, 31 July [1851]. Wellcome 9025/77. CW7, 526.

'In the evening': FN, Diary, 8 August [1851]. Wellcome 9025/78. CW7, 528.

'You will find': [?] to FN, 5 August [1851]. Claydon 40.

p. 158 'than the pleasure': FN to FaN, 8 August [1851]. BL 45790/138. CW1, 128.

'am perfectly well': FN to PN, 4 August [1851]. Wellcome 8993/44. CW1, 304.

'You don't think': FN to PN, 19 August [1851]. Wellcome 8993/45. CW1, 305.

'earnest affection ... path of life': FN to PN, 9 September [1851]. Claydon 124. CW1, 309.

'my pure': FN to FaN, 31 August [1851]. BL 45790/42. CW1, 130.

'some great absorption': WEN to FaN, [postmarked 30 July 1851]. Claydon 69.

p. 159 'This time': FaN to FN, 7 September [1851]. Claydon 274. The letter was sent from Franzensbad.

'in harness': FN, 'Death of Pastor Fliedner of Kaiserswerth', *Evangelical Christendom* (December 1864), CW7, 587.

'first-rate': FN to Samuel Howe, 20 June 1852. Richards, 'Letters of Florence Nightingale', 346. CW7, 581.

p. 160 'never in all': FN to Dr Sutherland, [January 1868]. BL 45753/3. CW7, 599.

'dangling': FN, Note, 7 December 1851. BL 43402/66.

CHAPTER 7: UNLOVING LOVE

p. 161 'a little': FN to FaN, 6 January [1852]. Wellcome 8993/69. CW7, 679. Johnson wrote a number of works on homoeopathy, the water cure and the nervous diseases of women.

p. 162 Clough's main problem: Recorded by BJ, commonplace book, 1880, Balliol College, Oxford. CW5, 762.

'indecent and profane': Quoted in Kenny, *Arthur Hugh Clough*, 149.

insufferably: Lothian Nicholson to PN, 12 December [1853]. Claydon 211.

'extremely': FN to FaN, 6 January 1852. Wellcome 8993/69. CW7, 679.

enlisting Monckton Milnes's: FN to Richard Monckton Milnes, 20 March 1851. Houghton Papers, Trinity College Cambridge, 18/126. CW1, 552-3.

'a fine': 'Chronology of Miss Smith', *Correspondence of Arthur Hugh Clough*, 2, 619.

'the friend . . . hard': A. H. Clough to Blanche Smith, [21 February 1852]. *Correspondence of Arthur Hugh Clough*, 1, 307.

p. 163 *'Service'* is everything: A. H. Clough to Blanche Smith, 1 January 1852. *Correspondence of Arthur Hugh Clough*, 1, 300.

'Love is fellow': 'Qui laborat orat' was the title of one of Clough's poems. FN quoted it to Clough's son Arthur in 1889. See CW1, 559.

'like two fools': FN to FaN, 8 January [1852]. Wellcome 8993/70. CW7, 680.

'Papa says': FN to FaN, 8 January [1852]. Wellcome 8993/71.

'quite full': FN to FaN, 9 January [1852]. Wellcome 8993/72.

'And if you': FN to FaN, 6 January [1852]. Wellcome 8993/69. CW7, 679.

p. 164 'a fancy place': FN to Hilary Bonham Carter, 28 March [1852]. BL 45794/150 [fragment].

'bundled out again': FN to FaN, WEN and PN [4 May 1852]. Wellcome 8993/124. CW7, 690.

'got her drinking over . . . convert': FN to FaN, WEN and PN, 16 May 1852. Wellcome 8993/124. CW7, 691, 694.

'unfulfilled hopes': FN to WEN, 12 May 1852. Wellcome 8993/85. CW1, 236.

p. 165 ' "formulas" ': Marian Evans to Sara Sophia Hennell [29 June 1852]. *The George Eliot Letters*, 2, 39-40.

p. 166 Aunt Mai continued to attend the Essex Street Chapel: See FN to PN, [February 1852]. Claydon 123. CW1, 312-3.

'having a family': FN to FaN, [mid-1840s]. Claydon 215.

'metaphysical mind': PN to Mary Mohl, [November 1852]. Quoted in O'Malley, 99.

'all she had taught': FN to FaN, WEN and PN, 17 January 1850. Wellcome 9017/16. CW4, 258

'. . . I have become': FN to Mai Smith, [1850]. BL 45793/75.

p. 167 'mere tea-drinkers': FN to Elizabeth Herbert, 4 September [1849]. BL 43396/7. CW3, 245.

'. . . One would think': FN to WEN, [summer 1851]. Wellcome 8993/46. CW3, 360.

'almost wholly uncared-for': FN to Henry Manning, 30 June [1852]. Pitts Theological Library, Emory University. CW3, 248.

p. 168 'perplexing mystery'; Dickens, *Hard Times*, chapter 5.

'I like anything': FN to FaN, [spring 1851]. Wellcome 8993/56.

'a west-end lady': Cook I, 120.

p. 169 'the most thinking': FN to Sir John McNeill, 17 May 1860. Quoted in Cook I, 120.

From her cousin Hilary: 'When you come back, you will tell me all about Comte . . .' FN to Hilary Bonham Carter, [1852]. BL 45794/150.

'any of my': FN to WEN, 12 May 1852. Wellcome 8993/85. CW1, 236.

'would look over': FN to Richard Monckton Milnes, 16 January [1853]. Houghton Papers, Trinity College Cambridge, 18/130.

a sixty-five-page proof: Bishop and Goldie, *A Bio-Bibliography of Florence Nightingale*, 119. This was the work on 'Religion' that FN referred to, some of which was later incorporated into the third volume of *Suggestions for Thought* (as opposed to the 'Novel' which became 'Cassandra' in the second volume). For a useful discussion of the chronology of the composition of FN's 'Works', see Calabria and Macrae (eds.), *Suggestions for Thought . . . Selections and Commentaries*, xxxvi.

p. 170 'With regard to health': Calabria and Macrae (eds.), *Suggestions for Thought . . . Selections and Commentaries*, 74.

a memorandum to herself: Quoted in O'Malley, 387.

p. 171 'deadly statistical clock': Dickens, *Hard Times*, chapter 15.

'I can never': FN to PN, 26 November 1847. Wellcome 9016/17. CW7, 115.

John Rickman: Rickman visited Embley in the 1840s. Correspondence at Claydon 47.

a study of the results of the 1841 Census: BL 43402/96–7. CW5, 92–5.

questionnaire: See letter from W. King of a hospital in Brighton to 'My Dear Sir', 25 November 1851 (BL 45790/143), which is perhaps one response to FN's circular of questions. Also draft circular, BL 45796/46.

Alphonse Quetelet: For an outline of Quetelet's work, see Stigler, *The History of Statistics*, 169–71, and 219–20. FN's copy of the two-volume 1869 edition of Quetelet's *Physique Sociale*, presented to her by the author in 1872, is now at University College, London. For a discussion of FN's relationship to Quetelet and of her marginal annotations to his work, see Diamond and Stone, 'Nightingale on Quetelet'.

p. 173 'a poor feckless': FN to Henry Manning, 29 June [1852]. Wellcome 8993/93[draft]. CW3, 247.

'After this': Henry Manning to Robert Wilberforce. Quoted in 'Henry Manning', *Oxford Dictionary of National Biography*.

'extinguished': FN to Elizabeth Herbert, 4 September [1849]. BL 43396/7. CW3, 245.

Mary Stanley . . . closer to conversion: 'I am afraid Mary's conversion is beginning to be talked about', FN to PN, [January 1852]. Wellcome 8993/74.

Florence's letters to Manning: Peter C. Erb and Elizabeth J. Erb, 'Florence Nightingale For and Against Rome', provides an excellent analysis of the correspondence.

p. 174 'All my difficulties': FN to Henry Manning, 30 June [1852]. Wellcome 8993/94 [draft]. CW3, 247–8.

'the uniformities': FN to Henry Manning, 13 July [1852]. Pitts Theological College, Emory University. CW3, 252.

'in the eyes': FN to Henry Manning, 22 July [1852]. Pitts Theological College, Emory University. CW3, 255.

'If you have': FN to Henry Manning, 19 August [1852]. Pitts Theological College, Emory University. CW3, 257.

'. . . My mission': FN to WEN, 29 August [1852]. Wellcome 8993/99. CW7, 714.

p. 175 'She has a great': Charlotte Clark to FN, [6 September 1852]. Claydon 300.

'. . . My dear Pop': FN to FaN, [13 September 1852]. Wellcome 8993/109. CW1, 130.

'absolutely no disease': Sir James Clark to FaN, 12 September [1852]. Claydon 300.

'The flood': PN to [?], 19 September [1852]. Claydon 23.

'fancies are more in number': FN to FaN, [20 September 1852]. Wellcome 8993/112. CW1, 131.

'not quite': PN to FaN [n.d.]. Claydon 300.

p. 176 'as nice': FN to FaN and WEN, 20 September 1852. Wellcome 8993/104. CW7, 707.

'a fine intellect': Sir James Clark to FaN and WEN, 7 October 1852. Claydon 300.

'awful warning': FN to Henry Manning, [29 September 1852]. Pitts Theological College, Emory University. CW3, 266.

'Sir JC's': FaN, Note. Claydon 274.

'bodily': FN to FaN and WEN, 30 September [1852]. Wellcome 8993/106. CW1, 106.

p. 177 'dim and dreary': Poem by PN, [1852–3]. Wellcome 9050/6. CW1, 313.

'by the conventional': FN to Henry Manning, 28 September [1852]. Pitts Theological College, Emory University. CW3, 260.

'something of the difficulties': FN, Draft novel. BL 45839/90.

'Cassandra': 'Cassandra' is named after the Trojan priestess to whom Apollo granted the gift of prophecy on condition that no one would believe her. Cassandra has individuality thrust upon her in infancy, and learns to fend for herself, and not rely on the teachings of others. She doesn't speak from received knowledge, but from a unique imagination of reality. She is a visionary, but her vision is not one that her fellow Trojans wish to hear. The name 'Cassandra' appears only once in the text of the version printed by Ray Strachey. But in the draft novel versions Cassandra appears as 'Aunt Cassandra', and Cassandra is also the name taken by Nofriani shortly before her death. FN's own identification with Cassandra is made clear in a letter to Hilary Bonham Carter of 8 January 1852 (quoted in Cook I, 116) in which she refers to herself as 'Poor Cassandra'.

'I must do something': Quoted in O'Malley, 175.

p. 178 March 1853: This suggests that the novel version was finally abandoned after the death of FN's grandmother Mary Shore, on 25 March 1853.

'very painful': The Letters of Mrs Gaskell, 117.

'self-indulgent': Stephen, Passages, 26.

'. . . she had no interest': ibid., 15.

'idle reverie . . . family': ibid., 77.

p. 179 'whether she did not like . . . aloud': FN, Draft novel. BL 45839/66–79. CW8, 116–17.

'the impossible': FN, Draft novel. BL 45839/66–79. CW8, 122.

'Of my life': FN, Draft novel. BL 45839/66–79. CW8, 118.

p. 180 'a stranded ship': FN to Henry Manning, [29 September 1852]. Pitts Theological College, Emory University. CW3, 266.

'a little strengthening': FN to FaN, 11 November [1852]. Wellcome 8993/116.

'eternal poor': PN to Mary Mohl, [November 1852]. Quoted in O'Malley, 99.

p. 181 'Flo you know': Mary Mohl to PN, [1852–3]. Claydon 35.

'self-forgetting': Quoted in Mayne, The Life and Letters of Lady Byron, 332.

'Poor sweet': Mai Smith to [?, n.d.]. Claydon 370.

'They also serve': Fanny Allen to PN, 2 May [1853]. Claydon 95.

a proposal of marriage: William Spottiswoode to WEN, 10 July 1854. Verney 10/327.

'. . . I hope I shall not ill requite your kindness in venturing to ask whether you would be willing to spare your eldest daughter, & she could be persuaded to exchange her home life for such a life as I could offer her.'

p. 182 'Ever since': Selina Bracebridge to Mai Smith, [1852]. Claydon 92.

'to follow out': Mai Smith to FaN, [1852]. Claydon 67.

'her Parents': Selina Bracebridge to Mai Smith, [n.d.]. Claydon 92.

'I do indeed': FN to FaN, [January 1853]. Wellcome 8994/2. CW1, 136.

p. 183 'She would never': Mary Mohl to PN, 16 February [1853]. Claydon 240.

'I think it': FN to FaN, 2 March [1853]. Wellcome 8994/9.

'Notre-Dame . . . effect': FN to FaN, [January 1853]. Wellcome 8994/4. CW7, 724.

'I have been': FN to PN, [5 February 1853]. Wellcome 8994/6.

p. 184 'The first snowdrops': FN to FaN, [14 March 1853]. Wellcome 8994/16. CW1, 417.

'diminished': WEN to FaN, [March 1853]. Claydon 390.

'Night nor day': FN to Hilary Bonham Carter, 25 March [1853]. BL 45794/153.

'so characteristic': FN to FaN, [1 April 1853]. Wellcome 8994/19.

'I was much touched': FN to FaN, 5 April [1853]. Wellcome 8994/23.

'first on': FN to FaN, WEN and PN, 8 April 1853. Wellcome 8994/24.

'I will call': Elizabeth Herbert to FN, [14 April 1853]. BL 43396/10.

p. 185 '... I hope the old': Lady Canning to Elizabeth Herbert, [18 April 1853]. Claydon 240 [copy].

Mrs Mary Clarke: For her acceptance of the post of 'Matron' (i.e. housekeeper), see Mrs Clarke to FN, 25 April 1853. BL 45796/15.

'impossible future ... in the air': WEN to FaN, [April 1853] (enclosing memorandums). Claydon 354.

p. 186 the strongest character: FN, Note, [1857]. BL 43402/182. CW5, 233.

'I do not wish': FN to Mary Mohl, 27 August [1853]. Quoted in Cook I, 138–9.

strains imposed ... by family tensions: see, for instance, FN, Notes on the family, c. 1857, in which she claims, in a cancelled phrase, to have 'first felt the symptom of the disease which is now bringing me to my grave' during a violent altercation with PN in 1851. BL 43402/178. CW5, 233.

'a thumbscrew': FN, [?]. Quoted in CW5, 623.

'unloving love': This phrase (aperōtos erōs) comes from Aeschylus's Cheophori, where the chorus sings of the terrible events produced in particular by female passion. For FN's use of it, see, for example, FN to PN, [1858–9]. Wellcome 8997/69. CW1, 321.

p. 187 'eccentric turn': FaN, Note, Claydon 280.

a bracelet: Now in the FN Museum (0028).

CHAPTER 8: IN THE HEY-DAY OF MY POWER

p. 188 formal acceptance: FN's acceptance of the post of 'Lady Superintendent of the Hospital for Invalid Gentlewomen' was made in a letter of 29 April [1853] to Lady Canning (BL 45796/17. Copy).

' "scrimmage" ': PN to Lothian Nicholson, [n.d.]. Claydon 283.

'behaved beautifully': [?]. BL 72826/97.

'absolute denials': PN to Lothian Nicholson, [n.d.]. Claydon 283.

'... but ... we are': PN to Hannah Nicholson, [n.d.]. Wellcome 9039/9.

p. 189 'paper wars': FN to Lothian Nicholson, 19 August [1853]. Wellcome 8994/36. CW1, 464.

'a comedy': FN to Mary Mohl, 8 April [1853]. BL 43397/306. CW8, 559.

'My Committee': Quoted in Cook I, 134.

'the gentlewoman': Establishment for Gentlewomen During Illness, 3.

p. 190 'wretchedly delicate': C. Brown to FN, 25 March [1854]. Claydon 240.

'... a Lady': 'Benevolent Institutions', 100.

'too good': Fanny Allen to PN, 21 October [1854]. Claydon 95.

'to the apparent eye': 'Memoir'.

p. 191 'Decayed Gentlewomen': Patty Smith to FaN, [summer 1853]. Claydon 283.

'most heartily': Elizabeth Blackwell to FN, 27 March [1854]. Claydon 240.

'volunteer': FN to Lady Canning, 29 April [1853]. BL 45796/17. [Copy].

'the Institution': FN to Lady Canning, 18 May 1853. BL 45796/33.

three-storeyed house: 90 Harley Street was demolished in 1909–10, and a stone plaque mounted on the new building to commemorate FN's association with the site. No photograph has come to light of the original building, though it's almost inconceivable that such a record of the house's appearance would not have been made.

p. 192 'instead of being': FN to FaN, [June 1853]. Wellcome 8994/23.

'... I have had': FN to FaN, 27 June [1853]. Wellcome 8994/28.

'You see': Selina Bracebridge to FN, [summer 1853]. Claydon 240.

'for stained': FN to PN, 24 July [1853]. Wellcome 8994/32.

'rat-eaten': *Florence Nightingale at Harley Street*, 1.

'converted': FN to Lady Canning, 5 June [1853]. BL 45796/40.

'I who never': FN to PN, 20 August [1853]. Wellcome 8994/37.

purchases: FN, Account book, 1 July 1853. BL 43403/A.

p. 193 'hermetically sealed': BL 43402/141.

'a turn': Mai Smith to FaN, [1853-4]. Claydon 303.

'... I so well': Lady Canning to PN, 20 June 1853. Claydon 315.

'dear Pop's': FN to WEN, 6 September 1853. BL 45790/148.

'You foolish': FN to PN, 19 October [1853]. Wellcome 8994/48.

'To settle': FN, Notes. Claydon 240.

p. 194 'went off': FN to WEN, 30 August [1853]. Wellcome 8994/38.

'John, the Cook': FN to Lady Canning, [c. August 1853]. BL 45796/50.

'nothing of the': FN to Lady Canning, 13 September 1853. Harewood Collection, 177/Z/5.

'our slovenly': FN to PN, 30 September [1853]. Wellcome 8994/44.

'salaried nurses': FN to Theodore Fliedner, 10 September 1853. Wellcome 9083/3.

[Copy. Translation from French]. For FN's plan, pre-Harley Street, for a private London hospital, run on non-denominational lines by nursing sisters, one of whom would be called the 'Mother', see *CW*8, 528-34.

'full of joy': FN to FaN, WEN and PN, 16 September 1853. Wellcome 8994/42.

'We are': FN to PN, 30 September 1853. Wellcome 8994/44.

'our new': FN to FaN, [11 October 1853]. Wellcome 8994/47.

'a good operation': FN to PN, 30 September 1853. Wellcome 8994/44.

'Rules for Patients': Wellcome 8994/80.

p. 195 'You are': Barbara Fleetwood to FN, 14 June [1854]. Claydon 240.

'Miss Nightingale's kindness': Christina Murray to [?, n.d.]. Claydon 240.

'care & kindness': Bessie Marks to FN, 13 May [1854]. Claydon 240.

'Sanatorium': Dante Gabriel Rossetti to William Rossetti, 14 May 1854, *The Correspondence of Dante Gabriel Rossetti*, 347. Rossetti's 'maniac aunt', Eliza Polidori, later managed the stores at the Barrack Hospital at Scutari. His sister Christina applied to accompany her aunt to Scutari but was rejected as too young.

'There is not': *Florence Nightingale at Harley Street*, 11.

'I had great': FN to FaN, WEN and PN, [November 1853]. Wellcome 8994/64.

p. 196 'observations': FN to WEN, 3 December 1853. BL 45790/152-5. CW1, 237.

'I regret': WEN to FN, [1853]. Claydon 240.

'constantly nursing': Anne Clarke to FN, 9 January [1854]. Claydon 240.

'an insane governess': FN to PN, 17 January 1854. Wellcome 8994/93.

p. 197 'bad pay': Elizabeth Herbert to FN, [1854]. Claydon 36.

'I had rather': FN, to WEN, [c. 26 May 1854]. BL 45790/158. CW1, 239 (where it is misdated to April 1854).

'... There have been difficulties': Mai Smith to FaN, [June 1854]. Claydon 289.

'They have asked': FN to FaN, 26 July 1854. Wellcome 8994/107.

p. 198 'Physical & Moral': Selina Bracebridge to FaN, 6 August [1854]. Claydon 240.

'as to good': *Florence Nightingale at Harley Street*, 33-6.

'devoted services': Lady Canning to FN, 8 August 1854. Claydon 315.

'leading Men': FN to PN, 25 August 1854. Wellcome 8994/110.

'where all received her': Claydon 276. See Smith, *Florence Nightingale*, 17: 'There is no evidence that Miss Nightingale ever revisited Harley Street or took any further interest in it.' This is just one example of Smith's tendency to make categorical statements to the detriment of FN's reputation without examination of the available evidence.

p. 199 'I ask': FN, *The Times*, 12 November 1901. See Bishop and Goldie, *A Bio-*

Bibliography of Florence Nightingale, 99, who suggest that the letter was written for FN by Elinor Dicey (née Bonham Carter).

Florence volunteered: Again, this is disputed by Smith, *Florence Nightingale*, 17, who states that the story of FN's work at the Middlesex is not supported by the hospital's archives. But it is confirmed in 'Memoir'.

'privatish' letter: Mrs Gaskell to Catherine Winkworth, [11–14 October 1854]. *The Letters of Mrs Gaskell*, 306–7.

p. 200 **'in every one's mouth'**: FaN to William Spottiswoode, [1855]. Claydon 286. ('Tomorrow I will make a holocaust of all remaining proof-sheets.' William Spottiswoode to FaN, 21 February 1855. Claydon 97.)

'does not care': Mrs Gaskell to Emily Shaen, [27 October 1854]. *Further Letters of Mrs Gaskell*, 114–16.

p. 201 **'If I were a Roman Catholic'**: Gaskell, *North and South*, chapter 15. A copy of Gaskell's novel was requested by FN at Scutari, in August 1855. Goldie, 144.

'thread of dark-red blood': Gaskell, *North and South*, chapter 22.

p. 202 **'We hope'**: Elizabeth Herbert to FN, 29 September [1854]. Claydon 204.

p. 203 **'Well, here we are'**: A. H. Clough to C. E. Norton, [February 1854]. *The Correspondence of Arthur Hugh Clough*, 2, 476.

'all buoyant': Quoted in Royle, *Crimea*, 178.

'but mentioned': 'Memoir'.

p. 205 **'than to march'**: FN to Selina Bracebridge, [15 October 1854]. Wellcome 8994/113. [Dictated]. Goldie, 21.

'to say': FN to Elizabeth Herbert, 14 October 1854. BL 43396/11.

p. 206 **a theory**: Smith, *Florence Nightingale*, 26. See Goldie, 22, for an efficient demolition of the idea.

'no military reason': Sidney Herbert to FN, 16 October 1854. Wellcome 8994/115. Goldie, 23.

p. 207 **'Government has asked'**: Quoted in Cook I, 154.

'in which all things': Quoted in Cook I, 155.

p. 208 **'to tamper'**: Sidney Herbert to FN, 20 October 1854. BL 43393/1. Goldie, 27.

49 Belgrave Square: Since 1936 this historic house has been the Argentinian Embassy.

surviving applications: PRO WO 25/264.

p. 209 **'sudden questions'**: Rickards, *Felicia Skene of Oxford*, 111. Skene writes that Mrs Bracebridge acted like the Duchess in *Alice in Wonderland* when she clearly means the Queen of Hearts.

'seeing nurses': PN, 'F's Journal'. Claydon 317.

'of no particular religion': Lesser, *Clarkey*, 99.

'in the centre': PN, 'F's Journal', Claydon 317.

p. 210 **'calm & self professed'**: FaN to Elizabeth Herbert, [October 1854]. Claydon 317.

her copy of Thomas à Kempis's: In the FN Museum. For the inscription, see CW2, 388.

'as I never loved': FN remembered these words in a letter written after the war. FN to WEN, 23 March 1857. BL 45790/177.

'with Miss F': Mary Watson to FaN, 19 October 1854. Claydon 240. I have silently changed Athena's sex here. Mrs Watson was under the impression that the owl was male.

'Her mistress': 'Memoir'.

CHAPTER 9: CALAMITY UNPARALLELED

p. 215 'the ugliest object': Terrot, *Nurse Sarah Anne*, 80.

'after climbing': Quoted in Shepherd, *The Crimean Doctors*, 1, 65.

Bracebridge . . . estimated: Charles Bracebridge to PN, 9 November 1854. Claydon 273 [Copy].

p. 216 In 1973: See correspondence about the museum at Scutari in Wellcome 8643.

sketches: These coloured sketches are now at the Royal Army Medical Corps Historical Museum at Aldershot. Several are reproduced in Goldie.

'so good': Maurice, *Life of Octavia Hill*, 431.

'a little': Charles Bracebridge to PN, 9 November 1854. Claydon 273 [Copy].

p. 217 'have any': Maurice, *Life of Octavia Hill*, 431.

'heroic dead': FN to PN, [8 March 1855]. Wellcome 8995/8. Goldie, 104.

Florence went ahead: This is clear from A. H. Clough to C. E. Norton, 21 October 1854. *The Correspondence of Arthur Hugh Clough*, 2, 490. W-S, 146, gives the impression that the party left London with FN. See also Terrot, *Nurse Sarah Anne*, 77, 'Miss Nightingale had preceded us to Paris.'

'feckless': Selina Bracebridge to [?], 22 October [1854]. Claydon 317.

'a very tasteful': Charles Bracebridge to PN, 26 October 1854. Claydon 52.

Marianne Galton: 'We met them at the steamboat & I have just been helping Mrs Bracebridge to set them down to a most magnificent banquet . . .' (Marianne Galton to FaN, 23 October 1854. Claydon 317).

binoculars: Now in the National Army Museum, London (NAM 1963-10-216).

'at the last': Sam Smith to FaN, [October 1854]. Claydon 317.

p. 218 'She lies': Charles Bracebridge to PN, 29 October 1854. Claydon 290.

'a very sensible . . . very suffering': Selina Bracebridge to PN, 3 November [1854]. Claydon 290.

p. 219 'in thick & heavy': FN to FaN, WEN and PN, 4 November 1854. Wellcome 8995/115. Goldie, 33.

'vast field': Osborne, *Scutari and Its Hospitals*, 12.

'the order': ibid., 15.

p. 221 'only two or three': Quoted by Richardson in Terrot, *Nurse Sarah Anne*, 85.

p. 222 'a humiliating contrast': Quoted ibid., 88.

unaware of the existence: 'When we came out we had not the slightest idea that there were two Hospitals . . .'. Selina Bracebridge to PN [November 1854]. Claydon 273.

'more like': Quoted in Shepherd, *The Crimean Doctors*, 1, 187.

'There is plenty': Quoted ibid., 1, 184.

'the sick . . . against us . . .': Quoted ibid., 1, 172. As Shepherd points out, Hall did not make the remark frequently attributed to him (e.g. W-S, 210) that the hospital establishment at Scutari 'has now been put on a very creditable footing and nothing is lacking'.

p. 223 'that intense': Fanny Allen to PN, 29 November [1854]. Claydon 302.

Alexander McGrigor: FN was later generous in giving credit to McGrigor for many of the improvements introduced to the Barrack Hospital. She recommended McGrigor's promotion to Sidney Herbert to ensure that he would not be superseded by a more senior officer.

p. 224 'regularity and comfort': Duncan Menzies to John Hall, 8 December 1854. Quoted in Mitra, *The Life and Letters of Sir John Hall*, 2, 338.

'Miss N.': Charles Bracebridge to Sidney Herbert, 8 November [1854]. Herbert Papers, Wiltshire Record Office.

'a wee room': Selina Bracebridge to PN, [November 1854]. Claydon 273.

'We tried': Terrot, *Nurse Sarah Anne*, 88.

p. 225 'to take': Richard Dawes to [?], 27 November [1854]. Claydon 290.

p. 226 'The great corridor': Charles Bracebridge to Sidney Herbert, 8 November [1854]. Herbert Papers, Wiltshire Record Office.

Bracebridge's figures: Charles Bracebridge to PN, 9 November 1854. Claydon 273 [Copy].

'Flo has not': Selina Bracebridge to FaN, 10 November [1854]. Claydon 273.

'700 were landed ... on the other': Charles Bracebridge to PN, 13 November [1854]. Claydon 273.

p. 227 'her breakfast': Selina Bracebridge to PN, [n.d.]. Claydon 52.

'cutting, cooking': Charles Bracebridge to PN, 15 November [1854]. Claydon 302 [Copy].

'of this appalling': FN to William Bowman, 14 November 1854. Private Collection. Goldie, 37.

p. 228 'Miss Nightingale': Lieutenant-General Sir John Burgoyne to Lord Raglan, 27 March 1855. National Army Museum, London (NAM 1968-07-293-9). See also Marianne Estcourt, MS Diary, Gloucestershire Record Office, D1571, F555-8. Marianne Estcourt, who travelled to the Crimea in 1854-5 to see her brother Major-General James Estcourt, reported on 29 January 1855, 'Capn. Jordan tells us that Miss Nightingale loves an operation to such a degree that she is always told what are going to be performed, has a list.'

flurry of controversy: See Shepherd, *The Crimean Doctors*, 1, 281–2.

p. 229 'This morning': FN to Sidney Herbert, 21 December 1854. BL 43393/41. Goldie, 52.

Francis Eyre: Francis Eyre, 9 January 1855. Claydon 286.

Mrs Gollop: Mrs Gollop, 2 April 1855. Claydon 319.

'I am really': FN to Sidney Herbert, 28 January 1855. BL 43393/113. Goldie, 79.

'a fine specimen': 'Extract from Mr Maxwell's ... letters to his wife', [1855]. Claydon 274.

p. 230 'for the systematic organization': FN to Sidney Herbert. 8 January 1855. BL 43393/75. Goldie, 73.

idea of officially appointing her: According to a letter from Elizabeth Herbert to FaN, 21 January [1855]. Claydon 302.

'What F does': PN, Note. Claydon 302.

as Aunt Mai was to report: 'She [FN] does no nursing work beyond going round to see the patients.' Mai Smith to FaN [August 1855]. Claydon 302.

p. 231 'for the love of': Selina Bracebridge to PN, 20 [January 1855]. Claydon 93.

'... We Cannot': [?] to Mary Jones, 4 December 1854. LMA HI/ST/SU/15.

'persons ... seldom sober': Quoted in Luddy (ed.), *The Crimean Journals of the Sisters of Mercy 1854-56*, xvi.

'somewhat brusque': FN to Council of St John's House, 11 January 1855. LMA HI/ST/NC.3/SU18. FN later admitted to Aunt Mai (16 April 1855) that Mrs Clarke 'either gets drunk or connives at the drunkenness of others'. Wellcome 8995/11.

'not Mix': Mary Ann Coyle to Mary Jones, 5 December 1854. LMA HI/ST/SU/16.

p. 232 'of every branch': PRO WO 25/264.

'With the greates': [?] to Mary Jones, 4 December 1854. LMA HI/ST/SU/15.

'very meek-looking': Quoted in Cope, *Florence Nightingale and the Doctors*, 47.

'Miss Nightingale is sweet': Luddy (ed.), *The Crimean Journals of the Sisters of Mercy 1854-56*, 86.

'a very ugly one': ibid., 64.

'uniform upper clothing': PRO WO 43/963.

p. 233 'not laced': Selina Bracebridge to PN 12 March [1855]. Claydon 273. A pair of moccasins said to have been worn by FN at Scutari, which were purchased by Henry Wellcome in 1929, are now part of the collection of the Wellcome Institute in London.

'She has one': Selina Bracebridge to PN, 22 February [1855]. Claydon 273.

'no time for long hair': Inscription on envelope containing a lock of hair cut off at Scutari in the winter of 1854-5. Verney 13/47.

'fonder of sketching': FN, Notes on Nurses. BL 43402/6-7.

'she does not': FN to Miss Gipps, 5 December 1854. LMA HI/ST/NC.3/SU14. Goldie, 42.

'of an infinitely': FN, Notes on Nurses. BL 43402/6–7.

'she was fit': Quoted in Sullivan (ed.), *The Friendship of Florence Nightingale and Mary Clare Moore*, 5.

p. 234 'speak soothingly': PRO WO 43/963.

'great disappointment': Emma Fagg to Mary Jones, 4 January 1855. LMA HI/ST/NC.3/SU22

'flibberty-gibbet': FN to Miss Gipps, 5 December 1854. LMA HI/ST/NC.3/SU14. Goldie, 42.

p. 235 'the fewer': FN, *Subsidiary Notes as to the Introduction of Female Nursing into Military Hospitals*, in Seymer (ed.), *Selected Writings of Florence Nightingale*, 73.

'very much': Quoted in Shepherd, *The Crimean Doctors*, 1, 280.

Greig's remarks: Quoted ibid. As it was, there were 38 nurses at Scutari for some 3,200 patients, which made each nurse responsible for 84 patients.

'Pray confirm': FN to Sidney Herbert, 25 December 1854. BL 43393/45. Goldie, 57.

p. 236 'Pray say': PN to WEN, [1854]. Claydon 305.

'overwhelmed': Elizabeth Herbert to FaN, [1854–5]. Verney 10/319.

'No wonder': Hilary Bonham Carter to PN, 4 December 1854. Claydon 209.

'entirely in the dark': PN to A. P. Stanley, [1855]. Claydon 302 [Draft].

p. 237 'We have painfully': Charles Bracebridge to PN, 15 December 1854. Claydon 273.

'air of comfort': Quoted in Rappaport, *No Place for Ladies*, 123.

'in great haste': FN to Sidney Herbert, 10 December 1854. BL 43393/22. Goldie, 48.

'itemizing': Hon. Jocelyn Percy to Emily Percy, 31 January 1855. Heber-Percy Archive.

'well knowing': FN to Sidney Herbert, 15 December 1854. BL 43393/34. Goldie, 50–51.

p. 238 'You have not stood': FN to Sidney Herbert, 15 December 1854. BL 43393/45. Goldie, 55.

'. . . There never was': Selina Bracebridge to PN, 21 December [1854]. Claydon 52.

p. 239 'which express': Charles Bracebridge to WEN, 5 February [1855]. Claydon 290.

'the perfect drudge': Quoted in Luddy (ed.), *The Crimean Journals of the Sisters of Mercy 1854–56*, xvi.

'an ardent': Quoted ibid., xii.

'lunch': ibid., 128.

'with a religious': FN to Sidney Herbert, 25 December 1854. BL 43393/45. Goldie, 55.

p. 240 'Dearest': FN to Mary Stanley, 20 December [1854]. Columbia School of Nursing, C-9.

'I confess': Quoted in Stanmore, *Sidney Herbert*, I, 375.

often partisan: The account most strongly in Stanley's favour is Stanmore, *Sidney Herbert*, I, 376–8. The diary of Marianne Estcourt (9 March 1855) provides an interesting commentary, from an unsympathetic contemporary observer, on the Nightingale–Stanley relationship. Marianne Estcourt, MS Diary, Gloucestershire Record Office, D1571, F555–8.

'Could Mrs Herbert': FN to Sidney Herbert, 28 January 1855. BL 43393/113. Goldie, 80.

'noble example': A. P. Stanley to PN, [1855]. Claydon 255.

'mutual affection': Mary Stanley to PN, 11 January [1855]. Claydon 290.

p. 241 'with an official': Elizabeth Herbert to FaN, 10 May [1856]. Verney 10/319.

'We long': Charles Bracebridge to PN, 13 March 1855. Claydon 273.

'So Mary': Quoted in Mitford (ed.), *The Stanleys of Alderley*, 95.

'from accepting': PN to Lady Canning, [1855]. Claydon 255.

a veiled threat: [?] to PN, 12 January [?1856]. Claydon 295.

p. 242 'for she is': Luddy (ed.), *The Crimean Journals of the Sisters of Mercy 1854–56*, 136.

'when she considered': ibid., 181.

p. 243 'the lady plan': FN to Sidney Herbert, 15 February 1855. BL 43393/154. Goldie, 92.

'scampering': Quoted in Summers, *Angels and Citizens*, 43.

'wandering': FN to Sidney Herbert, 12 February 1855. BL 43393/146. Goldie, 88.

'who promise': Quoted in Shepherd, *The Crimean Doctors*, 2, 351.

'betrayal': Selina Bracebridge to PN, 5 February [1855]. Claydon 93.

a staff sent to ... Balaclava: Martha Clough (no relation of A. H.), one of Mary Stanley's ladies, went to Balaclava in January 1855. She absconded in March, without FN's consent, to take charge of a regimental hospital with the Highland Brigade, and died of fever in September 1855. See Roxburgh, 'Miss Nightingale and Miss Clough. Letters from the Crimea'.

p. 244 outside the area: A point made by Summers, *Angels and Citizens*, 46.

'But I must bar': FN to Sidney Herbert, 19 February 1855. BL 43393/164. Goldie, 93.

'I regret': Mary Stanley to FN, 23 March 1855. Claydon 319 [Copy].

'Mary Stanley': *Collected Letters of Thomas and Jane Welsh Carlyle*, 256.

'treachery': FN to Lady Canning, [1855]. Claydon 255.

a jewel: This brooch, made by R. & S. Garrard & Co. in 1855, is now in the National Army Museum (NAM. 1963-10-280). It is described in the *Illustrated London News* for 2 February 1856.

'Do not be taken': FN to PN, 17 March 1856. Claydon 265.

p. 245 'The feeling': Stanley, *Memoirs of Edward and Catherine Stanley*, 344.

'formed one of': Russell, *The British Expedition to the Crimea*, 182.

'They stretch': Charles Bracebridge to PN, 14 January 1855. Claydon 93.

p. 246 '... The mortality': FN to Sidney Herbert, 5 February 1855. BL 43393/131. Goldie, 83.

'Can you suppose': FN to FaN, 1 February 1855. Wellcome 8995/3. Goldie, 81.

'an Originator': FN to FaN, 5 February 1855. Wellcome 8995/4. Goldie, 86.

p. 247 '... No one': FN to Sidney Herbert, 18 March 1855. BL 43393/192. Goldie, 107.

'Pray continue': Sidney Herbert to FN, 5 March 1855. Quoted in Stanmore, *Sidney Herbert*, I, 416.

'purify the hospitals': Cook I, 220.

p. 248 'marks of much': Quoted in Shepherd, *The Crimean Doctors*, 2, 397.

'The Sanitary Commission': FN to Sidney Herbert, 18 March 1855. BL 43393/192. Goldie, 108.

p. 249 'scarcely tenable': Shepherd, *The Crimean Doctors*, 2, 400.

'incompetent': Charles Bracebridge to WEN, 18 March 1855. Claydon 273.

'turned inside out': William Woodward Shore to FaN, 18 March 1855. Claydon 319.

'utterly ... in the dark': FN to Edwin Chadwick, 17 October 1860. Quoted in Cook I, 319.

'had received': Kinglake, *The Invasion of the Crimea*, 7, 485-6.

an older generation: For instance, a book I was raised on, Winston Churchill's *History of the English-speaking Peoples*, 4, 63.

'We pulled': FN to Elizabeth Herbert, 11 July 1885. BL 43396/45.

p. 250 'I would wish you': Charles Bracebridge to WEN, 24 March 1855. Claydon 273.

'all our arrangements': FN to Sidney Herbert, 26 February 1855. BL 43393/180. Goldie, 99.

'the bear-garden ... Robert Slow': FN to FaN, WEN and PN, 5 May 1855. Wellcome 8995/15. Goldie, 126-7.

CHAPTER 10: A VISIBLE MARCH TO HEAVEN

p. 251 'A Visible March': The phrase is Mrs Gaskell's. Mrs Gaskell to PN, [20 October 1854]. *The Letters of Mrs Gaskell*, 314.

Illustrated London News: On the *ILN* during the Crimean War, see Armstrong, 'Art and War Reportage in the Crimean War I: the *Illustrated London News*.'

p. 252 'day & night': Patty Smith to FaN, [1855–6]. Claydon 305.

'called up': Mai Smith to FaN, [1855]. Claydon 319.

' "the little lamp" ': Mai Smith to her children, 2 September [1855]. Claydon 290.

'She is a "ministering angel" ': Quoted in Cook I, 236–7.

'A dim': Taylor, *Eastern Hospitals and English Nurses*, 39.

p. 253 'The rats': Luddy (ed.), *The Crimean Journals of the Sisters of Mercy 1854–56*, 19.

lanterns with Crimean associations: See Attewell, 'Throwing light on Florence Nightingale. Of lamps and lanterns', and also Wellcome 8643.

'watered': Gwen Compton-Bracebridge to Margaret Stephen, 16 October [1913]. Wellcome 9077/69.

p. 254 'how inadequate': Henry W. Longfellow to PN, 25 January 1858. Verney 10/319.

'the true point': A. H. Clough to C. E. Norton, 23 November 1857. *The Correspondence of Arthur Hugh Clough*, 2, 536.

p. 255 'Nurses of Quality': *Punch* 27 (1854), 193.

p. 256 'the peculiar favour': Lady Maria Forester to PN, 17 November [1854]. Claydon 302.

'of that little': Quoted by PN in letter to Elizabeth Herbert, [December 1854–January 1855]. BL 43396/23.

'pretty good': Quoted in Smith, ' "A Noble Type of Good Heroic Womanhood" ', 63.

'without the possession': Osborne, *Scutari and Its Hospitals*, 25.

p. 257 'I can conceive . . . faith': ibid., 25–6.

'the frequent calls': Fanny Allen to PN, 30 March [1856]. Claydon 95.

p. 258 'an outpouring': PN to Arthur Stanley, [1855]. Claydon 280.

'the mother': C. Hamilton Gray to FaN, 23 October 1854. Claydon 305.

'The Queen': FaN to [?, n.d.]. Claydon 398.

'ventured out': FaN to [?, 1855]. Wellcome 9077/70.

'apotheosis': WEN to FaN, [1855]. Claydon 306.

'Surely it should': Hilary Bonham Carter to PN, [1855–6]. Claydon 56.

'They had just': WEN to FaN, 1 May 1855. Claydon 306.

p. 259 'inspiration': PN Note, [1855]. Claydon 296.

'You . . . are': Richard Monckton Milnes to PN, 8 September [1855]. Claydon 200.

'between 50 & 60': PN to Lady Elizabeth [?], [October–November 1854]. Claydon 302.

'12 or 13': PN to WEN, [1855]. Claydon 305.

'. . . the immense': PN to Bertha Smith, [1855]. Claydon 23.

'penworn': Sam Smith to PN, 18 December [1854]. Claydon 255.

'strictly Private': Elizabeth Herbert to PN, 21 January [1855]. Claydon 302.

'Her writing': PN to Elizabeth Herbert, [? 1856]. Claydon 296.

p. 260 'Miss Nightingale': Quoted in Cook I, 215.

'May we': PN to Elizabeth Herbert, 9 December 1854. BL 43396/14. [Copy].

'Nothing can': Lothian Nicholson to PN, 12 February 1855, Claydon 211.

'. . . if there': Private John Swains to Martha Swains and Mrs Ivernay, 3 April 1855. FN Museum (0523).

'. . . supposing . . . of course': Patty Smith to FaN (reporting on a Private of the 36th), [n.d.]. Claydon 314.

p. 261 'How did she look': Patty Smith to FaN, [October 1855]. Claydon 200.

Another man: PN, Note. Claydon 274.

'She's here': Unsigned note. Claydon 24.

'magic touch': Davies, *Florence Nightingale*, 9.

' "Miss Nightingale" . . . was to many': Hobson, *Catharine Leslie Hobson*, 48–9.

'The floating froth': *Punch*, 8 December 1855.

Poetry: There is a useful bibliography of FN-inspired poetry in Dereli, 'Gender Issues and the Crimean War: Creating Roles for Women?', 78–9, though it is far from complete. The album 'A Year at Scutari', Claydon 435, also includes a wide selection, as does the collection at the FN Museum (0507).

'the heroine': Cook I, 266.

'the Nightingale pedigree': Patty Smith to FaN, [October 1855]. Claydon 200.

p. 262 'Did you see': Patty Smith to FaN, 14 December [1855]. Claydon 303.

'Babies ad libitum': Mrs Gaskell to PN, 21 July [1855]. *The Letters of Mrs Gaskell*, 359.

'The mythical': PN to Richard Monckton Milnes, 12 September [1855]. Houghton papers, Trinity College, Cambridge, 18/151.

'come round again': Lady Dunsany to PN, [n.d.]. Claydon 278.

Mr Luck: Patty Smith to FaN, [n.d.]. Claydon 276.

Footnote: FN to PN, [September 1860]. Wellcome 8998/33.

p. 263 *Blackwood's Magazine*: Aytoun, 'The Conduct of the War', 15.

'. . . Let her': Ellen Tollet to PN, 6 November 1854. Claydon 317.

'your heroic sister': Elizabeth Barrett Browning to PN, [n.d.]. Verney 10/319.

'saintly nurse': Elizabeth Barrett Browning to Anna Jameson, 24 February 1855. *Letters of Elizabeth Barrett Browning*, 2, 189.

'revolution': Caroline Bathurst to PN, 16 July 1856. Claydon 295.

'Oh: Florence': Caroline Bathurst to PN, 26 January 1855. Claydon 302.

'degraded': Fanny Allen to PN, 12 August [1856]. Claydon 95.

p. 264 'What a veiled': Caroline Bathurst to PN, 16 July 1856. Claydon 295. On the same theme, Patty Smith to FaN, [1855–6], Claydon 23: 'I wish Mr Bracebridge or Mr Osborne could have touched even more plainly, on what is to me the brightest gem in Flo's diadem of martyrizing provocations, & that is her silence under so many odious abuses.'

'effigies & praises': FN to PN, 9 July 1855. Wellcome 8995/22. Goldie, 133.

Mary Stanley's assertion: Stanmore, *Sidney Herbert*, I, 374.

'How unlike': Selina Bracebridge to PN, [May 1855]. Claydon 93.

'two pictures': Fanny Wildgoose to FaN, 8 February 1855. Claydon 290.

prints . . . distributed: M. Fox to PN, 5 August 1856. Claydon 295.

'the article': Alfred Bonham Carter to [?], 29 January 1856. Claydon 307.

p. 265 Staffordshire factories: See Pugh, *Staffordshire Portrait Figures*, 259–62.

'Surely it would be': Patty Smith to FaN, [late 1855]. Claydon 319.

p. 266 her Bible: Annotation dated 6 December 1871. CW2, 166.

Steell's bust: The original marble bust, dated 1862, is in the National Army Museum (NAM 1963-10-193). There are bronze copies in the National Portrait Gallery and the FN Museum.

'soldiers, widows': Sir John Steell to WEN, 21 May 1861. Verney 10/143.

'serious inconvenience . . . show of': FN to Jerry Barrett, 18 July 1856. LMA HI/ST/SU193.

head and shoulders study: National Portrait Gallery (3303). Colonel Cadogan of the First Regiment Foot Guards also did two sketches of FN, dated 14 and 15 May 1856. These are now in the National Army Museum (NAM 1998-06-128-70/71).

p. 267 the Bracebridges: In 1859 Barrett would paint another canvas with a Crimean theme (though clearly not from life) of FN with Charles and Selina Bracebridge in a Constantinople street. This is now in the Wellcome Library in London (V0017966).

'looking at': Jerry Barrett to Thomas Agnew, 3 July 1857. National Portrait Gallery Archives.

Florence . . . never saw it: Despite Barrett's entreaties that she should. In May 1857, when she was hard at work on the Royal Commission on the Health of the Army, Barrett wrote to her, enclosing a photograph of the Barrack Hospital by James Robertson. 'My large picture of the arrival of the sick & wounded from Scutari will I trust soon be finished and I venture to hope that you will do me the <u>very great favour</u> of calling some time after the middle of next week in order that I may show it to you.' (Jerry Barrett to FN, 23 May 1857. Claydon 276). FN did later see the copy of the engraving of 'The Mission of Mercy' at Claydon. A note by her, *c.* 1877, identifies the figures in the picture. Claydon 431.

p. 268 **deposited at Buckingham Palace:** National Portrait Gallery (2939A) is a pen-and-ink diagram of the picture, drawn as an aid for Queen Victoria.

exhibited: A review in the *Athenaeum* (29 May 1858, 693) commented that 'an air of truthfulness pervades the whole scene'. Other large-scale paintings of FN at this time, painted from the imagination, included *The Wounded Soldier is Visited by Miss Nightingale* by Tomkins, exhibited at the Royal Academy. Album, 'A Year at Scutari'. Claydon 435.

p. 269 **'even had I':** FN to Lady Canning, 23 November 1856. Harewood Papers C177/23. Goldie, 288.

'flannel shifts': FN to Hilary Bonham Carter, 18 January 1863. BL 45794/205. CW3, 448.

'I did not like': Davis, *Autobiography*, II, 89.

repeated: Smith, *Florence Nightingale*. 38.

'odious <u>lying</u>': Selina Bracebridge to PN, [1857]. Claydon 307.

p. 270 **'Register of Nurses':** FN Museum (0073).

'extensive robbery': *Illustrated London News*, 15 September 1855.

'acquitted themselves': Palmer, *Florence Nightingale and the First Organized Delivery of Nursing Services*, 13.

p. 271 **'I often think':** FN to Mai Smith, [?1888]. Private Collection. Quoted in Small, *Florence Nightingale*, 32.

'Have you read': Patty Smith to FaN, 6 August [1857]. Claydon 309.

p. 272 **'an exemplary':** PRO WO/264.

'While the benevolent': *The Times*, 24 November 1856.

p. 273 **'that Englishwoman':** Seacole, *Wonderful Adventures*, 91.

p. 274 **'keenly observant':** ibid., 90.

'as I hear': Soyer, *A Culinary Campaign*, 269.

recently discovered evidence: 'At all events I was very glad that Florence appeared on the list of her [Mary Seacole's] subscribers. Whatever the other may be, or have been, it is one of F's privileges to sustain the publicans.' (Patty Smith to FaN, 6 August [1857]. Claydon 309. A list of subscribers to Seacole's Fund which includes FN's name has not come to light.

illegitimate teenage daughter: PN, Note, [?1857]. Claydon 110. For a discussion of this alleged daughter, and of FN's assertion that she was fathered by a Colonel Bunbury, see Robinson, *Mary Seacole*, 154–5. Robinson – and FN – assume that 'Sally Seacole', as this putative daughter was called, was Mary Seacole's child by one Henry Bunbury. Other sources suggest that the father was Thomas Bunbury, a Major-General in Jamaica from 1848 to 1854. I am grateful to Jane Robinson for elucidating this point.

'a "bad house" ': FN to Sir Harry Verney, [1870]. Wellcome 9004/60.

p. 275 **'The Path of Roses':** Quoted in Bakewell, *Lewis Carroll*, 75.

'Punch's . . . "Scutari" ': Published on 17 February 1855, this imagines FN as 'a bright star'.

Tupper's poem: 'To Florence Nightingale' in Tupper, *Lyrics* (1855), 159.

image of stability: I owe this idea to Dereli, 'Gender Issues and the Crimean War: Creating Roles for Women?', 66.

'. . . The people': Quoted in Cook I, 267.

p. 276 **'The men':** FN to PN, 10 May 1855. Wellcome 8995/16. Goldie, 130.

'packed like herrings': Charles Bracebridge to PN, 9 May [1855]. Claydon 93.

'a wonderful fancy': Charles Bracebridge to PN, [1855]. Claydon 24.

p. 277 'mustering & forming ... shell': FN to PN, 10 May 1855. Wellcome 8995/16. Goldie, 130.

13 May: Dated from account in letter of Mai Smith to FaN, [May 1855]. Claydon 290.

Colonel William Napier reported: Mai Smith to FaN, [May 1855]. Claydon 318.

CHAPTER 11: I SHALL NEVER FORGET

p. 278 as bad a case: Soyer, *A Culinary Campaign*, 133.

In one letter: FN to Sir John McNeill, 21 May 1855. BL 45768/1.

'which is called': Charles Bracebridge to Sidney Herbert, 22 May [1855]. Claydon 273 [Copy].

Panmure informed Herbert: Lord Panmure to Sidney Herbert, 25 May 1855. Claydon 273.

'convalescent': Charles Bracebridge, telegram, 26 May 1855. Claydon 273.

p. 279 'She was able': Charles Bracebridge to PN, 28 May [1855]. Claydon 273.

'from one': Charles Bracebridge to PN, 22 May [1855]. Claydon 273.

to 'quack': PN, Note, [?1857]. Claydon 110.

a call from Fanny Duberly: Duberly, *Mrs Duberly's War*, 174.

'And pray': Cook I, 259.

'jarring elements': FN to FaN, WEN and PN, 5 July 1855. Wellcome 8995/21. Goldie, 132.

'unconscious': FN to Mai Smith, 19 October 1855. BL 45793/106. Goldie, 166. The *Jura* does not appear on the 1855 shipping lists. See Shepherd, *The Crimean Doctors*, II, 501–2. For another account of the incident, see Soyer, *A Culinary Campaign*, 174–6. Soyer maintains that FN was transferred from the *Jura* because of its 'very disagreeable smell', which caused her to faint.

p. 280 'F looks': Selina Bracebridge to PN, [June 1855]. Claydon 52.

'Life and Death of Athena': The original is at Claydon. The FN Museum has a lithographed version.

'You have done': Fanny Allen to PN, 12 August [1856]. Claydon 286. See also Lady Canning to PN, 7 December [1856]. Claydon 286.

'& feeling so ill': Elizabeth Herbert to PN, 17 July [1855]. Claydon 255.

p. 281 'We all know': Sam Smith to FaN, 28 November [1855]. The services of the Bracebridges were due to be acknowledged the following day at the launch of the Nightingale Fund.

'lose the chance': Mai Smith to PN [1855]. Claydon 89.

'2 or 3 hours': FN to Mai Smith, 18 July 1855. BL 45793/104. On 31 August 1855, Mai Smith wrote to FaN that 'F's house is very pleasant, very airy & quiet', and that they breakfasted together at 7 before walking to the hospital at 9. Claydon 290.

'She looks pretty': Mai Smith to FaN, WEN and PN, [September 1855]. Claydon 52.

'Crimean Fever': See Young, 'Florence Nightingale's fever'.

'a compound': FN to FaN, WEN and PN, 18 June 1855. Wellcome 8995/17. Goldie, 131.

p. 282 brucellosis: For an analysis of the disease, see Spink, *The Nature of Brucellosis*.

'a great comfort': FN to the Bracebridges, 7 August 1855. Wellcome 8995/26. Goldie, 142.

p. 283 'When I lie ... two whole days': FN to the Bracebridges, 7 August 1855. Wellcome 8995/26. Goldie, 138–45.

ill-natured gossip: This was current before FN's illness, e.g. PN to Elizabeth Herbert, 8 May [1855], comments that the rumour originated 'in some malicious desire to complicate her already difficult position'. Claydon 293. See also Duberly, *Mrs Duberly's War*, xxv.

'hams, butter': FN to the Bracebridges, 7 August 1855. Wellcome 8995/26. Goldie, 138.

p. 284 'the education': Cook I, 283.

'... We have sent': PN to Ellen Tollet, [November 1855]. Quoted in Cook I, 280-81.

'I have never': Quoted in Cook I, 277.

p. 285 'I grieve': FN to Maria Hunt, 6 September 1855. LMA HI/ST/NC.1/55/4.

Florence sought Hall's assurance: See Goldie, 157-8.

p. 286 'It may be well': Rev. S. Woollett to Sir John Hall, 2 September 1855. BL 39867/28.

'the female element': FN to Sir John Hall, 21 September 1855. BL 39867/28. Goldie, 157.

p. 287 'at the beginning': Luddy (ed.), *The Crimean Journals of the Sisters of Mercy 1854-56*, 185.

'Really, Dr Hall': FN to Mai Smith, [October 1855]. Wellcome 8995/39. Goldie, 163.

'Knight of the Crimean': FN to Sidney Herbert, 3 April 1856. BL 43393/224. Goldie, 246.

'as that great': FN to WEN, 14 November 1855. Wellcome 8995/74. Goldie 174.

'Miss Nightingale appeared': Luddy (ed.), *The Crimean Journals of the Sisters of Mercy 1854-56*, 76.

p. 288 'papal aggression': Goldie, 159.

'Irish-Catholic': FN to Elizabeth Herbert, 17 November 1855. BL 43396/40. Goldie, 178.

'most difficult': Luddy (ed.), *The Crimean Journals of the Sisters of Mercy 1854-56*, 199.

'She wishes': ibid., 86.

'Christ was': FN to Mai Smith, 19 October 1855. BL 45793/106. Goldie, 165.

p. 289 'odd': Luddy (ed.), *The Crimean Journals of the Sisters of Mercy 1854-56*, 206.

'perfectly mad': Quoted in W-S, 188.

'neither kitchen': *The Times*, 16 October 1855. In a letter to *The Times*, 20 October 1855, Bracebridge claimed to have been misrepresented in certain respects.

'twaddling nonsense': Quoted in W-S, 230-31.

'a toady': Charles Bracebridge to WEN, 5 February [1855]. Claydon 290.

'active friend': FN to Charles Bracebridge, [October 1855]. BL 43397/171 [Typed copy].

p. 290 'her wasted': Hornby, *Constantinople during the Crimean War*, 150.

'Confidential Report': PRO WO 43/963. Reprinted in Goldie, 298-302.

'a malicious': FN to Lieutenant-Colonel Lefroy, 11 January 1856. BL 43397/205. Goldie, 194.

'only lower': FN to Sam Smith, 16 March 1856. BL 45792/20. Goldie, 234.

p. 291 'were definitely': FN to Lieutenant-Colonel Lefroy, 11 January 1856. BL 43397/205. Goldie, 202.

'I confess': Mr Prescott, PRO WO 43/963/223.

'The medical men': Lieutenant-Colonel Lefroy to F. Peel, [January 1856]. PRO WO 43/963/335.

'bruised & battered': FN to Lieutenant-Colonel Lefroy, 28 January 1856. Wellcome 8996/6. Goldie, 204.

'... The War Office': FN to Sidney Herbert, 21 February 1856. BL 43393/215. Goldie, 213.

p. 292 'an irritation': Sidney Herbert to FN, 6 March 1856. BL 43393/218. Goldie, 218.

'the rightful': Lord Panmure to Sir William Codrington, 25 February 1856. Goldie, 215.

'teapot and bracelet': Cook I, 268.

'People seem to think': FN to Sidney Herbert, 27 September 1855. Quoted in Cook I, 269.

p. 293 Dickens: Charles Dickens to Elizabeth Herbert, 21 October 1855. Claydon 304.

'... Our only wish'; Elizabeth Herbert to FaN, 25 November [1855]. Verney 10/319.

'universal oneness': Cook I, 270.

'sympathy': FN to Sidney Herbert, 6 January 1856. Quoted in Baly, *Florence Nightingale and the Nursing Legacy*, 19.

'a cut & dried': FN to Sidney Herbert, 6 January 1856. BL 43393/209. Goldie, 184.

p. 294 'is the only': FN to Henry Bence Jones, 1 March 1856. Wellcome 8996/15. CW 6, 234.

has been called: Baly, *Florence Nightingale and the Nursing Legacy*, 17.

'plenty of grimy': Mrs Gaskell to PN, [18 January 1856]. *The Letters of Mrs Gaskell*, 382–3.

p. 295 'a great deal': Mrs Gaskell to Richard Monckton Milnes, 16 December [1855]. *The Letters of Mrs Gaskell*, 377.

'a figure': Julia Smith to WEN, 30 May 1856. Claydon 210.

p. 296 'a sort of': Aunt Mai to FaN, WEN and PN, 18 [June 1856]. Claydon 209.

'quite prostrate': Quoted in Cope, *Florence Nightingale and the Doctors*, 68.

'rudeness': Luddy (ed.), *The Crimean Journals of the Sisters of Mercy 1854–56*, 224.

'. . . I cannot blame': Sir John Hall, to Lady Hall, [April 1856]. Quoted in Cope, *Florence Nightingale and the Doctors*, 55.

'Your pig sty': FN to Sam Smith, 17 April 1865. BL 45792/30.

'. . . This is one': Rev. Mother Bridgeman to Sir John Hall, 15 April 1858. Goldie, 254.

p. 297 'gratefully': FN to Mary Clare Moore, 29 April 1856. Sullivan (ed.), *The Friendship of Florence Nightingale and Mary Clare Moore*, 73.

'. . . She has a spirit': Mai Smith to FaN, WEN and PN, 7 July [1856]. Claydon 209.

'so must their': Mai Smith to FaN, WEN and PN, 18 [June 1856]. Claydon 209.

'privately': Mai Smith to FaN, WEN and PN, 6 July [1856]. Claydon 209.

'I think we': PN to [?], 30 July [1856]. Claydon 291.

'The curtain . . . fine spirited': Mai Smith to WEN, 18 June [1856]. Claydon 209.

p. 298 'a "Rooshan" trophy': FN to FaN, WEN and PN, 14 July 1856. Wellcome 8996/74. *CW* 1, 143

'mama': FN to FaN, [1856]. Wellcome 8996/68. *CW* 1, 144.

'A "nom de guerre" ': Richard Monckton Milnes to PN, 8 September [1856]. Claydon 200.

'I have many': Mai Smith to WEN, [?1856]. Claydon 290.

'Christian men': PN, Note, [1856–7] 'Dr Sutherland about F'. Claydon 274.

'Oh my poor': FN, Note, [end 1856]. BL 43402/166. CW 2, 390.

p. 299 'is just where': FN to Sidney Herbert, 3 April 1856. BL 43393/224. Goldie, 246.

'five pertaining': FN, Note, [end 1856]. BL 43402/166. CW2, 391.

'the laudation': Mai Smith to PN, 22 June 1856. Claydon 209.

'living skeletons': FN to Haldane Turriff, 22 April [1869]. BL 47757/107. [Incomplete letter that was not sent.]

p. 300 'I stand': Quoted in Goldie, 296.

CHAPTER 12: A TURBULENT FELLOW

p. 303 'dingy': FN to Hilary Bonham Carter, [? March 1847]. BL 45794/117. CW1, 441.

the apartment in Kensington Palace: In April 1861, the Queen offered FN the use of rooms in Kensington Palace. The offer was declined on the grounds that the Palace would be too far from Westminster during parliamentary sittings. FN to Sir Harry Verney, 22 April 1861. Wellcome 8999/11. CW1, 564–5.

p. 304 'private': FN to William Farr, 9 April 1861. BL 4339/10 [typed copy]. CW5,102.

'light lofty': Hilary Bonham Carter to FaN [postmarked 24 June 1857]. Claydon 276.

'& very much: FN to WEN, 23 March 1862. BL 45790/272. CW1, 251.

p. 305 a young girl: According to an account in the *Daily Telegraph*, 22 August 1910.

'noiseless': Lieutenant-Colonel Lefroy to FN, 28 August 1856. BL 43397/244.

return of her Crimean carriage: see the report in *The Times*, 18 August 1856.

'She came in': PN to Lady Canning, 2 September 1856. Claydon 23.

'a blessing': FaN to Miss Richardson, [August 1856]. Claydon 56.

'heaps': PN to Elizabeth Herbert, [August 1856]. BL 43396/50.

'a donkey': PN, Note, [1856]. Claydon 276.
p. 306 '... She is': PN to Elizabeth Herbert, [August 1856]. BL 43396//50.
'disturbing': Sidney Herbert to Elizabeth Herbert, 21 August 1856. Herbert Papers, Wiltshire Record Office, F4.
'constituted': Sidney Herbert to Sam Smith, 26 August 1856.
p. 307 'Facts': John Sutherland to FN, 25 August 1856. BL 45751/3.
'talked principally': Queen Victoria's Journal, 21 September 1856. Royal Archives. CW5, 413.
'Flo says': Blanche Clough to [?] Mai Smith [September 1856]. Balliol College, Oxford, 303.
'I don't': FN to PN, 25 September 1856. Wellcome 8997/4.
p. 308 'a rather cold': Queen Victoria's Journal, 21 September 1856. Royal Archives. CW5, 413.
'the least': From BJ's notes of conversations with FN. CW5, 415.
The Times: The Times, 20 September 1856.
p. 309 '... For the next': FN to FaN, WEN and PN, 13 October 1856. Wellcome 8997/7.
'great mind': PN to Ellen Tollet, [October 1856]. BL 45791/279.
p. 310 'were general': FN, Note, [16 November] 1856. Quoted in Cook I, 330.
p. 311 'You must': Quoted in W-S, 273.
'Gout': FN to Sir John McNeill, 15 December 1856. LMA HI/ST/NC. 3/SU/7.
'You will say': FN, Note [end 1856]. BL 43402/166. CW2, 391.
It has been plausibly argued: Small, Florence Nightingale, 59-60.
'crowds of students': FaN to WEN, [January 1857]. Claydon 308.
five hours at St Mary's: FaN to WEN, 22 March [1857]. Claydon 308.
p. 312 'The Sanitary reformers': John Sutherland to FN, 10 December 1856. BL 45751/9.
'You must think': FN to John Sutherland, [1857]. Wellcome 8997/59.
'one of your wives': Quoted in W-S, 290.
p. 313 'went off': FN to William Farr, Good Friday 1861. Wellcome 5474/37.
'Patron Saint': Eyler, Victorian Social Medicine, 160.
She felt like: FN to William Farr, 27 November 1871. BL 43400/269.
'sit at his feet': FN to William Farr, 14 February 1858. BL 43398/41 [copy].
'It has been held': William Farr to FN, [17 July 1857]. BL 43398/14.
p. 314 'in the attempts': William Farr to FN, [14 February 1857]. BL 43398/6.
'to have a mortality': FN, Notes on Matters..., 504. FN to Sir John McNeill, 1 March 1857. LMA HI/ST/NC.3/SU/75 repeats this statement verbatim.
'to affect': FN, Note, [1857]. BL 43397/3.
'line to line': FN to PN, 19 October 1858. Wellcome 8997/78.
'the dryer': FN, Note, [1861]. BL 43399/6.
p. 315 'How she collects': PN to Ellen Tollet, [October 1856]. BL 45791/279.
'in official life': FN to Sir John McNeill, 24 October [1856]. Wellcome 8997/9 [copy by PN].
'My dear Lady': John Sutherland to FN, 22 May 1857. Quoted in W-S, 290.
p. 316 'turbulent fellow': FN to Sir William Heathcote, 12 October 1861. BL 43398/7 [typed copy].
'a batch': Sidney Herbert to FN, 14 August 1857. BL 43394/135.
'suffer knowingly': John Sutherland to FN, 7 September 1857. BL 45751/42.
'I have been home': FN to John Sutherland, 9 February 1857. BL 45796/139.
'three months': Quoted in Stanmore, Sidney Herbert, II, 123.
p. 317 'the whole history': FN, Notes on Matters..., 81.
'will not answer': ibid., 11.
'separate pavilions': ibid., 477.
p. 318 'The administrative': ibid., xxv.
'the tears': ibid., 94.
'still some difference': ibid., 81.

'a historical': FN to Sir John McNeill, 11 May 1857. Wellcome 8997/42.

p. 320 'Dear Miss Nightingale': Sidney Herbert to FN, 12 July 1857. Claydon 308.

'pith': FN to Sir John McNeill, 27 June 1857. BL 45768/55 [typed copy].

'badger': FN to Sir John McNeill, 12 June 1857. LMA HI/ST/NC.3/SU85.

'broke down utterly': FN to Sir John McNeill, [July 1857]. Quoted in Cope, *Florence Nightingale and the Doctors*, 57.

'repugnance': Sidney Herbert to FN, 8 July 1857. BL 43394/100.

'treachery': FN to Sir John McNeill, 7 July 1857. LMA HI/ST/NC.3/SU87.

p. 321 'pestilential': FN to FaN, 13 June 1857. Wellcome 8997/44.

'Your ceaseless': FN to FaN, 14 December 1856. Wellcome 8997/13. CW1, 144.

'a public servant': FN to FaN, [25 March 1864]. Wellcome 9001/19. CW1, 166.

'contraband': Quoted in W-S, 285.

'inexorably': FN, Note, [1857]. BL 43402/178. CW5, 232.

p. 322 on a par: FaN, Note. Claydon 308.

'allowed to lift': FaN to WEN, 'Wed 7' [1857]. Claydon 308.

'The irritable': PN to WEN, 17 August [1857]. Claydon 308.

'soup, beef tea': Mai Smith to FaN, [1857]. Claydon 281.

'so entirely': FaN to WEN, 17 August [1857]. Claydon 308.

'for all': Sidney Herbert to FN, 14 August 1857. BL 43394/135.

'Last night': FaN to WEN, 17 August [1857]. Claydon 308.

CHAPTER 13: THORN IN THE FLESH

p. 324 'Thorn in the Flesh': FN's name for her illness. e.g. FN to PN, 4 May 1866. Wellcome 9002/11. CW1, 335.

commentators: For a discussion of the various theories about FN's illness, see CW1, 33-6.

'dilation of the heart': Cook I, 493. This had been the phrase used by WEN to describe his daughter's illness (WEN to FaN, [late 1850s]. Claydon 73). Pickering, *Creative Malady*, 165, pointed out that the description had 'no precise meaning', and that modern medicine would interpret it as a sign of 'psychoneurosis'.

the most damaging account: Smith, *Florence Nightingale*, 92.

compelling case: Young, 'Florence Nightingale's fever'.

p. 325 'one of the most': Spink, *The Nature of Brucellosis*, 175. Bone and joint difficulties are the second most common complication of brucellosis (the disease's impact on the nervous system being the first). Spink reproduces photographs of a number of X-rays demonstrating the destructive progress of brucellosis once its bacteria begin to invade the intervertebral disc.

'She always': Mai Smith to FaN and WEN, [June 1858]. Claydon 277.

'organic disease': 'Dr S said he still thought there was no organic disease'. Sir Harry Verney to PN, 16 March [1858]. Verney 10/271.

p. 326 'I fear': WEN to [?], 11 November [1857]. Claydon 274.

'go down': FN to Lady McNeill, 22 April 1857. LMA HI/ST/NC.3/SU/77.

'deceptive': Harriet Martineau to FN, 23 January 1865. LMA HI/ST/VI/65.

'one of the gayest': FN to Sir Harry Verney, 13 May 1861. Wellcome 8999/17.

'. . . Every stroke': Harriet Martineau to FN, 3 December 1858. *Collected Letters of Harriet Martineau*, 4, 139.

'entirely a prisoner': FN to Lady Harriet Ponsonby, 12 January 1866. Wellcome 9002/5.

p. 327 'quite alone': PN to WEN, [1857]. Claydon 308.

'. . . I was told': Quoted in Cook I, 322.

a Worcester newspaper: Patty Smith to PN, [1857]. Claydon 276.

attempting to obtain details: Walter Johnson to FaN, 10 September 1857. Claydon 276.

'it appeared': Quoted in Cook I, 368.

'long scold': John Sutherland to FN, 7 September 1857. BL 45751/42.
'what would': Quoted in Cook I, 368–9.
insisted on seeing him: FN to [?], 3 September 1857. Columbia School of Nursing, C-36.
'You know': Mai Smith to FN, [September 1857]. BL 45793/133.
p. 328 'She is extremely': Mai Smith to FaN, WEN and PN, 2 October 1857. Claydon 276.
'any more': A. H. Clough to FN, 6 September [1857]. *The Correspondence of Arthur Hugh Clough*, 2, 532.
'both the smallest': Mai Smith to FaN, [1857]. Claydon 74.
'porter's wife': FN, Notes on the family, c. 1857. BL 43402/178. CW5, 234.
'I am afraid': Mai Smith to FaN, [1857]. Wellcome 9049/11.
p. 329 'after sending': Hilary Bonham Carter to PN, [1857–8]. Claydon 85.
'selfishness': Mai Smith to Blanche Clough, [1857–8]. BL 72826/36.
'These things': A. H. Clough to PN, 16 May [1858]. Claydon 85.
gave Parthenope the impression: Mai Smith to FaN, [late 1850s]. Claydon 89.
'If I could give': FN to FaN, 6 January 1858. Wellcome 8997/60. CW1, 146.
to refuse to receive . . . visitors: See CW1, 34.
'an unnecessary': FN to W. E. Gladstone, 12 May 1879. BL 44460/33. CW5, 451.
'with inflammation': FN to W. E. Gladstone, 3 December 1884. BL 44488/196. CW5, 466.
p. 330 'a treat': Cook I, 500.
'a hard day': Hilary Bonham Carter to WEN, [1858]. Claydon 277.
'much fatigued': Hilary Bonham Carter to FaN, [June 1858]. Claydon 277.
'to do something': FN to PN, [? 14 July 1860]. Wellcome 8998/51.
'Stuffing': FN to PN, [July 1860]. Wellcome 8998/52.
'congestion': FN to Mary Mohl, 21 December 1861. Quoted in Cook II, 16.
Footnote: FN to Dr Lauder Brunton, 18 December 1887. Private collection.
p. 331 'fat': Lesser, *Clarkey*, 160.
portrait by . . . Watts: Cook II, 469, dates Watts's unfinished portrait to 1864. But see G. F. Watts to Sir Harry Verney, 30 June 1866, Claydon 200, which makes it clear that the sittings didn't begin until the summer of 1866.
Her personality was being transformed: Brucellosis at its most severe is associated with 'maniacal activity' (Spink, *The Nature of Brucellosis*, 173). One recorded case, discussed by Spink, was of a pleasant family man who become an alcoholic and then a drug addict. In a fit of mania he subsequently tried to murder his family before attempting suicide (ibid., 173–4).
'touching': Remarks of an unidentified member of the Clough family. BL 728832A/77.
'often cold': Mai Smith to 'Dearest', [autumn 1857]. Wellcome 9049/25.
'. . . the main part': FN to Sam Smith, 2 June 1861. Quoted in W-S, 360–61.
'was only too': WEN to FaN, [late 1850s]. Claydon 73.
'tells upon her': WEN to FaN, [?1860]. Claydon 72.
'weak footsteps': WEN to FaN, [1859]. Claydon 77.
'Who shall write': WEN to PN, 1 February 1859. Claydon 280.
p. 332 'The immediate': Thomas Southwood Smith, *A Treatise on Fever* (1830), quoted in Eyler, *Victorian Social Medicine*, 98–9.
member of the Nightingales' London circle: FaN, Diary, 26 March 1842, mentions dining with Chadwick. Wellcome 9040.
introduced new openings: FN to PN and FaN, [January 1852]. Wellcome 8993/54.
p. 333 'the great'; Edwin Chadwick to FN, 6 December 1858. BL 45770/91.
'Were "contagion" ': FN, *Notes on Nursing*. CW6, 104. See also Rosenberg, 'Florence Nightingale on contagion'. Rosenberg sees FN's ideas as typical of 'the accepted wisdom of her generation', though he fails to recognize FN's eventual conversion to germ theory.
'Do you': FN to WEN, 20 March 1857. Wellcome 8997/32. CW1, 242.
p. 334 'as conditions': FN, *Notes on Nursing*, CW6, 62.
'Medicine does not': FN, undated note. BL 45845/4. CW6, 510.

'All foul smell': FN, *Notes on Nursing*. CW6, 52. This phrase was itself a quotation from Chadwick.

'mere weeds': FN to William Farr, 26 January 1859. BL 43398/5.

'Chadwickize': William Farr to FN, 17 February 1859. BL 43398/14.

'. . . I do not': FN to William Farr, [?April 1859]. BL 43399/19.

p. 335 'germ theories': See Worboys, *Spreading Germs*, 2, for the range of theories current between 1865 and 1900.

Quain's Medical Dictionary: FN, 'Training of Nurses and Nursing the Sick', in Quain, *Dictionary of Medicine*, 1038–43.

p. 336 'to keep the wards': FN, *Notes on Hospitals*, 26.

'not even': FN, *Notes on Matters . . .*, 87.

p. 337 'discreet': FN to Sir Harry Verney, 5 October 1859. Wellcome 8997/102.

'It was longer': FN to Edwin Chadwick, 9 October 1858. BL 45770/55.

p. 338 'a head nurse': FN to Sir William Heathcote, 19 October 1863. BL 45798/185.

'obtain': Quoted in Taylor, *Hospital and Asylum Architecture Design*, 8.

'as from': FN to PN, [14 July 1860]. Wellcome 8998/57. For a list of hospitals whose construction FN advised upon, see Cook I, 423.

'a model': Thompson, *William Butterfield*, 116.

'the parlour': ibid., 117.

'terse phrases': *Lancet*, 27 February 1864.

p. 339 'rough treatment': *Medical Times and Gazette* (1864), i, 129.

a brave soldier: *Lancet* (1864), I, 248–50.

'In England': WEN to FaN, [1857–8]. Claydon 73.

p. 340 'unmanly': FN to Sir John McNeill, 10 October 1857. BL 45768/66.

'to keep': FN to Sir John McNeill, 15 November 1857. Quoted in Cook I, 366.

'which could hardly': *The Times*, 6 February 1858.

p. 341 'Not because': FN to Sidney Herbert, 12 March 1858. BL 44395/5.

'I had much': FN to Sidney Herbert, 27 March 1858. BL 44395/33.

p. 342 'a tie': Harriet Martineau to FN, 3 December 1858. *Collected Letters of Harriet Martineau*, 4, 139.

'The book': Harriet Martineau to Henry Reeve, 21 February 1859. *Collected Letters of Harriet Martineau*, 4, 153–4.

p. 343 '. . . We could have': Sidney Herbert to FN, [15 March 1858]. BL 44395/6.

'a great': FN to Elizabeth Herbert, 15 June 1859. BL 43396/63. CW8, 660.

p. 344 '. . . A cry': Quoted in Spiers, *The Army and Society 1815–1914*, 162.

'a nasty': Mai Smith to Blanche Clough, 6 September 1856. BL 72826/38.

p. 345 a room set aside: Will of Marianne Galton, 1909.

an extraordinary improvement: Skelley, *The Victorian Army at Home*, 40.

p. 346 'as the first': FN, 'Army Sanitary reform under the late Lord Herbert' [1861, draft]. BL 44395/40.

'on behalf': Cutting from the *Romsey Chronicle*. Claydon 37.

'lamentable': FN, *Notes on Matters . . .*, 565.

'4 Ladies': Patty Smith to FaN, [1857]. Claydon 306.

'anything': Quoted in Gourlay, *Florence Nightingale and the Health of the Raj*, 25.

'a great deal': FN, *Notes on Matters . . .*, 566.

CHAPTER 14: DYING BY INCHES

p. 347 'Dying by Inches': John Sutherland to FN, 7 September 1857. BL 45751/42.

'Poor F.': FaN to WEN, [1857]. Claydon 308.

'overwrought': Sir Harry Verney to FaN, 1 September 1857. Claydon 314.

'hot pursuit': FaN, Note, [1857–8]. Claydon 306.

p. 348 'her character': Sir Harry Verney to Edmund Verney, 10 May 1858. Verney 10/353.
    'that would make it safe': PN to Sir Harry Verney, [24 April 1858]. Verney 10/271.
    'Don't think': Sir Harry Verney to PN, [April 1858]. Verney 10/271.
    'independent existence': WEN to [?, June 1858]. Claydon 277.
    'constant & much loved': Sir Harry Verney to Edmund Verney, 11 May 1858. Verney
    10/353.
    'I never thought': PN to Mrs Gaskell, [May 1858]. Claydon 310.
p. 349 'whose life': Mrs Gaskell to PN, 29 May [1858]. Claydon 310.
    'a pompous': FN to Sidney Herbert, [n.d.]. Herbert Papers, Wiltshire Record Office. CW1,
    838.
    'on business': FN to Sir Harry Verney, 2 December 1857. Wellcome 8997/52.
    'ignorant': FN to Sidney Herbert, 9 February 1858. Herbert Papers, Wiltshire Record
    Office. CW1, 838.
    'mental qualities': Edmund Verney to Sir Harry Verney, 22 June 1858. Verney 10/44.
p. 350 'agreed with us': Emily Fremantle to [?, June 1858]. Verney 10/271.
    'as if': PN to FaN, [n.d.]. Claydon 397.
    'befitting': Sir Harry Verney to Edmund Verney, 11 May 1858. Verney 10/353.
    'God bless you': FN to PN, 22 June 1858. Wellcome 8997/67.
    'Nightingale Verney': Sir Harry Verney to PN, 23 April 1858. Verney 10/271.
    'a very delightful': FaN to [?, 1858–9]. Claydon 210.
p. 351 'A life': Elizabeth Waldegrave to PN, 22 December 1857. Claydon 89. In 1887 BJ
suggested that PN write a life of FN. BJ to PN, [1887]. Verney 10/171.
    'I have lived': 'Memoir'.
    'Those female': FN to Louisa Ashburton, 14 April 1861. National Library of Scotland.
    CW8, 720. Aunt Patty was evidently accused of having planned a biography of FN.
    She was affronted by the suggestion: 'I have never had an idea of attempting a memoir
    of F. Nobody can feel the impropriety more, let alone the pain to her. I avoid naming
    her, in letters & conversation . . .' (Patty Smith to FaN, [?1857]. Claydon 306). In 1857,
    the Shakespearian scholar Mary Cowden Clarke approached PN, informing her that
    she had been commissioned by a New York publishing house to write FN's biography.
    'I wish to collect all the most genuine and authentic scenes from which to depict my
    account' (Mary Cowden Clarke to PN, 10 April 1857. Claydon 307). PN, and Liz
    Herbert, who was also approached, refused to cooperate with Clarke. Nevertheless,
    Clarke's book World-Noted Women (1858) included a sketch of FN's life, though
    Clarke admitted the difficulty of trying to avoid 'wounding' FN's 'sensitive delicacy'.
    'fill the void': Fanny Allen to PN, 11 November [1858]. Claydon 95.
    'that little Flo': PN to FaN, [December 1858]. Claydon 397. PN suffered a miscarriage
    on or about 6 December 1858.
p. 352 'during which': A. H. Clough to Hilary Bonham Carter, [1858–9]. Bodleian MS Eng
Lett e.76/173.
    'take off': Hilary Bonham Carter to PN, [1858]. Claydon 277.
    'of the dust': FN to Elizabeth Herbert, 17 January 1861. BL 43396/110. CW8, 669.
    'a striking': FaN to PN, [1858–9]. Claydon 353.
p. 353 'Pray forgive': FN to WEN, 8 October 1858. Wellcome 8997/75. CW1, 243–4.
    'a kind of': FN to WEN, 9 October 1858. Wellcome 8997/76. CW1, 244.
    'one word': FN to WEN [c. 1861]. Wellcome 8999/53. CW1, 250.
    'unfeeling': FN to A. H. Clough, [n.d.]. Balliol College, Oxford, 303.
    'noiseless wheels': Invoice, February 1858. BL 45795/5.
    'no apparent': A. H. Clough to FN, 5 February 1858. The Correspondence of Arthur
    Hugh Clough, 2, 488.
p. 354 'blundering harasses': FN to Sir John McNeill, 18 November 1861. BL 45768/166
[typed copy].
    one of Clough's modern biographers: Biswas, Arthur Hugh Clough, 461.
    'ordinary': Quoted in Chorley, Arthur Hugh Clough: The Uncommitted Mind, 311.

'Some poor': Quoted ibid., 322.

'If I could give': FN to Sam Smith, [July or August 1858]. BL 45792/80. CW1, 476.

'suffering from severe': A. H. Clough, Note. BL 45795/11. The signed statement by FN is at BL 45795/9.

p. 355 'Wait on the Lord': A. H. Clough, 'Conversations with Florence Nightingale', [1859]. Wellcome 7204/7.

'. . . the mischief': A. H. Clough, 'Conversations with Florence Nightingale', [4 March 1859]. Wellcome 7204/3.

p. 356 anxious about him going home: Hilary Bonham Carter to FaN, 'Friday the 20th' [1860–61]. Claydon 37.

'very kind': Sam Smith to PN, [?1859]. Claydon 89.

'for each': Mai Smith to FN, [March or April 1857]. BL 45793/126.

'Do what I will': Lesser, Clarkey, 169.

p. 357 '. . . The very walls': FN, Notes on Nursing, CW6, 83.

sold 15,000 copies: For the publishing history of Notes on Nursing, see the introduction to Victor Skretkowicz's edition, ix–xl. Quotations from Notes on Nursing are taken from the text in CW6, 30–161.

'hints for thought': FN, Notes on Nursing, CW6, 30.

'If a patient': ibid., 31.

'hundred thousand': Edwin Chadwick to FN, 6 December 1858. BL 45770/89.

p. 358 'more preceptive': John Sutherland to FN, 10 February 1859. BL 45751/125b.

'A nurse': FN, Notes on Nursing, CW6, 63.

'Feverishness': ibid., 48.

'it is . . . certain': ibid., 98.

'great as those': Edwin Chadwick to FN, 9 June 1860. BL 45770/122.

The critics: See Bishop and Goldie, A Bio-Bibliography of Florence Nightingale, 18.

p. 359 'sadly large': FN, Notes on Nursing, CW6, 67.

'the acute suffering': ibid., 82.

'roguery . . . effect': FN to John Sutherland, 4 March 1860. BL 45751/153.

'What Is a Nurse?': FN, Notes on Nursing, CW6, 141–6.

p. 360 'Minding Baby': ibid., 146–51.

Mr Shields: FN to Edwin Chadwick, 21 April 1861. BL 45770/224.

'the parson': Harriet Martineau to FN, 8 May 1861. BL 45788/123.

'What would be': FN to William Farr, 20 May 1867. BL 43400/166.

'deaths by': William Farr to FN, 23 May 1867. BL 43400/175.

p. 361 'make our': FN, Note, [1875]. BL 45817/31. CW6, 161.

'every lady': Hoy, Chasing Dirt, 32.

Dix: For the missed meetings with FN, and the parallels between the two women, see Brown, Dorothea Dix, 230–38, 274–7.

p. 362 'diligent oversight': ibid., 290.

'with no bows': Hoy, Chasing Dirt, 47.

'meddler-general': Brown, Dorothea Dix, 291.

p. 363 'self-sealing': ibid., 312.

'Daily': In Louisa M. Alcott's Hospital Sketches (1863). Quoted in Brown, Dorothea Dix, 314.

'All our women': New York Herald, 5 April 1864.

'sanitary domestic': 'Florence Nightingale before the Army Medical Reform Commission', New York Times, 11 March 1858.

'the canons': Quoted in Hoy, Chasing Dirt, 48.

'cleanliness and order': ibid., 38.

p. 364 Florence Nightingale at Scutari: On Leutze's painting, see New York Evening Post, 22 March 1864.

p. 366 'if I can': FN to Sidney Herbert, 27 March 1858. Herbert Papers, Wiltshire Record Office.

p. 367 'among dense': FN, *Notes on Hospitals*, 26.

'to build': FN to R. G. Whitfield, 21 February 1859. LMA HI/ST/NC.1/59/1.

'It is not': FN to Sidney Herbert, 24 May 1859. Herbert Papers, Wiltshire Record Office.

p. 368 'sober': Baly, *Florence Nightingale and the Nursing Legacy*, 47.

'It is true': FN, *Notes on Nursing*, CW6, 157.

'snowy caps': Hall, 'Something of What Florence Nightingale Has Done and Is Doing', 38.

p. 369 'She is': Hilary Bonham Carter to WEN, [1859]. Claydon 77.

'neglected & weakly': Edwin Chadwick to FN, 9 June 1860. BL 45770/122.

'right': Edwin Chadwick to FN, 28 August 1860. BL 45770/151.

'most "faithful" ': FN to J. S. Mill, 5 September 1860. BL 45787/1 [copy]. CW5, 373.

p. 370 'No one': Sam Smith to FN, [1860]. BL 45792/123.

'God's scheme': FN, *Suggestions for Thought*, II, 54.

'a Being who': ibid., 88.

p. 371 'to unite': BJ to FN, [January 1861]. *Jowett Letters*, 3.

'Many sparks': Quoted in Cook I, 473.

two articles: Reprinted in CW3, 9–46.

'want of arrangement': FN to J. S. Mill, 28 September 1860. BL 45787/23 [copy]. CW5, 379.

'all of the arrangements': J. S. Mill to FN, 23 September 1860. BL 45787/13. CW5, 377.

p. 372 The surviving manuscript: BL 45839.

'Passion, intellect': FN, 'Cassandra', 398.

'never supposed': ibid., 401.

'the accumulation': ibid., 408.

p. 373 'the destruction': Quoted in Cook I, 499.

'rather impertinent': BJ to FN, 17 November [1861]. *Jowett Letters*, 13.

more like screaming: Woolf, *Women and Fiction*, 183.

p. 374 'the dinner parties': Mill, *The Subjection of Women*, chapter III.

'was heard': FN, *Cassandra*, 402.

'a celebrated': Mill, *The Subjection of Women*, chapter III. At the end of 1870 FN did complete an essay on 'The Family', unpublished in her lifetime, in which she delivers a devastating critique of the institution, and of a 'state of war' as being essential to a 'state of family'. BL 45843/1. CW3, 140–55.

'the rights': FN, *Notes on Nursing*. CW6, 157.

'what appear': J. S. Mill to FN, 10 September 1860. BL 45787/7. CW5, 374.

p. 375 'a dear & intimate': FN to J. S. Mill, 12 September 1860. BL 45787/9. CW5, 375.

Florence's . . . last two doctors: Caroline Keith and May Thorne were both graduates of the London School of Medicine for Women.

'much more hardly': FN to J. S. Mill, 11 August 1867. BL 39927 [draft]. CW5, 395–7.

p. 376 'and apparently effectually': J. S. Mill to FN, 31 December 1867. BL 45787/43. CW5, 398.

'a woman of': FN to Lemuel Moss, 13 September 1868. Published in *The Queen*, 21 November 1868.

'Women have': FN to Mary Mohl, 13 December [1861]. Quoted in Cook II, 13–16.

p. 377 'You know': FN to Sam Smith. Quoted in W-S, 388.

'neuralgic': Sidney Herbert to FN, 2 January 1858. BL 43394/27.

'was very sorry': FN to Elizabeth Herbert, 7 January 1858. BL 43396/54. CW8, 657.

'heartily ashamed': Sidney Herbert to FN, 16 March 1858. BL 44395/11.

'I really am not': Sidney Herbert to FN, [18 March 1858]. BL 44395/19.

p. 378 'by all his': FN to Sidney Herbert, 18 November 1859. Quoted in Stanmore, *Sidney Herbert*, II, 369. For FN's outline of War Office reform, see BL 44395/308.

'Sidney Herbert': FN to Douglas Galton, 24 April 1860. BL 45759/36.

'increasing sleeplessness': WEN to FaN, [1860–1]. Claydon 72.

'no statesman': FN to Harriet Martineau, 4 January 1861. BL 45788/103.

p. 379 '...I do hope': FN to Sidney Herbert, 8 December 1860. Herbert papers, Wiltshire Record Office, CW8, 664.

'an old Nurse': FN to Elizabeth Herbert, 5 December 1860. BL 43396/89. CW8, 663.

'not sauces': FN to Elizabeth Herbert, 10 April 1861. BL 43396/128. CW8, 674.

'that doctors': FN to Elizabeth Herbert, 13 December 1860. BL 43396/97. CW8, 665.

'after you': FN to Elizabeth Herbert, 14 May 1861. BL 43396/138. CW8, 679.

'Pray, pray': FN to Henry Bence Jones, 14 April 1861. Cambridge University Library. CW8, 677.

'travelling': FN to Sam Smith, [1861]. BL 45792/134.

p. 380 'There is': FN to Sam Smith, [end of May 1861]. BL 45792/163.

'There is an end': Sidney Herbert to FN, 7 June 1861. BL 44395/302.

'I consider': FN to Sidney Herbert, [June 1861]. BL 44395/305.

'I am disappointed': FN to Sidney Herbert, [June 1861]. BL 44395/308 [draft].

the only note of regret: See also FN's unsigned note, c. 1862, BL 43396/154, possibly addressed to the dead Herbert, in which she writes that 'I want you for my sake to forget any little quarrel or misunderstanding.'

'angelic temper': FN to Harriet Martineau, 24 September 1861. BL 45788/127.

p. 381 'That's the only': Stanmore, Sidney Herbert, II, 437.

'seemed very': Blanche Clough to A. H. Clough, 1 August [1861]. The Correspondence of Arthur Hugh Clough, 2, 595–6.

'the deepest': Mai Smith to FaN, [August 1861]. Claydon 89.

'some particulars': R. Chernside to FN, 10 August [1861]. BL 45797/250. These were supplied at Liz Herbert's request.

'Many men': W. E. Gladstone to FN, 10 August 1861. BL 44397/49 [copy].

'His last articulate': FN to PN, 7 August 1861. Wellcome 8999/33. CW1/327. 'Account of SH' by Elizabeth Herbert, among the Herbert papers, makes it clear that it was one of several messages to be delivered 'to different absent friends', and that the phrasing was 'Poor Florence! Who will carry on our joint work?'

p. 382 'a most rapid': FN to 'B', [September 1861]. BL 45797/27.

'the features': Blanche Clough to C. E. Norton, 29 November 1861. The Correspondence of Arthur Hugh Clough, 2, 610.

'all the money-making': Blanche Clough to C. E. Norton, 29 November 1861. The Correspondence of Arthur Hugh Clough, 2, 608.

'...If grief': Blanche Clough to C. E. Norton, 29 November 1861. The Correspondence of Arthur Hugh Clough, 2, 610.

CHAPTER 15: PHILOMELA

p. 383 'Philomela': One of BJ's epistolary names for FN. See Jowett Letters, 163, n.3.

'muff': FN to William Farr, 10 September 1861. BL 43399/41.

'He was my support': FN to Elizabeth Herbert, 12 December 1861. Herbert Papers, Wiltshire Record Office. CW8, 687.

'vehemently insisted': Mai Smith to Blanche Clough, 26 November [1861]. Balliol College, Oxford, 285.

'I hardly': Francis Newman to Blanche Clough, 23 November 1861. The Correspondence of Arthur Hugh Clough, 2, 606.

p. 384 'under such strange': FN to 'B', [September 1861]. BL 45797/27.

Elizabeth Blackwell . . . remarked: Quoted in Goldie, A Calendar of the Letters of Florence Nightingale, 6/182/26.

'at every waking': FN to Blanche Clough, [November 1861]. Balliol College, Oxford, 303.

'I know that his': Blanche Clough to FN [November–December 1861]. Balliol College, Oxford, 303 [draft].

'reverence & affection': Mai Smith to Blanche Clough, 25 November [1861]. Balliol College, Oxford, 303.

'overwrought': Mai Smith to Blanche Clough, 12 November 1861. Balliol College, Oxford, 285.

'in love': Mai Smith to Blanche Clough, 22 November [1861], Balliol College, Oxford, 285.

p. 385 'No Arts': FN to Sir Harry Verney. Wellcome 9000/55.

p. 386 'working just as': FN to Mary Mohl, 13 December 1861. Quoted in Cook II, 9.

'the reign of muffishness': FN to Elizabeth Herbert, 17 August 1861. Herbert Papers, Wiltshire Record Office. CW8, 684.

p. 387 'too indeterminate': FN to William Farr, 10 May [1860]. BL 43398/183 [copy].

'trash': FN to WEN, 23 March 1862. BL 45790/271. CW251.

'Agitate': Telegram, FN to Harriet Martineau, 16 April 1863. BL 45788/194.

The War Office Abstracts: W-S, 397.

p. 388 'unique collection': FN to WEN, 2 February 1862. BL 45790/247.

'could not bear': FN to Elizabeth Herbert, [17 October 1862]. BL 43396/187 [copy].

'a fashionable': FN to FaN, 7 March 1862. BL 45790/253. CW1, 152.

'Two VANS': FN to FaN, [19 April 1862]. Wellcome 9000/28. CW1, 155.

'Sometimes': FN to FaN, 7 March 1862. BL 45790/253. CW1, 151.

p. 389 'She is never': FN to FaN, 7 March 1862. BL 45790/253. CW1, 153.

'Few things': Quoted in W-S, 364.

twenty . . . small copies: One, for example, was placed, in 1865, in the Mechanics' Institute in Ambleside, near where Harriet Martineau lived. In June 1867, three of the statuettes arrived in Sydney, where their resemblance to representations of a saint fanned local suspicions of the Catholic sympathies of Lucy Osburn, the Nightingale nurse who had become Lady Superintendent at the Sydney Infirmary. See Godden, *Lucy Osburn*, 155–7.

'shocked at': FaN to PN, [n.d.]. Claydon 313.

'sewing': BJ to FN, [March 1862]. *Jowett Letters*, 14.

p. 390 'I do not': BJ to Archibald Tait, 21 October [1862]. Lambeth Palace Library. CW3, 524.

'a tender': *Essays and Reviews*, 363.

'patient': BJ to FN, [March 1862]. *Jowett Letters*, 14.

'a soft smooth': Allingham, *A Diary*, 98.

'something like': Faber, *Jowett*, 36.

'unhappiness': BJ to FN, [September 1861]. *Jowett Letters*, 11.

p. 391 'a sort of heaven': *Jowett Letters*, xxvi–xxvii.

'finding the better': ibid., xxiv.

'Forgive me': BJ to FN, 28 October [1862]. *Jowett Letters*, 23.

p. 392 in Derbyshire, he would go: Mai Smith to FaN, [?1863]. Wellcome 9049/45.

'the better': BJ to FN, 16 April [1865]. *Jowett Letters*, 51.

'to know': FN to BJ, 24 May 1865. ibid., 55.

'Bodily affliction': BJ to FN, 10 March 1865. ibid., 49.

'I mar': FN to BJ, 12 July 1865. ibid., 62.

p. 393 'Hardly anything': BJ to FN, [28 May 1865]. ibid., 56.

'Mr Jowett': ibid., xxxiii–xxxiv.

'Dear (tho' Perfidious)': FN to BJ, 8 August 1871. ibid., 213.

'the excitement': ibid., xviii.

p. 394 'struck dumb': Sorabji, *India Calling*, 31.

a print: Margaret Verney gave BJ the picture on his last visit to Claydon, not long before his death. See FN to Charlotte Symonds Green, 11, 18–21 November 1894. Wellcome 5477/19. CW8, 958.

'Benjamin Jowett came': Sorabji, 32.

diary . . . for . . . 1877: BL 45847. CW2, 434–93.

Footnote: Asquith, *Autobiography*, 75.

p. 395 'The great want': Faber, *Jowett*, 405.

'the natives': BJ to FN, [summer 1862]. *Jowett Letters*, 19.

'Governess': Cook II, 169.

'needed anything': *Amrita Bazar Patrika*, 29 June 1892. Quoted in Cook II, 27.

'really nothing': FN to J. Pattison Walker, 3 January 1865. BL 45781/260. CW9, 506.

p. 397 'a Queen's officer': CW9, 15.

'a deal better': FN to William Farr, 2 October 1861. BL 43399/54.

p. 398 'If we could': FN to Sir James Clark, 7 October 1863. BL 45772/173 [copy].

'We look': FN to William Farr, 2 October 1861. BL 43399/54.

'the biggest part': FN to FaN, 7 March 1862. BL 45790/253. CW1, 151.

'beginning': FN, 'Observations by Miss Nightingale on the Evidence Contained in the Stational Returns . . .' (1863). CW9, 135.

'At some stations': ibid., 142.

p. 399 'bed till': ibid., 154.

'the less': FN to Hilary Bonham Carter, 4 September 1862. BL 45794/183. CW9, 117.

'By dint': FN to Edwin Chadwick, 8 July 1863. BL 45771/28 [typed copy]. CW9, 219.

p. 400 'a certain': Quoted in W-S, 274.

'The suggestion': FN and John Sutherland, *Remarks . . . on a Report by Dr Leith* (1865). CW9, 416.

'as obstructive': Arnold, *Colonizing the Body*, 71.

p. 401 'The time': FN, 'How People May Live and Not Die in India' (1863). CW9, 191.

'. . . There is no': FN to Sir John Lawrence, [autumn 1863]. Quoted in Gourlay, *Florence Nightingale and the Health of the Raj*, 52.

p. 402 'Our great want': Sir John Lawrence to FN, 6 May 1864. BL 45777/33.

'the greatest figure': FN to Sir John Lawrence, 26 December 1864. BL 45777/49.

p. 403 'the fostering': Quoted in Gourlay, *Florence Nightingale and the Health of the Raj*, 69.

'long & anxiously': FN to Sir John Lawrence, 10 June 1867. BL 45777/97 [draft].

'Any foolscap': FN to Sir John McNeill, [1867]. BL 45768/217.

p. 404 'to suppose': FN to Sir John Lawrence, [1868]. BL 45777/172 [draft].

'unhealthy': FN, *The Sanitary Progress in India* (1870). Quoted in Gourlay, *Florence Nightingale and the Health of the Raj*, 80.

'For many ages': Quoted ibid., 83.

p. 405 'Mrs Butler & Co.': BJ to FN, 30 January 1870. *Jowett Letters*, 184.

'. . . The dreadful sin': FN to Sidney Herbert, [1861]. Herbert Papers, Wiltshire Record Office. CW8, 420.

'you actually have': FN to Douglas Galton, 12 April 1862. BL 45760/63. CW8, 420.

'Note on the Supposed Protection': CW8, 428–35.

'The great men': FN to Thomas Balfour, 10 December 1860. BL 45772/238 [copy]. CW8, 416.

'more than': FN to Douglas Galton, 25 June 1861. BL 45759/234. CW8, 422.

p. 406 ' "You may murder": FN to PN, [19 September 1863]. Wellcome 9000/130. CW8, 446.

'placing': FN to Sir Harry Verney, [July 1864]. Wellcome 9001/47. CW8, 452.

'I must say': FN, *Pall Mall Gazette*, 3 March 1870. CW8, 464.

'the doctrinaire': FN to Elizabeth Blackwell, 13 October 1870. Library of Congress. CW8, 477.

p. 407 'legal recognition': FN, *Pall Mall Gazette*, 18 March 1870. CW8, 470–71.

27 Norfolk Street: This address, together with 3 Upper Terrace, Hampstead, are the two of FN's London homes which still stand.

'the whole': FN to Mary Clare Moore, 12 May 1864. Sullivan (ed.), *The Friendship of Florence Nightingale and Mary Clare Moore*, 120.

'utter impracticality': FN to Harriet Martineau, [April 1864]. BL 45788/261. CW7, 335.

p. 408 '. . . The anxiety': FN to FaN, 16 August 1865. Wellcome 9001/148. CW1, 178.

'pale, broken': BJ to FN, [May 1865]. *Jowett Letters*, 55.

'beautiful softness': Mary Mohl to Selina Bracebridge, 9 September 1865. Claydon 85.

p. 409 'The golden bowl': Quoted in W-S, 437.

'truly a beautiful': FN to WEN, 17 June 1868. Wellcome 9003/32.

'to enable': FN to WEN, 27 October 1865. Wellcome 9001/170. CW1, 261.

'disgraceful': FN to Sir Harry Harry Verney, 3 January 1885. Wellcome 9010/53. CW1, 592.

'most vigorously': FN to Douglas Galton, 12 July 1879. BL 45764/264. CW6, 562.

'Florence Nightingale Street': FN to Sir Harry Verney, 15 December 1884. CW1, 591.

'It is very good': FN to PN, [1866–7]. Wellcome 9002/92. CW1, 336.

p. 410 'through the keyhole': Cook II, 301.

'There are some': FN to FaN, 7 March 1862. BL 45790/253. CW1/154.

'feeble': FN to PN, [?1870]. Claydon 371.

p. 411 'perennial': FN to FaN, [1860]. Wellcome 8998/42. CW1, 767.

'a very strict': FN to FaN, 22 July 1864. Wellcome 9001/44. CW8, 975.

'and everything': FN to FaN, 31 March [1862]. BL 45790/277.

'As Mrs N.': FN, Note, 16 March 1889. BL 45844/39. CW2, 507.

'the main thing': FN, 'Notes for the care of Mr Jowett when ill'. BL 52427/104.

soldiers should drink less, nuns more: The phrase is Lynn McDonald's. See the section on FN's 'Domestic Arrangements', CW1, 731–824.

p. 412 her allowance: After WEN's death in 1874, the allowance was increased to £2,000 a year.

'Dumb beasts': FN to FaN 7 March 1862. BL 45790/253. CW1, 755.

'the most sensitively': FN, undated note. BL 45845/236. CW1, 755.

'greatly to': FN to WEN, 18 June 1862. Wellcome 9000/51. CW1, 757.

p. 413 'If cats': FN to Mrs Turnham, 4 September 1888. BL 45808/202.

'. . . I have had': FN to Mary Mohl, 16 July 1870. Woodward Biomedical Library. CW1, 759.

'My present': FN to FaN, 25 April 1862. Wellcome 9000/31.

'altogether without': CW4, 94. FN's annotated copy of *The Imitation of Christ* is in the FN Museum.

p. 414 'worth all': CW5, 731.

'not striking': FN to Selma Björkenstam, 22 October 1843. Wieslander, 'Florence Nightingale', 49.

commiserated with Parthenope: George Smith to PN, 27 June 1873. Verney 10/321.

'as a religious': FN to WEN, [24 May 1862]. BL 45790/282. CW1, 254.

p. 415 'novel of genius': FN, *Fraser's Magazine*, May 1873. CW3, 12.

'an elderly': CW5,775.

'doctrine': FN to WEN, 23 May 1862. BL 45790/281. CW5, 778.

'defiance of conventionality': Lawrence, *Sword and Gown*, 65.

she asked Milnes: FN to Richard Monckton Milnes, 16 June 1861. Houghton Papers, Trinity College, Cambridge, 18/137. FN misattributed the poem to Currer Bell (Charlotte Brontë).

CHAPTER 16: A CRYING EVIL

p. 417 'A Crying Evil': Mary Jones to FN, 4 February 1864. BL 47744/20. CW6, 236.

'he ceases': FN to C. P. Villiers, [30 December 1864]. BL 45787/54 [copy]. CW6, 329.

'the poorest': FN to Henry Bence Jones, 1 March 1856. Cambridge University Library. CW6, 234.

p. 418 'great state': Quoted in Abel-Smith, *The Hospitals*, 46.

'these pitiable': FN to Sir Harry Verney, 11 February 1868. Wellcome 9003/7. CW5, 153.

p. 419 'soberly sensational': Abel-Smith, *The Hospitals*, 72.

p. 420 'who sees how much': FN to William Rathbone, 5 February 1864. Boston University. CW6, 237.

p. 421 'Is its foundation': CW6, 240. For Agnes Jones's early life, see Ross & Ross, *A Gifted Touch*.

'impertinent': FN to Theodore Fliedner, 19 July 1861. Kaiserswerth Diakoniewerth. CW6, 241 [translated from French].

'dreariness': Agnes Jones, Notes, 3 August [1865]. Liverpool Record Office [typed extracts]. CW6, 250.

'It almost': Quoted in Ross & Ross, *A Gifted Touch*, 40.

p. 422 'an apostle': FN to Agnes Jones, [before 30 July 1865]. BL 47752/249 [draft]. CW6, 249.

'your workhouse': FN to Agnes Jones, [10 August 1865]. BL 47752/162 [draft]. CW6, 251.

'unhappiness': FN, Note, [August 1865]. BL 47753/46. CW6, 254.

'can get on': FN to William Rathbone, 4 July 1866. Liverpool Record Office. CW6, 206.

p. 423 statistical evaluation: See the extracts from reports of the evaluation in CW6, 271–3.

'indefatigable exertion': Report by Robert Gee, [10 May 1866]. BL 45799/251. CW6, 273.

'inscribed': Report by J. H. Barnes, 21 March 1866. BL 45799/255. CW6, 271.

'. . . A great many': Quoted in Jones, *Memorials of Agnes Elizabeth Jones*, 36–9.

p. 424 '. . . I shall be': C. P. Villiers to FN, 31 December 1864. BL 45787/56. CW6, 331.

'always sensible': Greville, *The Greville Memoirs*, 7, 351.

'who can hold': FN to Sir Harry Verney, 12 June 1865. Wellcome 9001/128. CW6, 335.

'next year's': Henry Farnall to FN, [3 July 1865]. Quoted in Cook II, 132.

p. 425 'and, above all': FN, Note on Poor Law Reform [July 1865]. BL 45786/61. CW6, 337.

'a powerful protector': FN to William Farr, 19 October 1865. Wellcome 5464/95/1. CW5, 514–15.

'in the great': FN to W. Gathorne Hardy, [July 1866]. BL 45787/108 [draft]. CW6, 345.

'earned no common': W. Gathorne Hardy to FN, 25 July 1866. BL 45787/112.

p. 426 'to suffocate': FN to Douglas Galton, 28 October 1866. BL 45763/231. CW6, 355.

p. 427 'Very dearest friend': See Widerquist, ' "Dearest Friend", The Correspondence of Colleagues Florence Nightingale and Mary Jones', 25.

'a brace': FN to Mary Jones, 17 August 1866. LMA HI/ST/NC.1/66/14.

'A drive': FN to FaN, 3 February 1863. BL 45790/304. CW1, 160–61.

p. 428 '(quietly and sensibly)': FN to Douglas Galton, 17 December 1860. BL 45759/120.

'capacious ward': Baly, *Florence Nightingale and the Nursing Legacy*, 69.

'a want long felt': FN to Harriet Martineau, 24 September 1861. BL 45788/131. CW8, 161.

p. 429 'jawed away . . . men': FN to John Sutherland, [November 1867]. BL 45752/252. CW8, 182–3.

'the unhappy': Mary Jones to FN, 23 June 1867. BL 47744/125. CW8, 194.

p. 430 published research from mid-century: This included the work of Dr Ignaz Semmelweis at the Vienna General Hospital in 1847–8. Semmelweis published his findings in full in 1861. See CW8, 143–52, on Semmelweis and other indicators of high mortality rates connected to the spread of puerperal fever by doctors.

'deplorable': FN to William Farr, 3 March 1868. Wellcome 5474/116. CW8, 202.

'cultivating': FN to Sir John McNeill, 25 December 1868. LMA HI/ST/NC.3/SU159. CW5, 543.

'quick': FN to John Sutherland, [12 December 1868]. BL 45753/119. CW8, 542.

p. 431 'so laboriously': FN to John Sutherland, 19 September 1869. BL 45753/279. CW8, 222.

'With all': FN, *Introductory Notes on Lying-In Institutions* (1871). CW8, 276.

'between tragedy': Summers, *Angels and Citizens*, 67.

'memorable': Jane Shaw Stewart to FN, 18 October 1872. BL 45774/225.

'I shall serve': Jane Shaw Stewart to FN, 23 June 1856. BL 45774/22.

p. 432 'Breach of trust': Jane Shaw Stewart to FN, 26 May 1859. BL 45774/61.

Aunt Mai had stepped in: Jane Shaw Stewart to FN, 30 July 1870. BL 45774/214.

'to serve God': Jane Shaw Stewart to FN, 18 August 1856. BL 45774/8.

Things started to go wrong: For an authoritative account, see Summers, *Angels and Citizens*, 73–90.

p. 433 'it appears': *The Times*, 17 October 1866.

'rather than be subject': 'Evidence of Committee of Inquiry into the State of the Nursing Service at the Royal Victoria Hospital, Netley', May 1868. BL 45774/104.

'a Chief Justice': FN to Mary Jones, [May 1868]. LMA HI/ST/NC.1/64/24.

p. 434 'She will be': FN to John Sutherland, 11 November 1869. BL 45754/19.

p. 435 'the difficult': FN to Jane Shaw Stewart, 12 September 1882. BL 45774/250.

'whole system': Quoted in Summers, *Angels and Citizens*, 97.

'over & over': FN to William Rathbone, 20 February 1868. Liverpool Record Office. CW6, 282.

'the most disorderly': FN to PN, 8 March 1868. Wellcome 9003/13. CW6, 284–5.

p. 436 'a deadlock': FN to PN, [1870]. Wellcome 9004/29.

'a miserable business': FN to William Farr, 3 March 1868. Wellcome 5474/196. CW6, 284.

'the dearth': Martineau, 'Nurses Wanted', 410.

'We grew tired': ibid., 412.

p. 437 'the pioneer': FN, 'Una and the Lion' (1868), CW6, 290.

'All England': FN, ibid., CW6, 294.

'deeply touched': Harriet Beecher Stowe to FN, 20 March 1872. BL 45803 [typed copy]. CW8, 802–3.

'It is not her': FN to Harriet Beecher Stowe, 14 August 1872. Radcliffe College Library. CW8, 807.

'It was worse': FN to Emily Verney, 13 July 1871. Wellcome 9005/86. CW5, 306–7.

p. 438 'there *have* been . . . self-sacrifice': FN, 'Una and the Lion' (1868), CW6, 298.

so unwell: FN to Elizabeth Herbert, 12 January 1869. BL 43396/206.

'some unprofessional': BJ to FN, 28 May [1869]. *Jowett Letters*, 167–8.

CHAPTER 17: TAKING CHARGE

p. 443 'Are those': Quoted in Cook I, 427.

'its astounding': *Lancet*, 22 October 1870.

p. 444 'Telephonic': FN to Henry Bonham Carter, 5 July 1881. BL 47720/152.

'than that of': *Lancet*, 22 October 1870.

'boundless profusion': *The Builder*, 4 February 1871. Nevertheless, within seven years of the opening of the new hospital, a report on the sanitary state of St Thomas's would reveal it to be far from hygienic. Windows were difficult to open, chutes for soiled linen were not used, and chamber-pots left under beds were hidden by the pinned-down quilts.

'but a kind of': BJ to FN, 22 June [1872]. *Jowett Letters*, 229.

p. 445 'our dearly loved': Quoted in Cook II, 327.

'long hours': Cutting from *The Church Evangelical*, [1888]. BL 45774/254.

'Ward training': Quoted in Wake, *The Nightingale Training School*, 68.

'Harry Carter': FN to Sam Smith, 6 January 1856. BL 45792/1. Goldie, 185.

p. 446 'by her request': Henry Bonham Carter, Diary, 5 August 1873. Hampshire Record Office.

'Father often': Quoted in Bonham Carter, *In a Liberal Tradition*, 138.

'a dreadful': FN to FaN, 30 May 1866. Wellcome 9002/26.

p. 447 'to be obedient': Rappe, *God Bless you, My Dear Miss Nightingale*, 33–4.

'Kindness': Strong, *Reminiscences*, 5–6.

register of probationers: Baly, *Florence Nightingale and the Nursing Legacy*, 232–45.

p. 448 'I had rather': FN to Henry Bonham Carter, 24 June 1871. BL 47716/202.

'oftener tipsy': FN to Henry Bonham Carter, 18 May 1872. LMA HI/ST/NC.72/12a.

'governing': Henry Bonham Carter to FN, 3 February 1872. LMA HI/ST/V.3/72.

'were made': FN to Henry Bonham Carter, 12 May 1872. LMA HI/ST/V.13/71.

p. 449 'We were the making': Quoted in Godden, *Lucy Osburn*, 35.

'Lady of education': Quoted ibid., 50.

'as hard as': Quoted ibid., 63.

'the poor': FN to Henry Bonham Carter, 2 December 1867. BL 47715/120.

'prayer-ful': Quoted in Godden, *Lucy Osburn*, 75.

p. 450 'fair sisters': Quoted ibid., 98.

'How could': FN to Sarah Wardroper, 4 June 1868. BL 47730/267.

'They were not': Quoted in Godden, *Lucy Osburn*, 131.

'cast off': Quoted ibid., 207.

p. 451 'hopelessly unhealthy': FN to Henry Bonham Carter, [?] May 1875. BL 47719/107.

Footnote: Dock and Stewart, *A Short History of Nursing*, 154.

'a sheep's head': FN to Henry Bonham Carter, 18 January 1873. BL 47718/184.

'of any': FN to Henry Bonham Carter, 8 February 1873. BL 47717/226.

'the most utterly': FN to Henry Bonham Carter, 28 April 1873. BL 47718/69.

'her brain': FN to Henry Bonham Carter, 22 April 1873. BL 47718/59.

p. 452 'impertinent': Baly, *Florence Nightingale and the Nursing Legacy*, 153.

'unmanly wretch': FN to Henry Bonham Carter, 21 October 1872. LMA HI/ST/NC.1/72/25.

'all emotion': FN to Henry Bonham Carter, 9 November 1872. LMA HI/ST/NC.1/72/44.

p. 453 'an active': Quoted in Cook II, 248.

'all probationers': FN to Henry Bonham Carter, 16 February 1873. BL 47717/249.

'the counterpanes': Mary Cadbury, 'Ward Diary', 1873. Quoted in Smedley, Nightingale Nursing 1872–1890. The Practice Perspective', 10.

'at least four': *Mr Croft's Notes of Lectures* (1873). LMA HI/ST/N.73.

p. 454 'I would almost say': FN to Henry Acland, 20 July 1869. Bodleian Library, Oxford. CW8, 51.

p. 455 'excellent': Quoted in Baly, *Florence Nightingale and the Nursing Legacy*, 171.

'Always': FN, 'Training of Nurses and Nursing the Sick', in Quain, *Dictionary of Medicine*, 1038–43.

'Asceptik': FN, Note, [1896]. BL 47728/26.

'the last 6': FN to Mary Jones, 9 May 1873. LMA HI/ST/NC.1/73/2.

p. 456 'Queer and rough': Baly, *Florence Nightingale and the Nursing Legacy*, 173.

'cheerful': FN, Note, 14 November 1872. BL 47751/55.

p. 457 'that nursing': Cook II, 263.

'the vigour': FN to Rachel Williams, 22 October 1873. LMA HI/ST/NC.3/SU 180/9.

'old black': FN to Rachel Williams, 30 December 1876. LMA HI/ST/NC.3/SU/180/23.

p. 458 'my little': FN to Rachel Williams, 23 May 1873. LMA HI/ST/NC.3/SU/180/3.

'And life': FN to Rachel Williams, 2 May 1874. Quoted in Cook II, 255.

'I am so glad': Quoted in Cope, *Six Disciples of Florence Nightingale*, 36.

'a lawless': Quoted in Baly, *Florence Nightingale and the Nursing Legacy*, 161.

p. 459 'immersed': FN to Julius Mohl, 21 June 1873. Quoted in W-S, 521.

a large number: For a fuller list, see Cook II, 256.

'The new order': Abel-Smith, *A History of the Nursing Profession*, 24.

'at the end': Allingham, *Diary*, 99.

'I am grieved': FaN to PN, 30 November [mid-1860s]. Claydon 59.

'Carriage': WEN to PN, [n.d.]. Claydon 59.

p. 460 'the daily': FaN, Note, [1860s]. Claydon 404.

'You know': Harriet Martineau to Richard Monckton Milnes, 5 January 1867. *The Collected Letters of Harriet Martineau*, 5, 172.

'dilapidation': FN to [?] Julia Smith, 3 October 1871. BL 72832A/77.

'Upon me': FN to Mary Jones, 7 February 1873. BL 47744/210. CW1, 200.

p. 461 'It is the first': FN to FaN, 13 May 1868. Wellcome 9003/22. CW1, 192.

'in real memory: FN to WEN, [1870]. Wellcome 9004/50. CW1, 195.

'I do not feel': FN to Elizabeth Herbert, 8 January 1874. BL 43396/220. CW8, 703–4.

'Dearest': FN to Selina Bracebridge, 8 February 1873. Royal College of Nursing, Edinburgh. CW8, 538.

p. 462 'She was more': FN to PN and Sir Harry Verney, 4 February 1874. CW8, 541.

'very dear': FN to PN, 2 November 1874. Wellcome 9006/132.

'I am utterly': Quoted in W-S, 527.

'. . . I shall give': FN to Mrs Turnham, 24 August 1874. Claydon [unnumbered folder].

'I shall be very sorry': FN to Sir Harry Verney, 17 September 1874. Wellcome 9006/124. CW1, 583.

p. 463 'Either she drinks': FN to PN, 21 September 1874. Wellcome 9006/128. CW1, 206.

'like a new': FN to Sir Harry Verney, 12 August 1875. Wellcome 9006/164. CW1, 207.

'I am "out"': FN to Mary Mohl, 18 June 1875. Woodward Biomedical Library. CW8, 587–8.

CHAPTER 18: A TASTE OF HEAVEN IN DAILY LIFE

p. 464 A Taste of Heaven in Daily Life: BJ to FN, 18 April [1873]. *Jowett Letters*, 239.

'silent sympathy': FN to Mary Clare Moore, [? December 1857]. Vicinus and Nergaard (eds), *Ever Yours, Florence Nightingale*, 194.

'with watching': FN to a Sister of Mercy at Bermondsey, 12 December 1874. Sullivan (ed.), *The Friendship of Florence Nightingale and Mary Clare Moore*, 176.

'not like': FN to Mary Clare Moore, 22 July 1865. ibid., 140.

p. 465 'I am so': FN to Mary Clare Moore, 8 September 1868. ibid., 160.

'little cell': FN to Mary Clare Moore, 17 December 1866. ibid., 145–6.

'to have had': FN to Mary Clare Moore, 9 January 1865. ibid., 127.

'St Catherine': FN to Mary Clare Moore, 24 December 1863. ibid., 112.

p. 466 'in a state': FN, 'Notes from Devotional Authors,' [1872–3]. BL 45841. CW4, 20.

p. 467 'to the health': BJ to FN [24 September 1872]. *Jowett Letters*, 232.

'Notes from the Devotional Authors . . .': For the complete text of the surviving manuscripts, see CW4, 17–80.

p. 468 'too rhetorical': BJ to FN, 18 April [1873]. *Jowett Letters*, 239.

'spirituality of the active life': The phrase is Gérard Vallée's. CW4, 12.

'one of the': Underhill, *Practical Mysticism*, 102.

'under mystic': ibid., x.

p. 469 'This book': FN, 'Notes from Devotional Authors', [1872–3]. BL 45841. CW4, 18.

'If we . . . keep': ibid., 21.

'not to steal': FN, ibid., 33.

p. 470 brief diary ... for 1877: BL 45847. CW2, 433–93.

'Terrible night': FN, 17 March 1877. BL 45847. CW2, 447.

'Strong impression': FN, 16 February 1877. BL 45847. CW2, 441.

p. 471 'O God in Thee': FN, 9–10 November 1877, BL 45847. CW2, 482.

'O God, are you sure': FN, 18 November 1877. BL 45847. CW2, 484.

'Take O take': FN, 8–9 November 1877. BL 45847. CW2, 482.

'... can nothing': FN, 16–17 August 1877. BL 45847. CW2, 466.

'My mind': FN to Edwin Chadwick, 14 September 1877. BL 45771/158. CW9, 757.

Major famines: See CW9, 703–9.

p. 472 'walking in a dream': Roberts, *Salisbury*, 86.

'hundred-headed Hydra': FN, 'Life or Death in India' (1873). CW9, 713.

p. 473 '... one must live': ibid., 744.

p. 474 'the master': FN to Edwin Chadwick, 16 October 1877. BL 45771/159. CW9, 758.

'more frugality': Quoted in Gourlay, *Florence Nightingale and the Health of the Raj*, 126.

p. 475 'Lord Salisbury's worst': FN to Sir Louis Mallet, [1879]. Private collection.

p. 476 'individual and personal': FN to P. K. Sen, 4 April 1878. Sen (ed.), *Florence Nightingale's Indian Letters*, 1.

'English people': FN to P. K. Sen, 20 December 1878. ibid., 5.

'plain unvarnished': FN, 'The Dumb Shall Speak and the Deaf Shall Hear ...' (1883). CW10, 553.

p. 477 'the official': Quoted in Cook II, 289.

'advice': Minute paper, Revenue Department, 7 February 1878. BL 47779/77.

'the Government's': Gourlay, *Florence Nightingale and the Health of the Raj*, 124.

'jerky': BJ to FN, 11 August [1874]. *Jowett Letters*, 261.

p. 478 'shriek': Sir Louis Mallet to FN, 10 March 1879. Quoted in Cook II, 292n.

'We do not care': FN, 'The People Of India' (1878). CW9, 778.

'due to you': FN to William Shore Smith, 30 January 1893. Hampshire Record Office. CW1, 513.

p. 479 'protecting care': FN to Rosalind Shore Smith, 6 February 1880. BL 45795/49. CW1, 543.

'... Remember': FN to Rosalind Shore Smith, 5 December 1881. BL 45795/155. CW1, 546.

'our patients': FN to Christopher Dunn, 24 March 1879. Nightingale Collection, Derbyshire Record Office.

p. 480 'who is said': FN to Christopher Dunn, 27 October 1876. Nightingale Collection, Derbyshire Record Office.

'now & then': FN to Christopher Dunn, 30 November 1876. Columbia School of Nursing, C-9.

'Would you wish': FN to Christopher Dunn, 22 August 1877. Nightingale Collection, Derbyshire Record Office.

'in bodily fear': FN to Sir Harry Verney, 5 April 1879. Wellcome 9007/198.

p. 481 'the Nursing': FN to Christopher Dunn, 8 November 1879. Nightingale Collection, Derbyshire Record Office. For a full account of this episode, see MacQueen, 'Florence Nightingale's Nursing Practice'.

'strove for': FN to Sir William Webb, 10 February 1880. Royal College of Nursing, Edinburgh. CW1, 211

'She looked': FN to Sir William Webb, 10 February 1880. Royal College of Nursing, Edinburgh. CW1, 213.

CHAPTER 19: BATTLE OF THE NURSES

p. 483 'For six': FN to Sir William Webb, 20 February 1880. Royal College of Nursing, Edinburgh. *CW1*, 214.

'though it greatly': FN to PN, 11 February 1880. Wellcome 9008/14. *CW1*, 215.

'those ten': FN to Sir Harry Verney, 22 December 1883. Wellcome 9009/236. *CW1*, 541.

p. 484 'too London-y': FN to PN, 16 February 1880. Wellcome 9008/19.

'at high steam': FN to PN and Sir Harry Verney, 7 April 1880. Wellcome 9008/44.

'as no sick ... weak I am': FN to Mary Mohl, 30 June 1881. Woodward Biomedical Library. *CW8*, 595.

p. 485 '... Anyone might': Quoted in Cook II, 335-6.

'Not far': Queen Victoria's Journal, 4 December 1882. Royal Archives. *CW5*, 422.

the opening ... of the Royal Courts of Justice: Cook II, 339, says that FN declined the invitation. But BJ to FN, 26 May 1892, *Jowett Letters*, 321, makes it clear that she did attend.

'... I have only': FN to Sir Harry Verney, 23 April 1881. Wellcome 9008/145. *CW1*, 587.

Charles Bonham Carter: Bonham Carter, *In a Liberal Tradition*, 120.

p. 486 'We did not': Nash, 'I Knew Florence Nightingale', 62.

'the enjoyment': FN to Sir Harry Verney, 3 September 1881. Wellcome 9008/173. *CW1*, 588.

'I summoned': FN to PN, 22 September 1885. Wellcome 9009/205. *CW1*, 765.

'Great Western': FN to PN and Sir Harry Verney, 14 December 1887. Claydon [unnumbered folder].

p. 487 'self-denial': FN to PN, 1 May 1886. Wellcome 9011/20. *CW1*, 375.

'Sir Harry must': FN to PN, 28 August 1886. Wellcome 9011/49. *CW1*, 377.

'We have come back': The Nightingale Probationers, 7 July 1890. Claydon 404.

W. A. C. Egan ... recalled: Wake, *The Nightingale Training School*, 78. The year's intake were photographed at Claydon with FN.

'breathing hard': FN to Dr Benson, 26 September 1888. Wellcome 9012/55.

p. 488 'fipun': *CW8*, 877.

p. 489 'You understand': FN to Maude Verney, 14 June 1886. BL 68884/43. *CW8*, 891.

'Our maids': FN to PN and Sir Harry Verney, 1 April 1880. Wellcome 9008/42. *CW5*/346.

'I feel': FN to Edmund Verney, 14 January 1887. Wellcome 9011/74. *CW5*, 354.

p. 490 'his father': FN to Sir Harry Verney, 28 May 1891. Wellcome 9013/152. *CW1*, 606.

'She has had': FN to Sir Harry Verney, 6 November 1882. Wellcome 9009/104. *CW1*, 358.

William Ogle: For FN's relationship with Ogle, see Hubble, 'William Ogle of Derby and Florence Nightingale'.

'quack': FN to Margaret Verney, 2 March 1884. Wellcome 9010/9. *CW1*, 647.

'the safest': FN to PN, 19 October 1884. Wellcome 9010/36. *CW1*, 363.

p. 491 'outrageously': Quoted in W-S, 580.

'Grieved': FN to PN, 25 December 1888. Wellcome 9012/70.

'He's a good': FN to John Sutherland, 19 October 1868. BL 45753. *CW5*, 525.

'not only': FN to Sir Harry Verney, [February 1872]. Wellcome 9005/114. *CW5*, 526.

p. 492 'Dear Lord Ripon': FN to Lord Ripon, 14 April 1881. BL 43546/158.

p. 493 'morale-booster': Gourlay, *Florence Nightingale and the Health of the Raj*, 163.

'the interests': FN, 'The Dumb Shall Speak and the Deaf Shall Hear' (1883). *CW10*, 550.

p. 494 'that something': FN to Arnold Toynbee, 20 October 1882. BL 45807/14. *CW10*, 698-9.

'in some distant': Quoted in Gourlay, *Florence Nightingale and the Health of the Raj*, 179.

'long & busy': FN to Lord Ripon, 29 June 1883. BL 43546/197.

'pleasant': Lord Ripon to FN, 20 July 1883. BL 45778/88.

p. 495 '... that there are': FN, 'Our Indian Stewardship' (1883). CW10, 823. The article was a collaborative effort with Sir William Wedderburn, though it appeared in FN's name only.

'gracious Proclamation': FN to Queen Victoria, 6 August 1883. BL 45750/10 [draft]. CW5, 426.

'the powder': Quoted in W-S, 561.

p. 496 'a great': BJ to FN, 22 March [1888]. Jowett Letters, 309.

'"the Boy"': FN to Sir William Wedderburn, 2 November 1885. Quoted in Gourlay, Florence Nightingale and the Health of the Raj, 204.

'There are waves': FN, Notes, 30 July 1886. BL 45788/104.

p. 497 'We are watching': FN to Sir William Wedderburn, 27 November 1885. Quoted in Gourlay, Florence Nightingale and the Health of the Raj, 204.

p. 498 'India is not': FN to W. E. Gladstone, 4 December 1884. BL 44488/212.

'disinterestedness': Cook II, 323.

'I have had': FN to Sir Harry Verney, 25 April 1880. Wellcome 9008/50. CW5, 493.

p. 499 'I gained': Charles Gordon to FN, 29 April 1880. BL 45806/21. CW5, 493.

'a little book': Charles Gordon to FN, 8 May 1880. BL 45806/144. CW5, 494.

'My life': Charles Gordon to FN, 25 April 1881. BL 45806/136. CW5, 496–7.

'was literally': FN to Amy Hawthorn, 7 February 1885. BL 45776/114. CW5, 500.

'was the hospital': FN, 30 August 1886. BL 68884/131. CW5, 509.

p. 500 'We are still': FN to Rachel Williams, 27 March 1885. LMA HI/ST/NC.3/SU180/150.

p. 501 'not hopeless': FN to Rachel Williams, 3 July 1885. Quoted in Cook II, 350.

'far-off': FN to Rachel Williams, 17 July 1885. Quoted in Cook II, 351.

some former probationers refused: FN to PN, 3 June 1887. BL 52427/73.

'Do you': Angélique Pringle to FN, 1 December 1888. Quoted in Cope, Six Disciples of Florence Nightingale, 43.

'thinks that the': FN to Sir Harry Verney, 12 June 1889. BL 47721/224.

p. 502 'mystic religion': FN to BJ, [January 1889]. BL 47785/108.

'all that': FN to Henry Bonham Carter, 17 January 1873. BL 47717/179.

'We have fallen ...': FN to Frances Spencer, 16 August 1893. BL 47751/106.

p. 503 'and a refined': Helmstadter, 'Florence Nightingale's Opposition to State Registration of Nurses', 157.

'The idea': Quoted in Abel-Smith, History of the Nursing Profession, 65.

'We have exhausted': ibid., 66.

p. 505 'they are trying': ibid., 71.

'She has long': Lancet, 8 July 1893.

'a comparative': BJ to FN, 26 May 1892. Quoted in Cook II, 359.

p. 506 'to give herself': Cook II, 252.

'of a yet higher': Quoted in Baly, Florence Nightingale and the Nursing Legacy, 126.

In 1867 she had described: FN to Henry Bonham Carter, 4 June 1867. BL 47714/203. See discussion in CW6, 6–8.

p. 507 'box to hold': : FN, 'Sick-Nursing and Health-Nursing', 1893. CW6, 215.

'It is now': FN, Note, [n.d.]. BL 45820/12. CW6, 8–9.

'or rather': FN to William Farr, 22 May 1867. Wellcome 5474/115.

'it is no use': FN to Henry Bonham Carter, 4 June 1867. BL 47714/203.

CHAPTER 20: LUSTRE ON THE NAME

p. 508 'You contributed': Quoted in W-S, 581–2.
'Claydon is sad': FN to Louisa Ashburton, 12 August 1890. National Library of Scotland. CW8, 732.
'be chiefly remembered': Verney, *Memoirs of the Verney Family*, ii.
p. 509 'humble mind': BL 45793/225. CW1, 493.
'Let me say': FN to Mai Smith, 7 September 1888 [copy Balliol College, Oxford]. CW1, 490.
'. . . I was his pupil': FN to G. E. Buckle, 25 July 1891. Buckle Papers, News International. CW6, 676.
p. 510 'too much': BJ to FN, [October 1891]. *Jowett Letters*, 318.
'. . . You live on your head': FN to BJ, 10 November 1891. ibid., 319.
'You are never': BJ to FN, 26 May 1892. ibid., 321.
'How greatly': BJ to FN, 18 September 1893. ibid., 323.
'genius': FN, 6 October 1893. ibid., 323.
p. 511 'a substitute': ibid., xxxii. In May 1997, Oxford University inaugurated its Florence Nightingale Lecture on Statistics.
'Remember': FN to Sir Harry Verney, 27 November 1893. Wellcome 9014/130. CW1, 608.
'good & simple': FN to Margaret Verney, 12 September 1894. Wellcome 9014/171. CW1, 672.
'the three nearest': W-S, 585.
claimed unfairly: See CW1, 511–12.
p. 512 'six "vegetables"': FN to Rosalind Shore Smith, 9 November 1887. BL 46865/22. CW1, 547.
'except money': FN to Margaret Verney, 20 April 1892. Wellcome 9014/14. CW1, 668.
'that is': FN, Note. BL 45844/229. CW1, 561.
tiresome rather than painful: FN, Note, May 1900. BL 45844/205. CW2, 559.
'There is so much': Quoted in W-S, 585.
p. 513 'to nurse & to teach': FN to Dr G. H. De'Ath, 20 May 1892. Wellcome 5473/5. CW6, 591.
'collective cleanliness . . . conditions': Quoted in Gourlay, *Florence Nightingale and the Health of the Raj*, 212.
p. 514 'while the best nurse': FN, 'Sick-Nursing and Health-Nursing' (1893). CW6, 215–19.
p. 515 'a plague': FN to Margaret Verney, 13 February 1892. Wellcome 9014/8. CW1, 667.
'After being' Samuel Atkins to FN, 9 March 1887. University of British Columbia.
p. 516 'little': FN to WEN, 14 November 1855. Wellcome 8995/74. Goldie, 174.
'She says': Nicolson, *Diaries and Letters* 1939–45, 43. FN's recording is prefaced by a brief introduction from Mary Helen Ferguson. The second attempt can be heard on the British Library's *Voices of History* CD (2004). In a further gesture to raise money in support of the veterans, FN presented Colonel Gouraud with a print of the painting *The Return*, by Lady Butler, which showed the aftermath of the Charge.
'Oh the absurdity': FN to Maude Verney, 23 February 1897. BL 68889/6–7. CW8, 929–30.
p. 517 'all to pieces': Quoted in W-S, 588. In 1911 the carriage would be put on public display in Chesterfield, not far from Lea Hurst.
'relics': FN to Edmund Verney, 10 March 1897. Wellcome 9015/96. CW1, 696–7.
'typewriters': FN to Henry Bonham Carter, 22 March 1893. BL 47724/254.
'a want of memory . . . am dead': Quoted in Cook II, 404.
p. 518 'Louder & nastier': FN to M. Crossland, [November 1896]. BL 47741/267.

Alice Cochrane: Miss Cochrane became Mrs Crawley, and on her ninetieth birthday, in 1961, was interviewed about FN for *The Times*. See *The Times*, 12 January 1961.

'. . . When the nurse': Cook II, 417.

celebratory article: *Madame*, 20 December 1902, 733–5.

'to show': FN to Sibella Bonham Carter, 23 January 1901. Hampshire Record Office F583/5. CW8, 876.

p. 519 'He has always': Lord Knollys to Sir Henry Campbell-Bannerman, 12 June 1907. Campbell-Bannerman Papers, BL 41208/49.

'the more so': Sir Douglas Dawson to Elizabeth Bosanquet, 8 December 1907. Wellcome 9077/58.

'I do not think': Henry Bonham Carter to Miss Crossland, 5 April 1908. Claydon 363.

'to give her attention': Elizabeth Bosanquet to Margaret Verney, 24 September 1910. Claydon 363.

kindly sent: Sir Edmund Verney to Elizabeth Bosanquet, 6 November 1909. Claydon 329.

died in her sleep: FN's death certificate, dated 16 August 1910, gave old age and heart failure as the cause of death. The certificate was made out by Louisa Garrett Anderson, daughter of Elizabeth Garrett Anderson, the first English woman to be listed in the British Medical Register.

'immense activity': Quoted in Cook II, 402.

CHAPTER 21: A HARD NUT TO CRACK

p. 523 a scene: Described in *The Times*, 25 February 1915.

'any grand ceremony': L. Earle to Lord Knutsford, 14 January 1915. PRO Works 20/67.

p. 524 'I believe': Sydney Holland to L. Earle, 16 November 1912. PRO Works/67.

'The face': *The Times*, 12 January 1915.

'no excuse': S. K. McDonnell to Sydney Holland, 4 December 1911. PRO Works/67.

p. 525 'enclosed in a structure': Benson, *Diary*, 12 May 1916, 289.

'the bloody war': Gibbs, *The Pageant of the Years*, 261.

'treacherous': FN to Evelyn Abbott, 23 October 1894. Quoted in *Jowett Letters*, xxxvi.

'without my KNOWLEDGE': FN to Margaret Verney, 23 April 1896. Wellcome 9015/71.

'It is impossible': Stanmore, *Sidney Herbert*, I, 404.

p. 526 'The real': Cook I, 2.

accords a woman: In 1902, Sidney Lee had written an extended article on Queen Victoria for the *Dictionary of National Biography*, which was later reprinted in book form. But Cook's was the first full-scale biography.

p. 527 Cook's diary: Bodleian MS Eng d.3325. Cook had been recommended to FN's executors by the Liberal statesman and biographer John (Viscount) Morley.

Mrs Nash, once described: By Philip Radcliffe in his memories (*c.* 1976) of Rosalind Vaughan Nash and her brother Louis Shore Nightingale. FN Museum.

'Perhaps': Sir Edward Cook to Margaret Verney, 1 December 1913. Verney 10/555.

'F.N.'s strong dislike': Louis Shore Nightingale to Margaret Verney, 8 April 1914. Verney 10/555. The executors took legal advice to establish that the Verneys had no right to publish the letters from FN in their possession. See the memo by Louis Shore Nightingale, detailing the dispute between FN's executors and the Verney family, 20 February 1914. BL 72832A/91–3.

p. 528 'resolute and masterful': Cook II, 424–5

'the intolerable sister': Quoted in Saxon Mills, *Sir Edward Cook*, 229.

'Such a long': Flora Masson to Margaret Verney, 7 December 1913. Verney 10/554.

p. 529 'And so it happens': Strachey, *Eminent Victorians*, 119.

'immense energy': CW9, 990.

'written from': Strachey, *Eminent Victorians*, xi. BJ was at one point considered by Strachey as a potential subject.

'I have just been': Quoted in Merle, *Lytton Strachey*, II, 500–501.

'extremely interesting': Quoted ibid., 500.

p. 530 'rather a hard nut . . . off': Quoted in Holroyd, *Lytton Strachey*, II, 142–3.

'Last night': Virginia Woolf to Vanessa Bell, 22 April 1916, *The Letters of Virginia Woolf*, II, 91.

'would think': Strachey, *Eminent Victorians*, 120.

'recognised the greatness': Beerbohm, *Lytton Strachey*, 15.

p. 531 'a schizophrenic monster': Holroyd, *Lytton Strachey*, II, 290.

'absurd': Guppy, *Looking Back*, 248. Partridge believed that something of the austerity and practical efficiency of Strachey's older sister Pippa Strachey (1872–1968), who was for many years secretary to the London Society for Women's Service, had influenced his portrayal of FN.

no enormous liberties: However, Strachey does erroneously state that FN never believed in germ theory.

'fury': Nash, 'Florence Nightingale according to Mr Strachey', 261. Nash had published an abridged edition of Cook's *Life* in 1925. In 1937, she published *A Sketch of the Life of Florence Nightingale* for the Society for Promoting Christian Knowledge

'A large part': [?] BL 72832A/98.

p. 532 'adolescents to snigger': James Pope-Hennessy, *Spectator*, 182 (24 February 1949), 264.

'the events': Quoted in Spencer, *Dramatic Strategies in the Plays of Edward Bond*, 153.

p. 533 'without saying': Holmes, *Florence Nightingale*, 1.

emblazoned with 'Florence Nightingale': Lowndes's banner is now in the collection of the Women's Library, in London.

'The Warriors': See Cockin, 'Cicely Hamilton's Warriors', for a description of the *Pageant*.

as a separate booklet: There is a copy in the FN Museum (0780).

p. 534 'a protest': Brittain, ' "The Lady of the Lamp". Florence Nightingale as Feminist'.

'the founder': Brittain, *Testament of Youth*, 454.

Caroline Stephen: FN's letters to Caroline Stephen, from 1869 and 1870, are at BL 45802/12 and 45802/181.

'Women': FN, 'Cassandra', 402.

'great revolution': Woolf, *Women and Fiction*, 183–4.

p. 535 'a more personal': This was a phrase that Margaret Verney had used when advancing the case for her biography of FN to the Nightingale executors. Margaret Verney to Louis Shore Nightingale, 13 February 1914. BL 72832A/94.

'biographical rather than dramatic': See Kalisch, 'Heroine out of Focus', 2, 271.

erroneously . . . as the 'Founder of the Red Cross': Henri Dunant (1828–1910), a Swiss businessman, created the Red Cross after being appalled by the treatment of injured soldiers during the Battle of Solferino in 1859. But while Dunant credited FN as his inspiration – and she congratulated him on his 'noble work' – fundamentally she regarded the principle behind the Red Cross, of voluntary rather than governmental provision of nursing and medical care, as misguided and misdirected.

p. 536 'the highbrow . . . sheets': Kalisch, 'Heroine out of Focus', 1, 185.

the Broadway stage: The play enjoyed only a brief run on Broadway, despite receiving warm reviews, because of the economic slump experienced by New York theatres in 1931.

'of a propaganda': Quoted in Harben, *Twentieth-Century English History Plays*, 68.

p. 537 'St Joan': Quoted in Forbes, *Ned's Girl*, 136.

'entirely based': Quoted in Holroyd, *Lytton Strachey*, II, 627.

'No Henry, no': Berkeley, *The Lady with a Lamp*, 221.

'Liz, dear': ibid., 270.

'putting a premium': ibid., 246.

'in the prime': ibid., 263.

p. 538 'She's a saint': Kalisch, 'Heroine out of Focus', 1, 187.

'bloodless myth': *Daily Telegraph*, 7 January 1929.

'unaware of any': *The Times*, 13 February 1929. In fact Berkeley claimed to have consulted an unnamed member of the Nightingale family.

'the Nightingale Pledge': For the text of this pledge, see Dossey, *Florence Nightingale*, 391.

p. 539 'Now there seems': *Times Literary Supplement*, 1847 (26 June 1937), 472.

'She is a woman': Michael Sadleir to Ellin Salmon, 10 September 1943. Verney 10/703.

unflattering stories about Parthenope: See, for example, Sir Harry's extraordinary, and unfounded, claim that his mother Margaret Verney was the sole author of *Memoirs of the Verney Family*. 'Authorship of the Verney Memoirs'. Dorset Record Office Q(LBL)/1/V/1. In an address to mark the fiftieth anniversary of FN's death, given on 14 August 1960, Sir Harry recalled that PN was 'always cross ... and disliked children'. See Verney, 'The Perfect Aunt'.

p. 540 'an intolerable': Greenleaf, 'Biography and the "Amateur Historian" ', 202.

p. 541 'is infinitely': ibid., 193.

'the old fiction': Kalisch, 'Heroine out of Focus', 2, 273–4.

Athena the owl: Neagle, *An Autobiography*, 178. J. P. Mitchelhill had bought Lea Hurst with two friends in order to convert it into a convalescent home for nurses. Subsequently it became an RSAS Care Home (later AgeCare) for the elderly until its conversion into flats at the beginning of the twenty-first century. Embley Park is now an independent school.

p. 542 'almost bland': Cannadine, *History in Our Time*, 201.

close inspection of the citations: See McDonald, 'Florence Nightingale Revealed in Her Own Writings', for examples of Smith's practice.

'to promote an understanding': The Florence Nightingale Museum Trust, *Annual Report and Accounts*, 2004, 11. The collecting of Nightingale artefacts began at St Thomas's under the matronship of Alicia Lloyd-Still, but not until the formation of the FN Museum Trust in 1984 were plans made for the establishment of a museum.

p. 543 'an appropriate memorial': *British Journal of Nursing*, July 1932, 172.

p. 544 'You are an extraordinarily': Wake, *The Nightingale Training School*, 112.

p. 545 'All over': Unison press release, 1999.

as Patricia D'Antonio has said: Reported in *Washington Post*, 29 April 2003. D'Antonio is an Associate Professor of Nursing at the University of Pennsylvania, and editor of *Nursing History Review*.

Acknowledgements

My thanks to the Henry Bonham Carter Will Trust for permission to quote from unpublished Florence Nightingale material. I am very grateful also to Sir Edmund Verney and the Claydon House Trust for permission to use extensive unpublished Nightingale and Verney material from the Trust's collection.

One of my largest debts is to Alex Attewell, who, until October 2007, was the Director of the Florence Nightingale Museum in London. From the inception of this book, and throughout its research and writing, Alex has been tremendously supportive, discussing ideas, allowing me to draw on his fund of Nightingale knowledge, and alerting me to new discoveries and theories. I am also grateful to him for allowing me unfettered access to the Museum's collection. Other members of staff at the Museum have, over the years, proved unfailingly helpful: Caroline Roberts, formerly Curator, and her predecessor Susan Laurence; Daphne Fallows; Zoe Gilbert; Wendy Matthews; Kirsteen Nixon; and Penny Ritchie Calder.

Another major debt is to Susan Ranson, Archivist at Claydon House, who has made the long research days at Claydon, in the five years I have been going there, such a pleasure, facilitating my transport to the house, carrying endless supplies of documents to my desk, and drawing my attention to material I might otherwise have missed. One of the more interesting aspects of researching this biography has been the opportunity to study the voluminous papers of the Nightingale and Verney families that Claydon preserves in its archives, and I shan't quickly forget the thrill of coming across unpublished correspondence from Mrs Gaskell or Dickens in bundles of letters tied together in their pinkish-red ribbon; or of finding previously unknown portraits – and one photograph – of Florence Nightingale. Jennifer Bobrowski has been a regular companion on these visits while she researched her study of William Smith and the Smith family, Florence Nightingale's maternal relatives. I have relied heavily on her encyclopedic knowledge of members from the further reaches of the Nightingale family tree. Nigel Benford and Marjorie Brotherton, two of the National Trust's custodians at Claydon while I was working there, answered my questions, and allowed me to explore the house at times when it was closed to the public.

I have benefited enormously from the wisdom and encouragement of Pamela Norris, who took time away from her own writing to read and comment on my text. Her suggestions and corrections have been invaluable. My old friend Timothy Brittain-Catlin has advised me on innumerable matters of taste and technology, while I have derived much of lasting value from discussions with Lyndall Gordon about the nature of biography and approaches to the form. Margaret and Alastair Howatson, good friends for more than a quarter of a century, listened patiently to me and have always responded with sound common sense. I am particularly grateful to Margaret Howatson for the identification of the occasional classical allusion, and for her kindness in undertaking preliminary research on my behalf into the Clough and Jowett collections at Balliol College, Oxford. Frances Wilson has frequently boosted my confidence and provided useful advice.

Pat Smedley generously supplied me with the fruits of her research into the lectures of Dr

John Croft to the nursing probationers at St Thomas's in the 1870s, and talked about her own experiences as a Nightingale nurse at St Thomas's more than a century later. Michael Bresalier, formerly of Cambridge University, now at Bristol University, attempted to lighten the darkness of my ignorance about the development of germ theory in the final decades of the nineteenth century. Evelyn Barker and her husband Colin kindly gave me hospitality at their Norfolk home in the summer of 2006, and allowed me to examine the recently discovered photograph of Florence Nightingale, taken at Embley in May 1858, by William Frost, assistant to the Romsey chemist William Slater, before it was donated to the Florence Nightingale Museum. I am also grateful to Mrs Barker for her vivid reminiscence of her mother's disappointment at not being allowed to join the crowds of children following Florence Nightingale's funeral procession in August 1910.

Many friends, colleagues, acquaintances, as well as complete strangers, have answered inquiries, sent me information, or offered moral or practical support. I would like particularly to mention the following: Pauline Adams, for drawing my attention to the engraving of Florence Nightingale bequeathed to Somerville College, Oxford, by Benjamin Jowett; Beryl Bainbridge; Elizabeth Bonython (Cecil Woodham-Smith's daughter); Clive Brill; Myles Burnyeat; David Chapman, Headmaster of Embley Park School; Patricia D'Antonio; Belinda Drake; Suzi Feay; John Forrester; Rebecca Fraser; John Gaynor, for permitting me to see Nightingale material in his possession; Lennie Goodings; Luci Gosling at the *Illustrated London News* Picture Library; Claire Harman, especially for photocopying letters from Dorset Record Office which she knew would interest me; Brian Harrison, for giving me a copy of his research on Ida O'Malley; the late Jenifer Hart; Liz Hartford; Christopher Hilton at the Wellcome Institute; Michael Holroyd, for responding to questions about Lytton Strachey; David Horspool; Anthony Kenny, for his insights into the life and work of Arthur Hugh Clough; Mark Lomas, for sending, and allowing me to reproduce, the photograph of Florence Nightingale's funeral from his father, Stanley Lomas's collection; Father Dermot Morrin OP, for helping me to gain access to Florence Nightingale's birthplace at Bellosguardo; Peter Parker; the late Frances Partridge, for talking to me about Lytton Strachey and Florence Nightingale; Jane Robinson; Jean Seaton; Marion Shaw, for accompanying me on visits to sites in Derbyshire with Nightingale associations; Edi Smockum and David Owen; Ian Thomson; Katie and Scott Thomson, for their kindness while I was in New York working in the Auchincloss Collection at Columbia University; Claire Tomalin; Mark Walton; the late Bernard Williams and Patricia Williams; Shirley Williams and the late Richard Neustadt; Rebecca Williams and Christopher Honey; Ann Wroe, for supplying the cartoon from *The Economist* of Mrs Thatcher as the Lady with the Lamp.

I have been fortunate in having access to many different archives and collections. I would like especially to thank the respective staffs of the British Library, which houses the largest collection of Nightingale papers, and of the library at the Wellcome Institute in London, that extraordinary monument to one man's munificence. I am also grateful to the following institutions, and the librarians and archivists who work for them: Penelope Bulloch and Alan Tadiello at Balliol College, Oxford; the Bodleian Library, Oxford; Cambridge University Library; Stephen Novak at the Auchincloss Collection at Columbia University in New York; Neil Bettridge at Derbyshire Record Office; Rob Cowie at Edinburgh Academy; Gloucestershire Record Office; Hampshire Record Office; Marion Roberts at the Heber Percy Archive; Richard Bowden at the Howard de Walden Estate; the London Library; the London Metropolitan Archives; the National Archives at Kew; the Heinz Archive at the National Portrait Gallery in London; Leslie McGrath at Toronto Public Library; Trinity College, Cambridge; the Victoria and Albert Museum; Wiltshire Record Office.

My thanks to Dr Philip Mackowiak MD, of the University of Maryland School of Medicine, for inviting me to give a lecture in Baltimore, in May 2003, on Florence Nightingale's illness, and for helping me to understand the root causes of her disease. I am very grateful to Alexandre Toumarkine of the Institut Français d'Etudes Anatoliennes, in Istanbul, for asking me to take part in a conference in 2004 to mark the 150th anniversary of the outbreak of the Crimean War, and for his kindness in arranging my visit, across to the other side of the Bosphorus, to the closely guarded former Barrack Hospital at Scutari. And Hermione Lee's invitation, in 2006, to give a lecture to her biography seminar at Oxford University allowed me the opportunity to gather together some of the thoughts that form the basis of my final chapter.

Any individual attempting to write about Florence Nightingale cannot fail to owe a considerable debt to those writers and scholars, past and present, toiling in the same or related fields. I wish especially to acknowledge my own debt to the research of the late Monica Baly into the early years of the Nightingale School at St Thomas's; to Michael Calabria for his edition of Florence Nightingale's Egyptian and Greek diary, and to the same editor and Janet Macrae for their selections and commentaries on Florence Nightingale's Suggestions for Thought; to Sue Goldie for her exemplary edition of Florence Nightingale's Crimean War letters, and for her Calendar of the Letters of Florence Nightingale. I have learned much from John Shepherd's seminal work on the medical services in the Crimean War, from Carol Helmstadter's research into reformed nursing in nineteenth-century Britain, and from Jharna Gourlay's book on Florence Nightingale's involvement in reforms for health and social change in India.

Lynn McDonald's Collected Works of Florence Nightingale, published by Wilfred Laurier University Press, is one of the more important scholarly projects of recent years, and fills a significant gap among editions of writings of the major Victorians. I am very grateful to her for sending me material in advance of publication, and for the information contained in her commentaries, and in those of her associate editor Gérard Vallée. She will not agree with all my conclusions – any more than I always agree with hers – but I should like to salute her achievement here.

I was much aided in researching this book by grants from the Society of Authors, which helped with my travel expenses, and by the award of a Wingate Scholarship in 2003, and wish to record my gratitude to the trustees of both funds.

At Viking Penguin in London, I have drawn on the very welcome guidance, support and enthusiasm of my editor, Eleo Gordon, as well as on the assistance of Will Hammond. I am grateful, too, for the advice of Venetia Butterfield, Viking's editorial director. At Farrar, Straus & Giroux in New York, I have been well supported by Jonathan Galassi. Annie Lee copyedited the book with an eagle eye, and Debbie Hatfield saw it through production. Douglas Matthews was responsible for the index. My thanks also to my agent, Simon Trewin, at United Agents.

Robin Baird-Smith has been a stalwart in countless ways. Florence Nightingale may have inveighed against the institution of the family, but my own family has sustained me through thick and thin. I am grateful to my sister-in-law Lucasta Miller for her sympathetic interest and encouragement, to Ian and Charlie, and to the two O's, Oliver and Ottilie Bostridge. My love and respect go to my mother, who, decades ago, presented me with a copy of the Ladybird book on Florence Nightingale by the exotically named L. Du Garde Peach, and may therefore be said to have set the ball rolling.

Index

FN to relax, 438, 460;
favourite
undergraduates, 457;
encourages FN's book
of mystical writings,
467; criticizes FN's
paper on Indian land
tenure system, 477; on
Lansdowne, 486;
collaborates with FN on
education for Indian
Civil Servants, 493; and
Pringle's conversion to
Catholicism, 502; on
dispute over state
registration of nurses,
505; death, 510; letters
to FN published in
biography, 525
Jura (ship), 279, 281

Kaiserswerth, Germany:
Deaconess Institution,
97–9, 124, 127,
140–44, 146–7,
155–60, 163, 420–21
Karani, Crimea, 295
Katerina, Schwester (of
Kaiserswerth), 143
Keats, John, 125–6, 175
Keith, Dr Caroline, 375
Kempis, Thomas à:
Imitation of Christ,
210, 413, 499
Kensington Place: Queen
offers to FN, 303
Khartoum, 499–501
Kidd, Mr (Superintendent at
Liverpool workhouse
infirmary), 436
Kinglake, A.W.: The
Invasion of the Crimea,
249
King's College Hospital: FN
offered post of
Superintendent of
Nurses, 197–8; funding
of nurse training, 366,
428–30; midwifery,
428–9; St John's nurses
at, 428–9; puerperal
fever outbreak, 429–30
Kingsley, Charles, 415
Kiralfy, Imre, 516

Kirkland, Sir John, 209
Kneller, Private John, xx
Knollys, Francis, 1st
Viscount, 519
Knutsford, Sydney Holland,
2nd Viscount, 524
Koulali hospital, Turkey,
222, 242, 286
Kynsham Court,
Herefordshire, 20, 24

Ladies' Sanitary Association,
313
Lady with the Lamp, The
(film), 541
Lancet (journal), 339, 358,
443, 505
Land Transport Corps:
formed, 295; conveys
wounded men, 319
Lanfried, Martin, 516
Langston, Emma, 243
Lansdowne, Henry Charles
Keith Petty-Fitzmaurice,
5th Marquess of, 496
Lawfield, Rebecca, 231, 233
Lawrence, George Alfred:
Sword and Gown, 415
Lawrence, Sir John Laird
Mair (later 1st Baron),
401–4, 420, 472, 485,
491, 513
Lawson, Assistant-Surgeon
George, 289
Lea, Derbyshire: industries
and manufacturing,
26–7; Fanny
Nightingale's parish
activities in, 41
Lea Hall, Derbyshire, 23–4
Lea Hurst, Derbyshire,
23–30, 42, 67–8, 74–5,
89–90, 103, 105, 146,
199, 201, 258, 305,
309, 412, 460, 470,
478–9, 487
Lear, Edward, 115
Lee, James: The Holy Terror
(TV drama), 542
Lees, Florence, 506
Lefroy, Colonel John,
290–91, 307, 310
Leith, Dr Andrew
Henderson, 400

Leopold II, King of the
Belgians, 499
Lepsius, Karl Richard, 131
Leutze, Emanuel: Florence
Nightingale at Scutari
(painting), 364
Lewis, Sir Cornwall, 6
Lewis, Sir George, 383,
386–7, 392, 492
Liddell, Sir John, 311
Liggins, Joseph, 109
Light Brigade, Charge of,
219
Light Brigade Relief Fund,
516
Limb, Mrs (of Derbyshire),
480
Lincoln, Abraham, 362
Lind, Jenny, 294
Lister, Joseph Jackson, 335,
453
Liverpool: Brownlow Hill
Workhouse, 419,
421–3, 435–6, 465;
district nursing, 506
Lock Hospital, London, 153
Logan (surgical nurse), 328
London: social season, 66;
Nightingales in, 75; FN
praises, 81; German
Hospital (Dalston), 85,
153; teaching hospitals,
94n; cholera epidemic
(1854), 199;
workhouses, 419
London Library: FN
discontinues
membership, 192
London Nurses Institution,
King William Street,
197
Longden, Annie, 30
Longfellow, Henry
Wadsworth: 'Santa
Filomena', 254, 482
Louis XVIII, King of France,
23
Louis Napoleon Bonaparte
see Napoleon III,
Emperor
Louis-Philippe, King of the
French, 122
Lovelace, Ada, Countess of
(née Byron), 82

letters from FN in Rome, 115; takes cure at Malvern, 124; concern over FN's single state, 129–30; and Parthenope's ill-health, 149; visits Kaiserswerth, 155; and FN's second visit to Kaiserswerth, 156; accepts FN's nursing vocation, 158–60; in Germany for water cure, 159; and FN's liberal views on class, 168; and Parthenope's breakdown, 176; modifies opposition to FN's ambitions, 182; FN's devotion to, 187; supports FN's appointment to Upper Harley Street post, 188; opposes FN's move to King's College Hospital, 198; suppresses FN's letters from Egypt, 200; consents to FN's departure for Scutari, 206; letters from FN at Scutari, 246; relishes FN's celebrity, 257–8, 262; offers portraits of FN, 266; praises Barrett's portrait of FN, 267; cautions FN over impatience after illness, 280; and creation of Nightingale Fund, 293; on FN's return from Crimea, 305; with FN at Burlington, 321–2; and FN's invalid state, 324; visits FN at Oak Hill Park, 352; Jowett visits, 391; pet cats, 412; ageing and decline, 459–63; stays at Claydon House, 462; stays at Lea Hurst in old age, 478; final illness, death and funeral, 481–3

Nightingale, Florence:
funeral, xix–xx; public image and reputation, xx–xxii, 254–7, 261–4, 276, 292, 316, 515; seclusion, xxi–xxii, 325, 329–30, 351; chronic ill health, xxii, 76–7, 88, 100, 108, 324–6, 328, 330, 388, 438; birth in Florence, Italy, 3, 22; letters and papers, 4–8, 33–5; writing, 6–8, 33; condemns slavery, 11; breaks with family, 22; childhood ill-health, 23, 28; growing up at Lea Hurst, 25–6; holds Sunday Bible classes, 25; family network, 29; opposes Aunt Mai's marriage to Samuel, 30; devotion to Mai's son Shore, 31, 48–9, 89, 103; love of animals and pets, 32–3, 46–7; collects shells, 33, 43–4; interest in language, 33, 38; reading, 34–5, 60–61, 70, 140, 413–15, 466–7; evangelical influences on, 35; relations and tensions with Parthenope, 35–6, 49, 149, 154, 158, 174, 180–81, 186, 201, 491; serious-mindedness, 35–7; education and learning, 36–40, 44, 70; relations with parents, 40, 45, 321, 353, 459; supports Crich school, 42; and father's parliamentary ambitions, 43–4; bequest of shells from grandfather, 44; criticizes father's lack of ambition, 45; nurses sick dolls, 45; treats injured dog, 46–7; early caring for sick and

poor, 47–51, 58; religious beliefs and experiences, 51–5, 77, 80, 92, 113–14, 120–21, 138–40, 165, 169–70, 219, 333, 349, 355, 369–71, 464–71; continental tour with family (1837–8), 56–66; appearance, 57, 66, 140, 280–81, 290, 331; double portrait with Parthenope, 57; keeps journal, 58, 132, 147, 470; musical interests and activities, 60, 66–7, 70, 72; influenced by Mary Clarke, 64–5; presented to Queen, 66; studies mathematics, 70–72; Marmaduke Wyvill proposes marriage to, 72–3; concern for the poor, 74; amateur theatricals, 75; helps care for Reeve family, 75–6; relations with and reliance on Aunt Hannah Nicholson, 76–7, 79–80; rejects Henry Nicholson as suitor, 77–9; rift with Marianne Nicholson, 79, 188; on imaginary life, 80–81; social life and entertaining, 82; Bunsen's influence on, 84–5; plans nursing career, 85–7, 91, 98–101; gives up riding and sports, 88; nurses grandmother Shore, 89–90, 184; family opposition to nursing career, 99–101, 127–8, 147; frustration with limited family life, 101–2, 177–80, 186–7; dreaming, 102–3, 137, 154; courted by Monckton Milnes, 105–7, 126–8; view of marriage, 105–7;

Victoria, Queen – *contd.*
presenting jewels to FN
and Mary Stanley, 244;
invites Fanny to
Buckingham Palace,
258; gives brooch to
FN, 260; sends
encouragement to
Crimea wounded and
sick, 260; requests
photograph of FN, 266;
FN meets at Balmoral,
307, 362; view of Army
reform, 308; mourns
death of Prince Albert,
388–9; FN sends copy
of Indian Sanitary
Commission
Observations to, 399;
opens rebuilt
St Thomas's Hospital,
443; sends condolences
on Fanny's death, 483;
sees FN at review of
troops, 485;
proclamation to people
of India, 495; Golden
Jubilee (1887), 506;
Diamond Jubilee
(1897), 516; death, 518;
relations with FN in
Bond's *Early Morning*,
532
Villiers, Charles Pelham,
417, 423–5
Vincent de Paul, St, Order
of, 119, 132, 146, 184,
217
Vivian, Sir Robert, 397

Wakley, James, 419
Walker, A.G., 524
Walker, Dr J. Pattison, 395,
403
Walters, Catherine
('Skittles'), 409
Wantage, Harriet Sarah,
Lady (*née* Lloyd),
516–17
War Office: and FN's
position and authority
in Crimea, 291;
resistance to reform,
343; FN urges Herbert

to reform, 378, 380;
and threat of war with
USA, 386; consults FN
as adviser, 387; opposes
female nurses in army
hospitals, 433
Ward, Mrs Robert Plumer,
388
Ward, Thomas, Baron, 279
Ward, W.G., 162
Wardroper, Sarah Elizabeth,
366–8, 421, 434, 445,
447–52, 455–7, 470,
501
water cures, 124–5, 154–5
Waterloo Place, London,
523–4
Watson, Mary, 210
Watson, Assistant-Surgeon
Patrick, 243
Watson, Sir Thomas, 426
Watts, George Frederic, 331,
432, 486
Waverley Abbey, Surrey, 28,
69, 74, 76–8, 88
Wear, Margaret, 285–6
Webb, Beatrice, 103
Webb (Fanny Nightingale's
maid), 460
Webb, Sir William, 481
Wedderburn, Alexander, 527
Wedderburn, Sir William,
478n, 497
Wedgwood, Josiah II, 61
Wells, S.R.: *New System of
Physiognomy*, 265
Wesley, John, 53
West Wellow, Hampshire,
91
Westminster Abbey: annual
commemoration service
for FN, 545–6
Westminster, Hugh Lupus
Grosvenor, 1st Duke of,
409
Westminster, Hugh Richard
Arthur Grosvenor, 2nd
Duke of, 408n
Westminster Review, 341
Whatstandwell, Derbyshire,
41
Wheeler, Elizabeth, 235
White Angel, The (film),
538–9

White, William, 57
Whitfield, Richard, 366–8,
446, 448, 450, 452
Wilberforce, Samuel, Bishop
of Oxford, 259
Wilberforce, William, 11, 44
Wilbraham, Colonel, 433
Wilcox, Herbert, 541
Wildgoose, Fanny, 264
Wilding, Michael, 541
Wilhelm II, Kaiser, 7
Wilkinson, John Gardner:
Modern Egypt, 131,
134
William IV, King, 56
Williams, Jane, 269
Williams, Sir John Hay,
488
Willis, Irene Cooper, xix
Wilson, James, 124
Wilson, Laura, 453
Wilson, Mary, 217–18
Wilton House, Wiltshire,
116, 118, 122–3
Winifred, Sister: death from
cholera, 288
Winkworth, Catherine, 199
Wolseley, General Garnet
Joseph, Viscount, 500
women: education, 1, 14,
37; factory work and
conditions, 75;
restlessness and
frustration, 102–3, 145,
177–80, 186; in nursing
positions, 147; as
doctors, 151–4;
Anglican church's
attitude to, 167; surplus
of unmarried, 189–90;
military nursing, 206;
employment in military
hospitals, 255, 365; and
FN's public image, 256,
263–4; deaths from
clothing catching fire,
360; J. S. Mills's view of
condition of, 373–4,
376; FN on rights of,
374–6, 532; suffrage
question and
movement, 375, 532–3;
property rights, 376;
and Contagious